S0-APO-592

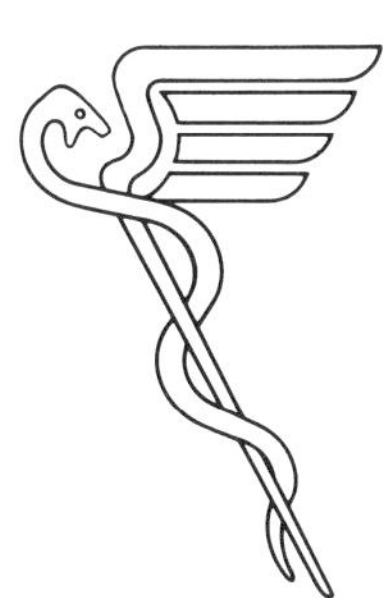

1984
YEAR BOOK OF
DERMATOLOGY®

THE 1984 YEAR BOOKS

The YEAR BOOK series provides in condensed form the essence of the best of the recent international medical literature. The material is selected by distinguished editors who critically review more than 500,000 journal articles each year.

Anesthesia: *Drs. Kirby, Miller, Ostheimer, Saidman, and Stoelting.*

Cancer: *Drs. Clark, Cumley, and Hickey.*

Cardiology: *Drs. Harvey, Kirkendall, Kirklin, Nadas, Resnekov, and Sonnenblick.*

Critical Care Medicine: *Drs. Rogers, Booth, Dean, Gioia, McPherson, Michael, and Traystman.*

Dentistry: *Drs. Cohen, Hendler, Johnson, Jordan, Moyers, Robinson, and Silverman.*

Dermatology: *Drs. Sober and Fitzpatrick.*

Diagnostic Radiology: *Drs. Bragg, Keats, Kieffer, Kirkpatrick, Koehler, Sorenson, and White.*

Digestive Diseases: *Drs. Greenberger and Moody.*

Drug Therapy: *Drs. Hollister and Lasagna.*

Emergency Medicine: *Dr. Wagner.*

Endocrinology: *Drs. Schwartz and Ryan.*

Family Practice: *Dr. Rakel.*

Medicine: *Drs. Rogers, Des Prez, Cline, Braunwald, Greenberger, Bondy, Epstein, and Malawista.*

Neurology and Neurosurgery: *Drs. De Jong, Sugar, and Currier.*

Nuclear Medicine: *Drs. Hoffer, Gottschalk, and Zaret.*

Obstetrics and Gynecology: *Drs. Pitkin and Zlatnik.*

Ophthalmology: *Dr. Ernest.*

Orthopedics: *Dr. Coventry.*

Otolaryngology: *Drs. Paparella and Bailey.*

Pathology and Clinical Pathology: *Dr. Brinkhous.*

Pediatrics: *Drs. Oski and Stockman.*

Plastic and Reconstructive Surgery: *Drs. McCoy, Brauer, Haynes, Hoehn, Miller, and Whitaker.*

Psychiatry and Applied Mental Health: *Drs. Freedman, Lourie, Meltzer, Nemiah, Talbott, and Weiner.*

Sports Medicine: *Drs. Krakauer, Shephard, and Torg, Col. Anderson, and Mr. George.*

Surgery: *Drs. Schwartz, Najarian, Peacock, Shires, Silen, and Spencer.*

Urology: *Drs. Gillenwater and Howards.*

The YEAR BOOK of

Dermatology®

1984

Edited by

ARTHUR J. SOBER, M.D.

Associate Professor of Dermatology, Department of Dermatology, Harvard Medical School

and

THOMAS B. FITZPATRICK, M.D.

Professor and Chairman, Department of Dermatology, Harvard Medical School

YEAR BOOK MEDICAL PUBLISHERS, INC.

CHICAGO

Printed in U.S.A.

International Standard Book Number: 0-8151-2670-0

International Standard Serial Number: 0093-3619

The editor for this book was Joan David, and the production manager was H.E. Nielsen.

Table of Contents

The material covered in this volume represents literature reviewed up to December 1983.

Contributing Editors . . . 7

Journals Represented . . . 9

Statistics of Interest to the Dermatologist . . . 11

Review Articles . . . 15

1. Acne and Disorders of Sebaceous and Apocrine Glands . . . 21
2. Bacterial and Miscellaneous Infections . . . 41
3. Bullous Diseases . . . 53
4. Collagen Vascular Diseases . . . 75
5. Atopic Dermatitis . . . 103
6. Contact Dermatitis . . . 117
7. Pharmacology and Drug Therapy . . . 125
8. Adverse Drug Reactions . . . 131
9. Fungal Infections . . . 145
10. Genodermatoses . . . 157
11. Hair and Nails . . . 165
12. Leprosy and Other Mycobacterial Diseases . . . 175
13. Melanocytic Nevi and Melanoma . . . 181
14. Nonmelanoma Skin Cancer . . . 217
15. Photobiology and Phototherapy . . . 247
16. Pigmentary Disorders . . . 267
17. Psoriasis and Related Disorders . . . 289
18. Urticaria and Mast Cell Disorders . . . 323
19. Vascular Lesions . . . 335
20. Viral Infections . . . 345
21. Miscellaneous Disorders . . . 363

Contributing Editors

Joseph C. Alper, M.D., *Assistant Professor of Medicine**

Richard W. Gange, M.D., *Assistant Professor of Dermatology***

Ernesto Gonzalez, M.D., *Assistant Professor of Dermatology***

Richard Masters, M.D., *Assistant Clinical Professor***

Martin C. Mihm, Jr., M.D., *Professor of Pathology***

Samuel Moschella, M.D., *Clinical Professor of Dermatology***

Peter Pochi, M.D., *Professor of Dermatology****

Rhonda Rand, M.D., *Clinical Assistant in Dermatology***

Arthur R. Rhodes, M.D., *Assistant Professor of Dermatology***

Nicholas A. Soter, M.D., *Professor of Dermatology*****

Robert S. Stern, M.D., *Associate Professor of Dermatology***

***Division of Dermatology,** *Brown University, Providence, R.I.*
***Harvard Medical School, Boston*
****Boston University*
*****New York University*

Journals Represented

Acta Cytologica
Acta Dermato-Venereologica
Acta Odontologica Scandinavica
Acta Parhologica et Microbiologica Scandinavica B. Microbiology
Allergy
American Journal of Clinical Pathology
American Journal of Diseases of Children
American Journal of the Medical Sciences
American Journal of Medicine
American Journal of Obstetrics and Gynecology
American Journal of Ophthalmology
American Journal of Pathology
American Journal of Roentgenology
American Journal of Surgery
Annales de Dermatologie et de Venereologie
Annals of Allergy
Annals of Internal Medicine
Annals of Rheumatic Diseases
Annals of Surgery
Archives of Dermatological Research
Archives of Dermatology
Archives of Disease in Childhood
Archives of Internal Medicine
Archives of Otolaryngology
Archives of Surgery
Arthritis and Rheumatism
Australasian Journal of Dermatology
Blood
British Journal of Dermatology
British Journal of Psychiatry
British Journal of Venereal Diseases
British Medical Journal
Canadian Journal of Surgery
Canadian Medical Association Journal
Cancer
Cancer Treatment Reports
Clinica Chimica Acta
Clinical Allergy
Clinical Endocrinology
Clinical and Experimental Dermatology
Cutis
Danish Medical Bulletin
Dermatologica
Deutsche Medizinische Wochenschrift
Diseases of the Colon and Rectum
European Journal of Clinical Investigation

Hautarzt
Head and Neck Surgery
Indian Journal of Dermatology
International Journal of Dermatology
International Journal of Leprosy
Journal of Allergy and Clinical Immunology
Journal of the American Academy of Dermatology
Journal of the American Medical Association
Journal of the American Podiatry Association
Journal of Applied Physiology: Respiratory, Environmental and Exercise Physiology
Journal of Clinical Endocrinology and Metabolism
Journal of Clinical Pathology
Journal of Cutaneous Pathology
Journal of Dermatology
Journal of Immunology
Journal of Investigative Dermatology
Journal of Laboratory and Clinical Medicine
Journal of Medical Genetics
Journal of Nuclear Medicine
Journal of Pediatric Surgery
Journal of Pediatrics
Journal of Trauma
Laboratory Investigation
Lancet
Leprosy Review
Medical Journal of Australia
Medicine
Nature
New England Journal of Medicine
New York State Journal of Medicine
Oral Surgery, Oral Medicine, Oral Pathology
Pediatric Research
Pediatrics
Plastic and Reconstructive Surgery
Postgraduate Medical Journal
Presse Medicale
Proceedings of the National Academy of Sciences
Revue Neurologique
Science
Southern Medical Journal
Surgery, Gynecology and Obstetrics
Thrombosis and Hemostasis
Tissue Antigens
Western Journal of Medicine

Statistics of Interest to the Dermatologist

MALIGNANT MELANOMA ESTIMATES FOR 1984[1]

Incidence	17,700 (8,700 men; 9,000 women)
Deaths	5,500

REPORTABLE COMMUNICABLE DISEASES WITH DERMATOLOGIC MANIFESTATIONS[2]

Disease	*Cases Reported*
AIDS	3,572[3]
Gonorrhea	898,936
Hepatitis B	22,292
Leprosy	229
Leptospirosis	45
Measles	1,436
Meningococcemia	2,645
Rocky Mountain spotted fever	1,132
Rubella	942
Syphilis	31,796
Toxic shock syndrome	382
Typhoid fever	436
Typhus (flea-borne)	48

COMMON SKIN DISORDERS ENCOUNTERED BY DERMATOLOGISTS AND PRIMARY CARE PHYSICIANS[4]

Disorder	*Percent of Visits*	
	Dermatologists	*Primary Care Physicians*
Tumors of the skin	21.8	19.1
Dermatitis and other dermatoses	19.6	18.5
Viral infections	10.2	6.8
Acne conditions	9.8	5.5
Disorders of epidermal proliferation	8.8	4.8
Bacterial infections	5	4.8
Fungal diseases	3.8	17.1
Alopecia	3	4.8
Xerosis	2	5.5
Urticaria	1.4	...
Parasites	1.4	...
Cutaneous manifestations of systemic diseases	1.2	...

MEMBERSHIP OF THE AMERICAN ACADEMY OF DERMATOLOGY—1984[5]

Top Ten States	*Rank*	*Number of Dermatologists*	*Percent of Total*
California	1	915	14
New York	2	579	9
Florida	3	359	5
Texas	4	352	5
Pennsylvania	5	279	4
Illinois	6	257	4
New Jersey	7	232	3
Michigan	8	221	3
Ohio	9	211	3
Massachusetts	10	165	2
Subtotal		3,570	53
Bottom Five States			
Maine	46	14	...
Delaware	47	12	...
Vermont	48	8	...
Wyoming	49	6	...
Alaska	50	2	...
Total		6,701	...

References:
[1]Silverberg, E.: *CA* 34:7–23, 1984.
[2]All data, except cases of AIDS, are for first 51 weeks of 1983; *MMWR* Dec. 30, 1983.
[3]Total number of cases reported in the United States up to Feb. 29, 1984; *Boston Globe,* Mar. 11, 1984.
[4]Branch, W.T., Jr., Wintroub, B.U.: *J. Am. Acad. Dermatol.* 9:281–282, 1983.
[5]In a personal communication with T. Stulka, American Academy of Dermatology, in April 1984.

Review Articles

Acne:

Cunliffe, W. J.: The conventional treatment of acne. *Seminars in Dermatology* 2:138–144, 1983.
Pochi, P. E.: Endocrinology of acne. *J. Invest. Dermatol.* 81:1, 1983.
Wilkin, J. K.: Rosacea. *Int. J. Dermatol.* 22:393–400, 1983.

Acquired Immune Deficiency Syndrome:

Daul, C. D., deShazo, R. D.: Acquired immune deficiency syndrome: an update and interpretation. *Ann. Allergy* 51:351–361, 1983.

Bacterial Infections:

Lyell, A.: The staphylococcal scalded skin syndrome in historical perspective: emergence of dermopathic strains of *Staphylococcus aureus* and discovery of the epidermolytic toxin. A review of events up to 1970. *J. Am. Acad. Dermatol.* 9:285–294, 1983.

Black Dermatology:

Brauner, G. J.: Cutaneous disease in black children. *Am. J. Dis. Child.* 137:488–496, 1983.

Bullous Disease:

Black, M. M., Meyrick, R. H., Bhogal, B.: The value of immunofluorescence technique in the diagnosis of bullous disorders: a review. *Clin. Exp. Dermatol.* 8:337–353, 1983.
Hietanen, J.: Acantholytic cells in pemphigus: a scanning and electron microscopic study. *Acta Odontol. Scand.* 40:257–273, 1982.
Patel, H. P., Anhalt, G. J., Diaz, L. A.: Bullous pemphigoid and pemphigus vulgaris. *Ann. Allergy* 50:144–150, 1983.

Cancer:

Adam, Y. G., Efron, G.: Cutaneous malignant melanoma: current views on pathogenesis, diagnosis, and surgical management. *Surgery* 93:481–494, 1983.
Bánóczy, J.: Oral leukoplakia and other white lesions of the oral mucosa related to dermatological disorders. *J. Cutan. Pathol.* 10:238–256, 1983.
Binnie, W. H., Rankin, K. V., MacKenzie, I. C.: Etiology of oral squamous cell carcinoma. *J. Oral Pathol.* 12:11–29, 1983.

Epstein, J. H.: Photocarcinogenesis, skin cancer, and aging. *J. Am. Acad. Dermatol.* 9:487–502, 1983.
Fukushiro, R.: Chromomycosis in Japan. *Int. J. Dermatol.* 22:221–229, 1983.
Goldschmidt, H., Sherwin, W. K.: Office radiotherapy of cutaneous carcinomas. I. Radiation techniques, dose schedules, and radiation protection. *J. Dermatol. Surg. Oncol.* 9:31–46, 1983.
Goldschmidt, H., Sherwin, W. K.: Office radiotherapy of cutaneous carcinomas. II. Indications in specific anatomic regions. *J. Dermatol. Surg. Oncol.* 9:47–76, 1983.
Kornbrot, A., Tatoiam, J. A., Jr.: Benign soft tissue tumors of the oral cavity. *Int. J. Dermatol.* 22:207–214, 1983.
Maize, J. C.: Primary cutaneous malignant melanoma: an analysis of the prognostic value of histologic characteristics. *J. Am. Acad. Dermatol.* 8:857–863, 1983.
Modlin, R. L., Crissey, J. T., Rea, T. H.: Kaposi's sarcoma. *Int. J. Dermatol.* 22:443–462, 1983.
Pawlowski, A., Lea, P. J.: Nevi and melanoma induced by chemical carcinogens in laboratory animals: similarities and differences with human lesions. *J. Cutan. Pathol.* 10:81–110, 1983.
Wagner, R. F., Jr., Wagner, K. D.: Cutaneous signs of coronary artery disease. *Int. J. Dermatol.* 22:215–220, 1983.

Collagen–Vascular Diseases:

Callen, J. P.: Mixed connective tissue disease: an overview. *South. Med. J.* 75:1380–1384, 1982.
Jorizzo, J. L., Daniels, J. C.: Dermatologic conditions reported in patients with rheumatoid arthritis. *J. Am. Acad. Dermatol.* 8:439–457, 1983.
Sibbitt, W. L., Jr., Williams, R. C., Jr.: Cutaneous manifestations of rheumatoid arthritis. *Int. J. Dermatol.* 21:563–572, 1982.
Sontheimer, R. D., Deng, J.-S., Gilliam, J. N.: Antinuclear and anticytoplasmic antibodies: concepts and misconceptions. *J. Am. Acad. Dermatol.* 9:335–343, 1983.
Weiss, R. A., Magavero, H. S., Jr., Synkowski, D. R., Provost, T. T.: Diagnostic tests and clinical subsets in systemic lupus erythematosus: update 1983. *Ann. Allergy* 51:135–146, 1983.

Contact Dermatitis:

Ahmed, A. R., Blose, D. A.: Delayed-type hypersensitivity skin testing: a review. *Arch. Dermatol.* 119:934–945, 1983.
Lemanske, R. F., Jr., Kaliner, M. A.: Late phase allergic reactions. *Int. J. Dermatol.* 22:401–409, 1983.
MacDonald, R. H., Beck, M.: Neomycin: a review with particular reference to dermatological usage. *Clin. Exp. Dermatol.* 8:249–258, 1983.
Stoner, J. G., Rasmussen, J. E.: Plant dermatitis. *J. Am. Acad. Dermatol.* 9:1–15, 1983.

Drug Reactions:

Commens, C.: Fixed drug eruption. *Australas. J. Dermatol.* 24:1–8, 1983.
Krumlovsky, F. A.: Drug-induced nephrotoxicity. *Arch Dermatol.* 119:681–682, 1983.

Portnoy, J. Z., Callen J. P.: Ophthalmologic aspects of chloroquine and hydroxychloroquine therapy. *Int. J. Dermatol.* 22:273–278, 1983.

Erythema Multiforme:

Binazzi, M., Papini, M., Simonetti, S.: Skin mycoses: geographic distribution and present-day pathomorphosis. *Int. J. Dermatol.* 22:92–96, 1983.
Huff, J. C., Weston, W. L., Tonnesen, M. G.: Erythema multiforme: a critical review of characteristics, diagnostic criteria, and causes. *J. Am. Acad. Dermatol.* 8:763–775, 1983.
McGinnis, M. R.: Chromoblastomycosis and phaeohyphomycosis: new concepts, diagnosis, and mycology. *J. Am. Acad. Dermatol.* 8:1–16, 1983.

Genodermatitis:

Graff, G. E.: A review of hereditary hemorrhagic telangiectasia. *J. Am. Osteopath. Assoc.* 82:412–416, 1983.
Hart, D. B.: Menkes' syndrome: an updated review. *J. Am. Acad. Dermatol.* 9:145–150, 1983.
Nusbaum, B. P., Frost, P.: Ichthyosiform dermatoses: Diagnostic and therapeutic aspects. *Seminars in Dermatology* 2:161–169, 1983.
Rand, R. E., Baden, H. P.: The ichthyoses: a review. *J. Am. Acad. Dermatol.* 8:285–305, 1983.

Graft-Vs.-Host Disease:

James, W. D., Odom, R. B.: Graft-*v*-host disease. *Arch. Dermatol.* 119:683–689, 1983.

Hair and Nails:

Callan, A.: Management of hirsutism. *Australas. J. Dermatol.* 23:97–104, 1982.
Jeanmougin, M., Civatte, J.: Nail dischromia. *Int. J. Dermatol.* 22:279–290, 1983.
Rentoul, J. R.: Management of the hirsute woman. *Int. J. Dermatol.* 22:265–272, 1983.

Immunopathology:

Keeling, J. H., Lewis, C. W.: In vitro analysis of lymphocytes: markers and functions. *J. Am. Acad. Dermatol.* 8:239–251, 1983.
Kung, P. C., Berger, C. L., Estabrook, A., et al.: Monoclonal antibodies for clinical investigation of human T lymphocytes. *Int. J. Dermatol.* 22:67–74, 1983.
Thivolet, J., Faure, M.: Immunohistochemistry in cutaneous pathology, *J. Cutan. Pathol.* 10:1–32, 1983.

Insects and Other Crawling Organisms:

Clausen, R. W.: Insect Stings. *J. Fam. Pract.* 15:969–976, 1982.
Henwood, B. P., MacDonald, D. M.: Caterpillar dermatitis. *Clin. Exp. Dermatol.* 8:77–93, 1983.

Krinsky, W. L.: Dermatoses associated with the bites of mites and ticks (Arthropoda: acari). *Int. J. Dermatol.* 22:75–91, 1983.

Keratinocytes:

Clausen, O. P. F.: Flow cytometry of keratinocytes. *J. Cutan. Pathol.* 10:33–51, 1983.

Leprosy:

Anderson, R.: The immunopharmacology of antileprosy agents. *Lepr. Rev.* 54:139–144, 1983.
Bjune, G.: Reactions in leprosy. *Lepr. Rev.* 61S–67S, 1983.
Nath, I.: Immunology of human leprosy: current status. *Lepr. Rev.* 31S–45S, 1983.
Shepard, C. C., Van Landingham, R. M., Walker, L. L.: Recent studies of antileprosy drugs. *Lepr. Rev.* 23S–30S, 1983.
Skinsnes, O. K.: Epidemiology and decline of leprosy in Asia. *Int. J. Dermatol.* 22:348–369, 1983.

Lyme Disease:

Meyerhoff, J.: Lyme Disease. *Am. J. Med.* 75:663–670, October 1983.

Percutaneous Absorption:

Franz, T. J.: Kinetics of cutaneous drug penetration. *Int. J. Dermatol.* 22:499–505, 1983.
Shellow, W. V. R.: The skin in alcoholism. *Int. J. Dermatol.* 22:506–510, 1983.
Suskind, R. R.: Percutaneous absorption and chemical carcinogenesis. *J. Dermatol.* 10:97–107, 1983.
Wester, R. C., Maibach, H. I.: Dermatopharmacokinetics in clinical dermatology. *Seminars in Dermatology* 2:81–84, 1983.

Photomedicine:

Epstein, J. H.: Phototoxicity and photoallergy in man. *J. Am. Acad. Dermatol.* 8:141–147, 1983.

Pityriasis Rosea:

Cavanaugh, R. M., Jr.: Pityriasis rosea in children: a review. *Clin. Pediatr.* 22:200–203, 1983.

Porphyria:

Eubanks, S. W., Patterson, J. W., May, D. L., et al.: The porphyrias. *Int. J. Dermatol.* 22:337–348, 1983.

Pregnancy:

Holmes, R. C., Black, M. M.: The specific dermatoses of pregnancy. *J. Am. Acad. Dermatol.* 8:405–412, 1983.

Psoriasis:

Ashton, R. E., Andre, P., Lowe, N. J., et al.: Anthralin: historical and current perspectives. *J. Am. Acad. Dermatol.* 9:173–192, 1983.
Bickers, D. R.: Position paper: PUVA therapy. *J. Am. Acad. Dermatol.* 8:265–270, 1983.
Farber, E. M., Abel, E. A., Cox, A. J.: Long-term risks of Psoralen and UV-A therapy for psoriasis. *Arch. Dermatol.* 119:426–431, 1983.
Wilkinson, J. D., English, J.: Psoralens. *Seminars in Dermatology* 2:85–100, 1983.

Psychodermatology:

Cotterill, J. A.: Biochemistry of anxiety, depression, itch, and the placebo response. *Seminars in Dermatology* 2:171–176, 1983.
Cotterill, J. A.: Clinical features of patients with dermatologic nondisease. *Seminars in Dermatology* 2:203–205, 1983.
Cotterill, J. A.: A psychodermatologic miscellany. *Seminars in Dermatology* 2:223–226, 1983.
Hardy, G. E.: Body image: the psyche and the skin. *Seminars in Dermatology* 2:207–211, 1983.
Lyell, A.: Delusions of parasitosis. *Seminars in Dermatology* 2:189–195, 1983.
Munro, A.: Delusional parasitosis: a form of monosymptomatic hypochondriacal psychosis. *Seminars in Dermatology* 2:197–202, 1983.
Musaph, H.: Psychogenic pruritis. *Seminars in Dermatology* 2:217–222, 1983.
Nutting, W. B., Beerman, H.: Demodicosis and symbiophobia: status, terminology, and treatments. *Int. J. Dermatol.* 22:13–17, 1983.
Seville, R. H.: Psoriasis, stress, insight, and progress. *Seminars in Dermatology* 2:213–216, 1983.
Sneddon, I. B.: Simulated disease and hypochondriasis in the dermatology clinic. *Seminars in Dermatology* 2:177–183, 1984.
Sneddon, I. B.: Simulated disease: problems in diagnosis and management. *J. R. Coll. Physicians Lond.* 17:199–205, 1983.
Sneddon, J.: Patients who do not want to get better. *Seminars in Dermatology* 2:183–188, 1983.

Retinoids:

Cunningham, W. J., Ehmann, C. W.: Clinical aspects of the retinoids. *Seminars in Dermatology* 2:145–160, 1983

Steroids:

Fritz, K. A., Weston, W. L.: Topical glucocorticosteroids. *Ann. Allergy* 50:68–76, 1983.

Surgery:

Apfelberg, D. B., Maser, M. R., Lash, H., et al.: The role of the argon laser in the management of hemangiomas. *Int. J. Dermatol.* 21:579–589, 1982.
Swanson, N. A.: Mohs surgery: technique, indications, applications, and the future. *Arch. Dermatol.* 119:761–773, 1983.

Sweet's Syndrome:

Storer, J. S., Nesbitt, L. T., Jr., Galen, W. K., et al.: Sweet's syndrome. *Int. J. Dermatol.* 22:8–12, 1983.

Urticaria and Angioedema:

Brickman, C. M., Hosea, S. W.: Hereditary angioedema. *Int. J. Dermatol.* 22:141–147, 1983.
Graham, J. A., Jouhar, A. J.: The importance of cosmetics in the psychology of appearance. *Int. J. Dermatol.* 22:153–156, 1983.
Ramesh, V., Reddy, B. S. N., Singh, R.: Onchomycosis. *Int. J. Dermatol.* 22:148–152, 1983.
Winton, G. B., Lewis, C. W.: Contact urticaria. *Int. J. Dermatol.* 21:573–578, 1982.

Viral Disease:

Bunney, M. H.: Wart treatments. *Seminars in Dermatology* 2:101–108, 1983.
Chang, T.-W.: Herpes simplex virus infection. *Int. J. Dermatol.* 22:1–7, 1983.
Levy, R. S., Fisher, M., Alter, J. N.: Penicillamine: review and cutaneous manifestations. *J. Am. Acad. Dermatol.* 8:548–558, 1983.
McElgunn, P. S. J.: Dermatologic manifestations of hepatitis B virus infection. *J. Am. Acad. Dermatol.* 8:539–548, 1983.
Robinson, T.: Antiviral agents and the skin. *Seminars in Dermatology* 2:130–137, 1983.
Simmons, P. D.: Genital warts. *Int. J. Dermatol.* 22:410–414, 1983.
von Krogh, G.: Condylomata acuminata 1983: an up-dated review. *Seminars in Dermatology* 2:109–129, 1983.

Vulvar Diseases:

Woodruff, J. D.: Vulvar disease: a spectrum of clinical pictures. *Postgrad. Med. J.* 73:232–245, 1983.

Wound Healing:

Bloom, S. R., Polak, J. M.: Regulatory peptides and the skin. *Clin. Exp. Dermatol.* 8:3–18, 1983.
Zitelli, J. A.: Wound healing by secondary intention. *J. Am. Acad. Dermatol.* 9:407–415, 1983.

1. Acne and Disorders of Sebaceous and Apocrine Glands

1-1 **Oral Treatment of Acne Conglobata With 13-*cis*-Retinoic Acid: Results of the German Multicentric Study After 24 Weeks of Treatment.** Results of the German Cooperative Study Group, with 198 acne conglobata patients treated with isotretinoin (13-*cis*-retinoic acid, Ro 4-3780) were reported by Wilhelm Meigel, Harald Gollnick, Heinrich Wokalek, Gerd Plewig, and 44 colleagues from 19 clinics. For the first 12 weeks (phase 1) there was an open assignment of patients to receive 0.2, 0.5, or 1.0 mg of isotretinoin per kg of body weight. This was followed by an additional 12 weeks of treatment (phase 2). If there was at least a 66% improvement of lesions, the 0.2-mg/kg dose was continued, and the 0.5-mg/kg dose was lowered to 0.2 mg/kg. If there was no such improvement, the dose was increased to 0.5 and 1.0 mg/kg, respectively. The initial high-dose group receiving 1.0 mg/kg was assigned after 12 weeks to receive 0.2 mg/kg of maintenance therapy or no therapy at all.

Noninflammatory and inflammatory acne lesions from the entire body were counted. Seborrhea was graded on a scale of 4 (0 to 3+). It improved from medium and severe to light and none. This was a definite advantage because patients with acne conglobata have chronic seborrhea which produces psychological stress. Subjective side effects were registered and found to be tolerable. Laboratory data included a hematologic profile with differential cell counts, creatinine, serum glutamic oxaloacetic transaminase, serum glutamic pyruvic transaminase, alkaline phosphatase, total bilirubin, serum cholesterol and serum triglyceride levels, and urinalysis.

For statistical analysis, 171 patients were available; 27 dropped out of the study, mostly for reasons unrelated to the drug. At least 75% improvement was observed in the 0.2-mg/kg group with 73.7% and 59.5%, respectively; in the 0.5-mg/kg group with 72.5% and 61.2%, respectively; and in the 1.0-mg/kg group with 85.4% and 92%, respectively. Sebum suppression was dose related. Subjective side effects were fairly well dose related, particularly those of skin and mucous membranes. Myalgia was rare. There was a dose-related elevation of triglyceride and cholesterol levels, but not significant for the mean in each group. Single patients did show significant elevation of blood lipids, but no other laboratory values changed significantly. A complete history and appropriate preexamination is recommended for patients at risk.

(1–1) Hautarzt 34:387–397, August 1982.

Isotretinoin is currently the most effective drug to control severe forms of acne and can produce long-lasting remissions.

▶ [This study is presumably an extension and expansion of one reported previously by these authors (*Hautarzt* 32:634, 1981) in which 127 patients with severe acne were assessed for their response to 12 weeks of oral isotretinoin with one of 3 dosages, viz. 0.2, 0.5, or 1.0 mg/kg/day. In the present report, 171 patients—apparently representing an addition of 44 patients– were treated with the same dosages which, however, could be changed upward or downward after the 12-week treatment period, depending on the patient's response to treatment. The additional treatment was for another 12 weeks. It is rather difficult to interpret optimal dosage regimens from studies in which midstream dose changes are made.

As had been the case before, lower doses were clinically effective although not as much as the highest dose, and most side effects were dose related. And as before, no data are made available on the incidence of recurrence vis-à-vis dosages received, based either on a daily or total amount of drug used.

It should be noted that the designation "acne conglobata" in the article's title may be inappropriate. The patient shown in the illustrations did not have acne conglobata but severe nodulocystic acne. The distinction is not one of mere quibbling. The response of patients with bona fide acne conglobata to oral isotretinoin is not as good cosmetically as that of patients with nodulocystic acne, because the interconnecting and deep sinus tracts and the frequent contractile-type scarring, which are characteristic of acne conglobata, are not affected materially by treatment.—P.E.P.] ◀

1–2 **Effect of Oral 13-*cis*-Retinoic Acid at Three Dose Levels on Sustainable Rates of Sebum Secretion and on Acne.** Mary Ellen Stewart, Allison M. Benoit, Anna M. Stranieri, Ronald P. Rapini, John S. Strauss, and Donald T. Downing (Univ. of Iowa) monitored changes in sustainable rates of sebum secretion in 20 patients, (18 males aged 17–26 and 2 women aged 19–28). All had active, severe nodulocystic acne, which had been resistant to previous therapy. Five patients received 0.1 mg of 13-*cis*-retinoic acid per kg per day; 7 received 0.5 mg/kg/day, and 8 received 1.0 kg/day. Half the dose was taken twice a day for 20 weeks.

Sebum secretion was measured at regular intervals by absorption of skin surface lipid into bentonite clay. The amount of absorbed sebum was estimated by measuring its wax ester component. Time courses for on-treatment suppression and posttreatment recovery of wax ester secretion are shown in Figure 1–1 for the 3 doses. Calculated as percentage of pretreatment values, the average wax ester secretion rates between 4 and 20 weeks for the three dosages were 23%, 12%, and 10%, respectively. The average pretreatment wax ester production in the study population was 1.13 mg/10 sq cm/3 hours, equivalent to a total sebum secretion rate of 4.52 mg/10 sq cm/3 hours or more than five times as high as the average for normal persons.

Reduction of sebum production rates by 13-*cis*-retinoic acid probably contributes importantly to its effectiveness against severe acne, and clearing continues after treatment with the drug has been stopped. Remissions are prolonged. Eight weeks after treatment, all subjects showed at least 60% clearing of cysts larger than 4 mm in diameter; 17 males were completely free from facial cysts, whereas women responded less well. Before treatment, all males had had chest

---

(1–2) J. Am. Acad. Dermatol. 8:532–538, April 1983.

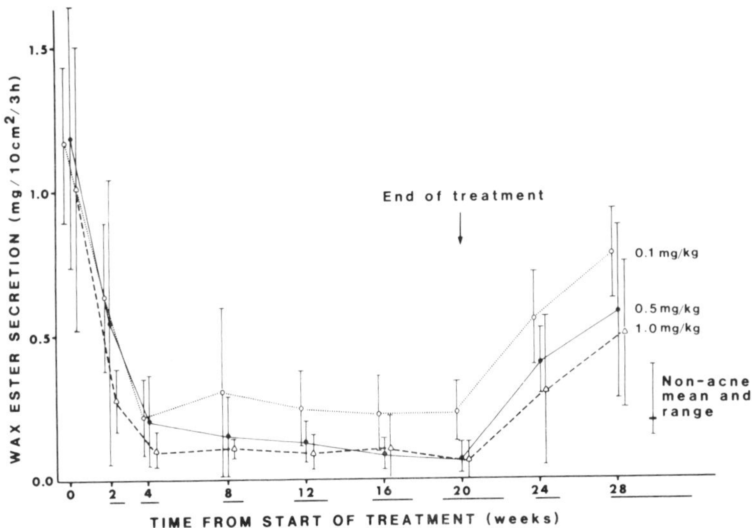

Fig 1–1.—Mean rates of wax ester secretion before, during, and after treatment of subjects with severe acne with 0.1, 0.5, or 1.0 mg of 13-*cis*-retinoic acid per kg per day for 20 weeks. Vertical bars indicate SD. Numbers on abscissa indicate nominal dates of measurements and horizontal bars show range. One subject receiving the 0.5-mg dosage was omitted because he failed to return for posttreatment measurements. His inclusion would have increased slightly on-treatment means for 0.5-mg group. Nonacne mean and range are from Harris, H.H., Downing, D.T., Stewart, M.E., and Strauss, J.S.: Sustainable rates of sebum secretion in acne patients and matched normal control subjects. J. Am. Acad. Dermatol. 8:203, 1983. (Courtesy of Stewart, M.E., et al.: J. Am. Acad. Dermatol. 8:532–538, April 1983.)

and back cysts; 8 weeks after treatment, these cysts were cleared in 6 men and greatly reduced in number in the rest.

Slow responders were not receiving the 0.1-mg/kg/day dose, and 1.0 mg/kg/day of the drug may have no advantage over this lowest dose although the larger dose has a significantly greater effect on wax ester production rates. Why some patients respond slowly, or not at all, remains to be determined.

▶ [Using the bentonite clay–absorption method of collecting sebum (see abstract 1–5) the authors confirmed the prior observations of several investigators, including themselves, that oral isotretinoin inhibits the synthesis of sebum rapidly and profoundly. Curves for the temporal and quantitative decrements in sebum values are virtually superimposable upon those demonstrated in earlier reports. Thus, the new technique of sebum collection seems comparable to the older paper-absorption method, at least in relation to the measured changes induced by oral isotretinoin. It remains to be seen if the methods differ from one another in the capacity to discriminate effects from treatment with less powerful sebostatic drugs, e.g. estrogen, glucocorticoid, or antiandrogens such as spironolactone.—P.E.P.] ◀

1–3 **Effects of Isotretinoin on Neutrophil Chemotaxis in Cystic Acne.** Isotretinoin improves several forms of acne including cystic acne; it has an anti-inflammatory action and causes sebaceous gland atrophy. Etritinate, another retinoid, leads to a marked reduction in

(1–3) Dermatologica 167:16–18, July 1983.

neutrophilic chemotactic activity in psoriasis. P. D. Pigatto, A. Fioroni, F. Riva, M. A. Brugo, A. Morandotti, G. F. Altomare, and A. F. Finzi (Milan) examined neutrophilic chemotactic activity in 8 males with cystic acne who received isotretinoin. Their average age was 23 years. Thirty-two healthy men, aged 19–32 years, were also studied. Isotretinoin was given in a dosage of 0.8 mg/kg daily, after a lipid-rich meal, for at least 15 days. Baseline neutrophil chemotactic activity in acne patients was in the range of that in normal subjects, but after 15 days of treatment the mean chemotactic activity was significantly lower.

Neutrophil chemotaxis in patients with acne is inhibited by isotretinoin, which impedes both sebaceous gland secretion and pustule formation. Other drugs used to treat patients with acne, including tetracycline, erythromycin, and clindamycin, also inhibit neutrophil chemotaxis. Retinoids appear to reduce chemotaxis not only by a keratolytic effect on chemoattractants in the stratum corneum but also by a direct action on polymorphonuclear leukocytes.

▶ [Oral isotretinoin administered for 2 weeks to 8 patients with cystic acne effected a statistically significant inhibition of in vitro chemotaxis of their polymorphonuclear leukocytes. From these results, the authors conclude that this effect plays an "important role" in the improvement of acne from isotretinoin treatment.

However, the overall decrease in chemotaxis was only 20%, with half of the patients showing a less than 10% inhibition. Unfortunately, no information is given about the clinical response of these patients who presumably were treated beyond the 2-week experimental period. Did those patients who demonstrated little chemotactic inhibition fare less well therapeutically than those who showed a greater reduction in chemotaxis?

Although these experimental results, as well as those of others, have indeed demonstrated that inhibition of chemotaxis of polymorphonuclear leukocytes occurs after retinoid administration, it has not yet been possible to determine the clinical significance of this in acne. For example, etretinate, which is not very effective in acne, also inhibits neutrophilic chemotaxis in vitro. With isotretinoin, chemotaxis inhibition probably results chiefly from the reduction of the number of *Propionibacterium acnes* organisms (as a result of the depletion of its substrate sebum) which elaborate a neutrophilic chemotactic factor.—P.E.P.] ◀

1–4 **Pyogenic Granuloma-Like Acne Lesions During Isotretinoin Therapy.** Isotretinoin is a vitamin A analogue that is highly effective in the treatment of severe cystic and conglobate acne. John H. Exner, Shamin Dahod, and Peter E. Pochi (Boston Univ.) report data on 3 men with severe cystic acne who received oral isotretinoin therapy; subsequently, inflammatory, hemorrhagic, pyogenic, and granuloma-like changes developed in previously crusted acne lesions, necessitating discontinuance of the drug in 2 of the 3 patients.

Man, 20, had very severe cystic acne since age 15. The disease responded poorly to treatment with oral antibiotics and topical agents, including tretinoin, but responded adequately to administration of oral prednisone with dapsone. Isotretinoin was given initially in a dose of 1 mg/kg daily in place of steroid-dapsone therapy. Lesion counts decreased slightly after a month, but existing lesions gradually became tender and inflamed, and large gran-

---

(1–4) Arch. Dermatol. 119:808–811, October 1983.

uloma pyogenicum-like nodules developed within several crusted areas (Fig 1–2). Crusting increased over 20 weeks of treatment, and gradual healing took place in the 8-week posttreatment period. Total lesion counts decreased to about a third of baseline. When therapy was resumed with isotretinoin in a dose of 1.5 mg/kg daily, no new erosions or crusts were observed, and all inflammatory lesions resolved within 8 weeks after treatment. Biopsy of a crusted lesion showed epidermal ulceration and dense inflammatory infiltration in the middle dermis and upper dermis. Mitotic figures were not noted in the cells of the infiltrate.

This reaction is characterized by ulceration, hemorrhagic crusting, and tenderness of preexisting acne lesions. Excess granulation tissue underlies many crusts, in some instances resembling pyogenic granuloma. Symptoms of acne fulminans did not occur in the present patients. The mechanism of the reaction is unknown, but skin fragility caused by isotretinoin and dermal factors may contribute. Changes in the vasculature may be involved. The reaction occurred in 3 of 66 acne patients treated with isotretinoin. Caution in using this drug

Fig 1–2.—Skin of patient 8 weeks after start of oral isotretinoin treatment; large, hemorrhagic crusts are seen. (Courtesy of Exner, J.H., et al.: Arch. Dermatol. 119:808–811, October 1983; copyright 1983, American Medical Association.)

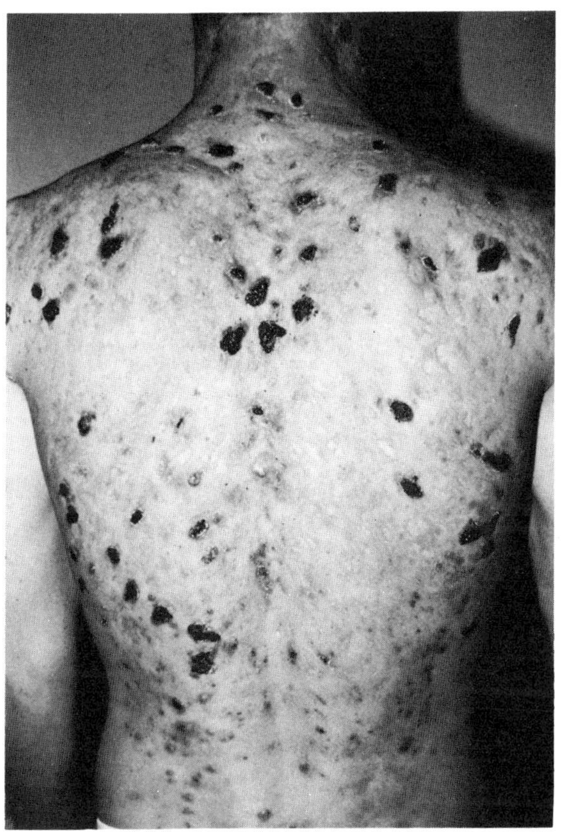

may be warranted, especially in patients who have even minimally crusted or ulcerated acne lesions.

▶ [Since the first account appeared of this vascular reaction in nodulocystic lesions of acne patients treated with oral isotretinoin (*Mayo Clin. Proc.* 58:509, 1983), a number of subsequent reports have been published describing the same side effect. Not clearly evident from any of the case reports is whether the individual sites where the reactions occur will heal with more scarring than if the acne lesions did not develop this hemorrhagic response. On the other hand, it appears that the occurrence of these lesions does not have an unfavorable prognostic indication of the ultimate response of the acne itself.—P.E.P.] ◀

1–5 **Sustainable Rates of Sebum Secretion in Acne Patients and Matched Normal Control Subjects.** Holly Hake Harris, Donald T. Downing, Mary Ellen Stewart, and John S. Strauss (Univ. of Iowa) measured sustainable rates of sebum secretion in 12 subjects with inflammatory acne and in 12 controls matched for age and sex who had no significant signs of acne. Measurements were made after the skin was depleted of an accumulation of previously secreted sebum by absorption into adherent layers of bentonite clay applied to the center of the forehead for 14 hours. Disks of fine Dacron mesh embedded in fresh clay were then applied to the forehead for 3 hours. Disks and adhering clay were removed and extracted with ether to recover collected lipids. Sebum recovered during the 3-hour period was measured by quantitative thin-layer chromatography.

All subjects with acne had significantly higher sebum secretion rates than their normal controls. In most cases the amounts from the right and the left sides were similar in individual subjects. As a group, subjects with acne had sustainable sebum secretion rates three times those of controls. Those with moderate inflammatory acne had sebum secretion rates almost twice as high as those with milder acne.

Sebum secretion may play a decisive role in the pathogenesis of acne, but other factors may also be involved.

▶ [A method for measuring surface sebum in which a 14-hour period of depletion of the follicular sebum reservoir precedes a 3-hour collection was studied in 12 patients with acne and 12 subjects without acne. The results disclosed that 10 of the 12 acne patients had sebum levels that clearly exceeded values for each of the normal subjects. The authors conclude that this method is an improvement over the standard 3-hour paper-absorption method (in which there is only a 30-minute depletion of sebum before collection), in that there is less overlap of sebum values between acne and normal subjects.

The author's interpretation of their results, although probably valid, must remain tentative until *(1)* many more subjects are studied to be able to determine that the segregation of acne sebum values from normal ones is maintained; and *(2)* a comparison of the "new" and the "old" methods of sebum collection shows distinctively less overlap with the former than with the latter technique. It is unfortunate that the usual 3-hour paper-absorption test was not done in the same subjects of the present study. This would probably have settled the issue beyond cavil.—P.E.P.] ◀

1–6 **Androgen Excess in Cystic Acne.** Samuel P. Marynick, Zaven H. Chakmakjian, David L. McCaffree, and James H. Herndon, Jr. (Baylor Univ.) measured hormone levels in 59 women and 32 men with long-standing cystic acne that was resistant to conventional

(1–5) J. Am. Acad. Dermatol. 8:200–203, February 1983.
(1–6) N. Engl. J. Med. 308:981–986, April 28, 1983.

therapy. The women had higher serum levels of dehydroepiandrosterone sulfate (DHEA-S), testosterone, and luteinizing hormone and lower levels of sex hormone–binding hormone than were found in controls. The men had higher levels of serum DHEA-S and 17-hydroxyprogesterone and lower levels of sex hormone–binding globulin than controls had. Therapy was aimed at lowering the DHEA-S levels. For this purpose, dexamethasone was chosen because of its ability to inhibit release of adrenocorticotropin hormone and lower adrenal production of androgen. Women received an initial dexamethasone dose of 0.125 mg daily, or an oral contraceptive pill, or both; the daily dose was increased by 0.125 mg of dexamethasone at monthly intervals until a total daily dose of 0.5 mg was reached, or the level of DHEA-S was lowered to less than 2.0 μg/ml, or remission of acne occurred. In the men, after an initial dose of dexamethasone of 0.25 mg daily, the dose was gradually increased by 0.125 mg daily at monthly intervals until there was resolution of acne, or the DHEA-S level was below 3.0 μg/ml, or a dexamethasone dose of 0.75 mg daily was reached.

Of patients treated for 6 months, 97% of the women and 81% of the men experienced resolution or marked improvement in their acne. The dose of dexamethasone required to reduce DHEA-S levels was low, rarely exceeding the equivalent of 20 mg of hydrocortisone daily.

Most patients with therapeutically resistant cystic acne have androgen excess, and lowering the elevated DHEA-S levels usually results in improvement or remission of the disease.

▶ [The findings in this study of abnormal hormone blood levels in patients with treatment-resistant cystic acne were not novel, but the high incidence of such deviations from normal certainly was, particularly in men in whom few abnormalities had been encountered in previous studies.

The most consistent abnormal finding was an increase in the adrenal androgen, dehydroepiandrosterone sulfate, occurring in 80%–90% of subjects studied. Treatment with oral dexamethasone in low dosage, i.e., 0.5 mg or less daily for 6 months, resulted in significant improvement or complete resolution of the acne in most subjects. Even without untreated or sham-treated patients for comparison, the clinical results were indeed striking.—P.E.P.] ◀

1–7 **Elevated Free Testosterone Levels in Women With Acne.** Acne vulgaris is considered to be an androgen-dependent disorder. Frank E. Schiavone, Robert L. Rietschel, Demetrios Sgoutas, and Russell Harris (Emory Univ.) evaluated data on female patients with varying grades of acne to determine whether the free testosterone level is a more sensitive indicator of hyperandrogenism than the total testosterone. About 99% of plasma testosterone is bound to serum proteins in normal women. Twenty-four females aged 16–37 years with varying grades of acne and 24 controls aged 17–32 years were included in the study. The use of oral contraceptives was discontinued at least 3 months before the study. No trial participant was using drugs known to alter albumin or sex hormone–binding globulin levels.

Two acne patients had mild and 1 had moderate hirsutism. Seven

---

(1–7) Arch. Dermatol. 119:799–802, October 1983.

patients with acne reported irregular menses or cycles lasting for more than 30 days. No patient had androgenic alopecia. The mean free testosterone level was higher in the acne patients when those with hirsutism were excluded. Total testosterone and dehydroepiandrosterone sulfate levels also were significantly greater in the acne group, but all patients had levels within the normal range. The mean free testosterone level was above the normal range in 11 patients. Four women with elevated total testosterone levels had abnormally elevated free testosterone levels. The 3 patients with hirsutism had free testosterone levels exceeding 0.93 ng/dl. Free testosterone levels could not be related to the severity of acne or its responsiveness to treatment.

The free testosterone level provides better distinction between women with acne and unaffected women than does the total testosterone level. Studies are underway to determine whether an increased free testosterone level is causally related to acne. If it is, more rational hormonal therapy may be possible.

▶ [In women with acne, the average serum concentration of both free (unbound) and total testosterone was found to be elevated, but elevations were more frequent for free testosterone than for total testosterone concentrations. These results are in agreement with those reported by Lucky et al. (see abstract below). Mean serum levels of dehydroepiandrosterone sulfate were also higher than normal, but the difference was not statistically significant. The patients in this study were not selected on the basis of severity of disease or resistance to conventional acne therapy. Thus, the endocrine abnormalities described seem to represent a general characteristic of female patients with acne.—P.E.P.] ◀

1–8 **Plasma Androgens in Women With Acne Vulgaris.** Anne W. Lucky, Joseph McGuire, Robert L. Rosenfield, Paul A. Lucky, and Barry H. Rich studied a group of women, with a mean age of 23.8 years, who had only acne (group A, 46 patients), only hirsutism (group H, 10), or acne plus hirsutism (group A + H, 19). Values for androgens, total and free testosterone, free 17β-hydroxycorticosteroids (17-β), dehydroepiandrosterone sulfate (DS), the androgen precursors 17α-hydroxypregnenolone (17-Preg) and 17α-hydroxyprogesterone (17-Prog), and testosterone-estrogen-binding globulin were determined in all patients. Plasma hormone concentrations of patients were compared with those of 23 controls whose mean age was 25.6 years and who had neither acne nor hirsutism.

The mean concentration of at least one hormone was elevated in every study group. In the 46 group A and the 19 group B patients, all steroids measured, except 17-Preg, had significantly elevated concentrations compared with those in controls. The total testosterone concentration was elevated in 13% of group A, 30% of group H, and 11% of group A + H. In contrast, the free testosterone concentration was elevated in 24% of group A, 50% of group H, and 26% of group A + H. Fifteen percent of group A had abnormal 17-α values. Free 17-β concentrations were more frequently elevated in hirsute patients. Follicular phase concentrations of 17-Prog were high in 31% of group

---

(1–8) J. Invest. Dermatol. 81:70–74, July 1983.

A, 67% of group H, and 40% of group A + H. Luteal phase 17-Prog values were rarely elevated. The most frequently abnormal androgen value was free testosterone concentration which was elevated in 24.6% of acne patients. The number of plasma hormone abnormalities per patient varied: 16 had one abnormality, 13 had two, 9 had three, and 4 had four abnormalities. Two had irregular menses.

There are plasma androgen abnormalities in a significant number of adult women with acne vulgaris. The patients in this study represent a selected population because of the persistence or appearance of acne in the third and fourth decades. Measurement of plasma free testosterone and DS concentrations in such patients may identify endocrine abnormalities potentially amenable to hormonal treatment.

▶ [Slightly more than half of 46 women with acne of moderate severity had one or more abnormalities of androgens or androgen precursors in their peripheral blood. There are a number of points of interest in this report: *(1)* the unbound or free fraction of testosterone was more frequently elevated than was the total amount; *(2)* when menstrual irregularities were present, they were not associated with a higher incidence of androgen abnormalities; *(3)* the degree of acne activity was not correlated with androgen levels; and *(4)* only one fifth of the acne patients had elevated dehydroepiandrosterone sulfate levels, compared with a very much higher incidence reported elsewhere (see abstract 1–6).

The findings suggest that endocrine alterations are of potential importance in the pathogenesis of acne in adult women. However, one should note that with any of the steroids measured in these patients, there were always more women who had normal rather than abnormal values. In addition, it remains to be determined whether normalization of the abnormal levels can reduce acne activity to any significant degree in such patients.—P.E.P.] ◀

1–9 **Low-Dose Prednisolone or Estrogen in Treatment of Women With Late-Onset or Persistent Acne Vulgaris.** C. R. Darley, J. W. Moore, G. M. Besser, D. D. Munro, and J. D. Kirby (London) studied 38 women with persistent or late-onset acne vulgaris. The women were allocated to either of 2 treatment groups: group 1 received prednisolone for 4 months, and group 2 received ethinyl estradiol and medroxyprogesterone acetate on days 1–7 of each calendar month for 4 months. Treatment dosage in group 1 was 2.5 mg of prednisolone on waking and 5 mg on retiring, and in group 2, 30 μg of ethinyl estradiol daily with 5 mg of medroxyprogesterone acetate on days 1–7 of each month. Group 1 patients were given low-dose prednisolone to suppress adrenocorticotropin hormone–dependent androgen secretion. Group 2 patients received cyclic estrogens with medroxyprogesterone to elevate the level of sex hormone–binding globulin (SHBG).

Of the 14 group 1 patients, 3 considered themselves improved, 7 considered the disease to be much better, and 4 reported no change. At the end of 4 months there was a significant improvement in observer assessment ($P < .01$). Testosterone, androstenedione, androstenediol, dihydroepiandrosterone (DHA), and DHA sulfate levels were significantly lower in all patients after 4 months' treatment. Four of 8 patients with irregular menses noted that their periods became more regular. In group 2, 10 patients completed 4 months' treat-

---

(1–9) Br. J. Dermatol. 108:345–353, March 1983.

ment. There was a significant improvement in observer assessment after this period ($P < .01$). Three patients reported that their acne was better, and 7 believed that it was much better. There was a significant increase in the SHBG level after 4 months; the testosterone level was significantly higher, but the androstenedione, androstenediol, and DHA values were not significantly different from baseline. Levels of DHA sulfate were significantly lower after 4 months' treatment. No serious adverse side effects developed. However, treatment was discontinued in 8 patients (2 in group 1, 6 in group 2) because of such side effects as did occur.

Improvement in acne in both groups did not correlate with the baseline androgen or SHBG levels. Thus, it is not possible to predict which patients will benefit from this form of therapy. However, certain guidelines can be suggested. For example, a suitable combined contraceptive pill containing ethynodiol diacetate should be prescribed for women with low SHBG levels or for any woman with acne who wishes this form of contraception. The serum testosterone assay should be repeated after 1 month to confirm that suppression has occurred. If a satisfactory response results, therapy should be continued for a year before attempts are made to withdraw the medication.

▶ [Women with acne and endocrine abnormalities were treated either with 7.5 mg of prednisolone daily (if serum testosterone levels were high) or with ethinyl estradiol 30 μg daily (if testosterone levels were normal but sex hormone–binding globulin was low). After 4 months of therapy, both groups showed significant improvement; specifically, 70% of the corticosteroid-treated patients and 90% of the estrogen-treated patients were improved.

The impressive response of the estrogen-treated group is all the more striking in view of the low dosage used, but it may reflect the authors' selection of patients whose level of sex hormone–binding globulin was subnormal.

In evaluating their results, the authors make no mention of a possible placebo effect or of an anti-inflammatory effect of the prednisolone. In fact, one wonders what the results would have been had the patients been treated at random with either of these two hormonal regimens. In this regard, the authors showed that the baseline levels of hormones could not be correlated with the clinical response.—P.E.P.] ◀

1–10 ***Propionibacterium acnes* Resistance to Antibiotics in Acne Patients.** James J. Leyden, Kenneth J. McGinley, Stephen Cavalieri, Guy F. Webster, Otto H. Mills, and Albert M. Kligman (Univ. of Pennsylvania) investigated *Propionibacterium acnes* resistance in patients receiving long-term systemic antibiotic therapy for acne. The patients included 40 men, mean age of 20, and 35 women, mean age of 19; all had long-standing inflammatory acne requiring systemic antibiotic therapy. The mean period of treatment was 21 months. Previously, 33 were treated with oral tetracycline, 14 with erythromycin, and 28 with both agents. No patient used a topical antibiotic during the 4 weeks before the study. Twenty-four patients with mild to moderate acne not treated with topical or systemic antibiotics, as well as 26 with other dermatologic disorders who had not received antibiotics were also studied.

The minimal inhibitory concentration (MIC) of *P. acnes* in the 75

(1–10) J. Am. Acad. Dermatol. 8:41–45, January 1983.

patients receiving long-term antibiotic therapy demonstrated the emergence of resistance strains. The mean MIC in 33 patients receiving tetracycline was 4–5 times higher than that found in acne patients not receiving antibiotic therapy and in controls free of acne. The average MIC for the erythromycin group was more than 100 times higher in those receiving long-term antibiotic therapy. In a second group of 62 patients, the clinical course and number of *P. acnes* were correlated with the presence of "resistant strains" defined as *P. acnes* with a 10-fold increase in MIC to tetracycline or erythromycin. Patients with resistant strains had higher counts of *P. acnes* and were not doing as well clinically as were those with sensitive strains.

Propionibacterium acnes resistance to antibiotics frequently develops in patients receiving long-term systemic antibiotic therapy. These results are in contrast with the results of previous attempts to find *P. acnes* resistance; most other studies were conducted many years ago. The present preliminary results indicate that antibiotic resistance is lost 1–2 months after the antibiotic is withdrawn, which is in accord with previous findings.

▶ [For years, an opinion prevailed that *Propionibacterium acnes* rarely, if ever, developed resistance to antibiotics. This belief was chiefly based on the clinical observation that acne can very often be controlled with antibiotic treatment for long periods of time. However, as demonstrated in this study and in an earlier one (Crawford, W. W., et al., *J. Invest. Dermatol.* 72:187, 1979), *P. acnes* can and, in fact, frequently does develop resistance, in varying degrees, to oral antibiotics. It appears, however, that such resistance can be lost after 2 months or more of antibiotic withdrawal, with antibiotic-sensitive wild strains replacing the resistant strains. As a clinical correlate, it is not uncommon for a patient's acne, controlled successfully with an antibiotic, to worsen later on, but then to respond well again to the reintroduction of the antibiotic months or years later.—P.E.P.] ◀

1–11 **Propionibacteria in Patients With Acne Vulgaris and in Healthy Persons.** M. Gehse, U. Höffler, M. Gloor, and G. Pulverer studied 375 anaerobic and microaerophilic coryneform rods, isolated from pilosebaceous ducts of 26 healthy persons (71 strains) and from comedones (93 strains), pustules (107 strains), and the unaffected skin (104 strains) of 36 acne patients. These specimens were classified according to the species key in *Bergey's Manual of Determinative Bacteriology,* the biotyping scheme of Pulverer and Ko, the serotyping schedule of Höffler et al., and the phage-typing schedule of Jong et al. The average age of the acne vulgaris patients was 19.1 years.

All isolates initially selected according to the microscopic and colony morphology on reinforced clostridial agar belonged to the family of Propionibacteriaceae. There was a new biotype, designated biotype Q, and 19 new phage types, designated XVIII to XXXVII. Results of species diagnosis showed that of 375 strains, 373 were *Propionibacterium acnes* or *Propionibacterium granulosum,* the remaining 2 strains being *Propionibacterium avidum.* The *P. granulosum* strains were isolated only from acne patients (21.4%). Of strains from unaffected follicles of acne patients, 7.7% were classified as *P. granulosum;* in comedones and pustules, this ratio increased to 30.1% and 27.1%, re-

---

(1–11) Arch. Dermatol. Res. 275:100–104, April 1983.

spectively. With regard to frequencies of *Propionibacterium* biotypes in different samples, biotype A was most common in healthy persons (52.1%). Biotype E was found in 21.1% and biotype D in less than 10% of the controls. In acne patients, only 17.2% of strains from comedones belonged to biotype A; 27.1% were from pustules and 38.5% from unaffected skin. Biotype C was found in 18.8% of acne strains. Of *Propionibacterium* strains from healthy skin, 97.2% were *P. acnes* serotype KB, as were 78.6% of strains from acne patients. The phage set used was specific for this species. Of the *P. acnes* strains in controls, 55.1% belonged to phage type I, whereas 73.2% of all *P. acnes* strains isolated from acne patients were classified in this group.

These results indicate that *P. granulosum* can be differentiated only in acne patients (50% of patients examined). Serologic examinations showed no difference in the distribution of *P. granulosum* serotypes in the test groups. By means of phage typing, a significant increase in lysotype I *P. acnes* strains was demonstrated in acne patients compared with healthy controls.

▶ [In the discussion section of this article, the authors state the "interesting result" that *P. granulosum* organisms were found in only 50% of acne subjects. If it is true that the acne follicles do not bear *P. granulosum* in 50% of patients with acne, then its role in the microbial etiopathogenesis of acne remains rather unsettled. *P. acnes,* on the other hand, was present 100% of the time; however, it was also present in normal subjects' skin, whereas *P. granulosum* was consistently absent in normal follicles. The data on the biotyping, serotyping, and phage typing of the propionibacteria offer, at present, little further help in affording any new insights into the role of these bacteria in acne.—P.E.P.] ◀

1–12 **Benzoyl Peroxide Versus Topical Erythromycin in Treatment of Acne Vulgaris.** B. Burke, E. A. Eady, and W. J. Cunliffe (Univ. of Leeds, England) conducted a double-blind clinical study in 94 persons to determine if a 1.5% (w/v) erythromycin lotion was as effective as 5% (w/v) benzoyl peroxide gel in significantly reducing the number of small inflamed lesions and overall acne severity. In addition to these 2 test formulas, the erythromycin base composed of SP alcohol 40 (0.5 ml/ml), propylene glycol (0.36 ml/ml), Laureth 4 (60.0 mg/ml), and perfume (W1942-1; 1 mg/ml) was used. Spot counts were made of blackheads and whiteheads (total noninflamed lesions, TNIL) and of pustules and papules (total small inflamed lesions, TIL).

Benzoyl peroxide treatment produced a significant reduction in TNIL at 4 and 8 weeks. The erythromycin-treated group showed a slight but significant reduction in TNIL after 4 weeks but not after 8 weeks. There was no change in TNIL counts in the group treated with erythromycin base. A between-group difference in favor of benzoyl peroxide was found at 4 weeks and 8 weeks. Both benzoyl peroxide and erythromycin produced a reduction in TIL at 4 and 8 weeks (the former by 33% and 37%, and the latter by 42% and 39%, respectively). These reductions were significant. No reduction occurred with the erythromycin base. Between-group comparisons showed no significant difference between the 2 active treatments. The only significant

(1–12) Br. J. Dermatol. 108:199–204, February 1983.

change in macule count was a decrease in the benzoyl peroxide–treated group at week 8. Mild erythema and scaling were observed in a small number of patients. In 2 patients clinical dermatitis developed, 1 in the erythromycin group and 1 in the benzoyl peroxide group.

These results confirm the clinical efficacy of benzoyl peroxide and topical erythromycin and show that both treatments are equally effective in reducing the number of superficial inflamed lesions. However, long-established, safe, and effective remedies should not be replaced by topical antibiotics until more comparative studies and investigations of bacterial resistance are completed.

▶ [The introduction in recent years of topical antibiotics for the treatment of acne has raised the question of whether they offer any particular advantage over benzoyl peroxide. The findings of this study do not provide an unequivocal answer. Although showing that benzoyl peroxide was no more effective than erythromycin, the investigators used different vehicles, i.e., a benzoyl peroxide *gel* and an erythromycin *solution.* Thus, the blinded nature of the experiment was in jeopardy from its conception. And since the authors have elsewhere raised concern over the use of oral or topical antibiotics in the treatment of acne, the results of the present study are made even more difficult to interpret.

Nevertheless, concern over the development of bacterial resistance cannot be dismissed lightly, so it would seem preferable, when a topical antibacterial agent is indicated for the treatment of acne, to begin with benzoyl peroxide. However, because of its irritant effect and the occasional development of allergic contact sensitization from its use, topical erythromycin and other marketed antibiotic antiacne preparations have provided a useful therapeutic alternative for many patients.—P.E.P.] ◀

-13 **Beneficial Effect of 15% Azelaic Acid Cream on Acne Vulgaris.** Azelaic acid is a competitive inhibitor of tyrosinase and has a cytotoxic effect on human malignant melanocytes. It has been shown to be effective in the treatment of various hyperpigmentary disorders. M. Nazzaro-Porro, S. Passi, M. Picardo, A. Breathnach, R. Clayton, and G. Zina undertook a preliminary study of a 15% azelaic acid cream in patients with acne because of observations of improvement in acne in patients treated for chloasma. A total of 100 unselected patients, aged 14–38 years, with acne of all types and of varying severity were treated for 3–9 months. The 15% azelaic acid cream was rubbed in thoroughly once a day and, after a week or so, twice daily. Several patients with acne conglobata were treated.

Most patients noticed mild inflammation in the first week of treatment. All observed significant improvement within 1–2 months. Comedones, papules, and pustules became less numerous, and the skin appeared less greasy. Nodules and cysts became softer and either discharged or were resorbed. Improvement was maintained, and the new lesions that developed in treated areas were more superficial. Eventually many patients applied the cream only to lesions as they appeared. Elevated red residua of previous nodular lesions became less prominent as treatment continued.

Topical azelaic acid therapy has a significant effect on acne vulgaris. Controlled trials of this treatment are warranted. Long-term

---

(1–13) Br. J. Dermatol. 109:45–48, July 1983.

treatment is necessary, although it can be interrupted once complete healing has taken place. Why this substance should be helpful in acne is unclear, but it inhibits some dehydrogenases of the respiratory chain, has a bacteriostatic effect on *Propionibacterium acnes* in culture, and inhibits conversion of testosterone to 5α-dehydrotestosterone by 5α-reductase in vitro.

▶ [One hundred patients with acne of varying severity were treated with topical azelaic acid for 3–9 months. All improved, but few details are provided. Moreover, the trial was an open study, such that double-blinded comparison with vehicle will be needed to establish the degree of efficacy attributable to the azelaic acid.—P.E.P.] ◀

1–14 **Indirect Evidence That the Action of Cyproterone Acetate on the Skin is Due to a Metabolite.** The antiandrogen cyproterone acetate inhibits sebum secretion in the rat and the sebum excretion rate (SER) in man, improving acne when given orally; however, topical treatment with antiandrogens has given disappointing results for reasons that are unclear. F. Lyons and S. Shuster (Univ. of Newcastle upon Tyne, England) examined the effects of topical cyproterone acetate therapy on the SER in 26 patients with acne. The chief metabolite of orally administered cyproterone, 17β-hydroxycyproterone acetate, was also evaluated. Patients made daily applications to the forehead skin of 1% 17β-hydroxycyproterone acetate in acetone; 1% cyproterone acetate in isopropyl myristate, a vehicle from which there is evidence of percutaneous absorption; and 1% cyproterone acetate in absolute ethanol, with which decreased sebaceous function has been described. The respective treatment periods were 4, 6, and 8 weeks.

Considerable personal variation in SER values was seen among patients. The values could not be related to treatment, sex, or pretreatment SER. No consistent clinical changes occurred in any of the three treatment groups.

The apparent lack of effect of topical cyproterone acetate therapy on acne does not seem to be due to inadequate absorption. It is concluded that cyproterone acetate itself has no direct effect on the sebaceous gland. Impaired sebaceous gland activity from systemic cyproterone therapy must be due to either a systemic action of the drug or the action of a systemically produced metabolite in the skin. Previous findings that the local stimulatory action of intradermal androgen injection is blocked by systemic cyproterone acetate administration indicates that a local antiandrogenic effect does occur in the skin when the drug is given systemically. The metabolite that competes with androgen locally is unlikely to be 17β-hydroxycyproterone acetate.

▶ [The antiandrogen cyproterone acetate has a significant sebum-inhibiting effect when administered systemically but has consistently failed to suppress sebum production when applied topically. In the present study, different vehicles were tried, as well as the 17β-hydroxy metabolite, still without a discernible effect. The authors' conclusion, which in essence is the title of the article, is probably correct, but the metabolite remains to be identified.

(1–14) Clin. Endocrinol. (Oxf.) 19:53–55, July 1983.

This circumstance is not unique to cyproterone acetate. 17α-Methyl-B-nortestosterone, another steroidal antiandrogen, was found to have a modest sebum-inhibiting effect when applied topically but a much greater effect when given orally (*J. Invest. Dermatol.* 52:95, 1969). It should be kept in mind that both cyproterone acetate and 17α-methyl-B-nortestosterone have an antigonadotropic action, so sebum reduction could be due, in considerable measure, to a decrease in androgen blood levels.—P.E.P.] ◀

1–15 **Pigmentation of Open Comedones: Ultrastructural Study.** Alvin S. Zelickson and Jess H. Mottaz (Univ. of Minnesota) note that the general consensus is that the black discoloration at the tip of the open comedo is melanin. To test this opinion, examination was made of the ultrastructure of 13 expressed open comedones obtained from the face, chest, and back of white and black individuals.

The general ultrastructural pattern was similar in all of the material studied. In the lowermost part of the comedo, loose, irregular arrays of horny cells were intermixed with sebaceous material and bacteria. The horny cells were not cohesive and were irregular in length and width. Frequently cells were disrupted and lacked internal structure. In the middle of the comedo, the horny cells were oriented in a more regular pattern; bacteria were present, but in relatively small numbers, and sebaceous material was observed between the horny cells. In the black outermost portion of the comedo, there were many tightly packed horny cells arranged in a regular longitudinal pattern, parallel to the infundibulum of the sebaceous follicle. The cells were cohesive, each being closely apposed to its neighbors in a regular pattern. Many bacteria were present between the horny cell masses. Sebaceous material was also present. No single melanosomes or melanosome complexes were observed in any of the tissue examined.

Thus, although this ultrastructural examination purposely included only very black comedones, no melanosomal material was observed. If any melanin or melanosomes are present, the amounts must be minimal. It seems unlikely that melanin is the source of the black color in open comedones. The dark color may be related primarily to the large number of densely packed, highly oriented, horny cells in the superficial infundibular region of the sebaceous follicle or possibly to numerous bacteria, bacterial breakdown products, and sebaceous material interspersed among these cells.

▶ [We have observed that albino patients with acne have unpigmented comedones and patients with skin type IV, V, and VI have black comedones. Yet these careful studies by an accomplished electromicroscopist fail to reveal melanin in black comedones. Certainly verrucous epidermal nevi and ichthyosis can be black, but the color is not caused by the presence of melanin at all.—T.B.F.] ◀

–16 **Favre-Racouchot Syndrome Associated With Radiation Therapy.** Stephen J. Friedman and W. P. Daniel Su (Mayo Clinic and Found.) describe a woman who developed Favre-Racouchot syndrome (nodular elastoidosis) involving the face and scalp primarily at sites of x-ray irradiation for therapy of an astrocytoma.

Woman, 56, had had progressive development of comedones around the

(1–15) Arch. Dermatol. 119:567–569, July 1983.
(1–16) Cutis 31:306–310, March 1983.

eyes and a rough, waxy plaque on the scalp for 1 year. She had undergone subtotal removal of a grade IV astrocytoma during the previous year and had received 6,000 rad of whole brain radiation therapy with the main target areas being the crown and temples. She was receiving phenobarbital and phenytoin for seizures. Three months after radiotherapy and chemotherapy, total scalp, eyebrow, and eyelash alopecia developed. At 6 months after therapy the patient noticed progressive comedone development. She denied excessive sun exposure. Biopsies of the crown and left zygomatic areas showed an atrophic epidermis with prominent follicular plugging and a large, keratinous mass. In the upper dermis and middermis there was basophilic degeneration of collagen bundles. Therapy was begun with retinoic acid gel 0.025% applied to the involved areas twice daily. Six weeks later the comedones were extracted manually, and the patient achieved excellent cosmetic results.

This is the first reported case of Favre-Racouchot syndrome developing after radiation therapy.

▶ [This syndrome of comedones and elastosis usually appears in older men and is associated with actinic damage. It is a bit surprising that it has not been reported among those who have received x-ray therapy for acne in the past.—R.M.] ◀

1–17 **Fume Inhalation Chloracne.** Chloracne, caused by exposure to chlorinated hydrocarbons, is a major industrial hazard, but it has not often been described as a result of fume inhalation. V. N. Sehgal and A. Ghorpade (New Delhi) report a case.

Man, 20, working in the manufacture of sodium pentachlorophenate, developed an eruption after having worked in the factory for nearly a year. Crops of dark lesions had appeared on the face, chest, and abdomen and had

Fig 1–3.—Multiple acneiform lesions on face and trunk. (Courtesy of Sehgal, V.N., and Ghorpade, A.: Dermatologica 167:33–36, July 1983.)

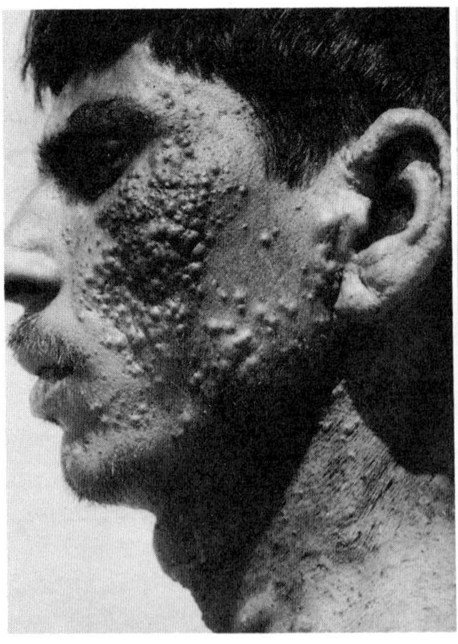

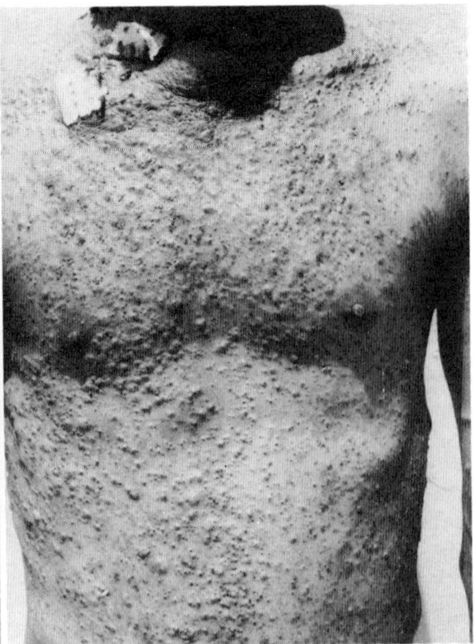

(1–17) Dermatologica 167:33–36, July 1983.

progressed, and several abscesses soon developed in the involved areas. There was no history of constitutional features, hematuria, or jaundice. The patient was often exposed to fumes when packing the material, but sudden leakage of gas from a closed cylinder containing phenol, through which chlorine gas was bubbled, had occurred about 3 months earlier. The patient had choked and felt giddy until he was removed to an open area. Multiple acneiform lesions were present (Fig 1–3). Some of the cysts and abscesses were fairly large and tender. Lesions predominated on the face, chest, abdomen, and proximal parts of the extremities. The mucous membranes and nails were uninvolved. No systemic abnormalities were found, but the sedimentation rate was 48 mm in the first hour. Renal and hepatic functions were normal. Biopsy showed large sebaceous cysts filled with keratinous material and impaction of the pilosebaceous orifices by keratotic plugs. A mild perifollicular chronic inflammatory infiltrate was seen in the dermis.

The extensive acneiform eruption in this patient was probably caused by repeated exposures to fumes of sodium pentachlorophenate during its packing. The disorder may have been triggered by inhalation of fumes during the process of bubbling chlorine gas through phenol. The hazard may be minimized by repeatedly washing the skin, wearing gloves, and using a face mask. The precise pathogenesis is obscure, but vitamin A deficiency due to liver disease, causing hyperkeratinization of the pilosebaceous apparatus, has been implicated.

▶ [Chloracne resulting from inhalation of acnegens is difficult to document. The case reported here is no exception. Suggestive evidence, which led to the presumptive title of this article, is that the patient developed chloracne one month after overexposure to a chlorinated phenolic compound. The appearance and distribution of the eruption was typical for chloracne. Although it is possible that the chloracnegen caused the skin eruption via systemic rather than epicutaneous exposure, the latter remains the more likely route of entry.—P.E.P.] ◀

1–18 **Double-Blind Study of 1% Metronidazole Cream Versus Systemic Oxytetracycline Therapy for Rosacea.** P. G. Nielsen (Boden, Sweden) undertook a double-blind comparison of 1% metronidazole cream and oxytetracycline in a daily dose of 500 mg in 51 patients (34 women) with rosacea, whose average age was 44 years. None had been treated with drugs active against rosacea in the preceding 3 months. Twenty-five patients applied 1% metronidazole cream daily for 2 months and received placebo tablets; 26 took 250-mg oxytetracycline tablets twice daily and applied placebo cream. The same cream base was used in the actively treated and placebo groups. Between the 25 metronidazole-treated patients and the 23 oxytetracycline-treated patients who completed the study, no significant clinical differences were apparent. Reductions in papules and pustules were comparable with both treatments. Numbers of telangiectases were unchanged. No side effects occurred in either group.

Improvement was observed in 90% of patients in this study treated with 1% metronidazole cream or orally with oxytetracycline for rosacea. There was no significant difference between the two treatments. No systemic side effects occurred. Transcutaneous absorption of met-

---

(1–18) Br. J. Dermatol. 109:63–65, July 1983.

ronidazole from the 1% cream results in a blood concentration that is, at most, 1% of that produced by the minimal effective oral dose for treatment of rosacea.

▶ [A high and similar rate of improvement in rosacea was observed in patients treated with metronidazole cream (plus placebo tablets) vs. oral oxytetracycline (plus placebo cream). If the results of this clinical drug trial and those of the author's prior report showing the same metronidazole cream to be more effective than placebo cream can be duplicated by others, this agent should prove a sorely needed addition to the topical treatment of rosacea. In the present study, the results would have been more illuminating had it been possible to include a third group of patients treated with placebo cream plus placebo tablets.—P.E.P.] ◀

1–19 **Advanced Hidradenitis Suppurativa: Review of Surgical Treatment in 23 Patients.** J. Ralph Broadwater, Robert L. Bryant, Robert A. Petrino, Charles D. Mabry, Kent C. Westbrook, and Robert E. Casali (Univ. of Arkansas) review their 15-year experience with the treatment of advanced hidradenitis suppurativa to delineate the nature of the disease and to outline important principles of its management.

The clinical course of hidradenitis suppurativa in 23 patients treated in Little Rock, Ark., are reviewed. Sixty-one percent of the patients were male; 78% were older than 20 years. Duration of disease at time of initial examination ranged from less than 1 year to more than 10 years (mean, 5.4 years). Multiple sites were involved in 65% of patients. Areas of involvement included the axilla (61%), groin (48%), perineum (48%), perirectum (22%), breast (13%), and others (13%). The most common bacterial organisms recovered were *Proteus* species, *Staphylococcus epidermidis,* and *Staphylococcus aureus.* Initial treatment was not aggressive in most patients: 5 were treated nonoperatively, and all had recurrences. Twelve patients underwent incision and drainage, with 10 recurrences (83%). Definitive treatment consisted of wide excision and appropriate closure. Wide excision with primary skin closure was performed in 10 areas, and only 3 abscesses (30%) recurred. Wide excision and coverage with split-thickness skin graft was performed in 24 areas, with only 3 recurrences (13%). Wide excision plus healing by secondary intention were performed on 4 lesions with 2 recurrences (50%). Three patients underwent a staged procedure consisting of colostomy, wide excision, and coverage with a split-thickness skin graft, with one recurrence (33%).

Hidradenitis suppurativa, characterized by recurrent painful abscesses that occur throughout the apocrine glands, remains a poorly understood disease. Local therapy and incision and drainage are associated with an unacceptable rate of recurrence. The authors recommend wide and deep excision of the area involved combined with individualized closure.

▶ [The authors describe their 15-year experience in the surgical treatment of 23 cases of treatment-recalcitrant hidradenitis suppurativa. It is difficult to know for certain how resistant these cases really were to nonsurgical management. For example, only 5 patients are described as having received oral antibiotic therapy, with no de-

---

(1–19) Am. J. Surg. 144:668–670, December 1982.

tails given as to which medications were used and whether treatment was based on the results of bacterial cultures. Moreover, it appears that none of the patients received intralesional steroid injections, a treatment most useful in quenching the inflammation of hidradenitis.

However, the major criticism of this retrospective report is that because such a variety of surgical procedures was performed, too few patients were subjected to a given modality to allow assessment of the superiority of one procedure over the other. What is abundantly clear, however, is that this frequently difficult therapeutic problem sometimes does require a definitive and aggressive surgical approach.—P.E.P.] ◀

2. Bacterial and Miscellaneous Infections

2-1 **Dermatologic Signs in Toxic Shock Syndrome: Clues to Diagnosis.** An eruption is one of the primary criteria for toxic shock syndrome (TSS), and other dermatologic abnormalities have been described, including bulbar conjunctival, oropharyngeal, and vaginal hyperemia and marked swelling of the palms and soles. Michael C. Bach (Maine Med. Center, Portland) reports data on two patients who had TSS with impressive dermatologic findings.

CASE 1.—Girl, 14 years of age, developed severe sore throat with low-grade fever followed by vomiting, shaking chills, and swelling in the hands and feet and vaginal area. She had used Tampax Super tampons for 2 years. Marked bulbar conjunctival inflammation and oropharyngeal inflammation were seen at admission, as well as a blanching, scarlatiniform rash over the entire body and brawny, indurated edema of the hands and feet. She improved rapidly on treatment with nafcillin.

CASE 2.—Woman, 24, developed shaking chills and a macular rash over the entire body 5 days after inguinal hernia repair. Swelling of the hands and feet followed. Regular tampons had been used during the menses. A diffuse, blanching, macular rash with some petechiae was observed, and the eyes were markedly inflamed, with a right bulbar conjunctival hemorrhage. The patient responded to nafcillin therapy and local wound irrigation with Betadine.

In both patients, desquamation occurred several days after onset of symptoms. Conjunctival hyperemia is a frequent finding in TSS, but it is not often observed in most other disorders. Edema of the hands and feet is also associated with TSS. The eruption resembles that of scarlet fever. The exotoxin isolated from *Staphylococcus aureus* strains in cases of TSS has an isoelectric point comparable with that of the pyrogenic exotoxin C of group A streptococci. The findings of conjunctival hyperemia and swollen hands in the presence of a rash should prompt a search for other features of TSS.

▶ [Some of the lesser known (but not uncommon) signs of TSS include bulbar conjunctiva erythema, erythema and edema of the palms and soles, and erythema and edema of the oropharyngeal and vulvovaginal mucosae. Petechiae may also be seen in skin and mucosa. The source of infection in one patient presented was surgical wound infection. In younger children, TSS may easily be confused with Kawasaki syndrome.—A.R.R.] ◀

2-2 **Toxic Shock Syndrome and Lysogeny in *Staphylococcus aureus.*** Steven E. Schutzer, Vincent A. Fischetti, and John B. Zabriskie (Rockefeller Univ.) note that toxic shock syndrome (TSS) is associated

(2–1) J. Am. Acad. Dermatol. 8:343–347, March 1983.
(2–2) Science 220:316–318, Apr. 15, 1983.

with *Staphylococcus aureus* and is characterized by fever, hypotension, and desquamating rash, among other symptoms. Lysogenic conversion is a process by which genetic material of the bacteriophage is incorporated into the DNA of the bacterium, thereby conferring certain characteristics on the host strain. It was postulated that the toxin(s) in TSS may be under the same genetic control. Screening for the presence of phage was done in each staphylococcal strain studied.

Eleven (92%) of 12 TSS-associated staphylococcal strains, upon irradiation, yielded plaques on at least 1 of the indicator lysogenic bacteriophage strains, 450 and 1830. Seventeen (94%) of 18 non-TSS-associated staphylococcal strains, including 4 vaginal isolates from young adults, did not release bacteriophage to which these indicators were sensitive. Lysogeny of both 450N(CSϕ) and 450N(Swϕ) strains was demonstrated by release of bacteriophage and subsequent plaque formation on the 450N indicator.

These findings add support to the theory that lysogeny by 1 or more bacteriophage in certain strains of *S. aureus* may be responsible for the pathogenesis of TSS.

▶ [This article demonstrates that *S. aureus* isolated from persons with TSS are more likely to demonstrate the presence of temperate bacteriophage than are *S. aureus* isolated from individuals without TSS (11 of 12 vs. 1 of 19). These studies do not answer the question of whether or not lysogenic bacteriophage in TSS-associated strains of *S. aureus* are responsible for the production of pyrogenic exotoxic C, enterotoxin F, or toxins not yet described that may be responsible for the pathogenesis of TSS.—A.R.R.] ◀

2–3 **Treatment of *Staphylococcus aureus* Infections in Children in Office Practice.** Infections caused by *S. aureus* continue to be treatment problems. Frank A. Disney and Michael E. Pichichero (Elmwood Pediatric Group., Rochester, N. Y.) reviewed experience with the treatment of 105 *Staphylococcus aureus* infections in 79 children in a private office practice. In all cases the infection was confirmed by culture, and the isolate was tested in vitro for antibiotic susceptibility. Vesicular pyoderma accounted for nearly half the cases. The next most common forms of infection were furunculosis, secondary pyoderma, and carbunculosis.

Treatment efficacies were comparable with orally administered erythromycin estolate and erythromycin ethylsuccinate, cefaclor and cephalexin, and clindamycin hydrochloride, and dicloxacillin sodium. Penicillin V potassium, ampicillin, and topical bacitracin therapy were generally ineffective. Twenty-three patients with 27 infections represented initial treatment failures. In all but 2 of these patients, disk susceptibility testing predicted the failure, showed what antibiotic would produce a clinical response, or both. Besides oral antibiotic therapy, topical therapy was used for pyodermas, and the carbuncles were surgically drained. Two children had drainage of a paronychia involving a finger. Three children initially received amoxicillin for suppurative otitis media resulting in tympanic membrane rupture; 2 required a change of antibiotic.

(2–3) Am. J. Dis. Child. 137:361–364, April 1983.

Several antibiotics are available that are effective in treatment of staphylococcal infections in children, and selection from among them may be based on factors such as side effects, patient acceptability, and cost. Initial treatment with erythromycin is preferred by the authors once the diagnosis is established. Failures can occur with any regimen, and in vitro antibiotic susceptibility data can be useful in these cases.

▶ [This article illustrates—on the basis of an outpatient pediatric practice in Rochester, New York, during the period from 1977 to 1980—that non-life-threatening *S. aureus* cutaneous infections generally responded to oral preparations of erythromycin, cephalothins, clindamycin, and dicloxacillin. Amoxicillin and topical therapy were usually ineffective.—A.R.R.] ◀

2–4 ***Pseudomonas aeruginosa* Serotype 0:9: New Cause of Whirlpool-Associated Dermatitis.** Rima F. Khabbaz, Thomas W. McKinley, Richard A. Goodman, Allen W. Hightower, Anita K. Highsmith, Keith A. Tait, and Jeffrey D. Band report that in a 5-day period dermatitis developed in nearly one fourth of the guests at a large Atlanta-area hotel. Within 24 hours of their arrival in Atlanta, severe dermatitis developed in several members of one hockey team. The disorder was classified as *Pseudomonas aeruginosa* dermatitis associated with the use of a whirlpool. This was the first outbreak in which *P. aeruginosa* serotype 0:9 was implicated. The authors inspected the recreational facilities of the hotel, including the swimming pool and whirlpool.

Of 310 persons who responded to a detailed questionnaire, 75 met the case definition. Age of these 59 male and 16 female patients ranged from 5 to 43 years. Mean duration of skin rash was 8 days. It primarily involved trunk and proximal extremities; associated symptoms included itching, earache, and malaise. Comparison of patients with control subjects who had used the hotel whirlpool during the same time but had not had a rash showed that patients had used the whirlpool significantly more often than control subjects, although mean duration of each use was the same for the 2 groups. Attack rates were higher in whirlpool users who were younger than age 10 years. Forty-one persons with infection sought care from a physician. Diagnoses included *Pseudomonas* rash in 12, staphylococcal infections in 3, insect bite in 2, allergy in 2. There was no diagnosis in 8. *Pseudomonas aeruginosa* serotype 0:9 was isolated from the whirlpool water and from a swab of the floor drain; *P. aeruginosa* serotypes 0:4 and 0:11 were isolated from the side of the whirlpool. Specimens from skin lesions in 20 persons were cultured, and *P. aeruginosa* was isolated from 13. Ten specimens showed serotype 0:9, and 3 could not be serologically typed. The whirlpool had been adequately chlorinated.

The findings indicate that this strain of *P. aeruginosa* may not be readily sensitive to recommended chlorine concentrations. Newly proposed guidelines for whirlpool maintenance have recommended higher levels of chlorine than for swimming pools (1–3 mg/L).

▶ [*Pseudomonas* dermatitis has been increasingly recognized among users of contaminated whirlpools, swimming pools, and hot tubs; and the Centers for Disease

(2–4) Am. J. Med. 74:73–77, January 1983.

Control have issued guidelines for the installation and use of these recreational and exercising facilities. It is not clear why this infection is more prevalent among whirlpool or hot tub users. Besides humidity that compromises normal barrier function, the high temperature of the water may also favor the growth of the organism. It is also possible that chlorination at those high temperatures is not adequate to prevent the growth of *P. aeruginosa,* as in the cases in this report.

Although the strains involved in this dermatitis are not the ones found most frequently in hospitalized patients and the infection is self-limited in otherwise healthy persons, it is conceivable that an immunocompromised host might not fare as well with this *Pseudomonas* dermatitis.—E.G.] ◀

2–5 **How Infectious is Syphilis?** P. C. Schober, G. Gabriel, P. White, W. F. Felton, and R. N. Thin (England) examined the sexual partners of patients with early-stage syphilis seen at three clinics to determine the prevalence of infection in these subjects. Index patients had either primary syphilis, diagnosed clinically and by the finding of *Treponema pallidum* in serum samples taken from a lesion, as well as positive serologic test results; or secondary syphilis, diagnosed from the clinical findings and strongly positive serologic results. In all of the latter cases, there was a rapid clinical response to treatment. Persons who were contacts of index patients during the preceding 12 weeks were sought for interview with health advisers. The 99 index cases yielded 127 contacts, 51% of whom were infected. The rate of infection of contacts was 49% for index homosexuals and 58% for heterosexuals. Fifty-eight percent of the contacts of patients with primary syphilis and 46% of those of patients with secondary syphilis were infected; the difference was not significant.

About half of the contacts of both heterosexual and homosexual patients with syphilis in this survey were found to be infected. The absence of infection in as many as half of contacts may be the most relevant finding. These findings are similar to what was reported from larger studies in the United States during the 1940s. Further studies are needed to elucidate host–*T. pallidum* relationships and to assess the risks associated with various forms of sexual contact.

▶ [The authors attempt to answer the question posed in the title by determining the prevalence of syphilis in named contacts of individuals with early syphilis. Although "contacts" could not be distinguished from the "source" of infection, it is interesting that only about half the named contacts had syphilis. Why doesn't everyone develop syphilis after exposure? The number of exposures, type of sexual activity, and types of exposure to infectious lesions may be some of the parameters responsible for the variable infectiousness of syphilis.—A.R.R.] ◀

2–6 **Spirochetal Etiology of Lyme Disease.** Lyme disease typically begins in summer with erythema chronicum migrans (ECM), which may be accompanied by headache, stiff neck, fever, myalgias, arthralgias, malaise, fatigue, or lymphadenopathy. Allen C. Steere, Robert L. Grodzicki, Arnold N. Kornblatt, Joseph E. Craft, Alan G. Barbour, Willy Burgdorfer, George P. Schmid, Elizabeth Johnson, and Stephen E. Malawista recovered a newly recognized spirochete from the blood, skin lesions (ECM), or cerebrospinal fluid of 3 of 56 patients with

(2–5) Br. J. Vener. Dis. 59:217–219, August 1983.
(2–6) N. Engl. J. Med. 308:733–740, Mar. 31, 1983.

Lyme disease and from 21 of 110 nymphal or adult *Ixodes dammini* ticks in Connecticut.

These isolates and the original one from *I. dammini* appeared to have the same morphological and immunologic features. In patients the specific IgM antibody titers usually reached a peak between the third and sixth week after the onset of disease; specific IgG antibody titers increased slowly and were generally highest months later when arthritis was present. Among 40 patients who had early disease only (ECM alone), 90% had an elevated IgM titer between the ECM phase and convalescence. Among 95 patients with later manifestations (involvement of the nervous system, heart, or joints), 94% had elevated titers of IgG. In contrast, none of 80 control subjects had elevated IgG titers, and only 3 control patients with infectious mononucleosis had elevated IgM titers.

Previously, diagnosis of Lyme disease was based on clinical and epidemiologic criteria and was heavily dependent on a history of ECM. Now antibody determinations can provide strong supportive evidence for diagnosis of this disease. Previous reports indicated penicillin or tetracycline given early in the illness can shorten duration of ECM and may prevent or attenuate subsequent arthritis. The authors conclude that the *I. dammini* spirochete is the causative agent of Lyme disease.

▶ [The story of Lyme disease continues to unfold thanks to the continuous and unrelenting efforts by the group of investigators from Yale and the State University of New York at Stony Brook. Since 1975 when the disease was described in a small town in Connecticut, we have followed new developments of this disease through periodic publications by these authors. Now, finally, they have been able to confirm the spirochetal nature of the causative organism. Interestingly, both groups of investigators were able to identify the spirochete of the *I. dammini* tick independently in the two most endemic areas: Lyme in Connecticut and Shelter Island in New York. Unfortunately, isolation of the spirochete requires rigorous and sophisticated laboratory procedures and at this point is not available for routine testing. Nonetheless, elevation of IgM and IgG levels during different stages of the disease seems to be specific enough so that such elevation in a patient with the clinical manifestations of Lyme disease should be sufficient evidence to institute therapy. As the authors pointed out, early therapy with tetracycline during the stage of ECM can prevent the late manifestations of arthritis as well as the more serious cardiovascular and neurologic complaints.—E.G.] ◀

2-7 **Treatment of the Early Manifestations of Lyme Disease.** Allen C. Steere, Gordon J. Hutchinson, Daniel W. Rahn, Leonard H. Sigal, Joseph E. Craft, Elise T. DeSanna, and Stephen E. Malawista (Yale Univ.) compared the efficacy of penicillin, erythromycin, and tetracycline in a series of 108 adult patients seen between 1980 and 1981 with early Lyme disease. Patients with erythema chronicum migrans received phenoxymethyl penicillin, erythromycin, or tetracycline in an oral dose of 250 mg 4 times daily for 10 days. The treatment groups were similar with regard to age, sex, and the duration of illness.

Fourteen percent of patients, generally those with more severe disease, had intensified symptoms during the first 24 hours of

---

(2–7) Ann. Intern. Med. 99:22–26, July 1983.

treatment. Erythema chronicum migrans and associated symptoms resolved significantly more rapidly in patients given penicillin or tetracycline (5.4 and 5.7 days, respectively) than in those treated with erythromycin (9.2 days). About twice as many erythromycin-treated patients required retreatment because of persistent symptoms or immediate relapse. In 3 of 40 penicillin-treated patients and 4 of 29 given erythromycin—but in none of the 39 given tetracycline—meningoencephalitis, myocarditis, or recurrent attacks of arthritis developed. Minor late complications were frequent in all of the treatment groups. Similar results were obtained with tetracycline, given for 10 or 20 days, in 49 subsequent adult patients. None had major late complications, and only 1 had to be retreated. Only 1 of 27 children treated with penicillin for 10 days required retreatment, although 3 children had major late complications. Late disease was more likely to develop in patients with severe initial symptoms.

Early Lyme disease may be treated with oral doses of tetracycline, given for at least 10 days and for as long as 20 days if symptoms persist or recur. Children can be given phenoxymethyl penicillin or, if allergic to penicillin, erythromycin. The dosage of penicillin is 50 mg/kg/day, with limits of 1–2 gm/day. Erythromycin is given in a dosage of 30 mg/kg/day for 15 or 20 days.

▶ [This article stresses the importance not only of early treatment but also the selection of the proper antibiotic therapy to prevent the complications of Lyme disease. Early diagnosis of erythema chronicum migrans therefore becomes of paramount importance to institute therapy; we should always be alerted to that possibility.

More recently the same group of investigators reported that for patients in whom Lyme meningitis developed, the most effective therapy was high doses of penicillin, e.g., 3.3 million units of sodium penicillin G intravenously every 4 hours for 10 days (*Ann. Intern. Med.* 99:767, 1983). Therefore, whereas tetracycline is the drug of choice to prevent meningitis (as well as other late manifestations), high doses of penicillin are required for therapy of this complication of Lyme disease.—E.G.] ◀

2–8 **Natural Distribution of *Ixodes dammini* Spirochete.** Edward M. Bosler, James L. Coleman, Jorge L. Benach, Darlene A. Massey, John P. Hanrahan, Willy Burgdorfer, and Alan G. Barbour isolated spirochetes believed to be the cause of Lyme disease from white-footed mice and white-tailed deer, which are the preferred natural hosts of *Ixodes dammini,* the tick vector. Lyme disease, an epidemic inflammatory disorder with a pathognomonic skin lesion that is often followed by joint, neurologic, and cardiac manifestations, was first recognized in 1975 in Lyme, Connecticut. Evidence suggests that nymphal *I. dammini* ticks transmit the causative agent of this disease to man.

Spirochetes believed to be the agents of Lyme disease were isolated only by culturing whole blood samples in BSK medium. Spirochetes were detected 10–31 days after the blood was added to the medium. Of 306 *I. dammini* subadults, 113 were infected with spirochetes. The infected ticks were removed from 33 (43%) of the tick-infested mice sampled. Spirochetes were isolated 2 days after aortic blood from a 2-

(2–8) Science 220:321–322, Apr. 15, 1983.

month-old female white-tailed deer was added to BSK medium. In addition, methanol-fixed smears of aortic blood drawn from 1 male fawn and from 8 of 11 deer captured on Shelter Island were shown by direct fluorescence to contain the spirochete. These deer had numerous *I. dammini* males and fewer engorged females.

Because deer host all stages of *I. dammini,* they may serve as a reservoir of the spirochete and provide an overwintering mechanism for both spirochetes and adult ticks. Some tick larvae may acquire the spirochete by transovarial passage, and the nymphal stage may transmit the disease to man.

▶ [Although the study identifies the white-footed mouse and the white-tailed deer as the preferred natural hosts of *I. dammini,* the tick vector that carries the spirochete causing Lyme disease, the authors also conclude that the vector may have a wider distribution than originally anticipated. In the future, other mammals may be identified as reservoirs for the parasite, and knowledge of these other reservoirs could be significant for further epidemiologic studies.

Interesting to note was the fact that the spirochetes were not easily identified by direct dark-field examination, and culturing the blood of host animals for a mean of 19 days was required for identification. This again is further testimony to the tenacity of these investigators to establish the identity of the cause of Lyme disease and fulfill Koch's postulates for a causal relationship (see abstract below).—E.G.] ◀

2–9 **Erythema Migrans Disease: A Contribution to its Clinical Features and Relationship to Lyme Disease.** K. Weber, A. Puzik, and Th. Becker (Munich) conducted a largely prospective 33-month study involving 30 patients with and 1 without (chronic) erythema migrans. Primary erythema migrans characteristics were observed in 97%, general complaints in 71%, and arthritis and neurologic and cardiac disturbances in 45%.

The focal points were located on the leg in 17 patients, the arm in 5 patients, the trunk in 7 patients, and the head in 1 patient; the average size was 23 cm. Twenty-two patients had generalized symptoms, and 15 had additional symptoms involving the joints, nervous system, heart, and nose, ear, and throat region. Difficulties were noticed by 4 patients before, 5 patients simultaneously with, and 13 patients after erythema migrans was diagnosed. In 1 patient the disease disappeared spontaneously; in 29 others it persisted as long as 6 months, but quickly responded to antibiotic treatment. An average of 7 months, measured from the occurrence of tick bite in 9 patients or from onset of erythema migrans, elapsed before arthritis and arthralgia appeared in 10 patients, and the symptoms persisted for an average of 10 months. In none of the arthritic patients, either from results of the authors' or other physicians' examinations, could causes other than erythema migrans be found. In 7 patients sensory disturbances appeared 3 weeks later, sometimes with signs of meningitis, which lasted an average of 4 months, whereas in 3 patients cardiac symptoms appeared a few weeks later and persisted an average of 4.5 months. In 1 patient tracheolaryngitis developed 2 months later and persisted for 3 months. These manifestations occurred in 7 patients despite antibiotic treatment.

(2–9) Dtsch. Med. Wochenschr. 108:1182–1190, August 1983.

Extradermal manifestations in 2 patients were successfully treated with high parenteral doses of penicillin; in one instance penicillin treatment was followed by administration of tetracycline. Erythema migrans disease, unlike Lyme disease, apparently cannot be successfully treated with low oral doses of penicillin, but can in certain circumstances be favorably influenced by high parenteral doses of penicillin G.

▶ [This prospective clinical study of the European version of Lyme disease gives a detailed account of its characteristics, which do not seem to differ substantially from those of its American counterpart. If the study had been supplemented by laboratory investigations to identify the spirochete that has been associated with Lyme disease, the authors probably would have found the same etiologic factor.—E.G.] ◀

2–10 **Single-Dose Therapy of Chancroid With Trimethoprim-Sulfametrole.** Frank A. Plummer, Herbert Nsanze, Lourdes J. D'Costa, Peter Karasira, Ian W. Maclean, Russell H. Ellison, and Allan R. Ronald conducted a randomized double-blind trial comparing the effect of a single dose of trimethoprim-sulfametrole (640–3,200 mg) with that of 5-day regimens of either trimethoprim-sulfametrole (160–800 mg twice daily) or trimethoprim alone (200 mg twice daily) in the treatment of men with chancroid. Of 95 patients, 78 had positive culture results for *Hemophilus ducreyi.* Twenty-seven, 23, and 28 patients, respectively, were assigned to the single-dose trimethoprim-sulfametrole, the 5-day trimethoprim-sulfametrole, or the 5-day trimethoprim alone regimens.

The mean numbers of days to healing (± 95% confidence intervals) were as follows: single-dose trimethoprim-sulfametrole, 10.3 ± 5.7; 5-day trimethoprim-sulfametrole, 11.0 ± 7.4; and 5-day trimethoprim, 11.9 ± 8.2. Three patients, 1 in each treatment group, had ulcer recurrence at the 28-day follow-up visit. Two treatment failures occurred in the 5-day trimethoprim group. *Hemophilus ducreyi* was eradicated from the ulcers by day 3 in all but 3 patients. The buboes in all 24 patients treated with either single-dose trimethoprim-sulfametrole or 5-day trimethoprim-sulfametrole, and those in 8 of 9 patients given 5-day trimethoprim alone, resolved by day 28; the mean numbers of days to bubo resolution were 10.5 ± 4.9, 11.8 ± 8.6, and 10.7 ± 10.6, respectively. Patient compliance with therapy was excellent.

These results demonstrate that single-dose trimethoprim-sulfametrole (640–3,200 mg) is highly efficacious in the treatment of chancroid. Ulcers, whether negative or positive for *H. ducreyi,* responded well to each of the 3 regimens. Single-dose trimethoprim-sulfametrole also was effective in treatment of the more severe manifestations of chancroid. In Kenya, where more than 90% of *H. ducreyi* infections are resistant to tetracycline and nearly 40% are resistant to sulfonamides, the treatment of chancroid with these agents results in failure rates of 70% and 30%, respectively. On the basis of high thera-

---

(2–10) N. Engl. J. Med. 309:67–71, July 14, 1983.

peutic efficacy and low cost, single-dose trimethoprim-sulfametrole may be the preferred treatment for chancroid.

▶ [This sounds too good to be true, but larger series may confirm the effectiveness of a single-dose therapy. As the authors mention, resistance by *H. ducreyi* to sulfamethoxazole and tetracycline is common, and for that reason the CDC recommends erythromycin and trimethoprim-sulfamethoxazole. The latter drug has a notorious record for inducing drug allergy, which is probably shared by trimethoprim-sulfametrole, but conceivably a single-dose regimen may reduce the possibility of sensitization.

Recently, Margolis and Hood (*J. Am. Acad. Dermatol.* 6:493, 1982) described a readily available technique for obtaining cultures of *H. ducreyi* from patients suspected of having chancroid. Serous exudate from the ulcerative lesion was inoculated in autologous culture medium obtained by clotting 5 or 10 ml of the patient's blood at room temperature and then incubated at 35 C for 48 hours in a 5% CO_2-enriched atmosphere. Read at 48 hours, the gram stain of these autologous media demonstrated clusters of the gram-negative rods. This simple technique may help in the identification of this fastidious organism.—E.G.] ◀

2–11 **Hemorrhagic Proctitis due to Lymphogranuloma Venereum Serogroup L2: Diagnosis by Fluorescent Monoclonal Antibody.** Stephen A. Klotz, David J. Drutz, Milton R. Tam, and Kevin H. Reed note that definitive diagnosis of lymphogranuloma venereum is impeded by difficulty in culturing the causative agent and by serologic cross-reactivity between *Chlamydia trachomatis* L1, L2, and L3, which can cause the disease, and the many other serotypes of *C. trachomatis,* which do not. An unusual case seen at Audie L. Murphy Memorial V.A. Hospital, San Antonio, Texas, is described below.

Man, 23, had painless rectal bleeding unrelated to bowel movements. Hematocrit value was 32%. He refused all diagnostic procedures and left the hospital against medical advice, but he returned 2 days later with profuse rectal bleeding and syncope. Blood pressure was 50/0 mm Hg in the sitting position and pulse rate was 150 beats per minute. Results of extensive gastrointestinal evaluation were normal. Repeat colonscopy disclosed a noncircumferential ulcer. Results of serologic tests showed the IgG titer of 1:2,048 as an absolute dilution end-point present against immunotype groups B; D, E; K, L3; and L1, L2, which is the typical pattern of serum from patients with lymphogranuloma venereum. The patient was treated for suspected lymphogranuloma venereum with tetracycline hydrochloride. Both monoclonal antibody 2C1 and antibody 2B6 stained chlamydiae that were intracellular or associated with phagocytic cells within the intestinal lumen.

The massive bleeding that occurred in this patient is rare for one with lymphogranuloma venereum. Confirmation of the presence of the organism associated with this disease was impossible until the tissue was subjected to a fluorescein-tagged monoclonal antibody directed against serotype L2 (lymphogranuloma venereum). This powerful test demonstrated the presence of lymphogranuloma venereum organisms within the lesion.

▶ [The importance of this report lies in the ability to establish a diagnosis of lymphogranuloma venereum with the use of monoclonal antibodies. Up to now the diagnosis has been by exclusion and by association of multiple parameters, including change in serologic titers. We hope that the technique will become available in the future so

---

(2–11) N. Engl. J. Med. 308:1563–1565, June 30, 1983.

that we can establish with certainty the diagnosis of this rare but severe and disfiguring disease.—E.G.] ◀

2–12 **Leishmanial Infections: A Consideration in Travelers Returning From Abroad.** James H. Maguire, Nelson M. Gantz, Samuel Moschella, and Steve C. Pan describe findings in 7 patients with leishmaniasis, including fatal visceral leishmaniasis in 1 and dermal leishmaniasis in 6. All 7 patients were seen in Boston during a 4-year period. Leishmaniasis comprises a group of clinically distinct diseases caused by the flagellated protozoan *Leishmania.*

CASE 1.—Woman, 78, was in good health except for chronic congestive heart failure requiring treatment with digitalis and diuretics. Three months after returning from a 6-week visit to Athens, Greece, and villages within 15 miles of the city, she experienced fatigue, anorexia, weight loss, and a nonproductive cough. She had neither lymphadenopathy nor rash. The bone marrow was hypercellular, and amastigotes of *Leishmania donovani* were seen in macrophages. Direct agglutination titers to *L. donovani* were 1:64 (greater than 1:32 is a positive result). After a 10-day course of sodium antimony gluconate, the patient began to feel well and gain weight. However, 2½ months later, direct agglutination titers for the organism yielded positive results. The patient died of renal and respiratory insufficiency.

CASE 2.—Man, 26, had a painless lesion of the right forearm after living in Afghanistan for a year. The results of impression smear and culture were positive for *Leishmania.* No treatment was given and the lesion healed after 2 years.

CASE 3.—Woman, 24, wife of case 2, had a lesion on the left elbow. The lesion had been aspirated by needle in Afghanistan, and amastigotes were identified. No treatment was required.

CASE 4.—Girl, aged 2 months, born in Israel, had a small nodule on her forehead at age 3 weeks. The results of impression smears and culture were positive for old world cutaneous leishmaniasis.

CASE 5.—Woman, 23, after camping in the Guatemalan forest, noted an enlarging lesion at the site of an insect bite on her hand. The results of culture from a skin slit were positive for *Leishmania.* The lesion healed after a 10-day course of sodium antimony gluconate, but scarring occurred.

CASE 6.—Man, 26, spent 6 months in the forests of Columbia. Three weeks before returning home, he noted painless ulcers on his forearm. Excisional biopsy was performed, and the lesions did not recur.

CASE 7.—Man, 62, from Brazil, had an ulcer on his face at age 40 that had healed. Several years later, when the site became ulcerated, he received several courses of parenteral antimony as well as intralesional corticosteroids. Results of a *Leishmania* test were positive. These findings represent leishmaniasis recidiva (or lupoid or tuberculoid leishmaniasis), an aberrant, nonhealing form of cutaneous leishmaniasis.

Case 1 is an example of visceral leishmaniasis, the diagnosis of which is often delayed because the onset of illness is insidious. Certain diagnosis requires isolation of the parasite. Cases 2, 3, and 4 are examples of *Leishmania tropica* infection, occurring in dry, rural areas. Treatment is not required because healing is spontaneous. Cases 5 and 6 are examples of *Leishmania mexicana* or *Leishmania braziliensis,* transmission of which occurs primarily in forests.

(2–12) Am. J. Med. Sci. 283:32–30, Mar.–Apr. 1983.

American physicians should be alert to the possibility of leishmaniasis in travelers from abroad. Leishmaniasis is resurgent in some areas in which insecticide spraying for malaria control has been discontinued.

▶ [In cutaneous leishmaniasis, the frustrating clinical problems are the inability to predict, in the "Old World" type, the eventual development of the lupoid or recidive type and its therapeutic resistance and the inability to predict, in the "New World" (American) type, the development of the mutilating mucocutaneous leishmaniasis and the lack of curative therapy.—S.L.M.] ◀

2–13 **Cutaneous Amebiasis.** Mary Ellen Rimsza and Robert A. Berg describe an infant admitted to Maricopa County General Hospital (Phoenix) with amebic liver abscess and vulvar ulcers.

Girl, aged 12 months, had a 3-week history of anorexia, fever, irritability, and weight loss. Examination of the external genitalia revealed 2 well-circumscribed, ulcerative lesions on the inner aspect of the labia majora. A whitish exudate was noted at the base of each ulcer (Fig 2–1). A Gram stain of this exudate showed only numerous neutrophils. Ultrasound scanning of the liver revealed a cystic mass (8 cm × 7 cm) with an air fluid level. Metronidazole therapy was begun. Concurrent epidemiologic evidence indicated a family cluster of amebiasis. The genital lesions, which had not improved with 8 days of meticulous local care, improved dramatically during the first 3 days of metronidazole therapy and were totally resolved by the tenth day. Because fever, abdominal distention, and diarrhea continued, the hepatic lesion was aspirated percutaneously. It yielded 12 ml of thick, odorless, greenish-yellow fluid. Results of Gram stain, trichrome stain, and fungal stains of the aspirate were negative, as were results of bacterial cultures.

The child, who improved clinically, was the first born to a 19-year-old woman. Nine people inhabited a crowded, filthy, 1-bedroom house with indoor toilet and bathroom facilities. All members of the family except for the grandfather were treated with metronidazole.

Fig 2–1.—Inspection of inner aspect of the labia majora shows ulcerative lesions. (Courtesy of Rimsza, M.E., and Berg, R.A.: Pediatrics 71:595–598, April 1983. Copyright American Academy of Pediatrics 1983.)

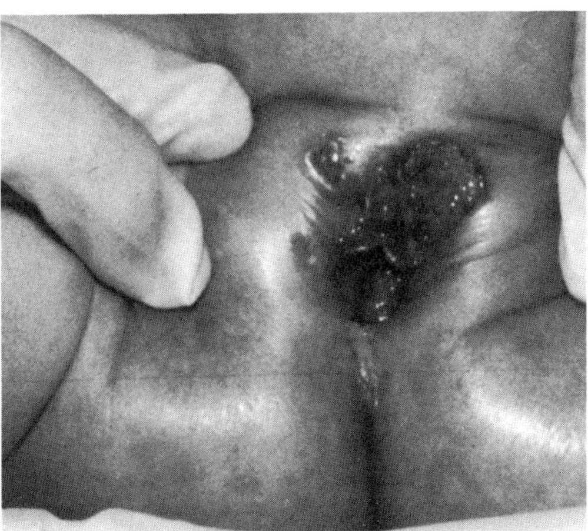

(2–13) Pediatrics 71:595–598, April 1983.

Cutaneous amebiasis is a rarely reported clinical manifestation of *Entamoeba histolytica* infections. But amebiasis is endemic in the United States, and cutaneous amebiasis should be considered in the differential diagnosis of perineovulvar or penile ulcers. The described patient appears to be the seventh with infantile cutaneous amebiasis reported in the world literature. Epidemiologic investigations and serologic studies may be crucial in establishing the diagnosis of invasive amebiasis.

► [Although the ulcers on the vulva or penis induced by *E. histolytica* have no specific characteristic, the appearance of such lesions in the perineal region in endemic areas should raise suspicion of this rare manifestation of amebiasis. Ulcers can also appear in the abdominal wall, frequently adjacent to a draining hepatic abscess.—E.G.] ◄

3. Bullous Diseases

3–1 **Transplacental Transmission of Pemphigus.** Nathan Wasserstrum and Russell K. Laros, Jr. (Univ. of California, San Francisco) present data on a case of pemphigus vulgaris (PV) in pregnancy which shows that PV is transplacentally transmitted in the manner of a tissue-specific autoimmune disease.

Woman, 30, had oral and cutaneous lesions in February 1980. Direct immunofluorescence studies showed IgG bound to the intercellular substance of the epidermis. Patient (gravida 4, para 1, spontaneous abortion 2) became pregnant in May 1980. In September 1980, prednisone therapy, 60 mg/day, was begun and continued for 2 months with good clinical result. Reduction to 40 mg/day resulted in a flare that remained uncontrolled. Patient was hospitalized at 30 weeks' gestation, with the PV refractory to corticosteroids. One week after admission, therapy was changed to azathioprine, 100 mg/day, and prednisone, 100 mg/day. Corticosteroid therapy was complicated by diabetes mellitus that was well controlled by insulin. Shortly after admission, fetal surveillance was begun. Four weeks after admission, patient reported absence of fetal movements for 24 hours, and a sonogram confirmed intrauterine death. Post partum, the patient's skin lesions continued to improve with azathioprine and prednisone therapy. Fetal autopsy showed 10% of fetal skin was denuded of epidermis. Histologic study demonstrated PV. Immunofluorescence of the skin was 4+ for IgG antibody in the intercellular substance. Also notable was hypoplasia of the fetal spleen and thymus.

The cause of fetal death in this case remains unknown. No pathologic abnormality could be identified. The occurrence of intrauterine death despite careful antepartum surveillance underscores the management problems encountered when pemphigus coexists with pregnancy.

▶ [This case report describes the intrauterine demise of a 2,770-gram fetus of a mother with PV. The fetus also had PV. The cause of fetal death was not clearly determined. The report provides additional evidence for the hypothesis that immunoglobulin deposition in the skin plays a causal role in the pathogenesis of PV. Skin lesions of PV are thought to be the result of epidermal cell proteinase activation in response to PV antibody binding. Documentation of more such "natural experiments" is required.—A.R.R.] ◀

3–2 **Pemphigus: Epidemiologic Study of Patients Treated in Finnish Hospitals Between 1969 and 1978.** Jarkko Hietanen and Osmo P. Salo (Univ. of Helsinki) reviewed data on 44 patients with pemphigus treated in Finnish hospitals between 1969 and 1978. The 36 new cases gave an annual incidence of 0.76 cases per million residents. The sex distribution was nearly equal. Half the patients had pemphigus erythematosus, and one fifth each had pemphigus vulgaris

(3–1) JAMA 124:1480–1482, Mar. 18, 1983.
(3–2) Acta Derm. Venereol. (Stockh.) 62:491–496, 1982.

and pemphigus foliaceus. Mean age at onset was 57½ years. Nine patients initially had oral lesions; most of them had pemphigus vulgaris. Most patients were first seen with moderate and restricted lesions, but those with pemphigus foliaceus more often had extensive initial lesions. The sedimentation rate was elevated initially in a majority of patients, except those with pemphigus vulgaris.

Systemic treatment usually began with prednisone or a derivative. The mean initial daily dose of prednisone was 61.4 mg. Patients with pemphigus vulgaris required doses greater than 50 mg longer than the other groups. Three patients did not require treatment when last seen, and about one fourth of the series were receiving topical treatment only. The mean duration of the longest continuous remission was 30½ months. Four patients had no remission. Three patients had osteoporosis, 2 had candidiasis, and 1 each had diabetes, pneumonia, and leukopenia. Pemphigus vulgaris was the immediate cause of 1 death. Three deaths in all were attributable in part to pemphigus or its treatment. The mean yearly number of hospital admissions was 0.7, and the mean number of days in the hospital was 16.

The low incidence of pemphigus in Finland may be in part a result of the small Jewish population. Most centers in Finland prefer to accept some lesions in place of vigorous systemic therapy, and this may explain the low frequency of side effects from systemic treatment.

3–3 **Juvenile Pemphigus.** Pemphigus is an autoimmune disease involving the skin and mucous membranes and characterized by the presence in the intercellular substance (ICS) and in serum of IgG antibodies to ICS. A. Razzaque Ahmed and Martin Salm (Univ. of California, Los Angeles) present data on 7 cases of juvenile pemphigus vulgaris and 1 case of pemphigus foliaceus.

CASE 1.—Girl, 16, of Hispanic descent, developed blisters on chest and arms initially. She later had multiple erosions in the buccal, gingival, and lingual mucosae as well as other areas of the body. Direct immunofluorescence (IF) of perilesional skin from the left arm showed IgG in the ICS. Patient was treated with and maintained on oral prednisone.

CASE 2.—Boy, 5, black, developed multiple blisters on arms and legs. Direct IF showed IgG and C3 in the ICS. Patient was treated with topical steroids only.

CASE 3.—Girl, 17, white, developed painful ulcerations of mouth and lips and scalp. Nine months later bullae and erosions spread over trunk, extremities, mouth, and vagina. Direct IF revealed deposition of IgG in the ICS. Serum titer of antibody to ICS was 1:320. She was treated with oral prednisone and has been symptom free during 15-month follow-up.

CASE 4.—Boy, 17, from Pakistan developed painful sores in mouth and blisters on the extremities. Indirect IF showed a titer of antibody to ICS of 1:640. Dapsone was increased to 200 mg/day and prednisone to 40 mg/day. Patient is now maintained on 100 mg/day of dapsone only.

CASE 5.—Boy, 12, white, developed blisters in and around the mouth, eyes, trunk, and extremities. Direct IF showed deposition of IgG in the ICS. Patient was treated with 100 mg/day of prednisone given orally and 500 mg/day of Solu-Medrol given intravenously. He was maintained for 2 years on pred-

---

(3–3) J. Am. Acad. Dermatol. 8:799–807, June 1983.

nisone, 20 mg on alternate days, and remained lesion free after therapy was discontinued.

CASE 6.—Man, 18, Hispanic, had a 2-month history of a bullous eruption on chest and back. Direct IF showed IgG deposition in the ICS. Treatment was begun with 20 mg/day of prednisone, then increased to 80 mg/day, and gradually tapered. This patient was lost to follow-up.

CASE 7.—Man, 18, black, developed multiple painful oral ulcerations that eventually spread to face, chest, and extremities. Direct IF showed IgG deposition in the ICS. Prednisone therapy was begun at 200 mg/day and increased to 1,500 mg/day. Later, Myochrysine, 50 mg intramuscularly, was given weekly. His condition improved, and prednisone was tapered. Later Myochrysine was discontinued, and 150 mg/day of azathioprine was given. Patient has been disease free for 7 years.

CASE 8.—Boy, 15, Hispanic, had pruritic eruptions on back, chest, face, and arms. Direct IF showed ICS deposition of IgG and C3 in the upper stratum malpighii. The disease was rapidly controlled by prednisone, and patient has been disease free for 4 years.

Morbidity and mortality in pemphigus are often due to complications of high-dose corticosteroid therapy. If a prednisone dose of greater than 120 mg/day is required, a second steroid-sparing drug should be given.

3–4 **Clinical and Cytologic Features of Oral Pemphigus.** The initial lesions of pemphigus reportedly occur in the mouth in at least half of cases. Jarkko Hietanen (Helsinki) examined the changes in acantholytic cells in smears in relation to the clinical state in 9 patients with pemphigus vulgaris and 1 patient with pemphigus vegetans. The di-

Fig 3–1.—Neutrophil-Tzanck cell rosette: acantholytic cell surrounded by polymorphonuclear leukocytes; original magnification, ×685. (Courtesy of Hietanen, J.: Acta Odontol. Scand. 40:403–414, 1982.)

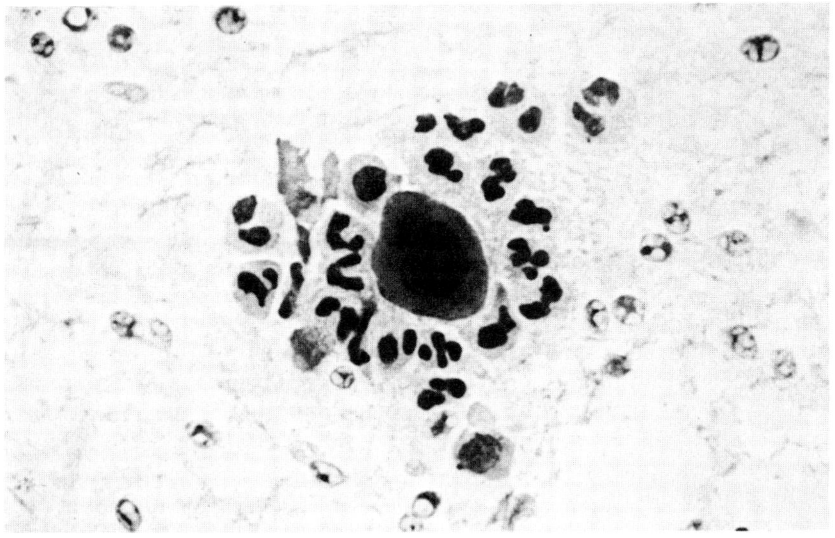

(3–4) Acta Odontol. Scand. 40:403–414, 1982.

agnosis was confirmed by biopsy in 9 cases. Smears were prepared from oral lesions of all patients and from the skin lesions of 1. Mean patient age was 55 years. All the patients had oral lesions, and 5 also had skin involvement. The usual oral lesions were denuded areas or erosions covered with whitish exudate. The oral lesions took longer to heal than did the skin lesions. Only 2 patients had prominent skin involvement. The 3 patients with severe disease had intercellular antibody titers of 160 and over, whereas 2 of the 4 with mild disease activity had undetectable antibody.

Acantholytic cells were present singly and in clumps in smears from oral and skin lesions. Neutrophil-acantholytic cell rosettes were sometimes observed (Fig 3–1). There were many binucleated epithelial cells and some binucleated acantholytic cells, and multinucleated giant cells also were found. Some of the giant cells appeared to be engulfing acantholytic-type cells. Neutrophils predominated in the inflammatory component. The number of acantholytic cells usually decreased when the clinical state improved. Acantholytic cells were absent from the smears of patients in remission and sometimes from smears of patients with mild disease activity.

The number of acantholytic cells in smears of oral and cutaneous lesions was usually correlated with the clinical state in this series of pemphigus patients, and clinical improvement was generally followed by a decrease in the number of these cells.

3–5 **Partial Purification and Characterization of Pemphigus-Like Antigens in Urine.** Richard I. Murahata and A. Razzaque Ahmed (Univ. of California, Los Angeles) note that present evidence implicates autoantibodies of the IgG class in the etiopathogenesis of pemphigus vulgaris, a rare disease characterized by superficial blisters on uninflamed skin. The detection and partial purification of pemphigus-like antigens from urine were accomplished using gel and ion-exchange chromatography. Urine, collected for 24 hours from each donor, was pooled. The 43 samples processed included some from patients with bullous pemphigoid, pemphigus vulgaris, and carcinoma of the urinary bladder.

Antigenic material was present in 12 of 40 urine samples obtained from 16 patients with bullous pemphigoid, cicatricial pemphigoid, or pemphigus vulgaris. Antigen was not detected in the urine of patients with bladder carcinoma. Antigenic activity was detectable in all fractions eluted from Sephadex G-200 in molecular weights of 90,000–180,000 daltons. Pemphigus-like antigens were glycoproteins with an apparent molecular weight of 75,000 daltons by sodium dodecylsulfate polyacrylamide gel electrophoresis. The antigens were immunogenic in mice, but were not detectable by double diffusion in agarose gels. They were water soluble and similar to those reported in the human esophagus.

The origin of the urinary antigen in pemphigus vulgaris is presently unknown. Its high molecular weight suggests local production

---

(3–5) Arch. Dermatol. Res. 275:118–123, April 1983.

in the urinary tract, although a distant origin cannot be excluded. Purified pemphigus-like antigens will be of great value in resolving the etiopathogenesis of the disease by aiding development of in vitro models of this condition.

3–6 **Identification of Chemoattractant Activity for Lymphocytes in Blister Fluid of Patients With Bullous Pemphigoid: Evidence for the Presence of a Lymphokine.** The lymphocyte, not the eosinophil, is the earliest infiltrating cell found in the dermis in bullous pemphigoid. David M. Center, Bruce U. Wintroub, and K. Frank Austen (Boston) have characterized a lymphocyte chemoattractant activity (LCA) in bullous pemphigoid blister fluids as being physicochemically identical to a recently described human lymphocyte chemoattractant lymphokine. Blister fluids from 6 patients were examined for LCA by a modified Boyden chamber method. Activity was found in all samples, but not in that of a patient with pemphigus vulgaris. The chemoattractant activity of the active fraction was predominantly chemokinetic by checkerboard analysis. Chromatography and studies of stability and function indicated that the activity resembles that of the human lymphocyte chemoattractant lymphokine.

The findings suggest that products of activated lymphocytes are present in the blister fluids of patients with bullous pemphigoid and may contribute to the early influx of lymphocytes seen in this disorder. Other products of activated lymphocytes may also be present in blister fluids of patients with bullous pemphigoid. A colony-stimulating factor-like activity for eosinophils has been described. Other investigators have found that mononuclear cells from bullous pemphigoid patients produce macrophage migration inhibitory factor in response to autologous epidermal extracts. This fact and the present findings support the theory that lymphocyte-mediated hypersensitivity have a role in the pathogenesis of bullous pemphigoid.

▶ [Analysis of spontaneous bullous fluid of patients with bullous pemphigoid has allowed the recognition of chemoattractant activity for lymphocytes and its identification as a lymphokine. This observation provides a possible molecular basis for the early tissue infiltration of lymphocytes. A time-course study of the stages of evolution of the tissue immunopathologic alterations with monoclonal antibodies could identify the subtypes of lymphocytes and provide additional information on the role of the lymphocyte as an effector cell in this disorder.—N.A.S.] ◀

3–7 **Heterogeneity of Pemphigoid Antigens.** Xue-Jun Zhu and Jean-Claude Bystryn (New York Univ.) studied the immunologic specificity of bullous pemphigoid (BP) antigens expressed in human skin by testing the reaction of serum samples from 34 patients with BP to several specimens of normal skin. Bullous pemphigoid antigen is a normal component of the basement membrane zone (BMZ) of human skin. The disease was confirmed histologically in all 34 patients. Normal human skin was obtained by punch biopsy or excision from 10 subjects.

(3–6) J. Invest. Dermatol. 81:204–208, September 1983.
(3–7) Ibid., 80:16–20, January 1983.

To study the expression of BP antigen in different individuals, a panel of serum samples from 16 patients with BP and from 2 normal individuals was tested with 5 specimens of normal allogeneic skin. Most (68.7%) serum samples reacted to antigens expressed in all 5 specimens of skin. Some skin had antibodies reacting to BMZ antigens expressed in some specimens of skin but not to others. Serum samples that were reactive with one skin specimen did not consistently give positive reactions with other specimens. Seven of 8 pemphigoid serum samples examined had antibodies to BP antigens in human skin when tested against 3 new specimens of skin. Usually, the antibody titer was low, but in 2 (25%) of the samples, BMZ antibodies were present in titers of 320 or more. In most instances there were differences in titer when the same serum was reacted with several specimens of allogeneic skin. Several studies indicate that 10% to 30% of BP patients lack BMZ antibodies. Of 10 serum samples from BP patients in this study tested against 5 new specimens of normal skin, one sample reacted to BP antigens with a low titer. The serum reacted to 4 of the 5 skin specimens, indicating that in a limited number of instances the apparent absence of BP antibodies in BP patients results from antibodies being directed to BP antigens with restricted expression.

These findings suggest that there is a heterogeneous population of BP antigens. Those having a different immunologic specificity may be present concurrently in the same specimen of skin. Both the type and the amount of individual BP antigens expressed in skin may vary from person to person. Most BP patients have antibodies to major BP antigen(s) that are expressed in the epidermis of most individuals. Some pemphigoid antibodies are directed to minor BP antigens with more limited distribution.

▶ [Recognition of the heterogeneity of antigens in bullous pemphigoid skin may be important in diagnosis in that the search for serum antibodies requires the use of skin from different species and multiple humans as substrates. Although differences in antigens may account for the range of clinical manifestations and the localization of the clinical lesions of bullous pemphigoid, the antigenic diversity may also provide a tool to explore the early alterations in the pathobiology of the tissue alterations.—N.A.S.] ◀

3–8 **Plasma Exchanges in Treatment of Bullous Pemphigoid.** The large doses of corticosteroids necessary to treat bullous pemphigoid, which primarily affects elderly patients, are frequently accompanied by major complications. The suggested use of plasma exchange (PE) offers the possibility of avoiding the risk involved in this mode of treatment. B. Guillot, D. Donadio, J. J. Guilhou, C. Courren, and J. Meynadier (Montpellier, France) present results of a study involving 10 patients (7 men and 3 women, aged 58–88 years) with bullous pemphigoid who underwent low-volume PE (33%–50% of the plasmatic mass), 3 times per week for 2–6 weeks, followed in some instances by maintenance corticosteroid therapy. The indication for the PE was determined by corticoresistance, corticodependence, or gen-

---

(3–8) Presse Med. 12:1855–1858, Sept. 3, 1983.

eral contraindication of corticotherapy (diabetes, major osteoporosis, etc.). Biologic efficacy of the treatment was surveyed by determination of circulating immune complexes.

Two groups of patients were distinguished: those initially treated with PE exclusively (7 patients), and those who received corticotherapy and PE simultaneously (3 patients). Complete control of the disease was obtained with PE alone in 3; low-dose corticosteroids were sufficient to procure remission in 2, and dosage could be reduced in 3 patients who had previously required high doses of corticosteroids. No serious side effects were observed; best results occurred in patients who had been ill less than 3 months.

Although this study involved only a limited number of patients, it showed that the institution of PE allowed considerable reduction of corticosteroid dosage. Moreover, the low volume of PE did not give rise to the rebound phenomenon sometimes observed after higher volume PE. Circulating immune complexes and pemphigoid antibodies usually decreased during treatment, but there was no close correlation between these changes and efficacy of treatment.

▶ [Low-volume plasma exchange therapy was used in a small number of individuals with bullous pemphigoid. Although there was a salutary clinical response in a small number of patients, it is important to note that some individuals experienced relapse and that the follow-up times were relatively short. Although the use of plasma exchange therapy is an exciting clinical experiment, it is doubtful that this expensive technique will achieve a prominent position as a therapeutic modality in bullous pemphigoid. Moreover, the long-term effects of chronic plasma exchange therapy remain unknown.—N.A.S.] ◀

3–9 **Positive Effect of "Etretinate" (Ro 10-9359) in a Case of Benign Familial Pemphigus.** Although dermabrasion has been reported to be helpful in certain cases, there is currently no truly effective treatment for benign familial pemphigus. Despite somewhat discouraging results with aromatic retinoids, J. L. Bonafé, B. Fontan, M. T. Pieraggi, and D. Divoux (Toulouse, France) report their results with Ro 10-9359, which they found clearly beneficial on a long-term basis.

Man, 54, had onset of symptoms 4 years prior to the current presentation. He had had no notable improvement despite various therapeutic trials with externally applied substances. Treatment with RO 10-9359 was instituted at 1 mg/kg of body weight per day, resulting in sharp decrease of cutaneous lesions within 3 days. The dosage was progressively decreased during the following 3-month period to a maintenance dose of 15 mg/day. Improvement has continued for 18 months to date; initial lesions are no longer visible and cutaneous manifestations have not recurred.

Ultrastructural study yields an explanation for the positive action of the aromatic retinoid. Its pharmacodynamic impact is manifested in the coupling "desmosomes-tonofilaments" which is restored after treatment and leads to reestablishment of epidermal cellular cohesion. In accordance with the theories regarding the action mechanism of retinoids, etretinate brings about the elimination of pathologic

(3–9) Ann. Dermatol. Venereol. 110:151–153, 1983.

acantholytic cells and the selection and proliferation of normal cellular clones.

▶ [These are not the usual results—one would expect decreased cellular cohesion with retinoids.—R.R.] ◀

3–10 **Clues to the Etiology and Pathogenesis of Herpes Gestationis.** The cause of herpes gestationis (HG) is unknown, but immunopathologic features are prominent. R. C. Holmes, M. M. Black, W. Jurecka, J. Dann, D. C. O. James, D. Timlin, and B. Bhogal (London) reviewed the findings in 25 patients affected by HG in 44 pregnancies. Each had a history of an extremely pruritic, urticarial, and bullous eruption in association with pregnancy, and all but 1 had confirmation by positive results in direct or indirect immunofluorescence assays for C3 at the basement membrane zone. The exception was not evaluated. Thirty-three women with normal pregnancies were also studied.

Ten patients developed HG in their first full-term pregnancy. In 5 others the onset coincided with a change in sexual partner. Clinical exacerbations occurred just after delivery in 55% of the pregnancies, and HG began post partum in 4 patients. Lesions developed sooner when patients breast-fed than when they bottle-fed their infants. Exacerbations were premenstrual in most instances. Oral contraception led to a clinical relapse in 4 of 8 patients. One neonate had a bullous eruption. Tests for HLA antibodies were positive in 50% of the 20 multigravidas examined, compared with 22% of multigravid controls. Five patients with HG developed Graves' disease, 2 had alopecia areata, and 1 had vitiligo. Thyroid autoantibodies were more frequent in the patients with HG than in controls.

Patients with HG exhibit a significant increase in the frequencies of the HLA antigens A1, B8, and DR3. Herpes gestationis has been described in association with hydatidiform mole and choriocarcinoma. Once HG develops, it usually recurs in all subsequent pregnancies. The activity of HG is undoubtedly hormonally modulated. Changes in activity are often apparent in relation to menstruation. It is possible that neonatal HG is mediated by cytotoxic T lymphocytes, which would cross the placenta less consistently than antibody.

▶ [Of interest is the reported increase in the frequencies of HLA antigens A1, B8, and DR3 in these patients with herpes gestationis, since DR3 has been noted previously in individuals with autoimmune and immunologic disorders, such as Sjögren's syndrome, myasthenia gravis, thyroiditis, and Addison's disease. This HLA association strengthens the argument for an immune pathogenesis for this idiopathic disorder that clinically is modulated by estrogens.—N.A.S.] ◀

3–11 **Herpes Gestationis: Clinical and Histologic Features of 28 Cases.** Jeff K. Shornick, Jerry L. Bangert, Robert G. Freeman, and James N. Gilliam (Univ. of Texas, Dallas) studied 28 patients with well-documented herpes gestationis (HG) to determine the frequency of complications and to review the histopathologic, immunopathologic, and clinical features of the disease. Herpes gestationis is an

---

(3–10) Br. J. Dermatol. 109:131–139, August 1983.
(3–11) J. Am. Acad. Dermatol. 8:214–224, February 1983.

autoimmune disease, which has been estimated to occur in 1 of 3,000 to 10,000 pregnancies.

CASE 1.—Woman, 39, developed HG during her sixth pregnancy. She had a recurrent course of the disease through her ninth pregnancy and terminated the tenth to avoid disease.

CASE 2.—Woman, 20, had HG during the first and third pregnancies, with recurrent disease during subsequent pregnancies by different husbands.

CASE 3.—Woman, 30, had HG during her third pregnancy. The boy born of this pregnancy also had HG.

CASE 4.—Woman, 17, developed HG during her first pregnancy. She also had the disease in subsequent pregnancies by different husbands, with more severe disease occurring during a subsequent gestation.

CASE 5.—Woman, 25, developed HG during her second pregnancy. A third pregnancy was not complicated by HG.

Review of 25 biopsy specimens from the 23 patients showed a highly variable spectrum of changes that seemed to parallel the polymorphic clinical patterns of disease. The most common epidermal findings included focal areas of liquefaction degeneration and a variable degree of spongiosis. Consistent changes in the papillary dermis included varied amounts of edema and perivascular infiltration by lymphocytes, histiocytes, and eosinophils. All 28 patients had linear deposits of C3 along the basement membrane of lesional or perilesional skin. Nine samples contained IgG. Other reactants included C4, C1q, properdin, and fibrin. Among the 28 patients there were 102 pregnancies, 42 of which were associated with cutaneous manifestations of HG. Maternal ages at initial onset ranged from 17 to 39 years. There were 13 spontaneous abortions in 10 women. The initial site of involvement was in or around the umbilicus in 12 patients and on the extremities in 15. Onset was usually gradual. Postpartum exacerbations occurred in 31 of 42 involved pregnancies and usually took place within 12–48 hours. Of 102 pregnancies, 79 were carried to parturition. Among 40 pregnancies carried to parturition and associated with HG, only 2 infants had cutaneous lesions.

Direct and indirect immunofluorescence studies appear to be the most reliable techniques for differentiation of this disease. The importance of correct diagnosis lies in the prediction of involvement during future pregnancies. Most patients choose definitive birth control when faced with the possibility of recurrent disease.

3–12 **Demonstration of Collagenase and Elastase Activities in the Blister Fluids From Bullous Skin Diseases: Comparison Between Dermatitis Herpetiformis and Bullous Pemphigoid.** Aarne I. Oikarinen, John J. Zone, A. Razzaque Ahmed, Urpo Kiistala, and Jouni Uitto examined possible mechanisms of blister formation by estimating proteolytic enzyme activities in blister fluids from 22 patients with various bullous disorders. The group included 6 patients with dermatitis herpetiformis (DH), 8 with bullous pemphigoid (BP), 2 with pemphigus vulgaris, 2 with chronic bullous disease of childhood (CBDC), 2 with burn blisters, and 1 each with bul-

---

(3–12) J. Invest. Dermatol. 81:261–266, September 1983.

lous drug eruption and toxic epidermal necrolysis. Samples were obtained from the DH patients after at least 3 days without suppressive therapy and from the others before specific treatment was given. Suction-induced blisters in 5 healthy subjects were also sampled. Collagenase activity was assayed by using ^{3}H-proline-labeled type I collagen as substrate, and elastase activity was tested by using either succinyl-(L-alanyl)$_3$-paranitroanilide or soluble tropoelastin C 14.

Collagenase activity was detected in most cases of DH, BP, and CBDC, but not in pemphigus vulgaris or control blister fluids. High elastase activity was found in all cases of DH, and lower activity was found in BP, CBDC, and pemphigus vulgaris. The active enzyme in BP appeared to be a metalloproteinase. Most of the elastase activity in DH blister fluids was due to a serine protease. Cells in DH blister fluids also contained high levels of elastase.

Blister fluids from lesions of various bullous disorders contain active proteases capable of degrading collagen and elastin. These enzymes may act in blister formation by degrading connective-tissue components of the dermis and dermoepidermal junction. In DH, the elastase activity is probably derived from the polymorphonuclear leukocytes that are abundant in the lesions.

3–13 **Increased Gliadin Antibodies in Dermatitis Herpetiformis and Pemphigoid.** Both dermatitis herpetiformis (DH) and pemphigoid are characterized by the formation of subepidermal blisters. Patients with DH have high titers of gliadin antibodies. Marianne Kieffer and R. StC. Barnetson have found that patients with pemphigoid also have elevated serum titers of gliadin antibodies. Thirty-four patients with bullous pemphigoid and 23 with DH, aged 20–96 years, were compared. None of the DH patients was receiving a gluten-free diet at the time of study. Nine patients with pemphigus vulgaris or pemphigus foliaceus and 23 healthy subjects were also evaluated. The control group included 13 subjects aged 22–65 years and 10 aged 65–81 years. Immunoglobulin G and IgA antibodies to gliadin were measured by an enzyme-linked immunosorbent assay.

Titers of IgG gliadin antibody were significantly higher in both the DH and pemphigoid groups than in the pemphigus patients or normal subjects. Titers of IgA gliadin antibody were significantly higher in the pemphigoid and DH groups than in normal subjects, but only the pemphigoid patients had significantly higher titers than the pemphigus patients. Titers of IgM and IgD gliadin antibodies did not differ in the bullous disease groups and control subjects. The titer of IgG β-lactoglobulin antibody was significantly higher in the DH group than in normal subjects. This was not true for the pemphigoid group, but 8 of the 28 patients tested had high titers, and 2 of them had extremely high titers. Titers of antibodies to cytomegalovirus, measles virus, and adenovirus did not differ significantly between pemphigoid patients and control subjects.

High titers of gliadin antibodies are observed in patients with bullous

(3–13) Br. J. Dermatol. 108:673–678, June 1983.

pemphigoid, as well as in those with DH, for reasons that are unclear. These patients may have increased intestinal permeability, as is suggested by the finding of increased β-lactoglobulin antibody levels in some cases, or gliadin may in some way precipitate the autoimmune process. There is good evidence that pemphigoid is an organ-specific autoimmune disorder, although the autoimmune process is often relatively transient, and the precipitating factors have not been identified.

▶ [The significance of the unexpected finding of elevated serum antibodies to gliadin in bullous pemphigoid remains to be clarified. Pemphigoid does not have an associated small bowel pathology, nor are there usually significant symptoms referable to the small bowel. The raised titers of β-lactoglobulin antibody suggests there may be an increased intestinal permeability.

A further study by Leonard et al. (*Br. J. Dermatol.* 110:307–314, 1984) has demonstrated that 6 of 27 patients with benign mucous membrane pemphigoid had serum gliadin antibodies (all IgG class), and 3 patients had homogeneous linear deposits of IgA in uninvolved skin. The interrelationships between linear IgA disease, bullous pemphigoid, benign mucous membrane pemphigoid, and DH remains clouded.—R.M.] ◀

3–14 **Renal Involvement and Circulating Immune Complexes in Dermatitis Herpetiformis.** Dermatitis herpetiformis (DH), a lifelong blistering skin disease, is characterized by IgA and complement deposit in the dermal papillae and an associated gluten-sensitive enteropathy in the small intestine. The antigen to the IgA bound in skin is unknown, though the IgA may originate in the form of immune complexes from the intestine. Timo Reunala, Heikki Helin, Amos Pasternack, Ewert Linder, and Kirsti Kalimo report the results of fine-needle kidney biopsy performed on 11 patients with DH who had no previous signs or symptoms of renal disease and were receiving a gluten-containing diet.

Glomeruli were not detected in the biopsy specimens of 3 patients. Of the other 8 patients with representative specimens, 5 had electron-dense mesangial deposits in glomeruli. These deposits were frequent and large and filled wide areas of the mesangium in 2 patients, but they were considerably smaller in the other 3. A conventional kidney biopsy specimen was obtained from 1 of the 2 patients with large deposits. Immunofluorescence microscopic examination of this specimen revealed IgA, C1q, and smaller amounts of C3 in the glomerular mesangial location; IgG and IgM were not observed. The demonstration of deposits in glomeruli was not related to the degree of jejunal villous atrophy or to the deposit of IgA and complement in skin. However, the glomerular deposits were associated with a high frequency of circulating IgA and IgG immune complexes and IgA antibodies to gliadin and reticulin. Serum concentrations of IgA, IgM, and C3 were within normal limits in all patients.

The results suggest that immune complexes or antibodies derived from the intestine can be deposited in the kidneys of patients with DH. Studies are needed to elucidate the similarities between these findings and those in IgA glomerulonephritis.

▶ [This article emphasizes a new aspect of DH: that of an autoimmune disease with possible reflections in other organ systems. Although there was no clinical evidence

---

(3–14) J. Am. Acad. Dermatol. 9:219–223, August 1983.

of renal disease in these patients, the authors are to be congratulated for their foresight and intuition in pursuing this issue and demonstrating that the DH problem is a more generalized one than we are accustomed to consider. One might almost begin to consider the skin as not a primary aspect of the DH spectrum but as an organ secondarily involved by virtue of some genetic or structural (chemical or immunologic) sensitivity, the primary defect lying in the gastrointestinal immune system. In this regard recent studies on the M cell (Wolf, J. L., Bye, W. A.: The membranous epithelial (M) cell and the mucosal immune system. *Annu. Rev. Med.* 35:95–112, 1984) may have a bearing.—R.M.] ◀

3–15 **Circulating IgA- and IgG-Class Antigliadin Antibodies in Dermatitis Herpetiformis Detected By Enzyme-Linked Immunosorbent Assay.** Cereal proteins, particularly wheat gluten and its fraction gliadin, appear to be involved in the pathogenesis of dermatitis herpetiformis (DH), and it has been proposed that the IgA deposited in skin is formed in the gastrointestinal tract and represents antigluten or antigliadin antibody (AGA), which cross-reacts with dermal reticulin or binds to gliadin attached to reticulin. Eeva Vainio, Kirsti Kalimo, Timo Reunala, Markku Viander, and Timo Palosuo devised an enzyme-linked immunosorbent assay (ELISA) that appears to be sensitive enough to detect both IgA- and IgG-class AGA. The assay was evaluated in serums from 24 patients with DH, 5 with celiac disease, and 75 normal subjects. Dermatitis herpetiformis was diagnosed on the basis of clinical, histologic, and immunofluorescence criteria, including IgA deposits in the papillary dermis. Ten patients with DH were receiving a gluten-free diet.

Antigliadin antibodies of the IgA class were detected in 71% of the patients with DH, all the patients with celiac disease, and 19% of control subjects. Antigliadin antibodies of the IgG class were found in 92% of the DH patients and all the celiac disease patients. No DH patient had IgM-class antibody. Mean levels of AGA in the DH group were significantly higher than those in the controls. Immunodiffusion studies showed precipitating AGA in 13 DH patients, 4 of whom had no IgA antibody on ELISA. Immunodiffusion tests showed AGA in 2 patients with DH and in 2 with celiac disease.

The finding of circulating IgA-class AGA in patients with DH is consistent with the suggestion that these antibodies can be deposited in the skin, possibly as immune complexes or because of cross-reactivity between gliadin and dermal reticulin. Factors such as genetic susceptibility or deviant immunologic reactivity may be critical in the manifestation of symptoms of DH. Study of the occurrence of AGA after treatment with a gluten-free diet may help elucidate the pathogenetic role of AGA in DH.

▶ [The demonstration that IgA antibodies to gliadin exist in the serum in DH supports the hypothesis that gluten-antigluten complexes may be deposited in the skin and contribute to the pathogenesis of DH. In previous studies, primarily IgG antibodies to gluten or gliadin were demonstrated in serum. However, it is not clear why patients with celiac disease or healthy subjects with circulating antibodies to gliadin do not develop skin lesions. The authors suggest that other factors such as genetically determined susceptibility or deviant immunologic reactivity or both may be involved.—R.M.] ◀

(3–15) Arch. Dermatol. Res. 275:15–18, February 1983.

3–16 **Dermatitis Herpetiformis: Relation Between Circulating Antibodies Against Reticulin and Gluten, Small Intestinal Mucosal Status, and Absorptive Capacity.** K. Ljunghall, L. Lööf, L. Grimelius, U. Forsum, J. Jonsson, A. Scheynius, and W. Schilling studied the status of the jejunal mucosa and of the intestinal absorptive capacity in 55 patients with dermatitis herpetiformis (DH); 28 were receiving a normal diet, 11 followed a gluten-reduced diet, and 16 had a gluten-free diet. Mucosal status was characterized on the basis of histopathologic findings and the numbers of intraepithelial lymphocytes present. Absorption was evaluated by 5-hour urine and 1-hour serum D-xylose tests.

A positive correlation was found between the degree of pathologic mucosal changes, malabsorption, and the occurrence of circulating antibodies to reticulin and gluten. Serum xylose tests were more sensitive than urine xylose tests in screening for the relatively mild enteropathy of DH, identifying 88% of the patients who had an abnormal mucosal status. The serologic test for antibodies to reticulin and gluten identified 80% of such patients. Among the 16 patients receiving a gluten-free diet, there was some discrepancy between results of the serum xylose test and the serologic test for antibodies, in that 5 of these patients had an abnormal serum xylose test result but no antibodies. In DH patients receiving a normal diet, the presence of antibodies to reticulin and gluten provided the same information about the presence of mucosal lesions as the serum xylose test did. In the entire series, a combination of tests for serum xylose and antibodies identified 24 of 25 patients who had an abnormal mucosal status.

Apparently, an interrelationship exists between an abnormal jejunal mucosal status, malabsorption, and circulating antibodies to reticulin and gluten. These factors were dependent on a gluten-containing diet. In these patients with dermatitis, the beneficial effect of gluten withdrawal supports previous findings. Both the serum xylose test and serologic test for antibodies were better in screening for an abnormal mucosal status in DH than was the usually employed urine xylose test.

▶ [The authors have demonstrated a relationship between jejunal pathology, malabsorption, and circulating antibodies to reticulin and gluten. Only 1 patient receiving a gluten-free diet had serum antibodies to gluten at the end of the study. It may be possible to measure antibodies to gluten to assess the degree of adherence to the gluten-free diet. A combined serum xylose test and determination of serum antibodies to gluten could identify almost all patients with an abnormal mucosal status.—R.M.] ◀

3–17 **Gluten Challenge in Dermatitis Herpetiformis.** Jonathan Leonard, Gerald Haffenden, William Tucker, Joseph Unsworth, Frances Swain, Robert McMinn, John Holborow, and Lionel Fry (London) conducted a study to determine whether the rash in dermatitis herpetiformis fulfills Frazer's criteria for gluten sensitivity and whether the gluten-free diet should be continued for life in these patients.

(3–16) Acta Derm. Venereol. (Stockh.) 63:27–34, 1983.
(3–17) N. Engl. J. Med. 308:816–819, Apr. 7, 1983.

Twelve patients with dermatitis herpetiformis whose rash had been controlled with a strict gluten-free diet for an average of 7.6 years were challenged with gluten. In 11 of the 12 patients the rash returned after an average interval of 11.9 weeks. A biopsy of the small intestine performed before challenge showed normal mucosa in 10 of 12 patients; after relapse a biopsy showed a deterioration in the mucosa of 7 of the 11 patients. Although deposits of IgA were absent from uninvolved skin in 3 of the 12 patients before gluten challenge, deposits of IgA returned to the skin in all 3 patients after challenge. Overall, IgG was not present in any of the biopsy specimens; IgM was present in 2 before and in 2 after challenge; C3 was present in 3 before and in 5 after relapse; and fibrinogen was found in 4 before challenge and in 8 at relapse. The degree of villous atrophy correlated with the appearance through the dissecting microscope. None of the patients had antigliadin antibodies before challenge, but 6 had these antibodies afterward.

This study shows that the rash in dermatitis herpetiformis is gluten dependent, and it refutes earlier claims that improvement on a gluten-free diet can be attributed to spontaneous remission. Current evidence indicates that a gluten-free diet should be continued indefinitely.

▶ [There is no longer much doubt about the efficacy of a gluten-free diet (GFD) in DH in clearing or improving the cutaneous lesions, improving the morphology of the small bowel, and removing or reducing the need for drug (sulfone) therapy. The authors have clearly demonstrated the recurrence of disease on reinstitution of a gluten-containing diet in a group of patients whose condition had previously been improved by eliminating dietary gluten. After relapse from gluten challenge, control of the disease was again obtained by reinstitution of a GFD in 8 of 11 patients. In 3 patients whose uninvolved skin was free of IgA deposits prior to gluten challenge, the IgA reappeared after gluten challenge. Two of the three redeveloped the cutaneous lesions, but the third patient did not. (It is curious that patients reported by Fry et al. [*Br. J. Dermatol.* 107:631–640, 1982] to have had spontaneous remissions after sulfone treatment and to no longer require any therapy still have IgA demonstrable in the skin.) IgG was generally not present in skin biopsy specimens, which is a curious finding because most of the serum antibodies to gliadin to both DH and celiac diseases are of the IgG class (Kreffer et al., *Arch. Dermatol. Res.* 276:74–77, 1984). In addition to recurrence of the cutaneous disease, most patients showed a relapse of previously cleared small bowel morphology. However, there are apparently varying degrees of gluten sensitivity and the involvement of one organ does not necessarily parallel the involvement of the other. Only 1 patient did not relapse and was assumed to have had a spontaneous remission, implying that most patients require indefinite maintenance of a GFD.—R.M.] ◀

3–18 **Long-Term Follow-Up of Dermatitis Herpetiformis With and Without Dietary Gluten Withdrawal.** Lionel Fry, J. N. Leonard, Frances Swain, W. F. G. Tucker, G. Haffenden, Nicola Ring, and R. M. H. McMinn (London) reviewed experience with a gluten-free diet (GFD) in the management of 78 patients with dermatitis herpetiformis (DH), 37 males and 41 females aged 15–64 years when first seen. Mean follow-up has been 7½ years. All patients had IgA deposits in the dermal papillae of uninvolved skin. All but 2 patients initially

(3–18) Br. J. Dermatol. 107:631–640, December 1982.

received dapsone in an initial dose of 100 mg daily. The dose was increased as needed until the rash was suppressed and was increased if a rash reappeared, whether or not a GFD was used. Sixty-two patients elected to try a GFD as part of their treatment, but 20 were unable to maintain the diet for as long as 1 year. A strict GFD was followed by 23 patients.

Drugs were not needed by 71% of patients receiving a GFD, and only 1 patient on a strict GFD required drug therapy. Patients in whom DH was controlled by a GFD alone reduced their drug use after a mean of about 8 months and stopped drug therapy after a mean of 29 months. Patients following a normal diet had a mean dapsone requirement of 728 mg weekly at the end of follow-up. Five patients, 4 with minimal disease, were not using drugs or a GFD at the end of the study. The mean dose of dapsone in patients receiving a GFD who also required drug therapy was 558 mg. Side effects occurred in one fourth of drug treated patients. Seven patients developed significant hemolytic anemia. Small bowel abnormalities and intraepithelial lymphocyte counts declined significantly in patients receiving a GFD but not in those receiving a normal diet.

The eruption of DH is gluten dependent and resolves on use of a strict GFD. The diet is difficult for some patients and is to a degree a social handicap, but it is effective if followed strictly and for a sufficient period. It has obvious advantages over drugs, which have a relatively high rate of side effects.

▶ [This is an excellent and interesting study which clearly shows that a GFD can produce remission of DH in 23 patients who follow it strictly; 22 (96%) were able to stop using medications. Of 17 patients following a modified GFD, only 8 (47%) could stop medications. A practical and important clinical observation was that it took an average of 8.2 months (range, 4–30 months) on a GFD before drug requirements could be reduced, and 29 months (range, 6–108 months) before use of drugs could be stopped. Clearly this needs to be explained to patients to secure maximal cooperation and compliance in following a diet which requires considerable effort and social inconvenience.

An additional incentive for following a GFD resides in the relatively high incidence of side effects (26%) from dapsone, including hemolytic anemia, headache, and lethargy. With respect to small bowel pathology, most patients reverted to or toward normal on a GFD, whereas dapsone did not alter the bowel pathology, as evidenced both by villous appearance and lymphocyte counts, even though it cleared the skin lesions. The presence or absence of bowel pathology did not influence the time of response to a GFD. The response of the skin lesions to a GFD does not insure complete restriction of the bowel pathology in all patients. Thus, although the skin and intestinal lesions are gluten dependent, the responses to a GFD are not necessarily parallel.

The authors raise an interesting point relative to the significance of IgA in the pathogenesis of the skin lesions. They point out that IgA is found in uninvolved skin, that it is found in patients who have undergone a "natural" remission, and that it is found in most patients whose condition is controlled with a GFD. Could continuous IgA then be an epiphenomenon or a secondary antibody to tissue damage? In line with this thinking is the observation that serum antibodies to gluten are primarily IgA.—R.M.] ◀

–19 **Dermatitis Herpetiformis: Effect of Gluten-Restricted and Gluten-Free Diet on Dapsone Requirement and on IgA and C3 Deposits in Uninvolved Skin.** Kerstin Ljunghall and Ulla Tjern-

(3–19) Acta Derm. Venereol. (Stockh.) 63:129–136, 1983.

lund (Uppsala, Sweden) studied 58 patients with classic dermatitis herpetiformis (DH). Seventeen were given a gluten-free diet (GFD) for periods varying from 6 to 47 months, and 11 received a gluten-reduced diet (GRD) for 7–29 months. The remaining 30 patients followed a normal diet.

The treated patients were able to reduce their dapsone requirement significantly compared with results in the 30 patients given a normal diet. In 7 of 17 GFD patients, dapsone could be withdrawn completely after diet periods of 4–38 months. No GRD patient could discontinue dapsone treatment. The occurrence and amount of IgA and of C3 in nonlesional skin were studied in the 3 diet groups during treatment. Initially, all patients had IgA deposits of the granular pattern, which remained unchanged during the follow-up period. The amount of IgA in the skin did not decrease more in the GFD group than in the normal-diet group. The occurrence of C3 diminished in all patient groups, but the decrease was most pronounced in the GFD group, in whom C3 disappeared completely. Deposits of IgA and C3 were not uniform throughout the skin. Slightly more IgA were found in skin from the buttocks than from the forearms. Patients receiving a higher dose of dapsone had less frequent C3 deposits in the skin than did those receiving a lower dose; this finding may indicate a suppressive effect of dapsone on C3 deposition.

Removal of gluten from the diet is the most satisfactory treatment of DH. For many patients, a strict diet seems difficult to follow, but those who can adhere to it report that, after acclimatization, the diet does not cause significant social or other problems. This diet gives most DH patients a new feeling of well-being and is a harmless form of therapy.

▶ [This is another clear demonstration that a GFD can reduce or eliminate the dapsone requirement in patients with DH. An interesting observation in the course of the studies on IgA deposits in the skin was that the granular linear deposits of IgA might appear in consecutive biopsy specimens as a papillary pattern or as mixed granular-linear and papillary patterns. No granular linear deposit of IgA ever appeared in subsequent specimens as a homogeneous linear pattern. This tends to support the observation by Leonard et al. (*Br. J. Dermatol.* 110:315–21, 1984) that the IgA in homogeneous linear IgA deposits is qualitatively different from the IgA in papillary deposits in DH, in that the latter has a J chain and is dimeric and possibly of mucosal origin, whereas the former lacks a J chain and has less frequent demonstrable small bowel pathology.

In this study, IgA deposits were not greatly influenced by the dietary program—they persisted in most patients. Deposits of C3, however, did decrease. There was no relationship observed between the size of the dapsone requirement and the amount of IgA in the skin.

The authors point out that remissions in patients following a GFD may take as long as 18 months, and they suggest that with longer dietary treatment even more remissions might occur. This again suggests that the keys to success with a gluten-free diet are strict observation and patient persistence.–R.M.] ◀

3–20 **Concurrence of Lupus Erythematosus and Dermatitis Herpetiformis: Report of Nine Cases.** Five cases of concurrent dermatitis herpetiformis (DH) and systemic or discoid lupus erythematosus (LE)

(3–20) Arch. Dermatol. 119:740–745, September 1983.

have previously been reported. J. R. Thomas III and W. P. Daniel Su report 9 further cases of sequential DH and LE occurring in the same persons that were encountered at the Mayo Clinic between 1950 and 1981. The clinical findings are summarized in the table. Seven patients acquired DH first and LE 1 to 14 years later. Two of the 4 patients treated with sulfapyridine for DH acquired discoid LE and 2 developed systemic LE. All 3 dapsone-treated patients developed systemic LE. Two of the patients with systemic LE had renal disease. Two patients developed systemic LE before DH; the intervals were 1 and 4 years. Only 1 of the 9 patients had gastrointestinal symptoms associated with DH. Three patients had definite renal involvement by systemic LE.

Five cases of DH associated with systemic LE and 1 with discoid LE have been reported previously. None of the Mayo Clinic patients in whom LE followed DH showed any definite relation between time of onset of LE treatment of DH, and none showed definite improvement in LE when treatment for DH was discontinued. Both LE and DH may be autoimmune disorders in which immune complexes have

CLINICAL DATA FOR NINE CASES REPORTED

Case No./Sex	First Disease/ Age at Diagnosis, yr	Second Disease/ Years Between Diagnoses	Comment
1/F	DH/27	DLE/14	Sulfapyridine and arsenic were given intermittently for DH, antimalarial agents for DLE of face and arm; DH was absent since age 42 yr; therapy for DLE was discontinued at age 47 yr; hyperthyroidism developed at age 54 yr
2/F	DH/24	SLE/14	DH was treated with sulfapyridine but drug was stopped at age 38 yr because of LE; sulfoxone sodium provided good control of DH
3/M	DH/18	SLE/5	Sulfapyridine was given for DH; at age 23 yr, prednisone was added for SLE; at age 26 yr, sulfapyridine was stopped, without flare of DH; LE nephritis was diagnosed
4/F	SLE/35	DH/4	Prednisone and hydroxychloroquine sulfate were given for LE, sulfapyridine was given for DH; at age 41 yr, nephrotic syndrome occurred, and LE nephritis was found at biopsy; patient died at age 47 yr of LE nephritis
5/F	DH/39	SLE/1	Raynaud's disease, rheumatoid arthritis, and sicca complex were diagnosed at age 38 yr; at age 39 yr, dapsone was started; at age 40 yr, hydroxychloroquine was added
6/M	DH/50	SLE/5	Dapsone was given at age 50 yr for DH; patient was also started on gluten-free diet because of daily diarrhea
7/F	SLE/66	DH/1	Patient had history of hypothyroidism; SLE was diagnosed at age 66 yr; creatinine clearance was decreased; hydroxychloroquine was started; topical steroids and gluten-free diet were started for DH; HLA typing showed A2, Aw30, B8, B13, DR4, and DR7
8/F	DH/21	SLE/2	Dapsone was given for DH; at age 23 yr, prednisone was added for SLE; at age 25 yr, hydroxychloroquine was added; dapsone was discontinued, diphenhydramine hydrochloride controlled itching of DH; renal biopsy showed lupus nephritis
9/F	DH/67	DLE/13	Sulfapyridine was stopped after 1 mo and nicotinyl alcohol was given for DH; it was discontinued at age 72 yr; topical steroids controlled symptoms of DH, at age 80 yr, DLE of left temple was diagnosed

(Courtesy of Thomas, J.R. III, and Su, W.P.D.: Arch. Dermatol. 119:740–745, September 1983; copyright 1983, American Medical Association.)

a role. That multiple other autoimmune disorders have been described in association with LE supports the hypothesis that there may be an immunologic relation between LE and DH.

▶ [A point of interest in this clinical review of the association of these 2 diseases is the fact the DH appeared first in most of the patients. The authors raise the question whether the use of sulfonamides or sulfones in the treatment of DH may have had an inductive or facilitating effect on the development of LE. This may be another argument for the use of a gluten free diet. Perhaps an antinuclear antibody titer should be part of a DH workup. The authors include a useful table of other autoimmune diseases associated with LE.—R.M.] ◀

3–21 **Skin Biopsies in Relatives of Patients With Dermatitis Herpetiformis.** J. N. Leonard, G. P. Haffenden, W. F. G. Tucker, D. J. Unsworth, A. Sidgwick, A. F. Swain, and Lionel Fry (London) investigated the possibility that IgA is present in the skin of relatives of patients with dermatitis herpetiformis (DH). They also report the incidence of overt DH in relatives of 109 patients with DH seen at St. Mary's Hospital since 1969. Twenty first-degree relatives of 10 patients with DH were studied. None had any symptoms suggestive of either DH or celiac disease. Average age of these 9 male and 11 female relatives was 32.4 years. Four-millimeter punch biopsy specimens of forearm skin were taken under local anesthesia.

Of the 109 patients only 1—a 33-year-old man who developed DH at age 32—has had a first-degree relative with DH. The study included the following members of this patient's family: father (aged 68) and mother (aged 65), neither of whom had the disease clinically; the patient's sister (aged 26), who developed DH at age 16; and an unaffected brother (aged 28 at time of study).

None of the 20 relatives studied had IgA deposits in the skin or antigliadin antibodies (AGA) in serum. In the family that included 2 siblings with DH, both affected members had IgA deposits in the papillary dermis of uninvolved skin. No other immunoglobulins and no C3 were found. Both affected members had AGA of IgA class, and both had macroscopically abnormal biopsy specimens from the small intestine. Neither parent, nor the unaffected sibling, had immunoglobulins or C3 in the skin biopsy specimen or AGA in the serum.

The findings of this study are consistent with previous reports of a low family incidence of DH, and they suggest that DH is caused by a combination of both genetic and environmental factors.

▶ [In view of the fact that both celiac disease and DH are gluten dependent, that the histocompatibility antigen HLA-B8 occurs in more than 80% of affected patients, and that celiac disease has a family incidence, the authors studied the incidence of IgA in the skin of relatives of DH patients. None was found, nor was antigliadin antibody found, results that support the previously reported low family incidence of DH.—R.M.] ◀

3–22 **Dermatitis Herpetiformis: Review of 119 Cases.** D. B. Buckley, J. English, W. Molloy, C. T. Doyle, and M. J. Whelton (Cork, Ireland) reviewed the findings in 119 patients with dermatitis herpetiformis (DH) whose disease was diagnosed in southern Ireland between 1954

(3–21) Acta Derm. Venereol. (Stockh.) 63:252–254, 1983.
(3–22) Clin. Exp. Dermatol. 8:477–487, September 1983.

and 1980. Dermatitis herpetiformis constituted 0.1% of all skin disorders seen during this period. Immunofluorescence study showed IgA in 94% of the 79 patients tested; it was usually in a granular distribution. Jejunal biopsies showed villous atrophy in 88% of the patients. Human leukocyte antigen typing studies showed HLA-B8 in 84% HLA-A1 in 74%, and HLA-B8 or A1 in 93%. Antinuclear factor was present in 19% of patients, thyroid antibodies in 6%, and gastric parietal cell antibodies in 8%. Two of 20 patients had antireticulin antibodies. Overall, 20% of the patients had a family history of atopy and 6% had a positive personal history of atopy. About 12% had a family history of celiac disease. In 1 patient, a man aged 70 with a previous diagnosis of celiac disease, Hodgkin's disease with predominantly lymphocytic histology developed.

The relationship between gluten enteropathy and skin lesions remains unclear, but circulating immune complexes are present in all patients with DH and celiac disease. It has been suggested that their deposition in the skin gives rise to the eruption. A gluten-free diet was unacceptable to most patients. About 20% of patients who rigorously maintained such a diet were able to reduce or discontinue dapsone after about 1–2 years. Most patients responded adequately to dapsone in a dose of 100 mg daily. Patients taking dapsone for a prolonged period was given iron and folic acid and, on occasion, vitamin B_{12}.

▶ [The authors review 119 cases of DH and emphasize several points: *(1)* Biopsies showed IgA in the skin of 93.6% of the patients; 90% granular IgA deposits, and 3 patients had linear IgA deposits. *(2)* In contrast to previous literature indicating little jejunal involvement in linear IgA disease, two thirds of the patients in this series who had linear IgA had jejunal involvement. *(3)* Ninety-three percent of the patients had HLA-B8 or A1 antigens, and the authors point out the previously reported strong association of DH with HLA-DRw3 antigen. *(4)* There was a significant association in this series between DH and other autoimmune disease. *(5)* Only 1 case of lymphoma (Hodgkin's disease) was noted in this series.—R.M.] ◀

3–23 **Increased Incidence of Malignancy in Dermatitis Herpetiformis.** J. N. Leonard, W. F. G. Tucker, J. S. Fry, Carmel A. E. Coulter, A. W. Boylston, R. M. H. McMinn, G. P. Haffenden, A. F. Swain, and Lionel Fry studied 109 patients who were followed up at St. Mary's Hospital, London, to determine whether there is an increased incidence of malignant disease in patients with dermatitis herpetiformis and, if so, whether there are any predisposing factors. Biopsy of the duodenal-jejunal flexure was performed by using a Crosby capsule in 96 patients (88%) at presentation. Patients were also graded with respect to their diet.

Seven (6.4%) of the 109 patients with papillary IgA dermatitis herpetiformis developed malignant disease between 1969 and December 1981, giving a relative risk of 2.38. Mean time from presentation to diagnosis of malignant disease was 41 months. Three patients later died. All three lymphomas would, until recently, have been classified as reticulum cell sarcomas, giving a relative risk for this disease of

---

(3–23) Br. Med. J. 286:16–18, Jan. 1, 1983.

100. In 6 of 7 patients who developed a malignancy, biopsy specimens of the small intestine were macroscopically abnormal, giving a relative risk for this feature of 4.22. Intraepithelial lymphocyte counts were obtained in 5 of 7 patients. Thirty-six (57%) of 63 patients with normal diet had a macroscopically abnormal small intestine compared with 24 (73%) of 33 patients following a gluten-free diet (an insignificant difference). Of the 7 patients who developed a malignancy, only 1 was following a gluten-free diet when the tumor first appeared. Relative risk in patients following a normal diet was 3.09 compared with 1.01 in those following a gluten-free diet. Of the 8 patients with linear IgA dermatitis herpetiformis, 3 developed malignancies; these 3 had macroscopically normal biopsy specimens.

This study has shown that patients with dermatitis herpetiformis have a signficantly increased risk of malignancy of 2.38. Comparison of this risk with the reported relative risk of malignancy of 4.16 in patients with adult celiac disease suggests patients with dermatitis herpetiformis are less at risk of developing a malignancy. Two of 3 patients with dermatitis herpetiformis who developed lymphomas had low intraepithelial lymphocyte counts in association with macroscopically abnormal mucosae of the small intestine. These findings suggest that patients with linear IgA dermatitis herpetiformis require careful follow-up and a gluten-free diet. The immune mechanisms of these patients should also be investigated.

► [The authors report 7 cases of malignant disease (3 lymphomas) in 109 cases of DH surveyed. This brings to approximately 20 the number of reported cases of lymphoma in association with dermatitis herpetiformis (Reunala et al.: *J. Am. Acad. Dermatol.* 10:526, 1984; Gawkrodger et al.: *Gut* 15:151, 1984). The association of lymphoma with celiac disease has been established; and in view of the similar small bowel pathology and gluten sensitivity, the association of lymphoma with DH seems most reasonable. The factor(s) responsible for this association remain unknown. Gluten sensitivity is a common etiologic factor in both disorders, but it is not yet clear whether a strict gluten-free diet (GFD) will prevent lymphoma, even though the clinical manifestations of both diseases may clear completely. A long-term detailed study will be necessary to answer this question. Although many of the patients who developed lymphoma were on a GFD, one needs to know the strictness of diet observance, the duration of the disease prior to institution of the diet, the duration of diet observance prior to the appearance of lymphoma, the fate of antigluten or antigliadin serum antibodies, the changes in appearance of the small bowel, and the changes in the cellular infiltrate of the bowel. Long-term observation of patients on a GFD would be especially useful. Although the answers are not available, it seems sensible to treat patients with DH with a GFD despite the inconvenience and possible expense. There are no intrinsic dangers to a GFD to my knowledge, and to the extent that it spares the use of potentially toxic drugs, it may be the safest path to take in the long run.—R.M.] ◄

3–24 **Prenatal Exclusion of Herlitz Syndrome by Electron Microscopy or Fetal Skin Biopsies Obtained at Fetoscopy.** L. Löfberg, I. Anton-Lamprecht, G. Michaëlsson, and B. Gustavii report the cases of 2 women, each of whom had previously had a child that died of epidermolysis bullosa astrophicans (Herlitz syndrome). In later pregnancies of both women, the syndrome was excluded antepartum by

(3–24) Acta Derm. Venereol. (Stockh.) 63:185–189, 1983.

ultrastructural study of fetal skin biopsy specimens obtained by fetoscopy. Fetoscopy was done at 19 weeks' gestation in both cases. (Fetoscopies were done at 16–21 weeks' gestation in 5 women scheduled for elective abortion by hysterotomy.) In both cases Herlitz syndrome was ruled out by the demonstration of the regular presence of normal hemidesmosomes with well-developed subbasal dense plates at the dermoepidermal junction. Both infants had normal skin after birth. The biopsy sites did not exhibit scarring.

The Herlitz syndrome is characterized by hypoplasia of hemidesmosomes with complete absence of the subbasal dense plates below the basal cell plasma membrane in the space of the lamina rara. It seems best to evaluate a fetus at risk of Herlitz syndrome or related skin disorders at 19–21 weeks' gestation. About 1 week is required for ultrastructural analysis. Biopsy under direct vision is much preferable to "blind" biopsy, which involves a risk of collecting fetal membranes or placental or uterine wall fragments and a risk of damaging the amniotic sac.

▶ [Nothing new is added to the literature by this paper, but it is a nice, concise review of the technique of fetoscopy. It stresses the need for direct visualization of the fetal skin while performing the biopsy.—J.C.A.] ◀

3–25 **Reduced Threshold to Suction-Induced Blister Formation in Insulin-Dependent Diabetics.** Diabetics may have an increased susceptibility to cutaneous blister formation that is clinically manifest as the bullous eruption of diabetes. Joel E. Bernstein, Lawrence E. Levine, Maria M. Medenica, Cheuk W. Yung, and Keyoumars Soltani (Univ. of Chicago) studied the mechanical force necessary to induce suction blisters in 15 insulin-dependent diabetics and 20 age-matched normal controls.

Mean suction blister threshold for the 15 insulin-dependent diabetics was 31.9 minutes, but threshold for the 20 controls was 68.0 minutes. This difference was statistically highly significant. In only 1 subject did the suction blister threshold exceed 45 minutes. Diabetes in this subject had been diagnosed only 12 months before the study. The suction blister threshold decreased with age in both subjects and controls. Histologic examination of suction blisters from both groups revealed a noninflammatory subepidermal separation. Ultrastructure studies demonstrated that this separation occurs in the lamina lucida between the cell membrane and basal lamina.

Insulin-dependent diabetics have a significantly reduced threshold to suction blister development. Whether this threshold varies with time or with control of diabetes remains to be determined.

▶ [A lower threshold to suction blister formation has been demonstrated in insulin-dependent diabetics. What correlation this finding has with clinical bulla formation and with control of diabetes remains to be explored.—R.M.] ◀

(3–25) J. Am. Acad. Dermatol. 8:790–791, June 1983.

4. Collagen Vascular Diseases

4-1 **The 1982 Revised Criteria for the Classification of Systemic Lupus Erythematosus.** Eng M. Tan, Alan S. Cohen, James F. Fries, Alfonse T. Masi, Dennis J. McShane, Naomi F. Rothfield, Jane Green Schaller, Norman Talal, and Robert J. Winchester discuss the revised classification of systemic lupus erythematosus (SLE), representing an update of the 1971 preliminary criteria. Variables were compared in 177 patients with SLE and 162 control patients from 18 clinics. The new criteria were found to be 96% sensitive and 96% specific when tested against the current patient data base. The strongest addition to the criteria appeared to be the fluorescence antinuclear antibody test, which was positive at some time in all but 1 of the 175 patients tested; however, positive results were also obtained in half the controls. Seven false-positive results were obtained by using the revised criteria and 8 by using the 1971 criteria. There were 7 and 22 false-negative cases, respectively.

The revised criteria for SLE include the fluorescence antinuclear antibody test and tests for antibody to native DNA and Sm antigen. Some criteria involving the same organ systems have been aggregated into a single criterion. Raynaud's phenomenon and alopecia are no longer included. The new criteria have sensitivity and specificity exceeding 95%, representing improvement over the 1971 criteria. The revised criteria are useful in discriminating SLE from rheumatoid arthritis, scleroderma, and dermatopolymyositis, but their performance in distinguishing SLE from other rheumatic disorders remains to be determined.

► [The revised criteria for the diagnosis of systemic lupus erythematosus include 11 elements. The prominence of alterations in the integument is especially noteworthy. Features of importance to the dermatologist are the presence of an erythematous malar eruption, atrophic plaques with follicular plugs, photosensitivity, and oral or nasopharyngeal ulcers. Alopecia and Raynaud's phenomenon were excluded owing to their lack of specificity and sensitivity as discriminating factors. Curiously, a skin biopsy is not included as a criterion. It should be noted that these revised criteria are used for the purpose of classifying patients and are not diagnostic criteria.—N.A.S.] ◄

4-2 **Antibodies to Native DNA and Serum Complement (C3) Levels: Application to Diagnosis and Classification of Systemic Lupus Erythematosus.** Arthur Weinstein, Bonnie Bordwell, Basil Stone, Clark Tibbetts, and Naomi F. Rothfield (Univ. of Connecticut) conducted a prospective study of 98 patients with systemic lupus erythematosus (SLE) for sensitivity and specificity of the presence of an-

---

(4-1) Arthritis Rheum. 25:1271–1277, November 1982.
(4-2) Am. J. Med. 74:206–216, February 1983.

tibodies to native DNA and low serum C3 concentrations. The patients were followed for a mean of 38.4 months. Hospitalized patients, patients with other connective tissue diseases, and subjects without disease served as controls.

Of the patients with SLE, 72% had a high DNA-binding value (more than 33%) initially, and another 20% had a high value later in the course of the illness. Similarly, C3 concentrations were low (less than 81 mg/100 ml) in 38% of patients with SLE initially and in 66% at any time during the study. High DNA-binding values and low C3 concentrations each showed extremely high predictive value (94%) for the diagnosis of SLE when applied to a patient population in which that diagnosis was considered. The presence of both abnormalities was 100% correct in predicting the diagnosis of SLE.

Antibodies to DNA measured by DNA binding and C3 concentrations determined by immunodiffusion are sensitive and specific markers for SLE. The antibodies have high predictive value for diagnosis of SLE in a population of patients with rheumatic diseases. The data suggest that the presence of both abnormalities is 100% predictive for the diagnosis of SLE. Both determinations should be included as major laboratory data in any revision of criteria for the diagnosis and classification of SLE.

4–3 **Pregnancy in Patients With Systemic Lupus Erythematosus.** Michael W. Varner, Richard T. Meehan, Craig H. Syrop, M. Paul Strottmann, and Clifford P. Goplerud (Univ. of Iowa) conducted a retrospective study of 31 patients with systemic lupus erythematosus (SLE) during 38 pregnancies. The patients were divided into 4 groups: (1) disease initially diagnosed during pregnancy; (2) disease exacerbated during pregnancy or within 6 weeks thereafter; (3) disease unchanged during pregnancy (with medication); and (4) disease unchanged during pregnancy (without medication).

Results of this study show a spontaneous or missed abortion rate of 7.9%, elective abortion rate of 10.5%, and a perinatal mortality of 12.9%. One maternal death occurred 5 weeks postpartum. The patients' ages ranged between 16 and 37 years. Range of parity prior to the index pregnancy was 0–6. Eleven patients had 24 pregnancies prior to diagnosis of SLE. These pregnancies resulted in 8 spontaneous abortions, 2 elective abortions, and 14 surviving live-born infants. Of the 38 pregnancies in all 4 groups, 2 ended in spontaneous abortion; 1, missed abortion; 4, elective abortion; and 2, stillbirth. Of the 29 infants born alive, 3 were small for gestational age, 1 was large for gestational age, and 25 were average. Patients in group 1 were more severely affected than those in all other groups. Thrombocytopenia and heavy proteinuria occurred more frequently in group 1. During most of the 20 pregnancies in groups 2 and 3, patients received anti-inflammatory therapy. Groups 2 and 3 had similar frequencies of serositis, CNS disease and hematologic manifestations. In group 4, there was a paucity of prior manifestations involving the

---

(4–3) Am. J. Obstet. Gynecol. 145:1025–1040, Apr. 15, 1983.

CNS and of renal or serosal disease compared with other groups. Serologic, cutaneous, and musculoskeletal symptoms were common among all groups and had no prognostic value.

Patients with SLE who become pregnant usually do well, provided the disease is in remission. Those requiring medical therapy at time of conception may either remain stable or require more intensive therapy. Management of the disease during pregnancy does not differ from that of the nonpregnant patient. Clinical parameters, renal function studies, and hematologic information were more useful than immunologic laboratory data in assessing the course of the disease during pregnancy and in indicating alterations in treatment. Antepartum fetal surveillance is advised. Timing of and route of delivery must be individualized.

4–4 **Neonatal Lupus Syndrome in Successive Pregnancies.** Neonatal lupus erythematosus is a rare, self-limited syndrome characterized by lupus skin lesions, congenital heart block, or both. The mothers sometimes have diagnosable systemic lupus erythematosus (SLE) but more often have mild symptoms of Sjögren's syndrome or SLE or are asymptomatic. The condition has been ascribed to transplacental passage of anti-SS-A(Ro) antibodies. Lela A. Lee, Patrick J. Lillis, Karen A. Fritz, J. Clark Huff, David A. Norris, and William L. Wes-

Fig 4–1.—Erythematous, scaly, atrophic papules on face. (Courtesy of Lee, L.A., et al.: J. Am. Acad. Dermatol. 9:401–406, September 1983.)

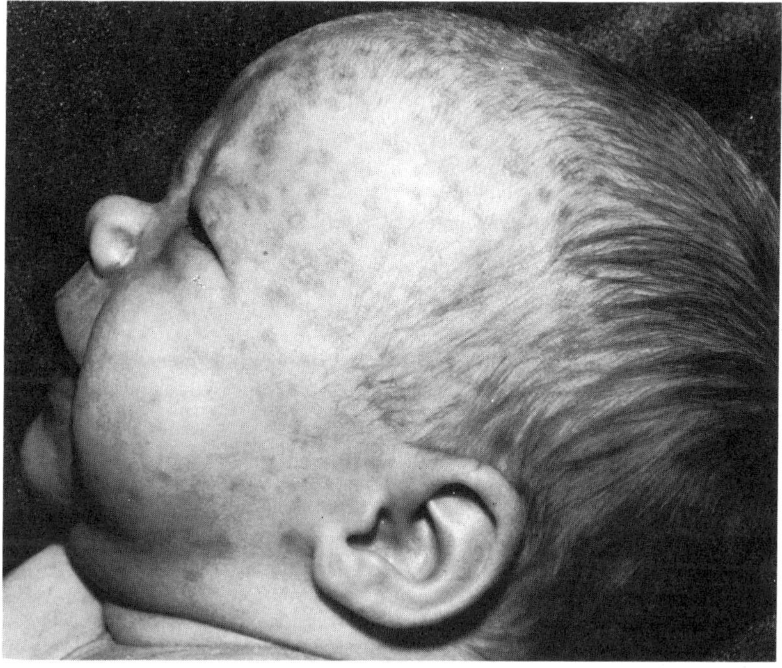

(4–4) J. Am. Acad. Dermatol. 9:401–406, September 1983.

ton (Univ. of Colorado) report the development of neonatal lupus in siblings born 15 months apart.

The first infant was born after an uncomplicated term pregnancy and developed skin lesions at age 8 weeks, after 2 weeks of deliberate sunbathing. The biopsy findings were consistent with lupus, and IgG deposits were confirmed. Speckled fluorescent antinuclear antibodies and anti-SS-A antibodies were demonstrated at age 4 months. The skin lesions faded by age 7 months but recurred during solar exposure. The appearance of the second infant is shown in Figure 4–1. Anti-SS-A antibody but not fluorescent antinuclear antibody was demonstrated in this case. The skin lesions resolved by age 15 months. The mother was asymptomatic but had anti-SS-A antibody. The maternal grandmother had Raynaud's phenomenon but no antibodies. Both the mother and the grandmother were DR3 positive on HLA typing, as was 1 of the children.

Organ systems other than the skin and heart may be involved in neonatal lupus erythematosus, but multisystem involvement is unusual. Nine other reports of congenital heart block or cutaneous lupus in sibling pairs have appeared. Children with neonatal lupus who developed multisystem connective tissue disease, notably SLE, later in life have also been described. The present cases indicate that neonatal lupus can occur in successive pregnancies, although the risk of having a second affected child is unknown.

▶ [Infants with neonatal lupus erythematosus may be asymptomatic except for the presence of a red, annular rash on the face and upper torso, often related to sun exposure. The most important complications of this syndrome include heart block, multisystem disease, and possibly progression to florid SLE later in life. Mothers are usually asymptomatic, and the diagnosis will be missed unless anticytoplasmic antibodies (anti-SS-A and anti-Ro) are specifically sought. Long-term follow-up of mothers and infants with this syndrome is required to fully appreciate the long-term consequences and frequency of disease in subsequent pregnancies. Until we know more, sun-protection is recommended for mothers and infants with this syndrome.—A.R.R.] ◀

4–5 **Neonatal Lupus Erythematosus: Five New Cases With HLA Typing.** Neonatal lupus erythematosus, an unusual manifestation of lupus erythematosus, can affect the cardiovascular, hematologic, and cutaneous sytems. Recent follow-up studies have demonstrated the potential for affected infants to develop severe lupus erythematosus during adolescence. Kirk A. Barber and Robert Jackson (Ottawa Civic Hosp., Ottawa) present data on 5 new cases of neonatal lupus erythematosus, examine the various clinical presentations, and report the results of HLA typing of the mother-child pairs.

Girl, aged 7 months, had had a skin eruption since age 2 months. Onset of the rash had been associated with her first direct exposure to sunlight. There were numerous, erythematous, scaling macules, 1–2 cm in diameter, on the center of the face and extensor aspects of the extremities. Atrophy or hypopigmentation was not observed. The hemoglobin concentration was 10.9 gm/dl, the leukocyte count was 6.5×10^9/L, and the platelet count was 420×10^9/L. An antinuclear antibody test was positive at a titer of 1:160 and

(4–5) Can. Med. Assoc. J. 129:139–141, July 15, 1983.

showed a speckled pattern. Tests for anti-DNA antibody and total hemolytic complement were normal. A biopsy of sun-exposed involved skin revealed changes compatible with lupus erythematosus. A test for antinuclear antibody in the mother was positive at a titer of 1:40 and showed a speckled pattern; an indirect Coombs test was also positive. Both the child and her mother had HLA antigens A1 and B8. The child also had antigens A2 and B13, and the mother had antigens A3 and B7. The child's rash had faded without sequelae at age 8 months, and an antinuclear antibody test at that time was negative.

It seems likely that transplacental transfer of maternal autoantibodies is responsible for the development of lupus erythematosus in neonates and accounts for its transient and multisystemic nature. In this study, 2 infants, both with the HLA antigens A1 and B8, did not develop the disease until after they had been exposed to direct sunlight, which suggests that an environmental factor, besides transient maternal antibodies, may be necessary in some cases for the disease to become manifest. Evidence for a genetic factor in the pathogenesis of neonatal lupus erythematosus has been supplied by studies of twins and is apparent from the increased familial incidence. Three of the mother-child pairs had the HLA antigens A1 and B8, though the significance of this finding is unclear.

▶ [An interesting clinical observation was the development of neonatal lupus in 2 infants only after exposure to sunlight.—N.A.S.] ◀

4–6 **Familial Systemic Lupus Erythematosus in Males.** Robert G. Lahita, Nicholas Chiorazzi, Allan Gibofsky, Robert J. Winchester, and Henry G. Kunkel (Rockefeller Univ.) report on 4 human kindreds in which systemic lupus erythematosus (SLE) occurred in males in 2 or more generations. In 1 family a father was dead, and in another a son was dead; data on these persons were derived retrospectively. Other family members were studied directly.

FAMILY 1.—Son had initial manifestations of SLE at age 16 years, with a positive lupus erythematosus (LE) test. Anti-DNA binding by radioimmunoassay was 100%. The patient was promptly treated with high-dose corticosteroids, and his disease is in remission. The father had influenza-like symptoms. Anti-DNA binding was 100%. He had had a positive VDRL test at marriage. Diagnosed hemolytic anemia and myositis responded to prednisone. A daughter had transient arthralgia and proteinuria, but DNA binding was normal.

FAMILY 2.—Son was seen at age 12 with nephritis and anti-DNA binding of 100%. He responded to large doses of prednisone. His brother, 3 years younger, developed fever, edema, acute renal insufficiency, and weight loss. Anti-DNA binding was greater than 60%. Plasmapheresis and corticosteroid therapy were transiently successful. The father had arthralgias and severe Raynaud's phenomenon. Concurrent with illness of the second son, 1 daughter had idiopathic thrombocytopenic purpura. Anti-DNA binding approached 100% while she was using oral contraceptives. After contraceptives were stopped, results of her serologic tests returned toward normal.

FAMILY 3.—Son, 36, had onset of Raynaud's phenomenon during the father's illness. The disease gradually progressed, but renal function remained

---

(4–6) Arthritis Rheum. 26:39–44, January 1983.

normal. The patient was maintained on high-dose prednisone and antihypertensive therapy. The father died at age 58, 2 years after diagnosis of SLE. He did well initially with corticosteroids. Renal function remained normal, but he developed a diastolic murmur of aortic insufficiency. He died shortly after aortic valve replacement. A brother and sister of the propositus are asymptomatic.

FAMILY 4.—Ten years before SLE was diagnosed in the father, it was diagnosed in the son. The son's renal function rapidly deteriorated, and he became severely nephrotic, dying shortly thereafter. The father, aged 69, had positive LE and VDRL tests. The disease in this father and son did not coincide. A history of rheumatoid arthritis existed in the paternal grandmother.

The presenting symptoms of SLE in males were similar to those observed in females. All males had normal karyotypes and had no obvious endocrinopathy. This situation is analogous to that in the BXSB mouse, in which the development of lupus-like syndromes occurs primarily in males.

▶ [This analysis of four kindreds in which SLE occurred in males draws attention to the familial aspect of the disease. Although the presenting symptoms of males were similar to those observed in females, the authors point out that many of the males developed the disease before puberty, whereas the disorder usually occurs in females after puberty.—N.A.S.] ◀

4–7 **Familial Systemic Lupus Erythematosus: Immunogenetic Studies in Eight Families.** John D. Reveille, Wilma B. Bias, Jerry A. Winkelstein, Thomas T. Provost, Carole A. Dorsch, and Frank Arnett (Baltimore) note that familial systemic lupus erythematosus (SLE) provides a unique opportunity to study the relationships between genetic factors (HLA and complement component deficiencies) and the occurrence of SLE, other immune disorders, and autoantibodies in families. Eight families were studied, each containing 2 or more affected members (22 total) with SLE, and 40 unaffected relatives; all were examined for HLA genotypes, complement components, and autoantibodies.

Among the 40 non-SLE relatives, 7 (18%) had other immune diseases, including thyroid disease in 2, rheumatoid arthritis in 2, immune thrombocytopenic purpura in 2, and Henoch-Schönlein purpura in 1. Four (18%) of the 22 SLE patients had other immune diseases, including thyroid disease in 3 and progressive systemic sclerosis in 1. Eleven (28%) non-SLE relatives had antinuclear antibodies (ANA), which were present at high titers in 5 (13%). Eleven (28%) had antibodies to ssDNA, and 1 had a biologic false-positive test result for syphilis. Only the SLE patients had antibodies dsDNA, Ro(SS-A), Sm, or nRNP. A heterozygous C2 deficiency (C2D) was found in 1 of 7 kindreds studied, and it followed an A25, B18, DR7 haplotype. Heterozygous C2D was inherited by only 1 of 3 family members with SLE. Also, HLA-DR2 occurred in 36% and DR3 in 36% of SLE patients, which was not significantly different from findings in non-SLE family members or in unrelated local controls. Similarly, other immune disorders and autoantibodies followed no consistent HLA hap-

---

(4–7) Medicine (Baltimore) 62:21–35, January 1983.

lotypes or DR specificities. Further, DR2 or DR3 was found in 5 (83%) of 6 patients having anti-Ro(SS-A) antibodies.

These data strongly suggest that genetic factors other than HLA and complement component deficiencies or environmental factors are necessary for the expression of SLE and other immune abnormalities in lupus families.

4–8 **Studies of Repeat Skin Biopsies of Nonlesional Skin in Patients With Systemic Lupus Erythematosus.** Naomi Rothfield and Cathy Marino (Univ. of Connecticut) studied 31 patients with systemic lupus erythematosus using repeat biopsy of nonlesional skin to determine whether there was a relationship between disease activity (clinical and serologic) and the presence and number of immunoglobulins and complement proteins in the dermal-epidermal junction. Patients included 3 males and 28 females, mean age of 45 years.

The 31 patients were divided into 6 groups based on the change in clinical disease activity between the first and second biopsies. Analysis of the presence of protein deposits revealed that, in each patient, IgG, IgA, and C3 were present more frequently during clinical disease activity of grades 1 to 3+ than during 0 activity. The number of proteins present in the dermal-epidermal junction correlated with degree of disease activity, increasing with increasing degree of activity. In 35 biopsies from patients with grades 1 to 3+ clinical disease activity, the mean DNA binding in patients with fewer than 3 proteins in the dermal-epidermal junction was significantly lower than that in patients with more than 3 such proteins. Patients with grade 0 activity had mean DNA binding in the normal range. The IgG and IgA deposits occurred in patients with high DNA binding and low serum C3 and C4 levels. Also, C3 and C1q deposits occurred in relation to high DNA binding; IgM and C4 deposits did not correlate with the serologic abnormalities. The presence of dermal-epidermal proteins appears to relate to an active process rather than to the presence or absence of renal disease at some time during the course of the disease.

This study found significantly fewer protein deposits in the skin of patients without disease activity than in the skin of patients with disease activity.

▶ [Direct immunofluorescence techniques have been applied to the study of the skin of patients with systemic lupus erythematosus as an aid in diagnosis and prognosis. In this study, the deposition of greater numbers of immunoreactants at the dermo-epidermal junction in clinically uninvolved deltoid skin of patients with active systemic lupus erythematosus was correlated with current clinically acute systemic manifestations rather than with the presence or absence of renal disease. Thus, the question of the relation of the deposition of immunoreactants in uninvolved non-sun-exposed skin to the presence of renal disease remains unresolved with studies both supporting (Gilliam, N. J., et al.: *J. Clin. Invest.* 53:1434, 1974; Dantzig, P. I., et al.: *Br. J. Dermatol.* 93:531, 1975) and refuting (Caperton, E. M., Jr., et al.: *JAMA* 222:935, 1972; Grossman, J., et al.: *Ann. Intern. Med.* 80:496, 1974) such a correlation.—N.A.S.] ◀

4–9 **ANA-Negative Systemic Lupus Erythematosus.** A. Razzaque Ahmed and Steven Workman (Univ. of California, Los Angeles) re-

---

(4–8) Arthritis Rheum. 25:624–630, June 1982.
(4–9) Clin. Exp. Dermatol. 8:369–377, July 1983.

NEGATIVE SYSTEMIC LUPUS ERYTHEMATOSUS NEGATIVE FOR ANA

Incidence	Unknown, approximately 4–13% of clinical SLE
Epidemiology	Age—average onset at 40 years (range 14–71 years)
Clinical features	Photosensitivity, oral ulcerations and malar rash. Relative sparing of arthritis, nephritis and haematologic involvement
Serological features	ANA-negative. Relative increase in antibodies to cytoplasmic antigens Ro and La
Histopathology	Light microscopy of lesional skin shows changes of lupus erythematosus. Direct immunofluorescence shows Ig or complement in lesional skin in 70%. Lupus band test positive on light-exposed uninvolved skin in only 10%
Course and prognosis	Relapses and remissions. Prognosis good
Treatment	Topical steroids and sunscreen for cutaneous manifestations. Systemic steroids, antimalarials if cutaneous involvement is extensive or systemic disease

(Courtesy of Ahmed, A.R., and Workman, S.: Clin. Exp. Dermatol. 8:369–377, July 1983.)

view data on a subset of patients who meet the ARA criteria for systemic lupus erythematosus (SLE) but whose sera lack antinuclear antibodies (ANA) when tested with various standard substrates. These patients have predominantly cutaneous involvement (table), and therefore are often seen initially by a dermatologist. The exact incidence of ANA-negative SLE is unclear, but it is about 5%–10% in several large series. Like ANA-positive lupus, the disorder is more frequent in women, and about 90% of the patients are white. The condition described as "subacute cutaneous lupus erythematosus" is clinically similar to ANA-negative SLE. The presence of antibodies to the cytoplasmic antigens Ro and La is important in identifying ANA-negative SLE patients. About 30%–40% of patients with ANA-negative SLE have reduced levels of total hemolytic complement, C3, and C4.

The histologic findings in cutaneous lupus in ANA-negative patients resemble those in ANA-positive patients. Treatment also is similar. Moderate doses of systemic steroids lead to rapid remission in patients with prominent systemic manifestations. Topical treatment, however, usually can be tried first. Sunscreens may also be helpful. Not many patients will require azathioprine. The clinical course is characterized by relapses and remissions. Apparently both the absence of ANA and the presence of anticytoplasmic antibodies are associated with a favorable prognosis, since these patients have less extracutaneous involvement. It is unclear whether the occasional conversion to ANA positivity represents a true change or whether ANA-negativity is a prodromal stage in the course of some SLE patients.

The subsets of SLE are not completely distinct. Serologic markers are both diagnostically and prognostically important in SLE. Further studies of changes in suppressor cells, which may underlie autoantibody production, may aid the development of specific treatment for SLE.

▶ [In patients with lupus-like syndromes and negative ANA study results, anti-native-DNA, anti-Ro, and anti-La antibody determinations are of value. This syndrome has also been described as subacute cutaneous lupus erythematosus (see Sontheimer,

R., et al.: *Arch. Dermatol.* 115:1409–1415, 1979). In this type of lupus the presence of annular lesions may be pronounced.—A.J.S.] ◀

4–10 **Clinical Significance of Anti-Sm Antibodies in Systemic Lupus Erythematosus.** Michel Beaufils, Fatma Kouki, Françoise Mignon, Jean-Pierre Camus, Liliane Morel-Maroger, and Gabriel Richet (Paris) analyzed the records of 34 patients (29 females) with well-established systemic lupus erythematosus (SLE) for the presence or absence of anti-Sm antibodies.

Of the 34 patients, 12 had both anti-DNA and anti-Sm antibodies (group I), and 22 had anti-DNA antibody with no antibody to an extractable nuclear antigen (group II). No patient had anti-Sm without anti-DNA antibody. There was no significant difference between the two groups in age, sex ratio, or duration of disease. Frequencies of erythema, arthritis, hemolytic anemia, leukopenia, and thrombocytopenia did not differ between groups. Raynaud's phenomenon was similarly frequent in the two groups. More severe manifestations of cutaneous vasculitis were almost exclusively observed in the Sm group (6 of the 12 in group I and 1 of the 22 in group II). Pleuritis and lupus pneumonia were more frequent in the Sm group. Pericarditis was relatively common in both groups. Neurologic symptoms included either unexplained seizures or transient paralysis of various sites (group I). Renal failure was present in 1 of the 12 patients in group I and in 4 of the 22 in group II. Ten patients in group I and 12 in group II required corticosteroid therapy with dosage equal to or greater than 1 mg of prednisone per kg per day. All patients in group II had a favorable outcome. In contrast, 4 patients in group I died.

In SLE, the presence of anti-Sm antibody is associated with a much higher incidence of vasculitis, resulting in peculiar visceral manifestations, which can be poorly responsive to therapy. Whether there is a direct association between anti-Sm antibody and vasculitis or whether the common denominator is a genetic selection remains to be determined.

▶ [Antibodies to Sm antigen, an extractable nuclear antigen, were noted in a high percentage of patients with SLE and systemic manifestations involving the heart, lungs, and skin. The dermatologic feature was described as a cutaneous vasculitis that appeared as purpuric lesions and digital necrosis. Regrettably, skin biopsies were not performed to document the histopathologic alterations.—N.A.S.] ◀

4–11 **Verrucous Lupus Erythematosus: Ultrastructural Studies on a Distinct Variant of Chronic Discoid Lupus Erythematosus.** Although lichen planus (LP), keratoacanthoma, and discoid lupus erythematosus (DLE) usually have distinguishing features, they may overlap. Daniel J. Santa Cruz, Jouni Uitto, Arthur Z. Eisen, and Philip G. Prioleau (Washington Univ.) report data on 10 patients with classic DLE of the face associated with verrucous, papulonodular lesions on arms and hands that were studied by electron microscopy.

The verrucous nodules on the extremities had two distinct histopathologic patterns. One consisted of focal acanthosis with deep der-

(4–10) Am. J. Med. 74:201–205, February 1983.
(4–11) J. Am. Acad. Dermatol. 9:82–90, July 1983.

mal projections, disruption of the epidermal plate, and the presence of cytoid bodies; these lesions resembled keratoacanthomas. The other histologic pattern was more flat, and the lesions were similar to hypertrophic LP.

By immunofluorescence microscopy, the verrucous lesions had IgG and C3 deposits along the basement membrane and globular deposits of IgM indicative of lupus erythematosus. The electron microscopic findings of apoptotic keratinocytes, intraepidermal lymphocytes, gapping, detachments, and reduplications of basal lamina were characteristic of ultrastructural findings in the chronic lichenoid reaction common to LP and DLE. Tubuloreticular inclusions in the endothelial cells of dermal vessels, if not diagnostic of DLE, were characteristic of the disorder.

On the basis of clinical, histopathologic, immunofluorescence, and electron microscopic studies, these cases represent a distinct subset of DLE.

▶ [These are important observations that emphasize the care one must take in evaluating squamous cell proliferation in lupus erythematosus. Without knowledge of the changes described, one can misdiagnose these lesions as neoplastic.—M.C.M.] ◀

4–12 **Histochemical Approach to the Differentiation of Lichen Planus From Lupus Erythematosus.** William Binkley, Janice Starsnic, Rafael Valenzuela, and Wilma F. Bergfeld (Cleveland Clinc Found.) describe a histochemical technique in which a maleimide-derived fluorochrome is used for the detection of disulfide bonds in subepidermal hyaline bodies. Lichen planus and the skin lesions of lupus erythematosus tend to demonstrate different patterns of reactivity with this reagent. Preserved frozen skin biopsy specimens from 4 patients with lichen planus, 10 with lupus erythematosus, and 10 with a variety of other dermatoses were studied.

The reaction of normal skin sections with N-(7-dimethylamino-4-methylcoumarinyl)-maleimide (DACM) showed strong fluorescence in the stratum corneum with little or no reactivity in the stratum malpighii and dermis. All 4 patients with lichen planus showed a type I pattern with moderate to large numbers of subepidermal hyaline bodies (SHB), all of which had a high content of disulfide groups. In contrast, 9 of 10 patients with lupus erythematosus had a type II pattern with few SHB. Although the number of patients evaluated is small, this difference in disulfide group distribution between lichen planus and lupus erythematosus is significant. Other inflammatory dermatoses that contained large numbers of SHB and stained strongly for disulfide groups by the DACM method included dermatomyositis, poikiloderma atrophicans vasculare, and lichenoid drug eruption.

Although DACM is commercially available, it is costly. The recent description of other similar fluorochromes suitable for detection of thiols in tissue sections may make routine application of such histochemical techniques to the differential diagnosis of inflammatory dermatoses more practical.

(4–12) Am. J. Clin. Pathol. 79:486–488, April 1983.

▶ [These are interesting observations which may eventually have practical applications.—M.C.M.] ◀

4–13 **Randomized Trial of Plasma Exchange in Mild Systemic Lupus Erythematosus.** Nathan Wei, David P. Huston, Thomas J. Lawley, Alfred D. Steinberg, John H. Klippel, Russell P. Hall, James E. Balow, and John L. Decker (Natl. Inst. of Health) evaluated the effects of intensive plasma exchange on the serologic and clinical manifestations of mildly active systemic lupus erythematosus (SLE) in 20 patients in a controlled, double-blind trial. Patients were randomly assigned to undergo either six 4-L plasma exchanges or a seemingly identical control procedure during a 2-week period. Properly performed plasma exchange was considered a low-risk procedure. Twelve of the 20 patients (18 women, 2 men) were receiving nonsteroidal anti-inflammatory drugs, and 15 took prednisone. Two patients were withdrawn as therapeutic failures and are excluded from analysis.

Results showed that plasma exchange produced significant reductions in serum levels of IgG, IgM, IgA, and circulating immune complexes as measured by ^{125}I-C1q binding assay. These serologic measurements returned to baseline 4 weeks after plasma exchange without a subsequent rebound above baseline values. Antibodies to DNA were reduced immediately after plasma exchange, but concentrations often returned to pretreatment levels before the next procedure. No changes in any serologic measurements were observed in controls. In 16 of the 18 patients who completed the trial, SLE activity had either remained stable or improved. Frequency and degree of clinical improvement was the same in both plasma exchange and control groups.

These results do not demonstrate that plasma exchange produces significant improvement in the clinical manifestations of mild acute SLE. Thus plasma exchange in mild SLE should continue to be considered an investigational procedure.

▶ [A controlled double-blind trial of plasma exchange therapy in patients with mild SLE proved ineffective despite the reductions in serum immunoglobulins, circulating immune complexes, and antibodies to DNA.—N.A.S.] ◀

4–14 **Linear IgA Dermatosis: Study of 10 Adult Patients.** Most bullous diseases can be separated into distinct entities on the basis of clinical, histologic, and immunologic features. However, the precise classification of skin disorders with clinical characteristics of both dermatitis herpetiformis (DH) and bullous pemphigoid (BP) is difficult because of the confusing terminology used to describe the immunologic findings. H. Mobacken, W. Kastrup, K. Ljunghall, H. Löfberg, L.-Å. Nilsson, Å. Svensson, and U. Tjernlund report the findings in 10 adults with homogeneous linear deposition of IgA along the basement membrane zone (BMZ).

The patients, 7 men and 3 women, aged 25–75 years at onset (mean, 46 years), were observed over a mean of 10 years (range, 3 months to 10 years). All had itching lesions. The lesions had a form

---

(4–13) Lancet 1:17–22, Jan. 1/8, 1983.
(4–14) Acta Derm. Venereol. (Stockh.) 63:123–128, 1983.

and distribution characteristic of DH in 3 patients, 1 of whom had urticarial lesions (table). Five patients had localized or disseminated vesicles and bullae suggestive of BP, and the other 2 patients had suddenly developing, large, annular, erythematous, confluent lesions primarily on the trunk, with peripheral blisters (Figs 4–2 and 4–3). Two patients had oral lesions. Scarring was not seen. Subepidermal blisters and neutrophilic papillary microabscesses were present in one or more skin biopsy specimens from all patients. The number of eosinophils in the upper dermis varied. Patients with homogeneous linear deposition of IgA did not differ histopathologically from those with granular, papillary deposition (classic DH). Immunofluorescence studies showed bandlike, homogeneous linear deposition of IgA along the BMZ in at least two biopsy specimens from each patient. Patients with BP-like lesions had linear IgA deposits less frequently in normal than in perilesional skin ($P<.05$). Neither IgG nor IgM was ever detected, nor was a granular linear (noncontinuous) pattern of IgA along the BMZ or in the papillary tips. Serum antibodies to BMZ and antinuclear antibodies were not found in any patient studied. Treatment with dapsone produced clinical improvement in 7 patients, though onset of relief was slow in 3. Three patients failed to improve, and 1 patient had new, itching vesicles, despite administration of 200 mg of dapsone daily. One patient required combined dapsone and

Fig 4–2 (left).—Acute, widespread, gyrate, itching eruption, mainly on trunk.
Fig 4–3 (right).—Close-up of peripheral blisters.
(Courtesy of Mobacken, H., et al.: Acta Derm. Venereol. [Stockh.] 63:123–128, 1983.

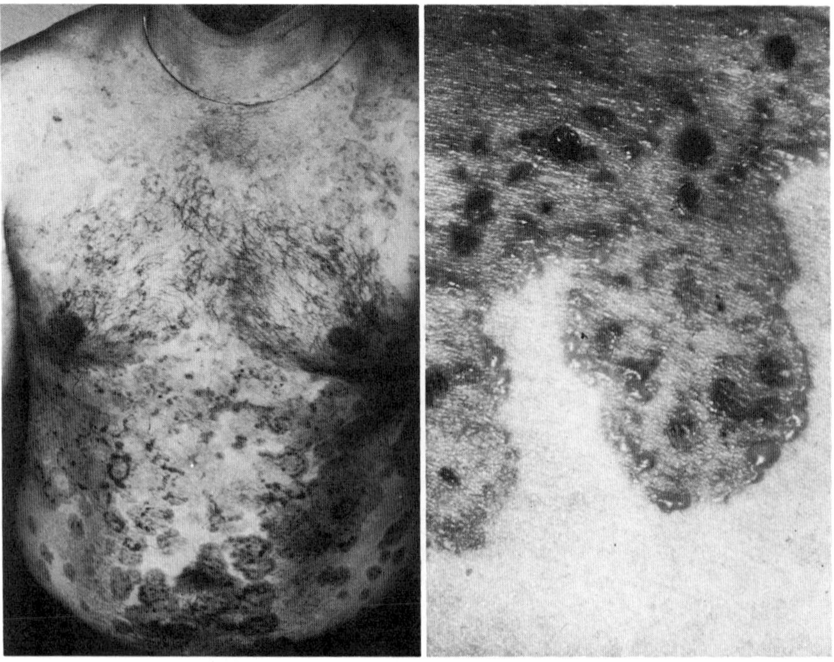

CLINICAL AND LABORATORY FEATURES OF 10 PATIENTS WITH LINEAR IgA DERMATOSIS (POSITIVE/STUDIED)

	Bullous pemphigoid-like	D. herpetiformis-like	Acute type
♂/♀	3/2	3/0	1/1
Mean age (y.)	55	45	32
Linear IgA (pos/total biopsies)			
Perilesionally	10/13	4/6	4/5
Normal skin	7/19	11/14	8/8
HLA-A1, B8, DR3	1/5	2/2	1/2
Glutensensitive enteropathy	0/4	1/2	0/2
Delayed or insufficient response to dapsone	4/5	1/3	1/2

(Courtesy of Mobacken, H., et al.: Acta Derm. Venereol. [Stockh.] 63:123–128, 1983.)

prednisolone therapy, and another required combined dapsone and azathioprine treatment to control the lesions. Seven of 8 patients from whom an intestinal biopsy specimen was obtained had normal villi. Five of 9 patients studied carried the haplotype HLA-A1, B8, DR3. Only 1 of the 10 patients showed a spontaneous remission, which occurred 5 years after onset of symptoms.

Patients with a homogeneous linear IgA pattern differ from those who have classic DH in that the clinical picture is heterogeneous, and small bowel biopsy findings are usually normal. The precise relation to DH and BP remains unclear.

–15 **Intensive Immunosuppression Versus Prednisolone in Treatment of Connective Tissue Diseases.** P. Hollingworth, A. De Vere Tyndall, B. M. Ansell, T. Platts-Mills, J. M. Gumpel, J. Mertin, D. S. Smith, and A. M. Denman (Harrow, England) compared intensive immunosuppression (IIS) with prednisolone alone during a 2-year period in the treatment of severe connective tissue diseases. Intensive immunosuppression consisted of 15 daily infusions of 750 mg of antilymphocyte globulin (ALG), 2.5 mg of azathioprine per kg per day, and prednisolone in an initial dose of 150 mg/day (reduced to 20 mg/day during a 10-day period). Maintenance therapy with azathioprine and prednisolone followed. The initial dosage for prednisolone by itself was 60 mg/day, and patients not responding to this regimen over a minimum of 1 month were then given IIS. Forty-one patients with life-threatening or severely disabling polyarteritis nodosa (PAN), dermatomyositis-polymyositis, or systemic lupus erythematosus (SLE) received one or the other treatment. The three treatment groups included patients receiving prednisolone alone, those receiving IIS with

(4–15) Ann. Rheum. Dis. 41:557–562, December 1982.

no prior prednisolone treatment or less than 60 mg/day for less than 1 month, and those receiving IIS after failure of prednisolone therapy (greater than 60 mg/day for more than 1 month).

All 11 patients receiving IIS for PAN had remissions. Ten of these had renal impairment, which was reversed or halted with IIS, and in 6, renal function had been deteriorating with prednisolone alone. One patient died of pneumonia in renal failure 9 months later but with PAN in remission. Two further patients, neither with renal involvement, achieved remission with prednisolone alone. Two patients with dermatomyositis-polymyositis entered remission with prednisolone alone. The other 12, in 5 of whom corticosteroid therapy had failed, received IIS. Improvement or halting of deterioration was achieved in all 12 with best results among those without marked muscle wasting consequent to prolonged disease. The IIS regimen was generally well tolerated, though infection occurred in 2 patients. Vertebral collapse or osteonecrosis of the femoral head occurred in 3 patients after IIS; all had been receiving long-term corticosteroid treatment.

The results suggest that IIS is more effective than prednisolone alone in treatment of PAN, particularly if there is renal involvement. Too few patients received prednisolone alone in this study for its role in initial treatment of dermatomyositis-polymyositis to be determined. Intensive immunosuppression appears to be no more effective than prednisolone alone in the treatment of SLE and particularly lupus nephritis.

4–16 **Methylprednisolone Pulse Therapy in Dermatomyositis.** Some patients with dermatomyositis (DM) fail to respond satisfactorily to corticosteroid therapy in usual doses and have been given methotrexate and other immunosuppressive drugs. T. Yanagisawa, M. Sueishi, Y. Nawata, T. Akimoto, T. Nozaki, T. Koike, H. Tomioka, and A. Kumagai (Chiba Univ., Japan) evaluated high-dose methylprednisolone therapy in 8 patients with uncontrolled, progressive DM. All had marked muscle weakness and a serum creatine phosphokinase (CPK) value exceeding 500 IU/L at admission. Patients received 1 gm of methylprednisolone intravenously each day for 3 consecutive days in 1 week. Two or three courses of pulse therapy were given each week, and prednisolone was then given orally in a dose of 60 mg daily. Three patients received pulse therapy, and 5 received prednisolone in a mean daily dose of 56 mg.

Serum CPK values declined rapidly during pulse methylprednisolone therapy and more gradually in patients treated orally with corticosteroid. Half the initial values were reached in mean periods of 1.2 weeks with pulse therapy and 3½ weeks with oral treatment. The respective mean intervals to normalization of serum CPK activity were 8.3 and 12.7 weeks. One patient receiving pulse therapy died of interstitial pneumonitis. Two controls died (1 of aspiration pneumonia and 1 of cerebral apoplexy) before the CPK value became normal. Muscle strength gradually improved with pulse therapy, but 2 pa-

(4–16) Dermatologica 167:47–51, July 1983.

tients receiving oral treatment did not recover muscle strength during follow-ups of 2 and 4 months.

High-dose pulse methylprednisolone therapy appears to be effective in the treatment of severe, uncontrolled DM. Symptoms can be rapidly controlled by this means in patients at risk of aspiration pneumonia, a common lethal complication of DM.

▶ [This study, which is based on the experience with three patients assigned nonrandomly to high-dose pulse steroid therapy, illustrates the possible utility and substantial hazards of high-dose pulse steroid therapy. Pulse therapy may also be useful in treating fulminant lupus and uncontrolled cutaneous pyoderma gangrenosum; however, sudden death can occur during high-dose pulse steroid therapy.—R.S.S.] ◀

4–17 **Serologic Evidence for Acute Toxoplasmosis in Polymyositis-Dermatomyositis: Increased Frequency of Specific Anti-*Toxoplasma* IgM Antibodies.** A number of case reports and two studies have suggested an association between acquired toxoplasmosis and polymyositis-dermatomyositis. Because the presence of IgM antibodies to *Toxoplasma* is indicative of acute infection, Steven K. Magid and Lawrence J. Kagen (New York) studied 58 patients with polymyositis-dermatomyositis for the presence of serum IgM antibodies by using a specific indirect immunofluorescent assay. The Sabin-Feldman dye test and complement fixation techniques were also used to examine serum samples for IgM antibodies.

Twenty-nine (50%) of the 58 patients had positive Sabin-Feldman dye tests and 14 (24%) had positive IgM immunofluorescent tests. All 29 patients with negative Sabin-Feldman tests also had negative IgM immunofluorescent tests. Thus, the results of the IgM immunofluorescent assay and the Sabin-Feldman dye test were strongly associated ($P<.01$). Titers of IgM ranged from 1:20 to 1:2560. Complement fixation could be assayed in serum samples from 9 of 14 patients with positive results in IgM immunofluorescent and Sabin-Feldman dye tests; 6 had positive complement fixation tests. Fourteen of 15 patients with negative IgM immunofluorescent tests but positive Sabin-Feldman dye tests could be assayed; 12 showed no complement fixation and 2 had positive complement fixation tests. Thus, the results of the IgM immunofluorescent assay and the complement fixation test were associated ($P = .023$). Further, the titers found on the Sabin-Feldman dye test and complement fixation also correlated with IgM positivity. The mean peak complement fixation titer was significantly higher in patients with positive results on IgM immunofluorescence than in those with negative results. The presence of antinuclear antibody or rheumatoid factor did not appear to influence the results. Of 30 control patients with muscular dystrophy and 58 with systemic lupus erythematosus (SLE), with or without myositis, all but 2 with SLE had negative IgM immunofluorescent tests.

The results reveal a high frequency of IgM immunofluorescent antibodies in patients with polymyositis-dermatomyositis, further supporting an association between recent infection with *Toxoplasma gondii* and polymyositis.

(4–17) Am. J. Med. 75:313–320, August 1983.

4–18 **Nailfold Capillary Abnormalities in Childhood Rheumatic Diseases.** Because distortion of the nailfold capillary pattern occurs in certain adult rheumatic disease populations, George Spencer-Green, Margaret Schlesinger, Kevin E. Bove, Joseph E. Levinson, Jane G. Schaller, Virgil Hanson, and William E. Crowe studied the nailfold capillary patterns in 84 children having a variety of rheumatic diseases and in 34 normal controls. Of the patients, 32 had childhood dermatomyositis, 22 had juvenile rheumatoid arthritis, 19 had scleroderma, 7 had systemic lupus erythematosus, and 4 had mixed connective tissue disease.

On capillaroscopy, a normal pattern at the nailfold was characterized by a uniform, homogeneous distribution of capillary loops; areas of capillary loop dropout or dilation were absent. Of the 118 patients and controls examined, nailfold capillary pattern abnormalities were found in 29, all of whom were children having scleroderma or dermatomyositis ($P<.001$). Of the 19 patients with scleroderma, 9 (all of whom had systemic disease) had nailfold capillary abnormalities. Twenty of 32 children with dermatomyositis had either dilation alone or dilation and dropout of nailfold capillary loops. In addition, 7 of the 20 had a highly arborized, tortuous nailfold capillary pattern. No other comparable nailfold capillary abnormalities were found in those with systemic lupus erythematosus, mixed connective tissue disease, or juvenile rheumatoid arthritis, nor were they observed in the controls.

Apparently, nailfold capillary abnormalities comparable to those seen in adults occur frequently in childhood dermatomyositis and systemic sclerosis. The pathophysiology of the vascular lesion in these diseases remains obscure. Those patients having a greater number of vascular lesions on biopsy seem to be more likely to have nailfold capillary abnormalities, further suggesting that these morphological abnormalities reflect an underlying vasculopathy. Nailfold capillaroscopy is useful in better characterizing certain types of rheumatic diseases and in providing an index of vascular involvement in dermatomyositis.

▶ [This article highlights an important but often neglected area of observation which may have significant diagnostic and prognostic value in the connective tissue disorders. The authors have examined the nailbed capillaries in 84 children with connective tissue disorders. Abnormal patterns were found only in the scleroderma (systemic) and dermatomyositis groups, both having the same morphological patterns. Futhermore, there was a correlation between the extent of capillary and vascular damage on muscle biopsy in DM and the nailfold capillary abnormality—patients having more vascular lesions on biopsy were more likely to have nailbed capillary abnormalities. Furthermore the presence of capillary abnormalities in childhood DM is more likely to be associated with persistent and chronic forms of the disease. Whether one can prospectively distinguish localized from systemic scleroderma by observed capillary changes remains to be established. The entire subject of nailfold capillary abnormalities has been reviewed by Maricq and Maize (*Clin. Rheum. Dis.* 8:455–475, 1982). The evolution of capillary changes in a case of childhood DM has been reported by Nussbaum, Silver, and Maricq (*Arthritis Rheum.* 26:1169–1172, 1983).—R.M.] ◀

(4–18) J. Pediatr. 102:341–346, March 1983.

4–19 **Systemic Scleroderma in Childhood: Report of 5 Cases and Review of Literature.** M. Larrègue, C. Canuel, J. Bazex, J. M. Bressieux, P. Ramdené, and B. Laidet (Poitiers, France) analyzed data on 62 cases of this rare disease. Cutaneous manifestations were identical to those seen in adulthood, whereas Raynaud's phenomenon was much more frequently absent. However, follow-up was limited to 4 years, and worsening of clinical symptoms must be expected during intercurrent infectious episodes. Exceptional radiologic bone anomalies and frequent involvement of the gastrointestinal tract were reported, particularly on the esophageal level. The small intestine may be latently affected. Normal thoracic roentgenograms may not rule out pulmonary involvement, and systematic respiratory function tests are imperative. All segments of the cardiac wall may be involved; the seriousness of this particular condition was clearly reflected in that 10 of 21 deaths were exclusively attributable to its presence. Renal involvement was rare.

In 2 of the cases a staturoponderal retardation was unexplained. In another instance a tumefaction of the left knee appeared when the patient was 6½ years of age and was followed after 6 months by the appearance of facial telangiectasias during the course of measles. This was followed in turn by ulceration of the tumefaction of the knee, which oozed a chalky substance. When the patient was about age 7, a Raynaud's syndrome of hands and feet was observed, and further tumefactions appeared on the interphalangeal articulations of the right knee (Fig 4–4).

Fig 4–4.—Calcifications of knees. (Courtesy of Larrègue, M., et al.: Ann. Dermatol. Venereol. 110:317–326, 1983.)

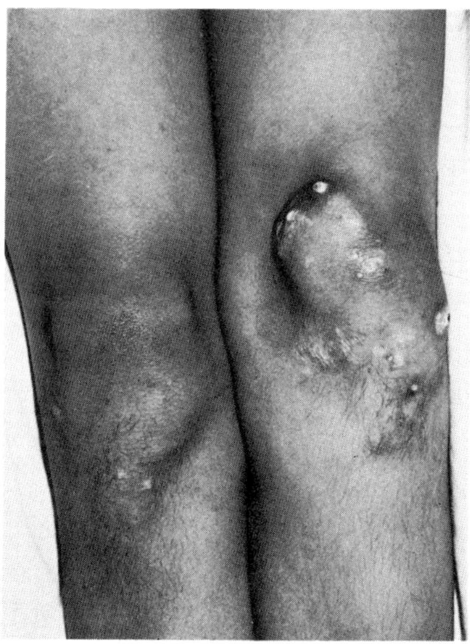

(4–19) Ann. Dermatol. Venereol. 110:317–326, 1983.

Familial forms are exceptions, although Mund (1978) documented 7 families in which parents and children were affected. Treatment remains poorly codified. Corticosteroids seem effective on the initial cutaneous fibrosis but show no action at all on older lesions. Primary indications are pulmonary or cardiac involvement, presence of a myositis, or major inflammation syndrome. An influence on the evolution of the illness was not evident. Immunosuppressive therapy does not alter the fatal course in cardiac involvement, although some success in amelioration of cutaneous and articular lesions has been reported. Colchicine was used in 1 instance, but its effect cannot as yet be evaluated owing to inadequate follow-up. Factor XIII was totally ineffective in the 1 case in which it was used. Only a better understanding of the physiopathology of this disease can lead to more efficient treatment.

▶ [Progressive systemic sclerosis (PSS) is as much a mystery in children as in adults. This article, written in French with an English abstract, reports 5 new childhood cases and reviews the literature. As in the adult cases, morbidity appears to be related to gastrointestinal, pulmonary, and cardiac involvement. Cardiac involvement accounted for 10 of the 21 deaths reviewed. Therapy and pathogenesis of PSS are still elusive.—A.R.R.] ◀

4–20 **Progressive Systemic Sclerosis (PSS, Scleroderma) Dermal Fibroblasts Synthesize Increased Amounts of Glycosaminoglycan.** Progressive systemic sclerosis is a systemic disorder of connective tissue that leads to inflammatory, fibrotic, and degenerative changes in the skin, vessels, and some internal organs such as the gastrointestinal tract, heart, lungs, and kidneys. The cause is unknown. Collagen is strikingly overabundant in PSS, and fibronectin and glycosaminoglycan (GAG) may also be present in excess. Robert B. Buckingham, Robert K. Prince, and Gerald P. Rodnan (Univ. of Pittsburgh) investigated whether fibroblast cultures derived from the lowermost parts of PSS dermis accumulate increased amounts of GAG as well as collagen. Fibroblast monolayers were established by explant culture of dermis from 7 women with early, rapidly progressive PSS and from 6 normal subjects. The respective mean ages were 48 and 48.5 years. Biopsy specimens were obtained within a year of onset of the illness. No patient was receiving drugs that affect collagen metabolism at biopsy. Net GAG synthesis was determined as ^{3}H-glucosamine incorporation into the polymer and as total uronic acid accumulation in culture.

Cultures from patients with PSS accumulated GAG in amounts as much as fivefold higher than those from normal subjects. This appeared to result from increased synthesis rather than from decreased degradation. Cultures from PSS patients also accumulated increased amounts of collagenase-sensitive protein. Study of several monolayers followed for as many as 10 generations indicated that the difference between PSS and normal cultures could be propagated. Apart from an increased total amount of GAG in PSS cultures, differences in the distribution of individual GAGs on a percentage basis were apparent between PSS and normal cell cultures.

(4–20) J. Lab. Clin. Med. 101:659–669, May 1983.

The findings indicate that GAG, as well as collagen, may be important in the development of connective tissue thickening and induration in PSS. Some in vivo event may irreversibly alter the normal cells, or fibroblasts producing large amounts of connective tissue may be selected for and may populate the involved tissues, leading to increased connective tissue accumulation. Immune mechanisms, vascular injury, or both may initiate connective tissue changes in vivo through fibroblast alteration or selection.

4–21 **Anticentromere Antibody: Clinical Correlations and Association With Favorable Prognosis in Patients With Scleroderma Variants.** Gale A. McCarty, John R. Rice, Mary L. Bembe, and Franc A. Barada, Jr. (Duke Univ.) report that the presence of antibody to the chromosomal centromere appears to be associated with findings in a subset of patients with the limited calcinosis, Raynaud's phenomenon, esophageal dysmotility, sclerodactyly, and telangiectasia (CREST) form of scleroderma. To define the prognostic value of this autoantibody, they studied 27 patients who were identified as having anticentromere antibody (ACA) by antinuclear antibody tests with HEp-2 substrates. The patients were followed up clinically and serologically for 2 years.

Discrete speckled patterns were confirmed as ACA on bone marrow chromosomal preparations in all 27 patients. The initial clinical association was with Raynaud's phenomenon. Eleven patients had Raynaud's phenomenon with another connective tissue disorder. Nine had various permutations of CREST. Of those with associated connective tissue disorders, 3 had systemic lupus erythematosus and 3 had rheumatoid arthritis. After 2 years none of the patients with isolated Raynaud's phenomenon or CREST variants had progressive systemic sclerosis (PSS)-diffuse or features of other connective tissue disorders. Nor did the 6 patients with secondary Raynaud's phenomenon have PSS-diffuse. During the study, renal disease attributed to scleroderma developed in 1 of 2 patients with ACA and PSS-diffuse. These data indicate that most patients with ACA did not develop major organ system involvement characteristic of PSS-diffuse during the 2-year study. There was a predominance of disease in females. Patients with ACA had a lower frequency of myositis and arthritis than did patients with speckled or nucleolar patterns, but this was not statistically significant.

The findings confirm the primary association of ACA with CREST variants of scleroderma and indicate that patients with ACA may exhibit certain clinical features distinct from those occurring with other variants of scleroderma. Patients with ACA had lower percentages of major renal, cardiac, pulmonary, and lower gastrointestinal tract involvement compared with patients with speckled or nucleolar antinuclear antibodies.

▶ [The speckled pattern of antinuclear antibody may represent an antibody to the chromosomal centromere. This anticentromere antibody was detected in patients

(4–21) Arthritis Rheum. 26:1–7, January 1983.

with Raynaud's phenomenon with and without associated collagen vascular disorders and in individuals with scleroderma and a low prevalence of major organ involvement, notably combinations of calcinosis, Raynaud's phenomenon, esophageal dysmotility, sclerodactyly, and telangiectases.

Although the follow-up time was only 2 years, the lack of involvement of critical internal organs is of interest. Moreover, the association between the presence of anticentromere antibody and Raynaud's phenomenon is noteworthy. The ultimate value of this antibody as a diagnostic or prognostic marker for subsets of patients remains to be determined.—N.A.S.] ◀

4–22 **Scleroderma With Progressive Crossed Atrophy Involving Left Side of Body and Right Side of Face.** J. Lapresle and M. Desi (Bicêtre, France) report the case of a 28-year-old woman who had chronic polyarthritis with a linear scleroderma and a crossed atrophy involving the left side of the body and the right side of the face and neck. This case raises once again the question of a possible connection between localized sclerodermic facial hemiatrophy and Romberg's syndrome. Review of the literature and the study of the present case do not provide a formal argument for differentiation of the 2 separate entities. The association of chronic polyarthritis with immunologic abnormalities would tend to favor the notion of a systemic disorder.

The patient first experienced polyarthritis at age 6, which resulted in considerable articular disability in the context of a febrile condition, adenopathies, and splenomegaly. From onset the patient had frequent and extremely painful muscular cramps in the left side of the body, which lessened in frequency with the appearance and progression of atrophy on the same side. At age 15 the patient began to experience similar cramping in the right face, followed by progressive right hemiatrophy. When the patient was age 28, examination disclosed the crossed atrophy associated with plaques on the skin in the atrophic areas, and circumscribed alopecia, as well as numerous joint sequelae with significant impairment of mobility and deformation. The laboratory data yielded immunologic abnormalities; brain scan, although grossly normal, showed right facial hemiatrophy involving the orbital region and pharynx. A muscular biopsy specimen showed inflammatory changes in the atrophic territory. Skin biopsy findings were consistent with scleroderma.

The strictly alternating topography of the atrophic syndrome was the most remarkable characteristic of this case and could not be explained by a disturbance of growth associated with a homolateral hemispheric lesion, nor by articular pathologic conditions associated with polyarthritis. The brain scan and radiologic examination of the cervico-occipital articulation did not reinforce these hypotheses. However, the perfect correspondence between the inferior level of the atrophy on the right and the superior level of the atrophy on the left suggests a focal lesion of the nervous system.

4–23 **Serum Eosinophilotactic Activity in Eosinophilic Fasciitis.** Stephen I. Wasserman, James R. Seibold, Thomas A. Medsger, Jr., and Gerald P. Rodnan determined the serum eosinophil chemotactic

(4–22) Rev. Neurol. (Paris) 138:815–825, 1982.
(4–23) Arthritis Rheum. 25:1352–1356, November 1982.

activity (ECA) in 20 patients with eosinophilic fasciitis (EF) by using the Boyden chamber technique. An additional 21 serum samples were tested in longitudinal studies on 8 of these patients. The group included 8 women and 12 men aged 23–70 years. All were evaluated at the University of Pittsburgh. Twenty individuals with systemic sclerosis and diffuse scleroderma served as matched controls.

All study patients had had rapid onset of pain and swelling of the extremities, which was soon followed by severe induration of the skin and subcutaneous tissues of the forearms and legs and in many cases the hands, feet, trunk, and face. The overlying skin was typically shiny and erythematous with a coarse peau d'orange appearance. All patients had total eosinophil counts greater than 600/cu mm at some point early in their illness, and in 10 instances eosinophilia greater than 2,000/cu mm was noted. Seven patients (35%) had an erythrocyte sedimentation rate (ESR) greater than 25 mm/hour. Five (25%) had a serum IgG concentration of 1,500 mg/dl or greater and 2 (10%) had a serum IgA concentration of 500 mg/dl or greater. None of the 20 had elevated serum levels of IgM or C3, C4. Elevated levels of circulating immune complexes were detected by Raji cell radioimmunoassay in 11 (55%). Increased serum ECA (greater than 125% of background) as found in all 20 patients with eosinophilic fasciitis. Results ranged from 150% to 575% of background. In contrast, serums of control subjects had increased ECA in only 6 of 20 cases (30%). Eosinophil chemotactic activity had a strong positive correlation with ESR and a negative correlation with disease duration.

All 8 patients studied longitudinally had the highest level of serum ECA early in the illness and showed progressive reduction in this activity during follow-up. Serum ECA became normal only in the 3 patients who achieved clinical remission after 32, 39, and 62 months of corticosteroid therapy. Four serums with high levels of ECA were fractionated by gel filtration. All 4 had a peak ECA coincident with material with absorbance at OD 280 and molecular weight 2,500–4,000.

These preliminary data suggest a common eosinophilotactic substance in patients with eosinophilic fasciitis. They also suggest that the underlying pathogenic abnormality in this disorder is of a chronic nature and may not be suppressed by corticosteroid therapy.

► [A chemoattractant activity for eosinophilic leukocytes has been recognized in the serum of each of 20 patients with eosinophilic fasciitis in contrast to systemic sclerosis and diffuse scleroderma. Although the origin of this partially characterized molecule is unknown, it is important to emphasize that this activity persists in some individuals despite therapy and clinical improvement, suggesting a relation to the chronicity of this clinical disease. A further physicochemical characterization of this molecule to identify its source may provide insights into the pathophysiology of this disorder.—N.A.S.] ◄

24 **Controlled Double-Blind Trial of Nifedipine in the Treatment of Raynaud's Phenomenon.** Raynaud's phenomenon can cause severe functional disability, and treatment may be difficult. Richard J.

(4–24) N. Engl. J. Med. 308:880–883, Apr. 14, 1983.

Rodeheffer, James A. Rommer, Fredrick Wigley, and Craig R. Smith (Johns Hopkins Univ.) evaluated the slow calcium-channel antagonist nifedipine, which causes vascular smooth muscle relaxation and relieves arterial vasospasm, in a prospective, double-blind, crossover trial in 15 patients with symptomatic Raynaud's phenomenon related to cold or stress. The 12 women and 3 men had a mean age of 34 years. Nine patients had systemic sclerosis, and 1 had systemic lupus erythematosus with cryoglobulinemia. Seven patients had had digital ulcers. Mean duration of Raynaud's symptoms was about 6 years. Patients received capsules containing either 10 mg of nifedipine or placebo. The initial dose of 1 capsule 3 times daily for 3 days was followed by 2 capsules 3 times daily if no severe side effects developed. The study lasted 7 weeks.

Patients preferred nifedipine over placebo. Nine reported moderate to marked improvement while receiving nifedipine and 2 while receiving placebo. The mean attack rate fell from 15 to 11 per 2 weeks with nifedipine. In some patients the fall in digital arterial systolic pressure and the digital pallor during cold exposure were ameliorated by nifedipine. Mean ambient temperatures were the same (39 F) during both phases of the study. Mild, transient headache occurred in 80% of nifedipine-treated patients and in 20% of those receiving placebo. Light-headedness occurred in 33% and 7%, respectively. There were no significant abnormalities in electrolytes or blood counts during treatment.

This study and two other double-blind trials have shown nifedipine to be effective in the management of patients with Raynaud's phenomenon. In the two studies, including the present one, in which personal responses were reported, subjective improvement in symptoms was reported by two thirds of patients. The drug is well tolerated. Further studies are needed to determine dose-response relations and the efficacy of long-term treatment and to identify predictors of clinical responsiveness.

▶ [This study demonstrates that in some patients nifedipine, a calcium-channel-blocking agent leads to subjective improvement in Raynaud's phenomenon. The therapeutic effect of nifedipine was most often noted in persons without systemic disease. Clinical improvement could not be correlated with any significant reduction in the cold-induced drop in digital artery systolic pressure. This finding may reflect the difficulty in eliciting Raynaud's symptoms in the laboratory among patients without systemic illness. Calcium-channel blockers are generally well tolerated. Their long-term effectiveness in treating Raynaud's phenomenon is not yet established. Other agents used to treat Raynaud's phenomenon include prazosin and griseofulvin.—R.S.S.] ◀

4–25 **Raynaud's Syndrome: Treatment With Sublingual Administration of Nitroglycerin, Swinging Arm Maneuver, and Biofeedback Training.** Larry Len Peterson and Catherine Vorhies (Portland, Ore.) evaluated sublingual administration of nitroglycerin, a swinging arm maneuver, and biofeedback for effectiveness in decreasing hand rewarming time after ice immersion in 6 patients with

(4–25) Arch. Dermatol. 119:396–399, May 1983.

Raynaud's disease and 4 with Raynaud's phenomenon. Ten patients with no history of disease or Raynaud's syndrome served as controls. All tests were performed twice by each participant; response curves were reproducible.

In all 10 controls, hand rewarming to baseline temperature occurred in less than 6 minutes; whereas in 9 of 10 patients with Raynaud's syndrome, more than 40 minutes was required to achieve rewarming. The remaining patient required about 35 minutes for rewarming. For the arm swinging maneuver, several older patients tired after about 30 seconds, but the younger patients had no difficulty in completing 60 seconds of this maneuver. However, objective or subjective improvement was found. In 2 of 10 patients in whom rewarming previously required 35–40 minutes, rewarming the digits took only 6 minutes or less after sublingual nitroglycerin was administered. However, the drug had no effect on the other 8 patients. During biofeedback training, several patients were able to raise their digital temperature by between 20 degrees and 88 Fahrenheit degrees after ice immersion. Also, in 8 of 10 patients, hand rewarming back to baseline levels occurred in 20 minutes or less after ice immersion; and in 2, rewarming occurred in 6 minutes or less. Six months later, all biofeedback responders reported a decrease in the number and severity of attacks, emphasizing new awareness of their hand temperatures.

As noted, no improvement occurred with the Mcintyre swinging arm maneuver. The clinician may want to try sublingual nitroglycerin in the patient who has infrequent attacks, because the drug is easy and convenient to use and causes few side effects. Biofeedback training is effective in the well-motivated patient who has no underlying structural abnormalities in the digital arteries. Training sessions, however, need to be tailored to the individual's ability to learn and must be continued for some months until a plateau of automaticity is reached.

▶ [The authors found that in Raynaud's syndrome, in the absence of organic pathology, nitroglycerin might help a few patients, but biofeedback was generally more successful and certainly longer lasting. It seems to be essentially free of side effects and therefore worth a try for the patient who is willing to spend the time and money to learn the technique.—R.M.] ◀

26 **Electrically Heated Gloves for Intermittent Digital Ischemia.** G. E. Kempson, D. Coggon, and E. D. Acheson (Southampton Genl. Hosp., England) note that intermittent digital ischemia (Raynaud's phenomenon) occurs in about one tenth of the general population. They describe the use of electrically heated gloves, which have recently been developed for patients with severe intermittent digital ischemia. The gloves are knitted from acrylic yarn with an interknitted electrical heating element that is exposed only on the inner surface of the glove, thus minimizing heat loss to the atmosphere. The gloves, indistinguishable from ordinary knitted gloves, are washable.

(4–26) Br. Med. J. 286:268, Jan. 22, 1983.

Electric power is derived from a low-voltage, rechargeable battery pack carried at the waist and connected to the gloves by flexible leads that pass along the arms. A fully charged battery pack will heat a pair of gloves for about 3 hours; patients are usually supplied with 2 battery packs.

Of 15 patients supplied with the system, 11 found the gloves helpful and wore them regularly. Two patients with chilblains were fitted with heated socks, which they found beneficial. Four patients found the gloves unsatisfactory; however, 2 of these patients had tried a more bulky prototype model. Although this prototype model kept the hands warm, the patients found it inconvenient to wear.

The heated gloves described are suitable for patients with incapacitating intermittent digital ischemia who wish to maintain and wear the apparatus.

▶ [A simple useful way to help minimize the adverse effects of chronic cold exposure. Reference to the supplier is given in the article, and a subsequent letter to the editor (*Br. Med. J.* 286:643, 1983) gives an alternate supplier. An additional letter (ibid, p. 694) indicates this type of device may be useful for patients with cryoglobulinemia and may be available for use in automobiles with adapters to obtain the necessary electric power from the car battery. For outdoor use rechargeable battery packs are available, and adapters for house current are available for indoor use.—R.M.] ◀

4–27 **Bowel-Bypass Syndrome Without Bowel Bypass. Bowel-Associated Dermatosis-Arthritis Syndrome.** A recurrent, episodic illness occurring in as many as 20% of patients who undergo ileojejunal bypass surgery for morbid obesity has been well characterized and involves inflammatory cutaneous lesions with a histologic appearance like that of neutrophilic vasculitis, a nondeforming polyarthritis, and other systemic manifestations. Current concepts of pathogenesis center on overgrowth of bacterial flora in the bypassed bowel segment with subsequent development of a circulating immune complex disease. Joseph L. Jorizzo, Prapand Apisarnthanarax, Paul Subrt, Adelaide A. Hebert, John C. Henry, Sharon S. Raimer, Scott M. Dinehart, and James A. Reinarz (Univ. of Texas, Galveston) report data on an identical clinicopathologic syndrome in 4 patients who have not had jejunoileal bypass surgery.

Case 1.—Woman, 46, had an acute syndrome of bouts of fever, myalgias, arthralgias, arthritis, and a vesiculopustular eruption on her trunk, arms, and hands. Acute episodes became more severe. Roentgenograms of the upper gastrointestinal (GI) tract disclosed almost complete obstruction of the duodenum just beyond the bulb. Oral prednisone was given. A later outbreak was treated with tetracycline hydrochloride. All signs and symptoms of the acute dermatosis-arthritis resolved. Skin biopsy was consistent with bowel-bypass syndrome or Sweet's syndrome. Patient has been treated with sulfamethoxazole and trimethoprim, with one recent flare-up.

Case 2.—Woman, 46, had cutaneous pustular lesions on purpuric bases with associated diffuse arthralgias, myalgias, and fever. Oral prednisone was given. Three weeks before admission she had experienced epigastric pain and GI symptoms similar to those of the dumping syndrome. Skin biopsy was interpreted as consistent with bowel-bypass or Sweet's syn-

---

(4–27) Arch. Intern. Med. 143:457–461, March 1983.

drome. Acute dermatosis-arthritis syndrome resolved with pulse corticosteroid therapy.

CASE 3.—Woman, 42, had acute fever, polyarthralgias, and a vesiculopustular eruption on the trunk. She had a previous diagnosis of granulomatous colitis (Crohn's disease). A dose of 60 mg of prednisone per day abolished symptoms. Skin biopsy showed bowel-bypass or Sweet's syndrome.

CASE 4.—Woman, 53, had nonspecific colitis for 1 year and fever polyarthralgias with acute arthritis of right index finger and a cutaneous eruption. Skin biopsy indicated bowel-bypass or Sweet's syndrome. Oral prednisone (60 mg/day) resolved symptoms. Patient later died of disseminated leiomyosarcoma.

The acute dermatosis-arthritis syndrome seen in these 4 patients is identical to the bowel-bypass syndrome except that these 4 patients had bowel disease and not jejunoileal bypass surgery. The cutaneous lesions are identical in character, progression, distribution, and histopathologic features; systemic symptoms are also identical.

▶ [The authors report 4 cases of a vasculitis-like dermatosis appearing on the upper arms and trunk, associated with bowel symptoms and arthralgias (in 2 patients). The pathology of the skin lesions resembled Sweet's syndrome and did not show fibrinoid necrosis, in contrast to a vasculitic process. The cutaneous features are similar to those reported in the jejunoileal bypass procedure for obesity, except that these patients had not had such surgery. However, 2 had diverticular and 2 had inflammatory colitis. The pathogenesis of this syndrome has not been clarified, though bacterial peptidoglycans and circulating immune complexes have both been implicated. The authors propose that this syndrome be called the bowel-associated dermatosis-arthritis syndrome.—R.M.] ◀

4–28 **Cutaneous Extravascular Necrotizing Granuloma (Churg-Strauss Granuloma) and Systemic Disease: Review of 27 Cases.** Marian C. Finan and R. K. Winkelmann (Mayo Clinic and Found.) reviewed information on 27 patients with skin biopsy findings of extravascular necrotizing granuloma. All had granulomas in the dermis or subcutaneous tissue with central necrobiosis of collagen, cells within the central necrobiotic area, a peripheral histiocytic reaction, and no evidence of abscess or another infectious process. There were 19 women and 8 men. Mean age at onset of associated systemic disease in 26 patients was 48 years, and mean age at onset of cutaneous disease in 25 was 49.5 years. Systemic disease occurred first in most patients. Only 1 patient had clinical features limited to the skin (Table 1). The most common skin lesion was a papule or nodule (Figs 4–5 and 4–6), distributed as shown in Table 2. Ten patients had skin lesions other than papulonodules. Peripheral palisading of histiocytes was observed in a large majority of specimens. Vasculitis was present in 10 specimens; it was usually of the necrotizing or leukocytoclastic type. Direct immunofluorescence microscopic examination yielded abnormal findings in 8 of 10 cases, usually showing deposit of complement and fibrin in the superficial vessels, with or without IgM.

Seven patients had allergic granulomatosis, and 7 had other forms of systemic vasculitis. Three of the latter had Wegener's granulomatosis. Six patients had connective tissue disorders; 2 had systemic lu-

(4–28) Medicine (Baltimore) 62:142–158, May 1983.

TABLE 1.—Cutaneous Extravascular Necrotizing Granuloma and Systemic Disease

	Patient No.		Patient %	
Systemic vasculitis	14		52	
Allergic granulomatosis		7		26
Wegener's granulomatosis		3		11
Periarteritis nodosa		1		4
Vasculitis (unclassified)		3		11
Connective tissue disease	6		22	
Systemic lupus erythematosus		2		7
Rheumatoid arthritis		4		15
Lymphoproliferative disease	3		11	
Acute myelomonocytic leukemia		1		3.7
Multiple myeloma		1		3.7
Lymphocytic lymphoma		1		3.7
Miscellaneous "immunoreactive" diseases	3		11	
Subacute bacterial endocarditis		1		3.7
Chronic active hepatitis		1		3.7
Chronic ulcerative colitis		1		3.7
Vasculitis involving skin only	1		4	
Total	27		100	

(Courtesy of Finan, M.C., and Winkelmann, R.K.: Medicine [Baltimore] 62:142–158, May 1983.)

Fig 4–5 (left).—Plaquelike lesion, formed by coalescence of papulonodules, with focal crusting, over extensor aspect of elbow in patient with multiple myeloma.

Fig 4–6 (right).—Discrete papulonodules over extensor aspect of knees in same patient.

(Courtesy of Finan, M.C., and Winkelmann, R.K.: Medicine [Baltimore] 62:142–158, May 1983.)

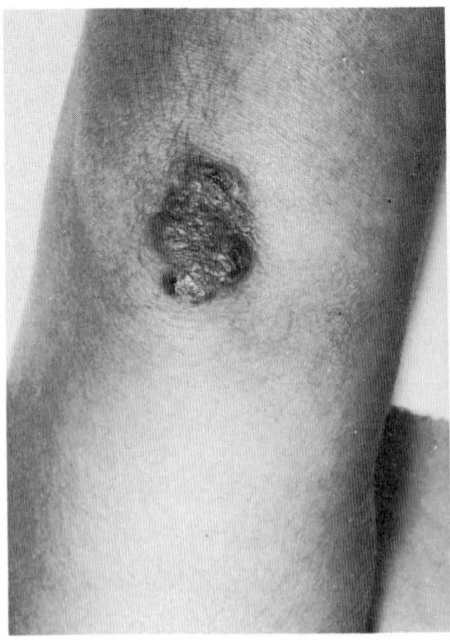

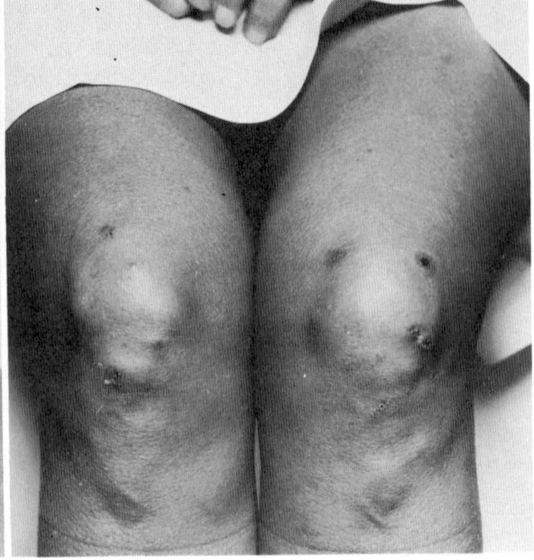

TABLE 2.—DISTRIBUTION OF PAPULONODULAR LESIONS (25 PATIENTS)

Site	No. of patients
Elbow	20*
Fingers/thumb	10
Buttocks	5
Scalp	3
Extensor aspect of knees	3
Hand	3
Dorsum of foot	2†
Neck	2
Forehead	2
Ear	2
Lower leg	2
Lower back	2
Toe	1
Thigh	1
Abdomen	1

*Bilaterally symmetric in 14.
†Bilaterally symmetric in 1.
(Courtesy of Finan, M.C., and Winkelmann, R.K.: Medicine [Baltimore] 62:142–158, May 1983.)

pus erythematosus and 4, rheumatoid arthritis. Three patients had lymphoproliferative disorders. Various other inflammatory disorders were seen in 3 patients. Most patients had laboratory evidence of inflammation or increased immunoreactivity. Six of the 23 patients followed died. Mean follow-up of survivors was 7½ years. Five deaths were due to associated disease. Most patients were treated primarily with systemic corticosteroid administration. Four patients received no specific treatment. Some of the patients who did not receive corticosteroids and who died probably would have benefited from corticosteroid therapy had it been available.

Cutaneous extravascular necrotizing granuloma is a distinct clinical and histopathologic entity and a cutaneous marker of systemic vasculitis and immunoreactive or autoimmune disorders. It may indicate a more favorable prognosis for patients with vasculitis, except those with severe toxic rheumatoid arthritis and moribund patients with a fulminant course in whom the lesions develop preterminally.

▶ [In 1951, Churg and Strauss (*Am. J. Pathol.* 27:277, 1951) defined the clinical syndrome of asthma, fever, hypereosinophilia, and multisystem vasculitis as an entity distinct from periarteritis nodosa which they termed "allergic granulomatosis." This disease is now termed "Churg-Strauss granuloma." In all cases of cutaneous extravascular necrotizing granuloma reported so far, systemic vasculitis and/or autoimmune or immunoreactive disease (which often occurs with vasculitis) has been a notable finding.—A.J.S.] ◀

-29 **Scleredema Adultorum and Diabetes Mellitus (Scleredema Diutinum).** Fiona McNaughton and Kalman Keczkes (Hull Royal Infirmary) describe findings in a patient with scleredema adultorum

(4–29) Clin. Exp. Dermatol. 8:41–45, January 1983.

associated with long-standing, poorly controlled diabetes mellitus.

Man, 55, obese and with an 11-year history of diabetes, complained of thickened, hard skin on his back and shoulders. Apparently, thc condition had begun 11 years previously, as noted by the patient's wife, but the patient himself was not aware of it until the gradual spread of the condition to the back of the neck, shoulders, and upper half of the back caused some restriction of neck movement. Initial treatment with oral hypoglycemic agents and diet, and treatment subsequently with increasing doses of insulin, failed to produce satisfactory control. On examination, there was an extensive area of very thick, indurated skin over two thirds of the back, as well as the neck, shoulders, and proximal halves of the upper arms. The results of blood chemistry studies were normal, but the ECG showed changes of ischemic heart disease and the blood sugar values were consistently elevated. Skin histology showed a normal epidermis and upper dermis; however, in the lower dermis there were numerous bundles of thickened, poorly cellular collagen fibers extending into the underlying adipose tissue. There was a slight perivascular and periappendicular infiltrate of nonspecific chronic inflammatory cells.

Patients with scleredema in association with diabetes mellitus are characterized by obesity and diabetes that is resistant to therapy. The onset of scleredema diutinum is insidious; there is no preceding viral or bacterial infection. There is a strong association with diabetes mellitus, and the diabetes is usually difficult to control. This disease does not resolve spontaneously. At present, however, no effective treatment has been found for it, and its cause remains obscure.

▶ [The authors report a case of scleredema associated with diabetes and discuss the differences between it and the classical scleredema of Buschke, which may occur at any age, usually follows an acute infection, and tends to remit completely or partially within 2 years. Scleredema associated with diabetes tends to occur in those with long-standing poorly controlled and complicated diabetes, occurs more often in middle age, and does not readily remit. A recent study by Christy et al. (*J. Rheumatol.* 10:595–601, 1983) showed an increased production of glycosaminoglycans (primarily hyaluronic acid) in fibroblast monolayer cultures from 2 patients with scleredema. They postulate that the increased glycosaminoglycans and the associated water bound between the side chains of the macromolecules produce the increased weight and thickness of the skin and the nonpitting edema and induration. One of their patients had IgG, IgM, and C3 demonstrated by immunofluorescence at the D-E junction.

In another case report of scleredema in a diabetic, Monk et al. (*Clin. Exp. Dermatol.* 8:389–391, 1983) postulate that persistent high levels of glucose are associated with nonenzymatic glycosylation of collagen, causing abnormal cross-linking and thereby impaired resolution of the disease.

Finally a third association of scleredema was reported by Clerici et al. (*Dermatologica* 166:240–246, 1983). They report 3 cases of scleredema and review 5 others that were associated with monoclonal gammopathy. Their 3 cases were associated with IgGκ, did not show evidence of multiple myeloma, and did not show IgGκ by immunofluorescence microscopy.—R.M.] ◀

5. Atopic Dermatitis

5–1 **Cellular Basis of Defective Cell-Mediated Lymphoysis in Atopic Dermatitis.** Impaired cell-mediated immunity has been described in a majority of patient with atopic dermatitis (AD). These patients are susceptible to disseminated infections by herpes simplex and vaccinia viruses, and most have elevated serum IgE levels that may result from a suppressor T-cell defect. Donald Y. M. Leung, Nancy Wood, Devendra Dubey, Arthur R. Rhodes, and Raif S. Geha (Harvard Med. School) examined the in vitro generation of alloreactive cytotoxic T cells in 19 patients with AD. Peripheral blood lymphocytes were examined for their ability to generate cytotoxic T cells in mixed lymphocyte culture. Studies also were carried out with cells from 14 patients with nonatopic skin diseases unrelated to AD who were matched with the study patients for age and with cells from 19 healthy subjects. No subject had received oral doses of steroids during the past 6 months or topically applied steroids for a week before the study.

Cell-mediated lympholysis (CML) activity was significantly reduced in AD, but proliferative responses in mixed lymphocyte culture were not. Regression analysis indicated a significant correlation between CML activity and the proportion of circulating $T8^+$ suppressor-cytotoxic T cells. Deficient CML activity was not corrected by recombining autologous $T4^+$ and $T8^+$ cells in a normal 2:1 ratio. Assessment of CML activity in cocultures of isolated $T4^+$ and $T8^+$ cells from 2 AD patients and their respective HLA-identical healthy siblings indicated that the defect in CML resided in both cell populations. Cocultures of AD and normal lymphocytes indicated that the defect was not due to excess suppressor activity.

Defective cytotoxic T-cell function may explain the increased susceptibility of patients with atopic dermatitis to severe viral infections. The exact nature of the defect in $T4^+$ cells in eczema is under study. The cells may prove to be defective in the generation of an inducer cytotoxic-differentiation factor.

▶ [This article explores the defect in cell-mediated lympholysis (CML) in atopic dermatitis. The defect could not be attributed to a failure of antigen recognition, nor to excessive suppressor activity. The numerical reduction of circulating $T8^+$ cells was not the sole cause of reduced CML. Mixing experiments suggested that $T8^+$ cells are selectively deficient in cytotoxic T lymphocytes and that there is also a $T4^+$ defect. The cell defects in atopic dermatitis may be responsible for the increased susceptibility to viral and bacterial infection. The dissection continues into the pathophysiology of atopic dermatitis.—A.R.R.] ◀

(5–1) J. Immunol. 130:1678–1682, April 1983.

5–2 **Characterization of the Mononuclear Cell Infiltrate in Atopic Dermatitis Using Monoclonal Antibodies.** Donald Y. M. Leung, Atul K. Bhan, Eveline E. Schneeberger, and Raif S. Geha (Boston) studied tissue sections from involved and uninvolved skin of 9 patients with atopic dermatitis (AD) by light microscopy, electron microscopy, and an immunoperoxidase method in which monoclonal antibodies to cell-surface antigens were used. The two male and 7 female patients had typical features of AD since early infancy, an elevated serum IgE level, and a personal or family history of other allergic disorders.

Five of the 9 patients had a significantly reduced percentage of circulating $T8^+$ suppressor-cytotoxic cells when compared with normal controls. The histologic appearance of sections 1 μm thick from involved skin of study patients was highly variable and depended on whether the biopsy specimen was taken from an acute erythematous lesion or a chronic lichenified plaque. Electron microscopy of 3 skin biopsy specimens (2 chronic, 1 acute) confirmed the observations made at light microscopy. In all sections examined there were large numbers of monocytes-macrophages in the papillary and reticular dermis interspersed with small lymphocytes.

Immunoperoxidase staining with anti-T3, anti-T4, anti-T8, anti-Leu-1, anti-Leu-2, and anti-Leu-3a monoclonal antibodies was restricted primarily to infiltrating lymphocytes. The staining was peripheral and consistent with cell membrane staining. Only occasional cells reacted with monoclonal antihuman IgM, suggesting that few B cells were present in the skin lesions. With the anti-T6 monoclonal antibody, diffuse staining of dendritic cells in the epidermis and dermis was obtained, with the cells considered to be Langerhans' cells. Two biopsies performed on clinically uninvolved areas of skin from 3 patients with AD showed a smaller degree of cellular infiltration than that seen in clinically recognizable lesions. Control skin biopsy specimens from 3 patients with no skin lesions showed the cellular infiltrate to be sparse.

The presence of increased numbers of Langerhans' cells and T cells of the helper-inducer phenotype may reflect increased antigen processing in diseased skin. In addition, the smaller number of $T8^+$ cells infiltrating into the skin suggests that the depression of circulating $T8^+$ cells observed in most patients with AD is not due to selective migration of these cells into the skin.

▶ [This is a very important observation in atopic eczema. Once again T4 helper cells predominate in an inflammatory dermatosis.—M.C.M.] ◀

5–3 **Isotopic and Enzymatic IgE Assays in Nonallergic Subjects.** The clinical value of the immunoassay for quantitating serum IgE depends importantly on its success in distinguishing allergic from nonallergic subjects. R. Stein, S. Evans, R. Milner, C. Rand, and J. Dolovich (McMaster Univ.) examined serums from 446 white Cana-

(5–2) J. Allergy Clin. Immunol. 71:47–56, January 1983.
(5–3) Allergy 38:389–398, August 1983.

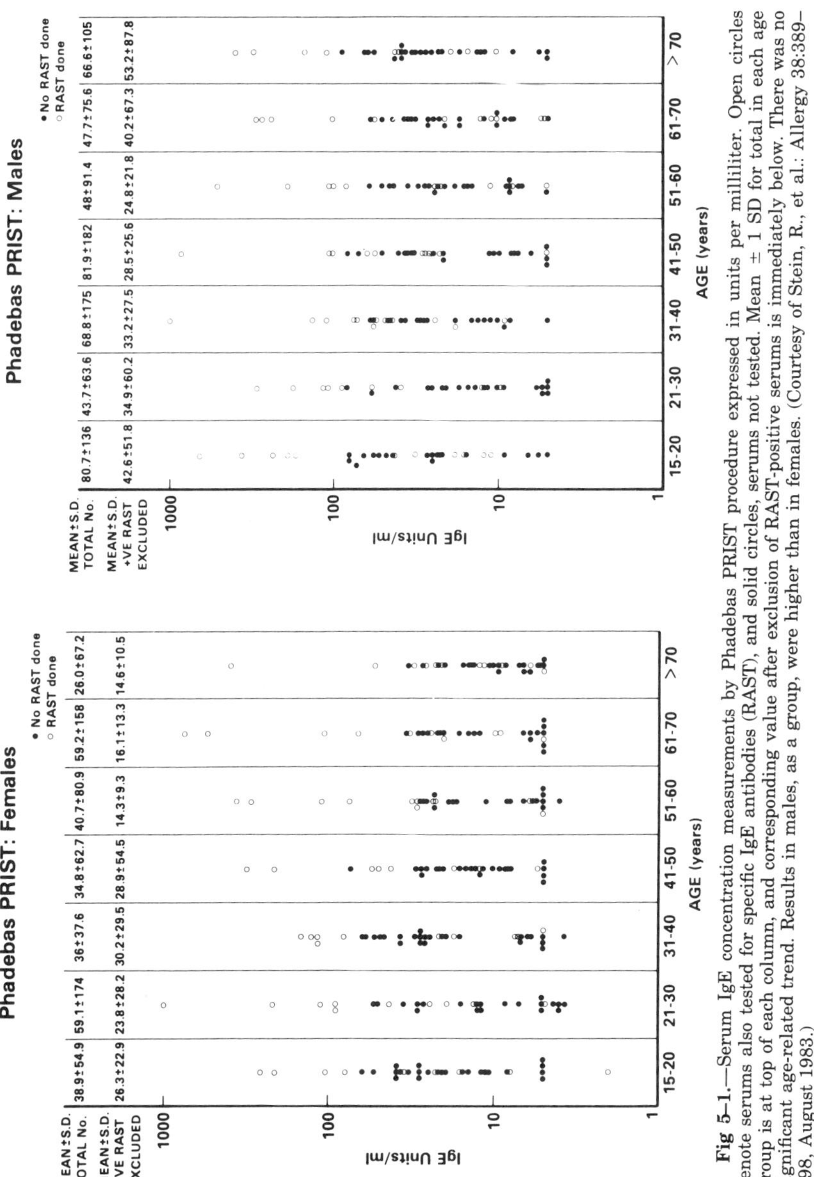

Fig 5–1.—Serum IgE concentration measurements by Phadebas PRIST procedure expressed in units per milliliter. Open circles denote serums also tested for specific IgE antibodies (RAST), and solid circles, serums not tested. Mean ± 1 SD for total in each age group is at top of each column, and corresponding value after exclusion of RAST-positive serums is immediately below. There was no significant age-related trend. Results in males, as a group, were higher than in females. (Courtesy of Stein, R., et al.: Allergy 38:389–398, August 1983.)

dians with no history of allergy to establish normal IgE values. The Phadebas paper radioimmunosorbent test (PRIST) was compared with its enzymatic counterpart, the Phadezyme PRIST.

Serum IgE concentrations determined by the Phadebas PRIST procedure are shown in Figure 5–1. No age-related change in IgE concentrations was observed. Men had higher levels than women. The median and 95th percentile values for women were 17.5 and 145 units/ml, respectively, and those for men were 25.5 and 275 units/ml. The mean values were 43 units/ml for women and 58 units/ml for men. Serums with IgE concentrations for more than 100 units/ml and some other samples were tested for specific Ige antibodies to 13 common allergens by the radioallergosorbent test (RAST). After RAST-positive serums were excluded, the mean values were 22 units/ml for women and 37 units/ml for men. The respective geometric mean values were 14.6 and 22.3 units/ml. The RAST explained serum IgE elevations to more than 100 units/ml in fewer than a third of cases. The radionuclide and enzymatic methods for IgG gave very similar results, with an overall correlation coefficient of 0.93. The proposed upper limits of normal for serum IgG concentrations are 66 units/ml for women and 135 units/ml for men.

▶ [Serum levels of IgE may be elevated in atopic diseases (asthma, allergic rhinitis, and atopic dermatitis), parasitic infection, IgE myeloma, hyperimmunoglobulinemia E syndrome, pemphigus, and Hodgkin's disease. This article by Stein et al. attempts to define the 95% upper limit of serum IgE in nonatopic adults. Exclusion of RAST-positive individuals increased the specificity of the test, which did not vary significantly according to age in adults. (Serum IgE is age-dependent in children.) Serum IgE was dependent on sex (higher levels in men) and on smoking history in men (higher levels in smokers). Perhaps you should let your laboratory know about this article.—A.R.R.] ◀

5–4 **IgE Production In Vitro by Human Blood Mononuclear Cells: Comparison Between Atopic and Nonatopic Subjects.** Zuhayr Hemady, Fred Blomberg, Stephen Gellis, and Ross E. Rocklin examined in vitro IgE synthesis by blood mononuclear cells (MNC) from atopic patients and nonatopic subjects to clarify discrepant results that have been reported. Patients included 6 subjects with atopic dermatitis (mean age, 14.18 years) and elevated serum IgE levels (greater than 2,000 kU/L) and 33 adult subjects with atopic asthma or hay fever, or both, without eczema and with positive skin tests. Control subjects were 40 adults with no history of atopy. A modified Phadebas IgE paper radioimmunosorbent test was used for quantitation of supernatant IgE concentration.

Net IgE synthesis increased from time 0 until day 7 of culture at which time the highest concentration of spontaneously produced IgE was reached. In 40 normal nonatopic subjects, there was no difference between IgE level in supernatants of unstimulated 7-day MNC cultures and their cycloheximide-treated counterparts. In contrast, supernatants of 7-day MNC cultures from 6 of 6 patients with atopic dermatitis and elevated serum IgE contained significantly higher levels of IgE than analogous cycloheximide-treated cultures. Spontaneous de novo IgE synthesis also occurred in supernatants of 7-day MNC cultures from 22 of 23 atopic subjects without eczema. Most of the latter patients were studied during their allergy season. In all atopic patients, polyclonal stimulants appeared to have a variable inhibitory effect on spontaneous in vitro IgE production. No induction

(5–4) J. Allergy Clin. Immunol. 71:324–330, March 1983.

of de novo IgE synthesis occurred when polyclonal activators were added to cultures from nonatopic controls. Only Concanavalin-A in relatively high concentrations significantly interfered with measurement of IgE in radioimmunoassay when the polyclonal stimulants used were added at various concentrations to known quantities of polyclonal IgE.

Blood MNC from a large group of nonatopic donors do not spontaneously produce de novo IgE in vitro. Blood MNC from atopic eczema patients and from most atopic patients without eczema during their allergy season do spontaneously secrete IgE in vitro. Polyclonal activators such as pokeweed mitogen, *Staphylococcus aureus* strain Cowan I, Concanavalin-A and phytohemagglutinin failed to induce or enhance in vitro IgE synthesis in normal and atopic subjects. These findings indicate that the study of immunoregulation of IgE synthesis in human beings will be difficult until new methods are developed that allow induction of the IgE response in vitro in nonatopic subjects.

▶ [This is yet another article demonstrating that regulation of in vitro IgE production is altered in atopic dermatitis (AD) and other atopic states without dermatitis. Blood mononuclear cells from nonatopic controls did not spontaneously produce de novo IgE in vitro. The number of patients with AD was small ($N = 6$), and eczema patients were selected for having increased IgE production. The implications of these findings in the pathogenesis of AD is not discussed, nor can these data be taken as evidence that spontaneous production of IgE in vitro is a marker of AD.—A.R.R.] ◀

5–5 **Quantitative Assessments of IgG and IgE Antibodies to Inhalant Allergens in Patients With Atopic Dermatitis.** Whether IgE antibodies to inhalant allergens are relevant to atopic dermatitis is uncertain. M. D. Chapman, S. Rowntree, E. B. Mitchell, M. C. Di Prisco de Fuenmajor, and T. A. E. Platts-Mills (Harrow, England) used antigen-binding radioimmunoassays to measure class-specific antibodies to two major inhalant allergens, antigen P_1 from *Dermatophagoides pteronyssinus* and Rye I from grass pollen, in serums from 69 patients with atopic dermatitis who had a characteristic rash. The age range was from less than 1 to 60 years. Moderate to severe eruptions were present. The 38 patients aged 11 and older were compared with 26 patients with perennial rhinitis, 24 with asthma, and 19 controls with either seasonal rhinitis only or no allergic symptoms.

Serums from 46 study patients contained IgE antibody binding activity (BA) to the dust mite allergen (P_1). These serums also contained IgG BA to the same antigen. Antibody titers were higher than in the patient control groups. All but 3 of 32 patients with atopic dermatitis who had positive skin tests to grass pollen had IgE BA for Rye I. The same serums also contained IgG BA for Rye I, and 6 serums contained IgG BA for Rye I but no IgE BA. In many instances, IgE antibodies to these allergens contributed significantly to the total serum IgE concentration. Total IgE and specific antibody levels to P_1 antigen in 11 adults with atopic dermatitis alone were closely similar to those in patients who had both atopic dermatitis and asthma. Neither study pa-

(5–5) J. Allergy Clin. Immunol. 72:27–33, July 1983.

tients nor controls had serum IgE diphtheria antitoxin, although most of them had been immunized with diphtheria toxoid in the past.

Many patients with atopic dermatitis have IgE antibody to house dust allergen. These IgE antibodies are part of an immune response that includes IgG antibodies. It remains unclear whether the antibodies can mediate eczematous skin lesions, but the patients appear to have some form of cellular immunity to the same allergens. Both positive skin tests and serum IgE antibody can be considered as markers for a complex form of hypersensitivity. In patients with IgE antibody who are exposed to the relevant allergens, the latter should be considered a potential cause of skin lesions.

▶ [Chapman et al. demonstrate the presence of IgE and IgG antibodies and positive skin reactions to common antigens in atopic dermatitis. It is not at all clear what role these antibodies play in the pathogenesis of disease. Immune responsiveness, rather than being nonspecific, may be a "marker" for disease. The utility of these observations in the management of patients with atopic dermatitis requires additional study.—A.R.R.] ◀

5–6 **Early Diagnosis of Infantile Seborrheic Dermatitis and Atopic Dermatitis: Total and Specific IgE Levels.** The difficulty of distinguishing clinically between atopic and infantile seborrheic dermatitides in young infants has been proved. Victoria M. Yates, Rebecca E. I. Kerr, K. Frier, S. J. Cobb, and Rona M. MacKie (Glasgow) measured total and antigen-specific IgE levels in young infants suspected of having these disorders. Thirty-seven consecutively seen infants younger than age 6 months who appeared with a clinical diagnosis of atopic or infantile seborrheic dermatitis were evaluated. They were followed up closely for 1–2 years, and a diagnosis was made on purely clinical grounds. Total IgE level was measured, and a radioallergosorbent test (RAST) screen for 7 allergens was carried out at initial examination (aged 3–4 months), at ages 6 months and 12 months, and, when appropriate, at age 2 years.

Nine infants received a clinical diagnosis of atopic dermatitis, and 27, infantile seborrheic dermatitis. One child's condition has not yet been definitively diagnosed. Eight infants with atopic dermatitis had a total IgE level higher than 80 units/ml at first visit, and all 9 by age 1 year; 4 had levels exceeding 1,000 units/ml. Two infants with seborrheic dermatitis had significantly elevated total IgE levels, but levels were normal at age 6 months. At age 1 year, 3 other infants had elevated IgE levels, but 24 had normal levels. The RAST screening for egg white and milk antibodies was helpful in distinguishing between the disorders. Elevated titers were noted initially in the atopic infants, whereas most infants with seborrheic dermatitis had a completely negative RAST screen initially. In nearly all of the atopic infants, further IgE antibodies had developed by age 1 year, but 23 of the 27 infants with seborrheic dermatitis had a negative RAST screen at this time. Positive titers in this group were in the low range. Eosinophil counts were quite variable, and no group differences in serum IgA, IgG, or IgM levels were evident.

(5–6) Br. J. Dermatol. 108:639–645, June 1983.

A RAST screen to egg white, cow's milk, and possibly fish is helpful in distinguishing atopic dermatitis from infantile seborrheic dermatitis as early as age 3–4 months. Estimation of total IgE levels also may be helpful. The findings support the view that atopic dermatitis and infantile seborrheic dermatitis are distinct entities.

▶ [Although the sample sizes were small in this report (9 children with atopic dermatitis and 27 with seborrheic dermatitis), the best distinguishing features appeared to be total IgE level and a positive RAST score to an average of 4 allergens. Although these laboratory tests may be helpful in some cases, and may give us a clue to the etiology of atopic dermatitis, this sort of laboratory testing cannot be recommended in the routine evaluation of patients suspected of atopic dermatitis vs. seborrheic dermatitis. Positive tests do not clinch the diagnosis of atopic dermatitis—there was some overlap—nor do negative tests exclude the diagnosis.—A.R.R.] ◀

5–7 **Early Diagnosis of Infantile Seborrheic Dermatitis and Atopic Dermatitis: Clinical Features.** Victoria M. Yates, Rebecca E. I. Kerr, and Rona M. MacKie (Glasgow, Scotland) undertook a prospective study of the clinical manifestations of atopic dermatitis and infantile seborrheic dermatitis in 37 infants younger than age 6 months who were seen consecutively with extensive dermatitis. The 23 male and 14 female infants had a mean age of 14 weeks at initial examination. Five met the criteria for atopic dermatitis initially, while 12 received a firm diagnosis of infantile seborrheic dermatitis. At age 1 year, a firm diagnosis of atopic dermatitis was made in 9 cases, and that of seborrheic dermatitis was made in 27; 1 infant remains without diagnosis. Twenty-five infants have been followed up for 2 years or longer.

The two diagnostic groups did not differ significantly in the mean age at onset of skin lesions. The face and napkin area were affected initially in both groups of infants. Seborrheic infants had more lesions in the axillae, and atopic infants had more lesions on the forearms and shins. Pruritus was more common in the group with atopic dermatitis. A little more than half of the atopic infants and a third of the seborrheic infants had a family history of atopy. Clearance times with treatment did not differ significantly in the two groups, but all of the atopic group had relapses. Only 3 of 27 seborrheic infants had significant further skin lesions. The bacterial flora in skin cultures was similar in the two groups. One atopic infant had evidence of definite food intolerance.

There are few useful clinical measures for distinguishing between atopic dermatitis and infantile seborrheic dermatitis in young infants. A "wait and see" approach is appropriate if the distinction is not evident initially. A definitive diagnosis can nearly always be made confidently on clinical grounds by age 1 year. Estimates of total and antigen-specific IgE levels may be diagnostically helpful. These observations confirmed the much better prognosis of infantile seborrheic dermatitis.

▶ [Infants with chronically relapsing red rashes present a formidable challenge to the practicing physician. The authors of this article investigated features that might

(5–7) Br. J. Dermatol. 108:633–638, June 1983.

be useful in establishing an early diagnosis of atopic dermatitis (vs. infantile seborrheic dermatitis) among individuals presenting with either of these two diseases early in life and followed long enough to ultimately establish the diagnosis. The "ultimate" diagnosis for the two disorders was based on clinical criteria, the most useful of which for the diagnosis of atopic dermatitis appeared to be irritability or pruritus, or both, skin lesions distributed on "exposed" surfaces of the extremities, and a positive family history of atopy. Total numbers were too small to justify a more definitive statement about the usefulness of these criteria.—A.R.R.] ◀

5–8 **Does Infant Feeding Affect the Risk of Allergy?** Michael L. Burr (Cardiff, Wales) discusses the still controversial assertion that withholding cow's milk from infants reduces the risk of allergic disease. The chief fault of prospective observational studies, whether of infants selected by medical history or of unselected infants, is that mothers who decide to breast-feed their infants are likely to differ from others in ways that could affect the risk of allergic disease developing in their children. Grulee and Sanford reported a striking association between bottle-feeding and eczema in a large study, and the conclusions have been challenged but not rejected. Retrospective studies rely on the mother's memory. Random, controlled trials have given conflicting results, but the best study tends to support the hypothesis. Most other intervention studies have shown a relation between cow's milk and allergic disease.

Allergic disease has been positively associated with cow's milk or mixed feedings in early infancy in about half of a total of 24 reported studies. In only one study was allergic disease positively associated with breast-feeding. Many studies failed to monitor early supplementary feeds in breast-fed infants, although it is likely that small amounts of foods could influence the development of allergy. The issue remains unsettled, but the balance of available evidence tends to favor the hypothesis that feeding cow's milk or solids to infants increases their risk of developing allergic disease. A convincing answer could be obtained from two or three carefully conducted, random, controlled trials with reasonable numbers of subjects and "blind" assessments. There is little reason to conduct further observational studies.

▶ [This article is a comprehensive and critical review of the relationship between early introduction of solid foods and cow's milk and the development of atopic disease. The author concludes that only randomized trials and blinded clinical assessments are required to finally settle the issue. Easier said than done!—A.R.R.] ◀

5–9 **Role of Immediate Food Hypersensitivity in Pathogenesis of Atopic Dermatitis.** Hugh A. Sampson (Duke Univ.) evaluated 26 children with atopic dermatitis (AD) and markedly elevated serum IgE levels for clinical evidence of hypersensitivity to foods; a double-blind, placebo-controlled food challenge was used. Selection of foods for challenge was based on positive responses to prick skin tests or a convincing history. Median age was 11 years.

Half of the children had the classic triad of AD, asthma, and allergic rhinitis, whereas 5 had AD alone. Twenty-four children had at least 1 positive response on skin testing at time of admission. Fifteen

---

(5–8) Arch. Dis. Child. 58:561–565, July 1983.
(5–9) J. Allergy Clin. Immunol. 71:473–480, May 1983.

children demonstrated 23 positive responses to food challenges, 9 reacted to only 1 food, 4 reacted to 2 foods, and 2 reacted to 3 foods. There was no significant difference between the patients with positive responses to food challenge and those with negative responses with regard to sex, age, diagnosis, serum IgE levels, or number of positive skin test results. All symptoms developed within 10 minutes to 2 hours of the challenge. Of 23 positive responses to food challenges, 21 involved cutaneous symptoms consisting of pruritus and erythematous macular or maculopapular rash involving 5% or more of the body surface. Nine food challenges resulted in skin symptoms alone, whereas the remainder caused concomitant gastrointestinal tract or respiratory tract symptoms. Of 63 food challenges, 43 (68%) in patients with positive skin test results and a history of possible intolerance were negative, suggesting that skin test reactions were clinically insignificant. Foods most often eliciting hypersensitivity reactions included egg, milk, wheat, and peanut.

Apparently, in some children with AD, food can lead to an immediate hypersensitivity reaction of the skin. Although food hypersensitivity may represent only 1 of several pathogenic factors in AD, removal of an offending food may result in marked improvement in skin symptoms. History is often unreliable in determining specific food hypersensitivities, and skin testing may also be unreliable in this regard. At present, double-blind, placebo-controlled food challenges are the only definitive means of diagnosing food hypersensitivity in AD.

▶ [Are elimination diets and routine skin testing for food allergy worthwhile in the standard evaluation of individuals with AD? One must conclude from the above article that if double-blind food challenge is the ultimate test of food sensitivity for a given individual, then elimination diets and routine skin testing are not useful in AD. Positive skin tests predict significant cutaneous reaction to food challenge in only 23% of cases, and negative skin tests do not exclude food sensitivity. Double-blind food challenge may be the only reliable way of documenting a role for food sensitivity in patients with AD. History should be the guide in deciding which patients are tested. Food-related reactions usually occur within 2 hours of food challenge.—A.R.R.] ◀

5–10 **Oral Evening-Primrose-Seed Oil Improves Atopic Eczema.** S. Wright and J. L. Burton (Bristol, England) conducted a double-blind, controlled crossover study of the effect of various oral doses of evening-primrose oil in 99 patients with atopic eczema. Patients included 60 adults (aged 15–58 years) and 39 children (aged 8 months to 14 years). Disease was moderate or severe, and all patients continued their normal treatment during the trial. Each patient received evening-primrose-seed oil (Efamol) for 12 weeks and a placebo for 12 weeks, in random order. Each Efamol capsule contained 360 mg of linoleic acid and 45 mg of γ-linoleic acid. Patient group A received 2 capsules twice daily, group B received 4 capsules twice daily, and group C had 6 capsules twice daily. Among the children, group D received 1 capsule twice daily and group E received 2 capsules twice daily.

(5–10) Lancet 2:1120–1122, Nov. 20, 1982.

Of the 60 adults in the trial, 16 (26%) dropped out before completing the 6 months (8 during treatment with Efamol and 89 during administration of placebo). Only 3 of the 39 children dropped out. In the low-dose groups (A and D), itch was the only symptom responding better to Efamol than to placebo. In the high-dose groups (B, C, and E), however, patient assessment showed that Efamol was significantly superior to placebo for itch, scaling, and general impression of severity. Physicians' assessments also showed a significant beneficial effect of active treatment on the overall severity of the condition. An analysis of the mean symptom scores for all 99 patients showed that Efamol produced an improvement of about 30% in overall severity of the eczema, with adults responding better than children. For patients in the high-dose groups, overall improvement in severity was about 43%. No side effects occurred.

This study has shown that larger doses of linoleic and γ-linoleic acid, in the form of evening-primrose oil (Efamol), significantly improve symptoms of atopic eczema, particularly in adults. The mode of action of Efamol is uncertain, but essential fatty acids may be involved in the maintenance of skin health.

▶ [The hallmark of atopic dermatitis is extremely sensitive, hyperreactive, itchy skin. The cause for this reactivity and itchiness is still a mystery. The observations of Burton and Wright require confirmation, and if they are valid, the mechanism of action of the "drug" must be elucidated.—A.R.R.] ◀

5–11 **Atopic Hand Dermatitis: Comparison With Atopic Dermatitis Without Hand Involvement, Especially With Respect to Influence of Work and Development of Contact Sensitization.** Margit Forsbeck, Erik Skog, and Eva Åsbrink (Stockholm) compared findings in 77 patients without atopic hand eczema and those in 136 atopic dermatitis (AD) patients with hand involvement. Age distribution was identical in the 2 groups, peaking at 25–39 years; and in both groups females were predominant. The 2 groups were comparable with respect to atopic heredity, occurrence of other atopic manifestations, and distribution of serum IgE values.

The first appearance of hand eczema was unrelated to any change in occupation. However, in both sexes, significantly more patients with hand eczema had changed occupation compared with those free of hand lesions. In both groups, change of occupation resulted in significant improvement of the eczema. Of the 136 patients with hand eczema, 82 (60%) were first employed performing wet or unclean jobs; 52 (63%) of these changed occupations. In the 77 patients without hand involvement, 47 (53%) had wet or unclean jobs and 7 (17%) changed to another occupation. The prevalence of positive results on patch testing was high in both groups. High and low quantities of serum IgE were equally distributed between the 2 groups. However, significantly more patients with IgE values of less than 120 units/ml had positive patch test reactions than did those with IgE values of more than 1,000 units/ml.

(5–11) Acta Derm. Venereol. (Stockh.) 63:9–13, 1983.

These results do not support the hypothesis that any established contact sensitization is of major significance for the development or persistence of hand eczema. However, they do support the finding that patients with relatively high serum IgE levels have a significantly lower incidence of positive patch test reactions than do those with lower IgE levels.

▶ [The concept that atopic patients with chronic hand dermatitis will be at higher risk of becoming sensitized by exposure to sensitizers at work is not confirmed by this study, since atopic patients without hand involvement showed the same high incidence of allergic contact dermatitis as the ones with hand eczema. It follows therefore that the problems encountered by atopic patients with hand involvement are secondary to the irritant effect of environmental exposure. From the disability standpoint this is an important concept, since certain third-party carriers will only award disability payments if an allergic contact dermatitis is proved.—E.G.] ◀

5–12 **Oral Disodium Cromoglycate Treatment of Atopic Dermatitis.** Rune Lindskov and Lone Knudsen (Finsen Inst., Copenhagen) conducted a double-blind, crossover study of the effect of oral disodium cromoglycate (DSCG) in 14 adults and 10 children with active atopic dermatitis. Oral DSCG and placebo were given for 6 weeks in random order. Adults received 200 mg of DSCG 4 times daily, and children were given 100 mg of DSCG 4 times daily.

No significant differences between DSCG treatment and placebo were detected with regard to daytime itching or severity of eczema. In adults who began the study with placebo, itching during the night was significantly diminished within the first 3 weeks of DSCG treatment compared with results in the corresponding period of placebo treatment. In adults who began the study with DSCG, itching during the night was significantly diminished within the second 3 weeks of placebo treatment compared with results when taking DSCG. No significant effects were detected except for eczema in all patients after 6 weeks' treatment; DSCG treatment produced significantly better results than placebo. No differences were found between food-allergic patients and non-food-allergic patients. The results of radioallergosorbent and skin tests were not significantly different in the 2 treatment groups. Possible side effects reported by 2 patients included joint pain in an adult and unexplained urticaria during DSCG therapy in a child.

Although oral DSCG caused few side effects, further clinical studies are necessary to assess its usefulness in the treatment of atopic dermatitis.

▶ [The oral administration of disodium cromoglycate appears not to be an effective therapy in patients with atopic dermatitis as had been documented previously in a controlled study (Atherton, D. J., et al.: *Br. J. Dermatol.* 106:681, 1982). The oral administration of this therapeutic agent has not been convincingly associated with side effects with the possible exception of rare instances of mild degrees of nausea. Other reported symptoms and signs, such as headache, urticaria, arthralgia, and gastrointestinal tract manifestations, may be specious attributions or may be related to the disorder being treated. However, patients sensitive to lactose, milk, or milk products may be allergic to the capsule dosage form, since the capsule contains a lactose vehicle.—N.A.S.] ◀

(5–12) Allergy 38:161–165, April 1983.

5–13 **Thymopoietin Pentapeptide (TP-5) Improves Clinical Parameters and Lymphocyte Subpopulations in Atopic Dermatitis.** Kefei Kang, Kevin D. Copper, and Jon M. Hanifin (Oregon Health Sciences Univ.) conducted a double-blind prospective study in 20 patients with atopic dermatitis (AD) using thrice-weekly injections of 50 mg of thymopoietin pentapeptide (TP-5) or placebo for 6 weeks. The recent availability of monoclonal antibodies provided a means of evaluating the distribution and function of peripheral blood mononuclear leukocyte (MNL) subpopulations and showed that the OKT8-positive ($T8^+$) suppressor-cytotoxic cell subset was significantly reduced in AD. A potent synthetic pentapeptide known as TP-5 represents residues 32–36 of thymopoietin, induces maturation of thymocytes, and influences T-cell and B-cell differentiation in vitro and in vivo.

Eighteen of the 20 patients completed the 6-week trial. Of the 2 patients discontinuing, 1 was dropped because of his history of carcinoma, and in the other generalized pruritus and erythema developed for 24 hours, starting 2 hours after the first TP-5 injection. Clinical parameters, lymphocyte subsets defined by monoclonal antibodies, and serum IgE levels were modified. Younger patients (age less than 34) responded to TP-5 with much greater improvement in severity scores than did TP-5-treated patients older than 34 years or those given placebo regardless of age ($P<.05$). Both absolute lymphocytes and $T8^+$ cytotoxic-suppressor cells were significantly increased ($P<.05$) in the TP-5 group, whereas they were not significantly increased in the placebo group ($P>.05$). Conversely, Ia^+ cells were significantly increased in the placebo group ($P<.05$), but remained the same in the TP-5 group ($P>.05$). Serum IgE levels were not significantly altered in either group.

Thus, based on clinical and in vitro data, TP-5 may have a beneficial effect in some patients with AD and may fulfill a need for safe, systemic treatment in those with widespread, recalcitrant disease.

▶ [In a small number of patients with atopic dermatitis (AD) assessed before, during, and after a 6-week period, there appeared to be a beneficial response in 5 of 8 patients treated with a compound of thymopoietin, compared to a good response in only 2 of 10 patients treated with placebo. Cutaneous infections, extent of involvement, and the dependence on other oral and systemic medications would be other useful parameters to study during therapy in a larger number of patients.—A.R.R.] ◀

5–14 **Extensive Pityriasis Alba: Histologic, Histochemical, and Ultrastructural Study.** S. T. Zaynoun, B. G. Aftimos, K. K. Tenekjian, N. Bahuth, and A. K. Kurban (American Univ. of Beirut, Lebanon) note that pityriasis alba is a relatively common skin disorder, usually seen in children. The lesions are frequently limited to the face. Seven females and 2 males with extensive pityriasis alba were examined using histopathologic and histochemical techniques and electron microscopy. All except 1 were adults (age range, 6–27 years). The duration of the eruption ranged from 2 weeks to 6 years.

(5–13) J. Am. Acad. Dermatol. 8:372–377, March 1983.
(5–14) Br. J. Dermatol. 108:83–90, January 1983.

Histopathologic examination showed the epidermis to be mildly to moderately hyperkeratotic in 4 patients and parakeratotic in 1; a significant reduction in amount of melanin in the epidermis in the clinically affected skin was noted in all patients except 1; and focal exocytosis and spongiosis were seen in the affected skin in 2 patients. A mild perivascular inflammatory infiltrate was observed in the upper dermis in both affected and apparently normal skin in 4 patients. Light microscopic examination revealed a decrease in melanocyte density in the affected skin of all patients. The shape and size of melanocytes and dendrites in affected skin and in normal skin appeared not to differ. Electron microscopy indicated a significant degree of intercellular edema in the affected skin in 4 patients, no edema in 1 patient, and mild edema in 4 patients' control skin. The melanocytes in the affected as well as control skin appeared normal when examined by electron microscopy. No apparent differences in shape and degree of melanization of melanosomes between the affected and normal skin were found.

The main microscopic findings consisted of a decreased number of functional melanocytes and a reduction in the amount of melanin in the affected hypopigmented skin without any appreciable change in shape, size, and cytoplasmic activity of the melanocytes or the number and length of dendrites. Although various microscopic abnormalities were present in the affected skin in nearly all patients, none of these findings alone would explain all of the changes in the pigment cell or its product. The patients in this study differed clinically from those with classic pityriasis alba in that they were predominantly adults and the condition was of a longer duration. Disease in these patients may represent a new entity of undetermined etiology.

▶ [Zaynoun et al. describe clinical, light-microscopic, and ultrastructural features of an extensive form of leukoderma that for want of a better term is called extensive pityriasis alba (EPA). Antecedent inflammatory diseases are excluded on the basis of history, although mild inflammation is noted histologically. Although some of us may have (mistakenly) attributed similar conditions to antecedent inflammatory processes of various types (but for unknown causes), perhaps EPA is indeed a unique entity worthy of further consideration. It would be ideal to compare EPA to ordinary postinflammatory hypopigmentation.—A.R.R.] ◀

6. Contact Dermatitis

6–1 **Epidemiology of Work-Related Skin Disease in South Carolina.** Julian E. Keil and Edward Shmunes (Univ. of South Carolina, Columbia) examined problems associated with occupationally related skin disease by reviewing the charts of all closed cases of skin disease processed by the South Carolina Industrial Commission from July 1, 1978, through June 30, 1979.

Financial settlements were awarded to 958 persons because of skin disease in the period studied. The condition in 898 (93.8%) of these claimants was diagnosed as contact dermatitis, indicating some type of chemical or plant exposure. As shown in the table, contact dermatitis caused by oils, solvents, and other chemicals accounted for 42.7% of all affected persons. The average age of the claimants with settled cases was 33.4 years; 66% were men. Metal and machinery workers collectively had the highest proportion of dermatoses. Employees of governmental agencies represented the largest single segment of patients. The average incidence of dermatoses for all industries was 10.8 per 10,000 employees. Ten industries exceeded this average, but 3 (transportation equipment, machinery, and furniture products) had

DISTRIBUTION OF CLOSED CASES BY ICDA* NOMENCLATURE FOR CONTACT DERMATITIS AND OTHER DERMATOSES

Diagnosis and Attributive Cause	%	n
Contact dermatitis†		
Detergents	5.7	55
Oils and grease	8.1	78
Solvents	11.1	106
Drugs	0.2	2
Other chemicals	23.5	225
Food	1.9	18
Plants	14.3	137
Other and unspecified	11.2	107
Other eczemas and dermatitis	17.8	171
Other dermatoses	6.2	59
Total No. of Cases	**100.0**	**958**

*ICDA = *International Classification of Diseases Adapted for Use in the United States,* ed. 8.

†The subtotal in 899 claimants (93.8%).

(Courtesy of Keil, J.E., and Shmunes, E.: Arch. Dermatol. 119:650–654, August 1983; copyright 1983, American Medical Association.)

(6–1) Arch. Dermatol. 119:650–654, August 1983.

incidences more than double the average for all industries. Almost 90% of all cases reported indicated that the claimants' hands were affected. With regard to case severity, 43.4% were considered minor, 24.4% were moderate, 16.8% were moderately serious, and 15.3% were serious. Serious cases accounted for 48% ($20,521) of medication costs, 82% ($20,756) of the clincher payments, 70% ($101,489) of total fees, and 96% (2,028) of all days lost from work. Cost of all medical, legal, and other settlements provided claimants of closed cases totaled $142,925. Total days lost from work were 2,102. The greatest number of cases among male workers occurred during June, whereas in female workers the greatest proportion occurred during September. In both sexes, the greatest number of cases were reported on Mondays, which is significantly higher than for other weekdays. Identification of factors characterizing the small number of cases with disproportionate economic impact deserves greater attention and investigation.

▶ [The proportion of industrial compensation cases involving the skin in this report (less than 1%) is surprisingly low. Not surprisingly, the hands were most frequently involved. The authors fail to differentiate between allergic and irritant dermatitis. Could the relatively nonunionized nature of the work force explain in part the low rate of claims?—R.S.S.] ◀

6–2 **Contact Dermatitis Caused by Diphenhydramine Hydrochloride.** Ralph J. Coskey (Wayne State Univ.) reports 3 cases of contact dermatitis caused by an ethanolamine antihistamine, diphenhydramine hydrochloride (Benadryl).

CASE 1.—Child, 10, developed erythematous, scaly plaques on the right antecubital space and dermatitis on left arm and back. The eruption started on the right antecubital space from an insect bite. Diphenhydramine hydrochloride lotion (Caladryl), Benadryl cream, and first-aid cream and ointment containing neomycin, bacitracin, and polymyxin B (Neosporin) had been applied to the eruption. Therapy consisted of Burow's solution compresses, methylprednisolone by mouth, and topical betamethasone valerate (Valisone cream) application. Patch tests showed reactions to Benadryl cream and Caladryl lotion.

CASE 2.—Man, 60, had an eczematous, weeping eruption of the hands. He had applied Zemo, Dermamycin, bacitracin, Caladryl, and Ziradryl. Contact dermatitis was diagnosed. The patient was treated with Burow's solution compresses, topical corticosteroid preparations, and antihistamines. Two days after patch tests, the patient had a strong reaction to Ziradryl, Caladryl, and Benadryl cream.

CASE 3.—Man, 54, had generalized dermatitis on the trunk and extremities. He had first developed localized dermatitis after exposure to a vine and was treated orally with Benadryl. He had applied Caladryl topically. He felt faint during the office visit for 3 hours. Treatment consisted of intramuscular methylprednisolone and oral prednisone, Aveeno colloidal baths, and 0.025% triamcinolone applied topically. Patch tests were positive for Caladryl lotion and injectable diphenhydramine hydrochloride.

Review of the literature indicated that contact dermatitis from diphenhydramine hydrochloride is probably not uncommon. Patients who have become sensitive to topical use of the drug may develop a

---

(6–2) J. Am. Acad. Dermatol. 8:204–206, February 1983.

flare of dermatitis if they use it orally or parenterally. Sensitive patients should avoid cough mixtures and other preparations containing this drug.

▶ [The author comments that allergic contact dermatitis to diphenhydramine hydrochloride is probably more common than the reports in recent medical literature indicate. This is probably owing in part to the fact that most dermatologists avoid its topical use because of the notorious stigma of sensitization that has accompanied this topical preparation for many years.

Besides the ethanolamine-derived antihistamines such as Benadryl and Dramamine, the other important sensitizers among antihistaminics are the ethylenediamine-derived drugs such as Atarax and Vistaril. Several cases of exacerbation of contact dermatitis in ethylenediamine-sensitized patients while receiving Atarax have been reported.—E.G.] ◀

6–3 **Hypersensitivity Angiitis Caused by Fumes From Heat-Activated Photocopy Paper.** John R. Tencati and Harold S. Novey describe a patient with recurrent palpable purpura that was suspected of having an occupational origin. A job site visit and challenge studies confirmed the suspicion and permitted identification of the probable causal agent.

Woman, 53, had had weekly episodes of palpable purpura on the lower extremities for 22 months. Lesions appeared 3 months after she began working as an industrial librarian. Purpura typically developed after 4–6 hours at work and was preceded by intense burning and itching. Laboratory studies indicated no underlying disease. Lesions resolved completely during vacations but recurred within hours of return to work. Evaluation of the job site showed that three photocopy machines for microfilm files were near the patient's desk and were often used. No other workers had similar lesions.

The patient underwent a series of challenges in which she was seated in an enclosure and exposed to fumes released from heat-activated photocopy paper, its chemical components, or control paper. Purpura did not occur after exposure to fumes of control paper, undeveloped photocopy paper, or three of four chemical components. Fumes released from developing (heated) photocopy paper produced purpura beginning 4 hours after exposure and continuing for 4 hours after exposure was ended. Chemical component challenges produced an equivocal reaction to behenic acid. Challenge with behenic acid produced purpura after 3 hours. No significant changes occurred in the physiologic studies from challenge with photocopy paper fumes.

Contact dermatitis to paper additives is common, but palpable purpura had not been reported. Inhalation of chemical fumes with absorption through the respiratory mucosa was the likely route of entry of the offending agent. This belief is supported by the observation that the patient always had upper respiratory tract symptoms. Behenic acid is a naturally occurring C22 fatty acid present in the oils of many plants, marine animals, and some bacteria. Physicians should be aware that fumes liberated by heat-activated photocopy papers are potentially harmful and that palpable purpura may result from their inhalation.

▶ [This case report is unique because patch testing to the offending agent was negative and cutaneous contact with the fumes did not reproduce the vasculitis, suggesting that sensitization was through inhalation of the fumes. Purpuric eczematous

(6–3) Ann. Intern. Med. 98:320–322, March 1983.

allergic contact dermatitis has been described previously with antioxidants used in the rubber industry, such as paraphenylenediamine; but patch testing has been positive, and the sensitization is believed to have occurred exogenously.—E.G.] ◀

6–4 **Allergic Contact Dermatitis to Garlic (*Allium sativum* L.): Identification of the Allergens. The Role of Mono-, Di-, and Trisulfides Present in Garlic: Comparative Study in Man and Animal (Guinea Pig)** is reported by C. Papageorgiou, J.-P. Corbet, F. Menezes-Brandao, M. Pecegueiro, and C. Benezra. Positive patch tests to garlic have been described in patients with hand contact dermatitis related to vegetables, and allergic contact dermatitis to garlic is now a recognized entity. Garlic water- and ethanol-soluble extracts were purified and tested on both guinea pigs and garlic-sensitive patients. The allergenic component was well localized to a few column chromatographic fractions. Diallyldisulfide was detected in the fractions that effectively sensitized guinea pigs given water-soluble extracts. Animals were sensitized to this product and cross-reacted with garlic; those sensitized to garlic extracts cross-reacted with diallyldisulfide. Both groups reacted to allicin, an oxidized derivative of diallyldisulfide present in garlic. Garlic-sensitive patients had positive tests with diallyldisulfide, allylpropyldisulfide, allylmercaptan, and allicin.

Reactions to garlic in both guinea pigs and man are allergic, although some skin reactions to garlic may also be irritant. The allergens identified to date include diallyldisulfide, allylpropyldisulfide, and allicin.

▶ [This study leaves no doubt that contact dermatitis to garlic can be allergic although there is no question that irritant reactions are not uncommon. The difficult cases are seen in Italian chefs who are exposed continuously to garlic and develop an irritant dermatitis which predisposes them to become sensitized.—E.G.] ◀

6–5 **Evaluation of Immune Status in Vivo By 2,4-Dinitro-1-Chlorobenzene Contact Allergy Time (DNCB-CAT).** Immunologic mechanisms are of pathogenetic significance in many dermatoses, and neoplastic disorders have been related to impaired immune defenses. Bernhard Przybilla, Günter Burg, and Christian Thieme (Munich), determined the interval from the start of continuous application of DNCB epicutaneously to the appearance of an allergic contact reaction, or "contact allergy time" (CAT), in 73 patients with malignant melanoma. In 34 patients (group I) 2% DNCB ointment was used for 2 days, after which 0.05% DNCB ointment was applied daily. In the other 39 patients (group II) only the 0.05% ointment was used. In group I the 2% ointment was applied to the extensor surface of an upper arm and the 0.05% ointment to the flexor surface of the ipsilateral forearm. Thirty-two patients had superficial spreading melanoma, and 30 had nodular melanoma.

No dissemination of dermatitis occurred in patients with positive DNCB skin tests. The median DNCB-CAT was 11.2 days in group I and 22.3 days in group II. The CAT was significantly longer in pa-

---

(6–4) Arch. Dermatol. Res. 275:229–234, August 1983.
(6–5) Dermatologica 167:1–5, July 1983.

tients older than age 55 than in younger patients. Median values did not differ in males and females. No significant differences were found between patients receiving cytostatic drugs and those not so treated.

In contrast to conventional DNCB sensitization procedures, the CAT method permits quantitative estimates of the induction and the elicitation phases of sensitization. False-negative results may be obtained with the conventional threshold method before the induction phase is completed. Threshold testing permits quantitation of only the elicitation phase. The amount of DNCB applied is important when the CAT method is used, but some variation in the amount of ointment used will not result in considerable change in the amount of DNCB per unit of skin.

▶ [The standard method of DNCB sensitization requires that the skin of the subject be exposed to a toxic dose of the chemical during the induction phase and to a subtoxic dose of DNCB 14 days after to elicit the immunologic response. The DNCB-CAT is a new method to assess elicitation response by an original application of a toxic dose (2% DNCB) followed by a daily application of a subtoxic dose of the chemical until a contact dermatitis is elicited. The advantage of this new method is that it minimizes the false-negative reactions of a fixed-time evaluation, since some subjects were shown to react after 14 days. It also provides a more quantitative method to measure induction and elicitation phases. One of the obvious disadvantages of this new method is that it transfers the responsibility of the application of the contactant to the subject where compliance may be more difficult to assess; furthermore the authors admit that this method depends greatly on the proper administration of the ointment by the patient. Since this study was carried out on melanoma patients, it requires confirmation on other population of patients.—E.G.] ◀

6–6 **Effect of Repeated Delayed Hypersensitivity Skin Tests on Skin Test Responses.** N. V. Christou, J. B. Pietsch, and J. L. Meakins (McGill Univ.) conducted a retrospective analysis of 426 skin tests on 107 patients, who had a mean of 4.3 weekly tests with 5 recall antigens, to determine whether repeated skin tests can augment a previously weak delayed hypersensitivity response or convert previously nonreacting tests and thus yield false-positive data. They also skin tested 10 healthy volunteers weekly for as long as 6 weeks. Reactions (induration measured in millimeters) were recorded, and a regression and correlation analysis was carried out.

The 107 patients included those responding to 2 or more antigens (reactive), 1 antigen (relatively anergic), or none of the antigens (anergic). The only antigen showing a weakly significant correlation between diameter of induration and time was *Candida*. None of the other 4 antigens (mumps, purified protein derivative [PPD], *Trichophyton*, and Varidase) showed an increase in induration diameter with time. No patient showed subsequent reactions to antigens to which they were initially nonreactive. All volunteers were reactive. Two reacted to all 5 antigens, 2 reacted to 4, 5 to 3, and 1 to 2. Conversion to reactivity was defined if 3 consecutive responses with no induration were followed by 1 or more responses with induration greater than 5 mm. Three such conversions took place, all to PPD. One occurred after 3 weeks, 1 after 5 weeks, and 1 at the end of 6

(6–6) Can. J. Surg. 26:139–142. March 1983.

weeks. Varidase was the only antigen to show a weak positive correlation.

The slight augmentation in the delayed hypersensitivity response seen in this study is not significant enough to interfere with the usefulness of repeated tests to monitor a patient's clinical course. On the basis of these results, sequential delayed hypersensitivity skin testing can be used to monitor the clinical course of surgical patients, and false-positive reactions due to a booster effect of repeated testing will be minimal.

▶ [This reassuring study puts to rest the concern of many immunologists that false-positive reactions could develop from frequent skin testing.—E.G.] ◀

6–7 **Dermatoses Associated With Brominated Swimming Pools.** A small but increasing number of public swimming pools in the United Kingdom have been disinfected with a solid brominated agent rather than chlorine. The product, which is available under the proprietary names Di-halo and Aquabrome, has 1-bromo-3-chloro-5,5-dimethylhydantoin as its active constituent. R. J. G. Rycroft and P. T. Penny summarize the strong circumstantial evidence that swimming pools disinfected with this product are associated with dermatoses, primarily eczematous, and they present 2 case reports.

Case 1.—Man, 32, developed widespread, itchy, red papules after swimming in a pool that had changed from a chlorine gas disinfectant to Di-halo 1 month previously. Eczema subsequently developed on the hands and in patches on the body. This improved when the patient was away from work as attendant of the pool, but it rapidly relapsed when he returned. He was asymptomatic when swimming in a chlorinated pool, but a rescue dive into the brominated pool resulted in an itchy, red, papular eruption within 20 minutes. There was no medical or family history of eczema, asthma, or hay fever. Examination showed a discoid eczema of the trunk and limbs and a vesicular eczema of the palms and fingers. Patch tests with the International Contact Dermatitis Research Group standard series of allergens and with Di-halo were negative, as were prick tests with Di-halo (1% in water and 1% in petrolatum).

Case 2.—Woman, 40, a swimming instructor, had similar history and symptoms. When the pool she worked in changed to a solid chlorine disinfectant, her rash cleared, but it returned when she began to work in another pool treated with Di-halo.

Visits to 19 brominated pools revealed that at least 5% of users of a pool treated with Di-halo had recently experienced pruritus and subsequent rashes. High proportions of the staffs were found to have been affected, suggesting that frequent exposure was a relevant factor. Older persons were also affected more often than children. A mail survey uncovered 70 reports from persons who had experienced more than trivial rashes associated with pools, 65 of which were associated with pools treated with Di-halo. Other reported symptoms include soreness of the mouth, throat, vulva, female urethra, and breasts. Most of the symptoms occurred within 12 hours after swimming.

When mixed with water, bromine and chlorine ions are released

---

(6–7) Br. Med. J. 287:462, Aug. 13, 1983.

from 1-bromo-3-chloro-5,5-dimethyl-hydantoin to leave 5,5-dimethylhydantoin (DMH). Accompanying reactions with contaminants such as urea and creatinine produce various chemicals, including bromamines, chloramines, and complex organic bromine and chlorine compounds. It is unlikely that allergy to the parent compound or DMH is responsible for the rashes. As the rashes usually occur within 12 hours after swimming, *Pseudomonas aeruginosa* infection is also unlikely. The evidence suggests that these dermatoses may be forms of cumulative irritant contact dermatitis subject to acute exacerbations.

▶ [The authors do not indicate why these brominated compounds are replacing chlorine in England, but it is conceivable that it's either more effective or less expensive. If that is the case, we may see the same trend in the United States, and we should be alerted to the possibility of seeing similar skin eruptions in our population.—E.G.] ◀

6–8 **Dermal Glycosaminoglycans Characterize the Primary Irritant Dermatitis in Psoriatics and Healthy Individuals.** Primary irritant dermatitis involves an inflammatory process of connective tissue. To characterize this process biochemically, J. H. Poulsen and M. K. Cramers (Univ. of Aarhus, Denmark) investigated the response of 4 dermal glycosaminoglycans (GAGs) and hydroxyproline to primary irritant dermatitis induced by 10% aqueous benzalkonium chloride patches in 8 psoriatic patients and 7 healthy controls.

Before induction of irritant dermatitis, the skin of the controls and the unaffected skin of the psoriatics showed exactly the same concentrations of hydroxyproline, hyaluronic acid, dermatan sulfate, chondroitin 4/6-sulfate, and heparan sulfate. On day 3 after the chemical injury, the mean concentrations of hyaluronic acid were significantly decreased by 56% in the controls and 59% in the psoriatics. These decreases were still present in both groups at day 6. The controls showed a 34% decrease in the mean concentration of dermatan sulfate by day 3, followed by an increase to the initial value at day 6. However, this pattern was not observed in psoriatics, in whom a decrease of 23% by day 3 was not followed by an increase. Chemical injury produced an increase in the concentration of chondroitin 4/6 sulfate in both groups. By day 3 the mean concentrations of chondroitin 4/6 sulfate had increased by 54% in the controls and by 43% in the psoriatics. By day 6 the increases were 84% and 88%, respectively. Whereas the controls showed an initial 48% increase in concentration of heparan sulfate, which was sustained through day 6, no increase was observed in the psoriatics during the study period. Hydroxyproline concentrations remained constant in both groups throughout the study. Age did not influence any of the GAG responses, and both groups showed similar clinical degrees of inflammation.

Dermal metabolism of GAGs in primary irritant dermatitis is different from that of the wound-healing process, including granuloma formation. This specificity of the dermal GAGs as a marker in inflam-

---

(6–8) Clin. Chim. Acta 130:305–315, June 15, 1983.

mation is encouraging, and interest in them should not be limited to the detection of mucopolysaccharidoses.

▶ [This study opens a new dimension in the identification of chemical changes in inflammatory processes of the skin. The authors compare these changes with changes in wound healing. It would be interesting to perform similar chemical determinations in allergic contact dermatitis to see how they differ from the irritant reactions.—E.G.] ◀

7. Pharmacology and Drug Therapy

7–1 **Evidence for Anti-Inflammatory Activities of Oral Synthetic Retinoids: Experimental Findings and Clinical Experience** are reviewed by C. E. Orfanos and R. Bauer (Free Univ. of Berlin). There is increasing evidence that the synthetic retinoids exert a direct anti-inflammatory effect, which contributes to their value in the treatment of various skin disorders, besides their beneficial effect on keratinizing epithelia. The reduction in temperature of psoriatic skin lesions described with Ro 10–9359 suggests a decrease in microcirculation in the diseased skin. Changes in the dermal papillary vessels in psoriasis are largely absent after 3 weeks of treatment, and the lumina are markedly smaller. Activity of neutrophils in tissue appears to be reduced in conjunction with oral retinoid therapy. Clinical studies have shown that oral retinoid therapy inhibits leukocytotaxis and migration of inflammatory cells into the epidermis in vivo. Long-term oral retinoid therapy apparently can increase the number of peripheral blood monocytes. Stimulation of Langerhans cells in psoriatic skin has been observed. Synthetic retinoids may also inhibit mitogen-induced DNA synthesis of peripheral blood lymphocytes.

Inhibition of neutrophil migration into the psoriatic epidermis is one of the earliest cellular events associated with oral retinoid therapy, and it appears to be important in the antipsoriasis efficacy of these drugs. Retinoids may have clinical value in many skin disorders characterized by dermal inflammation and secondary epidermal involvement, such as cutaneous disseminated lupus erythematosus, Behçet's syndrome, bullous pemphigoid with eosinophilia, and necrotizing vasculitis with eosinophilia. The retinoids used orally exhibit some similarities to corticosteroids. Retinoids are conversion products or synthetic derivatives largely corresponding to natural metabolites of the body. Both groups of drugs have broad, nonspecific effects on skin disorders. Neither specificially counteracts pathogenic factors in given dermatoses, but retinoids appear to have anti-inflammatory properties affecting only the cell-mediated pathways of inflammation.

▶ [Orfanos and Bauer have reviewed the vascular and immunologic effects that are characteristic of retinoids in addition to their well-known antikeratinizing effect. Their anti-inflammatory properties have perhaps been previously overlooked as a major therapeutic mechanism in the treatment of a variety of dermatoses. The authors note similarities between retinoids and corticosteroids and suggest that retinoids (like corticosteroids) may act as a modified hormone.—R.R.] ◀

7–2 **Comparison of Miconazole Nitrate and Selenium Disulfide as Antidandruff Agents.** Rekha A. Sheth (Bombay, India) compared

(7–1) Br. J. Dermatol. 109(Suppl. 25):55–60, July 1983.
(7–2) Int. J. Dermatol. 22:123–125, March 1983.

the antidandruff efficacy of two shampoos containing 2% miconazole nitrate (15 subjects) and 2.5% selenium disulfide (8 subjects), respectively. No other antidandruff medication had been used in the preceding 3 months.

In the miconazole group, 9 subjects had definite clinical amelioration of symptoms, which could be confirmed by a reduction in clinical grades by 50% of the original score. In 4 subjects the condition remained the same, and the other 2 patients improved moderately. However, the corneocyte count paralleled clinical improvement in only 6 of the former 9 subjects. In the selenium group, 4 of 8 subjects improved clinically. Among these 4, the corneocyte count showed an increase in 1 and remained almost the same in another; in 2 the counts and clinical grades corresponded. Simple cytologic examination of Giemsa- and Gram-stained smears was more useful in assessing factors underlying the pathogenesis of dandruff.

Dandruff is a symptom complex with many different causal factors. That miconazole, with antifungal and antibacterial properties, was effective in 9 of 15 subjects is not surprising, because fungal and bacterial infections may be two of the more common causal factors.

7–3 **Suppression of Alcohol-Induced Flushing by a Combination of H_1 and H_2 Histamine Antagonists.** Alcohol-induced flushing of the face and neck is probably a genetically determined state and is a result of individual differences in alcohol metabolism. As many as one fourth of white subjects in England and the United States are affected, and the condition is even more frequent in Orientals. O. T. Tan, T. J. Stafford, I. Sarkany, P. M. Gaylarde, C. Tilsey, and J. P. Payne (London) examined the influence of blood alcohol concentrations on flushing in 7 sensitive women aged 23–50 years. Three of the 5 whites and the 2 Chinese women had marked facial flushing after they ingested alcohol. Oxygen concentrations were recorded transcutaneously at the site of maximal flushing as the subjects drank sherry in amounts of 0.5–3 ml/kg. The effects of chlorpheniramine and cimetidine on flushing and blood alcohol concentrations were examined in 3 of the alcohol-sensitive subjects and 1 control.

Flushing occurred in susceptible subjects at blood alcohol concentrations of 20–35 mg/dl. Controls did not flush even with a concentration of 80 mg/dl. A combination of 4 mg of chlorpheniramine and 200 mg of cimetidine, given 30 minutes before ingestion of 1 ml of sherry per kg, prevented blood alcohol concentrations from reaching control values. Concentrations remained at less than 20 mg/dl, and flushing did not occur. One of 2 subjects flushed after 2 ml of sherry per kg and the other after 3 ml/kg. Lower blood alcohol concentrations followed ingestion of equivalent amounts of ethanol in water rather than sherry. No flushing followed ingestion of freeze-dried extract of sherry in water or histamine in water.

Facial flushing occurs in sensitive persons above a threshold blood alcohol concentration of 20–35 mg/dl. Both peak blood concentration

(7–3) Br. J. Dermatol. 107:647–652, December 1982.

and rate of alcohol absorption are reduced by a combination of H_1 and H_2 receptor antagonists, and flushing is abolished.

▶ [This study strongly suggests that H_1 and H_2 antagonists together suppress alcohol-induced flushing by their effect on alcohol levels and not by a direct effect on cutaneous vasculature. Somewhat surprisingly, the H_1 antagonists alone appear to increase alcohol absorption. Because of the CNS effects of H_1 antagonists, their use with alcohol may lead to extreme drowsiness.—R.S.S.] ◀

7–4 **Effects of Potent Topical Corticosteroids on Adrenocortical Function.** Miki Aso (Yonago, Japan) treated 37 males and 11 females, mean age 51.3, with 9 potent corticosteroid ointments and examined their adrenocortical function during treatment. The 9 topical steroids included 0.025% beclomethasone 17,21-dipropionate ointment, 0.12% betamethasone 17-valerate ointment, 0.05% fluocinonide ointment, 0.1% diflucortolone 21-valerate ointment, 0.025% budesonide, 0.1% halcinonide, 0.05% clobetasol 17-propionate (CBP), 0.25% desoximethasone, and 0.05% diflorasone 17,21-diacetate. Each patient was treated with a single ointment only by simple application twice a day in doses of 10–60 gm/day for 7 consecutive days. Serum cortisol levels were measured before and during treatment. Results in 54 healthy male volunteers receiving various doses of oral betamethasone were compared with those in the 48 patients.

All 48 patients had normal levels of serum cortisol before treatment, but these decreased during treatment. Adrenocortical function was not suppressed by beclomethasone dipropionate, betamethasone valerate, or fluocinonide. It was moderately suppressed by diflucortolone valerate, budesonide, and halcinonide and was markedly suppressed by CBP, desoximethasone, and diflorasone diacetate. When the dose relationship between topically applied CBP and orally administered betamethasone for adrenocortical suppression was examined, it was found that CBP in a topical dose of 10 gm/day was equivalent in effect to betamethasone in an oral dose of less than 0.75 mg/day. Further, CBP, 20 gm/day, was equivalent to betamethasone, 0.375–1.0 mg/day; CBP, 30 gm/day, to betamethasone, 0.75–1.0 mg/day; and CBP, 40 gm/day, to betamethasone, 0.5–0.75 mg/day.

These results suggest that excessive application of strong topical corticosteroids has much the same effect as systemic administration of small doses of corticosteroids. Topical corticosteroids and methods of application should be selected according to the severity and location of skin lesions, as well as the age of patients, to prevent the occurrence of severe adverse effects.

▶ [The authors compared 9 steroids applied topically twice daily in doses of 10–60 gm for 7 days with respect to their capacity to suppress serum cortisol levels. The results indicated that the topical steroid preparations could be divided into 3 groups of 3 steroids each: *(1)* clobetasol 17-propionate (.05%), desoximetasone ointment (0.025%), and diflorasone 17,21 diacetate ointment (0.05%) (adrenal suppression at 20 gm/day); *(2)* diflucortolone 21-valerate ointment (0.1%), budesonide ointment (0.025%), and halcinonide ointment (0.1%) (adrenal suppression at 40 gm/day but not at 20 gm/day); *(3)* beclomethasone 17,21-dipropionate ointment (0.025%), betamethasone 17-valerate ointment (0.12%), fluocinonide ointment (0.05%) (no suppression at

---

(7–4) J. Dermatol. 10:145–149, April 1983.

40–60 gm/day). The moral of the story is to choose the least potent steroid necessary to achieve the effect you are aiming for.—R.M.] ◀

7–5 **PUVA Treatment in Lymphomatoid Papulosis.** Lymphomatoid papulosis is a continuing, self-healing eruption that is clinically benign; however, histologic malignancy has been described in some patients. Psoralen and ultraviolet A (PUVA) therapy has proved to be useful in the treatment of cutaneous T-cell lymphomas. G. Lange Wantzin and K. Thomsen (Finsen Inst., Copenhagen) evaluated PUVA therapy in 5 patients who had had classic lymphomatoid papulosis for 1–13 years. All responded to PUVA therapy. Fewer lesions developed, and the duration of individual lesions declined from a range of 3–6 weeks to 1 week. One patient with the disease for 1 year had a complete remission; the other 4 patients had partial remissions. One of these had only a few lesions but continued PUVA therapy because of erythroderma. No changes in the histologic pattern were observed on sequential lesion biopsies.

Therapy with PUVA may be useful in controlling lymphomatoid papulosis. Further study is needed to determine whether PUVA therapy influences the long-term prognosis of lymphomatoid papulosis or the development of malignancy.

▶ [PUVA appeared to be an effective and useful treatment in this series of patients, resulting in both fewer and more short-lived lesions.—R.W.G.] ◀

7–6 **Dapsone Treatment of a Brown Recluse Bite.** Corticosteroids, antibiotics, antihistamines, and excision have all been used to treat the skin ulcer produced by the venom of the brown recluse spider. Lloyd E. King, Jr., and Riley S. Rees (Vanderbilt Univ.) describe a patient with a documented bite from the brown recluse spider who responded dramatically to dapsone therapy.

Man, 27, killed a spider that had bitten his right leg. An 8 × 8-cm lesion was present 24 hours later, with erythema, itching, and pain. The spider was identified as *Loxosceles reclusa.* The bite became worse despite treatment with antihistamines and dicloxacillin sodium. At 48 hours a tender, 32 × 14-cm lesion was present and showed evidence of early blister formation and incipient cutaneous necrosis. Two violaceous papules were present within the major lesion. Right inguinal adenopathy was present. The leg was elevated, ice packs were applied, and the patient was given 100 mg of dapsone orally twice a day. Pain was absent by the second day, and erythema and induration had decreased markedly. The lesion resolved completely during 2 weeks of dapsone therapy. No lesion was seen on follow-up 2 months later.

This patient probably would have developed an indolent ulcer if not treated. Dapsone is effective in skin disorders in which polymorphonuclear leukocytes are important. Drugs that inhibit polymorphonuclear leukocyte function ameliorate the effects of the venom in experimental loxoscelism. Dapsone has been shown to be effective when used to pretreat guinea pigs before intradermal injection of a spider venom fraction. The judicious use of dapsone, starting with a low dose, should help eliminate necrotic skin ulcers produced by the bite

---

(7–5) Br. J. Dermatol. 107:687–690, December 1982.
(7–6) JAMA 250:648, Aug. 5, 1983.

of the brown recluse spider, although not all patients will require such treatment.

▶ [The effectiveness of dapsone administered 48 hours after a bite seems surprising. Still, since there is no good alternative treatment for brown recluse spider bite and since at these doses dapsone has limited toxicity (except for occasional toxic epidermal necrolysis) therapy with dapsone for such bites is worth considering. Early intervention would seem essential if dapsone is to arrest the effects of a recluse spider bite.—R.S.S.] ◀

7–7 **Clinical Experience With Pimozide: Emphasis on Its Use in Postherpetic Neuralgia.** Pimozide has been shown to be effective in the treatment of delusions of parasitosis and other monosymptomatic hypochondriacal conditions. Elgin E. Duke (Ottawa) describes the clinical experience of 12 patients who were treated with the drug for a variety of conditions.

The first 2 patients had monosymptomatic hypochondriasis and benefited within weeks from pimozide therapy. The next 2 patients treated with this drug had neurotic excoriations, with lesions clearing during 1 month of therapy. The rest of the patients had postherpetic neuralgia; 3 had a positive result, 4 had a negative result, and 1 showed initial benefit lasting about 3 months. In 9 cases pimozide was initially given in doses of 2 mg twice daily. Pimozide is thought to act on central aminergic receptors. It has been shown to inhibit pituitary-releasing factors in rats.

Pimozide is contraindicated in central nervous system insufficiency, blood dyscrasias, depressive disorders, and Parkinson's disease. Its safety has not been established in pregnant women or children. Side effects include hypotension, sedation, and lowering of convulsive threshold. The main adverse effects of pimozide include extrapyramidal symptoms consisting of akathisia, dystonia, and parkinsonism.

Pimozide, which is used to treat schizophrenia, appears to benefit patients with postherpetic neuralgia who have neurotic excoriations or clinical symptoms suggestive of localized parasitosis. The drug seemed to be of limited benefit for those whose only symptom is severe pain.

▶ [A positive clinical effect of an antipsychotic agent for delusions of parasitosis and "neurotic" excoriations hardly seems surprising. This open drug trial provides little new information. Pimozide is a potent agent. Extrapyramidal side effects may be severe and persistent. If it becomes available in the United States, this drug should not be used casually.—R.S.S.] ◀

(7–7) J. Am. Acad. Dermatol. 8:845–850, June 1983.

8. Adverse Drug Reactions

8–1 **Retinoid Hyperostosis: Skeletal Toxicity Associated With Long-Term Administration of 13-*Cis*-Retinoic Acid for Refractory Ichthyosis.** Richard A. Pittsley and Frank W. Yoder (Ohio State Univ.) describe 4 of 9 consecutive patients receiving long-term 13-*cis*-retinoic acid for ichthyosis who developed an ossification disorder resembling diffuse idiopathic skeletal hyperostosis.

CASE 1.—Woman, 33, developed arthralgias 2 years after beginning treatment with 13-*cis*-retinoic acid (3 mg/kg/day) for lamellar ichthyosis. The arthralgias were relieved by temporary discontinuation of the drug. X-ray films of the spine revealed ossification in the anterior longitudinal ligament, thoracic spine, and several other areas.

CASE 2.—Man, 43, began losing extension of the cervical spine 2 years after beginning treatment with 13-*cis*-retinoic acid (3 mg/kg/day) for congenital psoriasiform ichthyosis. Rheumatic evaluation revealed a moderately advanced thoracic kyphosis. Six months after discontinuation of the drug all musculoskeletal symptoms disappeared.

CASE 3.—Man, 23, developed vague aching soreness in the neck, shoulders, and back 2 years after beginning treatment with 13-*cis*-retinoic acid for lamellar ichthyosis. X-ray films showed small, bony, spikelike projections on anterior aspects of vertebral bodies of lumbar spine.

CASE 4.—Girl, 16, presented with bilateral heel pain 6 years after beginning treatment with 13-*cis*-retinoic acid (4 mg/kg/day) for lamellar ichthyosis. X-ray films showed ossifications resembling idiopathic skeletal hyperostosis at the greater and lesser trochanters of the hip and plantar fascial insertions of the calcanei.

Irreversible skeletal toxicity may result from administration of 13-*cis*-retinoic acid. Large doses and long-term use of this synthetic retinoid and possibly others should be approached with great caution until the scope and magnitude of the ossification disorder can be defined. The authors believe retinoid hyperostosis is a distinct rheumatic disorder and speculate that patients with ichthyosis are perhaps more vulnerable to this disorder because of the need for high daily doses and long-term use of this drug.

▶ [Fortunately, 13-*cis*-retinoic acid–associated skeletal hyperostosis appears to occur principally in persons who use this drug for a substantially longer period than that required for a single therapeutic course for cystic acne. It is not established whether continuous long-term treatment alone puts patients at risk for developing this syndrome, or whether patients using multiple shorter courses of isotretinoin during an extended period may also be at risk for the development of this severe and irreversible condition. Idiopathic skeletal hyperostosis and tetratogenesis appear to be the most serious toxicities associated with the use of 13-*cis*-retinoic acid.—R.S.S.] ◀

(8–1) N. Engl. J. Med. 308:1012–1014, Apr. 28, 1983.

8–2 **Chronic Vitamin A Intoxication: Portal Hypertension Without Hepatic Cirrhosis in a Patient With Chronic Vitamin A Intoxication.** Hepatomegaly and abnormal liver function have been described in children and adults taking large amounts of vitamin A over a long period, and cirrhosis has been documented in a few instances. O. Baadsgaard and N. Holmgaard Thomsen (Copenhagen) describe a patient with chronic vitamin A intoxication and portal hypertension but without cirrhosis.

Woman, 35, had ingested 60,000 IU of vitamin A daily for about 4 years because of psoriasis. Eyelashes, brows, and axillary and pubic hair were lost, but the dose was increased to 100,000 IU/day. Alcohol abuse during a 6-month period was managed with disulfiram. Fatigue, anorexia and weight loss, brittle nails, oral fissures, conjunctivitis, and episodes of headache developed, as well as nausea and vomiting, and examination revealed ascites, hepatomegaly, and a pleural effusion. Marrow examination showed hyperplasia with active erythropoiesis and normal iron stores. Hepatic alkaline phosphatase was increased. The serum vitamin A concentration was 7.9 μmole/L. A liver biopsy specimen showed a few focal necroses, slight focal Kupffer cell proliferation, and an increased iron content. The symptoms resolved after vitamin A was discontinued and a diuretic was given. The patient was well 2 months later. Portal hypertension of the postsinusoidal type was observed at this time. Liver function was normal 6 months later, when a liver biopsy showed no pathologic changes.

Pronounced liver abnormalities did not develop in this case of chronic vitamin A intoxication, and both the clinical and the pathologic changes resolved when vitamin A ingestion was discontinued. Portal hypertension of the postsinusoidal type was present in this case, and it also resolved. The morphological liver changes induced by high-dose, long-term vitamin A intake are sometimes reversible.

▶ [Although higher doses of vitamin A can cause hepatic dysfunctions, it seems unusual for 100,000 IU of vitamin A to induce hepatic cirrhosis in an otherwise well woman. There is little evidence to suggest that vitamin A therapy at this dose level has a substantial beneficial effect on psoriasis. Its use in the face of the acute side effects described here hardly seems justified.—R.S.S.] ◀

8–3 **Skin Necrosis as Consequence of Coumadin Therapy.** Elethea H. Caldwell and Scott Stewart (Univ. of Rochester) report that skin necrosis is an unexpected consequence of Coumadin therapy, and the more common complication after use of this drug is cutaneous hemorrhage. It is essential to differentiate these 2 conditions because treatment and prognosis are different in each case.

Woman, 57, had a 1-year history of crescendo angina and hypertension. She underwent a 4-vessel coronary artery bypass procedure and was given Coumadin, 10 mg orally. On the fourth postoperative day, after receiving a total of 22.5 mg of Coumadin, the patient experienced pain and tenderness in the right breast and both hips. On the fifth postoperative day, these areas were ecchymotic with a halo of erythema (Fig 8–1). Coumadin therapy was discontinued. The lesions overlying the right and left trochanters progressed to blistering and frank skin necrosis with dry gangrene (Fig 8–2). The eschars were debrided and spontaneous healing occurred over a 5-month period.

(8–2) Dan. Med. Bull. 30:51–52, February 1983.
(8–3) Plast. Reconstr. Surg. 72:231–233, August 1983.

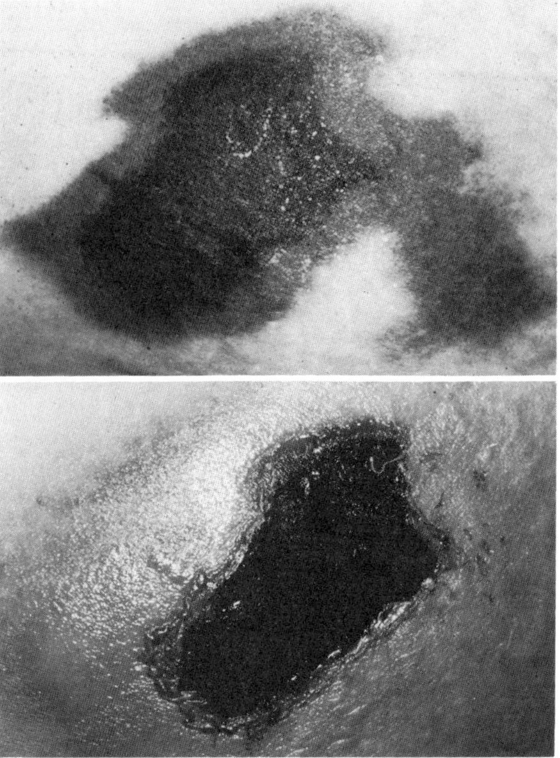

Fig 8–1 (top).—Initially, the lesions appeared ecchymotic with a halo of erythema.
Fig 8–2 (bottom).—Subsequently, the lesions progressed to skin necrosis.
(Courtesy of Caldwell, E.H., and Stewart, S.: Plast. Reconstr. Surg. 72:231–233, August 1983.)

Skin necrosis as a complication of Coumadin therapy is rare. At present, it is not possible to predict which patient will experience such an event secondary to Coumadin-congener therapy. No method of treatment has been effective.

▶ [Coumadin-induced necrosis is an infrequent, but not rare, side effect of Coumadin therapy. This case is relatively typical. Reactions typically start 3–5 days after beginning treatment with the drug. Women appear to be more frequently affected than men. Areas most often affected include the breasts, abdomen, buttocks, and flanks. Skin hemorrhage rarely gives as impressive and deep necrosis as does Coumadin necrosis. Coumadin-induced necrosis can usually be arrested with cessation of the drug. Therefore, rapid recognition of the condition is the key to therapy. A case of Coumadin-induced penile gangrene has been recently reported. (Weinberg, A., et. al.: Warfarin necrosis of the skin and subcutaneous tissue of the male external genitalia. *J. Urol.* 130:352–354, 1983.)—R.S.S.] ◀

8–4 **Repeated Occurrence of Skin Necrosis Twice Following Coumarin Intake and Subsequently During Decrease of Vitamin K–Dependent Coagulation Factors Associated With Cholestasis.** Coumarin necrosis is a rare, usually early complication of oral anti-

(8–4) Thromb. Haemost. 3:245–246, Dec. 27, 1982.

coagulation therapy, characterized by lesions in fat-abundant regions that represent thrombotic occlusion of venules and capillaries. The cause is not known. V. Hofmann and P. G. Frick (Univ. of Zurich) describe a patient who experienced two episodes of coumarin necrosis after acenocoumarol intake and a third episode, independent of oral anticoagulation therapy, during cholestasis associated with low levels of vitamin K–dependent coagulation factors.

Woman, 36, experienced left calf tenderness shortly after a therapeutic abortion at 16 weeks' gestation. Phlebography showed phlegmasia cerulea dolens, and heparin and acenocoumarol were administered after thrombectomy and fasciotomy. Severe pain developed in the right breast and left thigh during full oral anticoagulation therapy. The Quick test result was 17%. Erythematous areas and blue-black nodules appeared at the sites of pain. The lesions resolved within a few days when heparin was substituted for acenocoumarol, but necrosis developed in the right thigh after oral anticoagulation therapy was resumed. Subsequently colicky pain developed in the right upper quadrant, and the presence of gallstones was confirmed sonographically. Necrosis developed in the right breast following cholecystectomy. No traces of acenocoumarol were found in the serum. The Quick test result was now 24%. Heparin and vitamin K_1 were given for 6 days until the skin lesions resolved. The Quick test result 2 days later was 60%. The total bilirubin and alkaline phosphatase levels remained elevated for several weeks.

Three episodes of typical "coumarin necrosis" occurred in this patient within 6 months. The first two were related to intake of a coumarin derivative, but the third episode could not be attributed to drug use. The decrease in vitamin K–dependent clotting factors noted at this time was presumably related to cholestasis, fasting, and influence of antibiotic therapy on the vitamin K–producing intestinal flora. Individual hypersensitivity to decarboxylated clotting factors may be involved in coumarin necrosis and may help to explain both its possible occurrence with administration of all coumarin and indanedione derivatives and its appearance in only a few patients.

▶ [This is an interesting but not well-supported hypothesis. We have no proof that the third episode was "coumarin necrosis" rather than simply purpura associated with bleeding disorders. A biopsy and more complete clotting studies would be helpful.—R.S.S.] ◀

8–5 **Heparin-Induced Cutaneous Necrosis Unrelated to Injection Sites: Sign of Potentially Lethal Complications.** An instance of heparin skin necrosis in which development of lesions was unrelated to sites of injection is reported by Lawrence E. Levine, Joel E. Bernstein, Keyoumars Soltani, Maria M. Medenica, and Cheuk W. Yung (Univ. of Chicago).

Woman, 32, with chronic renal failure and insulin-dependent juvenile-onset diabetes, was admitted for treatment of pericarditis, hyperkalemia, fluid overload, and hypertension. Hemodialysis therapy had been instituted earlier elsewhere. The patient was given a 2,400-calorie diet and isophane insulin coverage. Elevated serum potassium concentrations returned to normal after dialysis and treatment with polystyrene sodium sulfonate. As part of dialysis

---

(8–5) Arch. Dermatol. 119:400–403, May 1983.

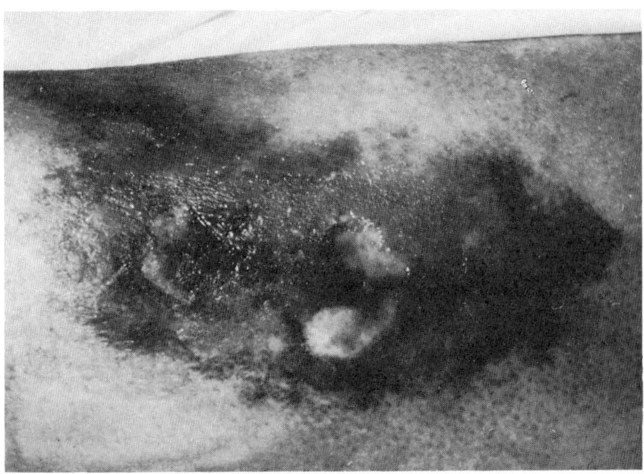

Fig 8–3.—Eroded hemorrhagic bullae on left thigh. (Courtesy of Levine, L.E., et al.: Arch. Dermatol. 119:400–403, May 1983; copyright 1983, American Medical Association.)

treatment, heparin was given for 4 hours daily in an intravenous dose ranging from 650 to 2,000 units (average, 1,200). Recurrent arteriovenous shunt failure complicated therapy and required several embolectomies. The platelet count dropped from 379,000 to 76,000/cu mm after the last shunt revision. Because of the complications, peritoneal dialysis was substituted for hemodialysis, but peritonitis developed after 11 days. To forestall thromboembolic disease, 5,000 units of heparin sodium was injected subcutaneously in the arms every 12 hours. After about 2 weeks, a tender, bullous eruption developed on the lateral surfaces of the thighs and progressed to deep-seated hemorrhagic bullae within a few days (Fig 8–3). Anticoagulation necrosis was diagnosed. Subcutaneous heparin therapy was discontinued. Warfarin had never been given. Death occurred within a few days. Autopsy demonstrated an acute myocardial infarction with extension to the right septum as the cause of death.

Skin necrosis, a rare complication of heparin therapy, has been reported in 16 patients, usually in middle-aged women; it has a predilection for heparin injection sites on the thighs, buttocks, and abdomen. Burning pain begins within 6–13 days of the start of treatment, and well-delineated necrotic lesions develop 12–24 hours thereafter. Lesions are black, with a well-defined border and a surrounding zone of erythema. Pain and erythema usually resolve within 5 days but may require debridement and grafting.

An immunologic basis has been suggested for heparin skin necrosis. In this patient, skin necrosis was preceded by thrombocytopenia and followed by myocardial infarction, an association frequently reported. Patients sensitized to heparin may produce immunoglobulins that can predispose them to necrosis, thrombocytopenia, and thromboembolic events. Diabetes, obesity, and treatment with broad-spectrum antibiotics seem to augment this potential. When necrosis or thrombocytopenia develops, heparin therapy should be discontinued and oral anticoagulation therapy considered.

8–6 **Captopril Drug Eruptions: Frequency During 1,321 Months of Treatment** was reported by F. Daniel, C. Foix, M. Barbet, A. Schwebig, F. Plouin, J. Ménard, and A. Baviera (Paris). Captopril (D-3-mercapto-2-methylpropanoyl-L-proline) is an oral angiotensin-converting enzyme inhibitor which has been found effective in most hypertensive conditions. Cutaneous manifestations are the most frequent side effects. The present study is based on a series of 123 patients followed up from December 1978 to December 1981, and it focuses on clinical aspects and triggering mechanisms.

In terms of clinical features, 3 types of cutaneous manifestations can be distinguished: *(1)* pruritus, the most frequent manifestation with 10.5%, may appear between 1 and 4 months of treatment, in most cases with a dose of 1–7 mg/kg; *(2)* rashes, reported with variable frequency (largest series, 11.3%; see table), were seen in the present study with a frequency of 2.4%, which was considered to be mainly influenced by the smaller doses administered; and *(3)* occasional cases of aphtha and pemphigoid-like manifestations.

The cutaneous eruptions triggered by captopril are characterized by a certain polymorphism; pruriginous urticarial lesions, macular, maculopapular, maculosquamous, or lichenoid forms may generally be seen. The areas of the body most frequently involved are the torso, nape of the neck, face, and upper extremities. Prognosis is favorable. The rash usually clears up within 1 week after reduction of drug dose.

The angiotensin-converting enzyme plays a hypertensive role based on a double mechanism. At the level of the kidneys it promotes the synthesis of angiotensin II, whereas on the peripheral level it aids the hydrolysis of bradykinin into inactive derivatives. Thus, the antihypertensive effect of captopril, an angiotensin-converting enzyme inhibitor, is based on this same double mechanism. The elevation of kinin levels will result in vasodilatation, augmentation of capillary permeability with diapedesis and exoserosis, and edema and perivascular infiltrates responsible in turn for the cutaneous lesions observed. The hypothesis of an immune mechanism has been proposed. Captopril may provoke modifications of intercellular substance, conferring it with antigenic properties, which results in the induction of antibodies to intercellular substance.

8–7 **Bilateral Abdominal Lipohypertrophy After Continuous Subcutaneous Infusion of Insulin.** A. Mier, J. Weerakoon, and P. Dandona (Royal Free Hosp., London) describe a patient who developed appreciable bilateral abdominal lipohypertrophy at sites of insulin infusion within 5 months of the start of treatment.

Woman, 58, was referred for stabilization of diabetes. Continuous subcutaneous infusion of insulin was begun via a battery-operated pump and resulted in excellent control of the patient's blood glucose and hemoglobin A_1 levels. During the 6 months after subcutaneous insulin infusion was begun, no episodes of hypoglycemia occurred. However, the patient noted soft, painless swellings (10 × 7 cm) at the sites of insulin infusion.

(8–6) Ann. Dermatol. Venereol. 110:441–446, 1983.
(8–7) Br. Med. J. 285:1539, Nov. 27, 1982.

CLINICAL MANIFESTATIONS OF CAPTOPRIL-INDUCED ERUPTIONS

Auteur	Année	Fréquence	Aspect clinique de l'éruption				
			Urticarienne Angio-œdème	Morbilli-formes	Maculo-papuleuse	Rash non précisé	Lichénoïde
Brunner (5)	1978	1/7				+	
Gavras (10)	1978	1/12			+ diffus		
Squibb (*)	1978	9/80		+	+		
Case (6)	1978	2/19			+		
Bravo (4)	1979	2/17		+			
Wilkin (18)	1980	7/12	4		6		
Daniel	1982	3/123	1		1		1

*Data supplied by Squibb Laboratories.
(Courtesy of Daniel, F., et al.: Ann. Dermatol. Venereol. 110:441–446, 1983.)

Subcutaneous insulin infusion is extremely useful and effective in managing insulin-dependent diabetics with recurrent hypoglycemia. Low-dose continuous delivery of insulin does not protect against development of local lipohypertrophy. Rapid development of bilateral lipohypertrophy within a short time of starting subcutaneous insulin infusion points to the extraordinary sensitivity of this patient's abdominal subcutaneous fat to insulin. The authors note the patient had not had local cutaneous lesions during the previous 30 years of insulin injection into her thigh. Presently they are investigating the sensitivity to insulin of fat from various sites in this patient.

▶ [This is an interesting observation. It would not be surprising to find some metabolic differences between abdominal fat and thigh fat. The abdominal fat deposits are more labile, on the basis of simple gross observations, than fat in the extremities, and I would assume this implies some sort of chemical difference. In addition, major functions of insulin lie in the conversion of glucose to long-chain fatty acids and their esterification to triglycerides. Furthermore, insulin has an inhibitory effect on lipolysis. Therefore, one might assume that the slow continuous infusion of insulin produces a continuous high concentration of insulin in a localized site and that this state leads to a rather continuous synthesis of fat and inhibition of lipolysis. The net result would be lipohypertrophy.—R.M.] ◀

8–8 **Hepatic Reactions During Ketoconazole Treatment,** both silent and symptomatic, are reviewed by Paul A. J. Janssen and Jan E. Symoens (Janssen Pharmaceutica Beerse, Belgium). Silent hepatic reactions were investigated in 1,074 patients with various deep and superficial mycoses who had been treated with daily doses of ketoconazole (usually 200 mg) for as long as 15 months. Liver enzyme data were screened for elevations of 50% above the upper limit of normal range of serum glutamic oxaloacetic transaminase, serum glutamic pyruvic transaminase, γ-glutamyl transferase, alkaline phosphatase, or more than one of these before or during ketoconazole treatment. Elevations were found in 148 (14%) patients. Enzyme elevations had preceded treatment in 8% of patients. Levels increased during treat-

SYMPTOMATIC CASES REPORTED

Country	Total Reported	Icteric Reaction	Anicteric Reaction
United States	14	13	1
United Kingdom	6	5	1
Sweden	2	1	1
Japan	2	0	2
Netherlands	2	2	0
Denmark	2	2	0
Switzerland	1	1	0
Germany	1	0	1
Columbia	1	1	0
Total	31	25	6

(Courtesy of Janssen, P.A.J., and Symoens, J.E.: Am. J. Med. 75:80–85, Jan. 24, 1983.)

(8–8) Am. J. Med. 75:80–85, Jan. 24, 1983.

ment and dropped below pretreatment values toward the end of treatment. Transient liver enzyme elevations during treatment often paralleled healing of the fungal disease.

Estimated prevalence of symptomatic hepatic reactions during ketoconazole treatment was 1/12,000 (table). Hepatic reactions were classified as icteric (jaundice, dark urine, or pale stools) or anicteric (fever, fatigue, weakness, malaise, anorexia, nausea, or vomiting). Patients with onychomycosis may be more prone to develop symptomatic reactions to ketoconazole than patients with other mycoses. Median time of onset of icteric reactions was 6 weeks; it was 11 weeks for anicteric reactions. A history of hepatitis or drug idiosyncrasy and previous treatment with griseofulvin may predispose patients to symptomatic reactions.

If symptoms of a hepatic disorder are detected in a patient during ketoconazole treatment, medications should be discontinued promptly. Delayed recognition and inadequate follow-up probably led to the two deaths reported in this series.

▶ [Written by one of the manufacturer's executives, this study provides relatively imprecise information about ketoconazole's hepatotoxic risk. The 1,074 patients who received laboratory tests were treated for a myriad of conditions and varying time periods. No mention is made of the use of a central laboratory or fixed intervals for retesting. Therefore, relatively little can be said from these data. The 31 cases with icteric signs or anicteric symptoms were ascertained through spontaneous reports. Given the relatively low proportion of adverse reactions that are reported, the author's estimate of an incidence of 1 per 10,000 patients is probably a substantial underestimate, especially for patients such as those with onychomycosis, who receive prolonged ketoconazole therapy. Given its potential toxicity, ketoconazole is rarely indicated in the prolonged treatment of onychomycosis. Any therapeutic advantage over griseofulvin is not well established. Ketoconazole's cost and risks are certainly higher than those of griseofulvin or of topical agents.—R.S.S.] ◀

8–9 **Review and Controlled Study of Cutaneous Conditions Associated With Lithium Carbonate.** Lithium has been the subject of numerous studies of side effects (table). Dimocritos Sarantidis and Brent Waters (Royal Ottawa Hosp., Ottawa) compared the occurrence of a variety of cutaneous states in 91 patients treated with lithium carbonate and 44 given other nonneuroleptic maintenance medications for affective disorder or anxiety. The lithium-treated patients had unipolar or bipolar manic-depressive disorder, and the controls received either minor tranquilizers or tricyclic antidepressants, or both, for anxiety.

Thirty-one of the 91 lithium-treated patients reported a cutaneous condition possibly secondary to lithium therapy, compared with 6 possible treatment-related disorders in the control group. An acneiform eruption was seen in 10 lithium-treated patients and 2 controls. Two lithium-treated patients had psoriasis possibly related to lithium. Three others had atopic dermatitis, 1 had seborrheic dermatitis, and 1 had exfoliative dermatitis. Two patients had alopecia areata. The study patients had received lithium for a mean of 52 months, whereas the controls had received their medications for a mean of only 18

(8–9) Br. J. Psychiatry 143:42–50, July 1983.

CUTANEOUS CONDITIONS SECONDARY TO LITHIUM REPORTED IN THE LITERATURE

	Number of cases	Relation to lithium			Sex		
		New condition	Exacerbated	Not ascertained	Male	Female	Not ascertained
Psoriasis	28	15	13	—	17	11	—
Acne and acneiform eruptions	17	5	2	10	4	8	5
Other dematoses							
Alopceia	2	—	1	1	—	1	1
Exfoliative dermatitis	1	—	—	1	1	—	—
Maculopapular rash	7	5	—	2	4	2	1
Ulcer	3	2	1	—	3	—	—
Folliculitis	12	12	—	—	2	10	—
Stomatitis	1	1	—	—	1	—	—
Ichthyosis	1	—	—	1	—	1	—
Xerosis	1	1	—	—	—	1	—
Eczema	1	—	—	1	—	—	1
Dematitis herpetiformis	1	—	—	1	—	1	—
Pruritus	2	—	—	2	—	1	1
Unspecified eruption	10	—	—	10	—	—	10
Total	87	41	17	29	32	36	19

(Courtesy of Sarantidis, D., and Waters, B.: Br. J. Psychiatry 143:42–50, July 1983.)

months. More of the patients with secondary cutaneous disorders were female, had a history of allergies, and had had cutaneous reactions to other medications. There was no significant sex difference in latency between the start of lithium or other medication and the onset or worsening of a secondary cutaneous condition.

Women may be particularly disposed to develop secondary cutaneous disorders when receiving lithium therapy. Presumably some nonspecific mechanism activates different cutaneous disorders at different stages of the life cycle. Lithium-induced inhibition of adenylate cyclase–cyclic adenosine monophosphate systems is a possibility. A controlled prospective study of the cutaneous disorders associated with long-term lithium therapy is warranted.

▶ [That lithium can exacerbate underlying dermatologic diseases including psoriasis and acne and cause exfoliative erythroderma either as a result of exacerbating an underlying skin disorder or by inducing a hypersensitivity reaction is unquestioned. The relation to eczema, alopecia areata, and seborrheic dermatitis (if not just a forme fruste of psoriasis) is less well established. The authors argue that suggestability may explain the higher frequency of lithium cutaneous side effects among females. This study provides few new data. It is not surprising that persons with other risk factors for a skin disease are most likely to develop that condition when exposed to lithium.—R.S.S.] ◀

8–10 **Fatal Polymyositis in D-Penicillamine-Treated Rheumatoid Arthritis.** Deborah R. Doyle, Thomas L. McCurley, and John S. Sergent (Vanderbilt Univ.) describe a patient who developed polymyositis with predominant clinical and pathologic cardiac involvement while receiving penicillamine therapy and who died.

Woman, 59, developed seropositive rheumatoid arthritis and was treated

(8–10) Ann. Intern. Med. 98:327–330, March 1983.

with gold, which was discontinued. She then received D-penicillamine, 250 mg/day. One month later, profound weakness with myalgias, nausea, and diarrhea developed. The ECG showed complete heart block with idioventricular rhythms. The hospital course was characterized by progressively severe cardiac arrhythmias and renal failure. Despite vigorous medical management, the patient died on the seventh hospital day of intractable ventricular tachycardia. D-Penicillamine had been discontinued 2 days before death. Postmortem examination of the right and left ventricles showed widespread muscle necrosis. Skeletal muscle showed widely scattered foci of degenerating fibers.

Thirteen other cases of polymyositis-dermatomyositis associated with D-penicillamine therapy have been reported. Eleven patients were being treated for seropositive rheumatoid arthritis, 1 for progressive systemic sclerosis, and 1 for Wilson's disease. Dosages of D-penicillamine ranged from 250 to 1,200 mg/day. Duration of therapy ranged from 3 days to 2 years. Two patients had clinical cardiac involvement: 1 had S4 gallop and mild arrhythmia, and the other died of cardiac complications 3 days after beginning D-penicillamine therapy.

The temporal association of D-penicillamine therapy with onset of polymyositis-dermatomyositis was strong enough in all instances reviewed to suggest a causal relation. D-Penicillamine has an important place in the treatment of rheumatoid arthritis, but its toxicity severely limits its use. Treated patients must be monitored closely for development of rash, nephritis, hematologic disorders, and other less common toxicities, including dysphagia and muscle weakness.

▶ [Penicillamine is a potent agent with potentially serious side effects. In addition to the adverse effects described in this report, thrombotic thrombocytopenia, purpura, pemphigus, a lupuslike illness, myasthenia gravis, nephropathy, eosinophilia, and necrotizing vasculitis have all been described in association with this drug's use.—R.S.S.] ◀

8–11 **Zomepirac-Induced Serum Sickness: Report of Two Cases.** Reza Kiani and Mark Kushner (Univ. of Illinois, Chicago) describe two patients who had serum sickness associated with the use of zomepirac sodium.

CASE 1.—Man, 57, developed low-grade fever, rhinitis, and mild, nonproductive cough, as well as generalized pruritic rash and burning sensation of tongue and hands. He had a history of anaphylactic reaction to penicillin, hypertension for 8 years, and long-standing osteoarthritis. Two months before admission he began taking zomepirac sodium (100 mg, 4 times per day) for arthritic pain. The extremities revealed tenderness of all joints to palpation, with swelling of wrists and fingers. Laboratory studies showed eosinophilia. A chest roentgenogram showed bilateral platelike atelectasis and hilar fullness. Use of zomepirac was discontinued. Biopsy of a right cervical lymph node showed reactive hyperplasia. Four weeks after discharge, the patient was asymptomatic.

CASE 2.—Man, 32, experienced patchy pruritic rash on the extremities and low-grade fever 3 months after beginning to use zomepirac (100 mg, 1 to 3 times per day) for back pain. He had tenderness of multiple symmetric joints to palpa-

---

(8–11) JAMA 249:2812–2813, May 27, 1983.

tion and palpable, nontender anterior and posterior lymph nodes. Results of laboratory tests were generally normal. Zomepirac therapy was discontinued on admission, and 3 weeks after discharge the patient was asymptomatic.

These two patients exhibited signs and symptoms of a multisystem disease process with acute toxic eruption, fever, lymphadenopathy, arthralgias, angioedema of hands and feet, and eosinophilia—all of which are consistent with a type 3 allergic reaction. Laboratory investigation failed to demonstrate an infectious cause for their symptoms.

▶ [The diagnosis of serum sickness in these patients must be questioned. The time course (2–3 months) for the development of symptoms in these two patients is longer than the usual 2–3 weeks for developing serum sickness. Hepatitis or nephritis frequently accompanies serum sickness, and only equivocal findings in one of these patients support involvement of either organ. Other nonsteroidal anti-inflammatory agents that have been described as causing a serum sickness include sulindac and naproxen. Anaphylaxis remains the most important and most frequent side effect of zomepirac acids. Because of anaphylactic reactions, this drug is no longer available in the United States.—R.S.S.] ◀

8–12 **Seborrheic Dermatitis in Neuroleptic-Induced Parkinsonism.** Renee L. Binder and Frank J. Jonelis (San Francisco) note that an increased prevalence of seborrheic dermatitis has been reported in patients with idiopathic Parkinson's disease or postencephalitic parkinsonism. Eighty-nine patients were studied to determine whether neuroleptic-induced Parkinson's disease is also associated with an increased prevalence of seborrheic dermatitis. The patients were divided into 2 groups, 42 patients with and 47 without parkinsonian symptoms. Those with symptoms had a median age of 31.5 years, and those without symptoms, 30 years. The sex ratio in the symptomatic group was 4 men to 1 woman; in the group without symptoms, it was 3 men to 1 woman.

The 2 groups differed in type of neuroleptic drug prescribed and in use of antiparkinsonian agents. More symptomatic patients received haloperidol and more patients without symptoms received chlorpromazine and thioridazine hydrochloride. Of the symptomatic group, 57% received antiparkinsonian agents, as did only 15% of those without symptoms. Of the 42 patients with parkinsonian symptoms, 25 (59.5%) had seborrheic dermatitis, whereas only 7 (15%) of the 47 patients without parkinsonian symptoms had seborrheic dermatitis.

Thus, a strong association was found between neuroleptic-induced parkinsonism and the prevalence of seborrheic dermatitis. The cause of seborrheic dermatitis is unknown, and the reason for its association with postencephalitic, idiopathic, and neuroleptic-induced parkinsonism is also unknown.

▶ [This is an interesting observation showing an increase in seborrheic dermatitis in drug-induced parkinsonism in hospitalized patients. No mechanism is known for seborrheic dermatitis in association with parkinsonism of whatever etiology.—R.M.] ◀

8–13 **Injectable Collagen Implants.** Injectable collagen implants have been a major aid to the management of soft-tissue deformities, partic-

---

(8–12) Arch. Dermatol. 119:473–475, June 1983.
(8–13) Ibid., pp. 533–534.

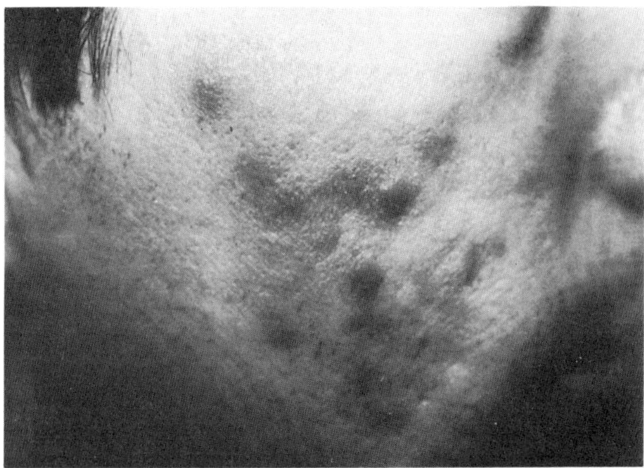

Fig 8–4.—Erythematous nodules at collagen implant injection sites on cheeks 2 weeks after second series of injections. (Courtesy of Hanke, D.W., and Robinson, J.K.: Arch. Dermatol. 119:533–534, June 1983.)

ularly postacne scars and wrinkle lines in older patients. Skin testing, however, will not always identify patients who are hypersensitive to these implants. C. William Hanke and June K. Robinson (Northwestern Univ.) report data on 2 patients who had positive responses to collagen implant skin tests and 2 others who became sensitized to implants in the course of treatment.

Man, 25, with wide-based postacne scars on both cheeks, had a negative collagen implant skin test on the forearm at 2 and 4 weeks and had a total of 2 ml of implant injected into the scars 4 weeks after skin testing and again 4 weeks later. Cystic nodules appeared at injection sites 2 weeks later (Fig 8–4). There were no systemic symptoms, and the initial skin test site remained unreactive. There was no personal or family history of connective tissue disease. The facial nodules resolved after 10 weeks. Laboratory studies including antinuclear antibody and latex tests were negative.

Patients may be so eager to have collagen implant therapy that they conceal a family history of connective tissue disease. Patients with questionable skin test responses should be retested at a different site before treatment is instituted. It is possible that patients with a negative history and negative skin test will nevertheless become sensitized to collagen implant during treatment. Nodular reactions may resolve spontaneously; further implant therapy is contraindicated. Necrobiotic granulomas unresponsive to topical steroid have been described at test implant sites.

▶ [This is one of the earlier articles published on adverse reactions to Zyderm. Two previous reports have described granulomatous reactions at the skin test site (Brooks, N. J.: *Dermatol. Surg. Oncol.* 8:111–114, 1982; Barr, R., et al.: *J. Am. Acad. Dermatol.* 6:867–869, 1982). Approximately 3% of patients undergoing skin testing with Zyderm will have a positive reaction. Of those with negative skin patch tests, an additional 1.3% will have adverse reactions. (Cooperman, L., Michaeli, D.: *J. Am. Acad. Dermatol.* 10:638–646, 1984). These adverse reactions are grouped into 4 categories: *(1)* herpes infection; *(2)* bacterial infection; *(3)* localized immune reaction (erythema, induration, and/or urticaria); *(4)* overlooked positive patch test, i.e., slight erythema for 1–2 days. All localized immune reactions thus far have resolved. Of note are the anti-implant collagen antibodies that have been detected in individuals with localized responses at implant sites. These antibodies did not cross-react with human dermal collagen, nor did they result in elevated levels of circulating immune complexes in the two patients tested (*J. Am. Acad. Dermatol.* 10:638–646, 1984).—R.R.] ◀

9. Fungal Infections

9-1 ***Trichophyton mentagrophytes* Granulomas: Unique Systemic Dissemination to Lymph Nodes, Testes, Vertebrae, and Brain.** Masaki Hironaga, Naoki Okazaki, Koji Saito, and Shohei Watanabe describe findings in a patient with *Trichophyton mentagrophytes* infection that ultimately involved the lymph nodes, testes, vertebrae, and central nervous system.

Man, 43, had contracted at age 6 years a dermatophyte skin infection, first affecting the feet and subsequently the toenails. The skin lesions gradually became generalized and persistent. In February 1971, a diffuse, edematous swelling developed on the patient's right leg; in May 1971, numerous cutaneous nodules of various sizes appeared on the right thigh. In November 1971, upon the patient's hospitalization, annular scaly plaques were observed scattered on the face, neck, trunk, groin, and lower extremities. The inguinal and femoral lymph nodes were notably enlarged and confluent bilaterally. There was a strong immediate hypersensitivity reaction to a skin test with *T. mentagrophytes* antigen. The patient could not be sensitized to dinitrochlorobenzene.

Histologic examination disclosed a well-delineated, granulomatous infiltration with central suppuration and necrosis throughout the entire dermis. The epidermis was flattened and thinned over the greater part of the affected area. Regional lymph nodes were abnormal. The right testis, later removed at surgery after enlargement, was a cavity of necrotic material. The third to fifth lumbar vertebrae showed several suppurative lesions of the bone. Cerebral and cerebellar abscesses, which developed during the patient's terminal course, had histologically well-delineated borders and showed softening necrosis. The patient's mycologic isolates were most compatible with *T. mentagrophytes interdigitale.*

The patient was consistently anergic to delayed intradermal skin testing with purified protein derivative and trichophytin; lymphocytes cultured only in homologous or in autologous plasma never responded to trichophytin. No decreased phagocytosis by mononuclear leukocytes was observed. The serum IgE level was increased, but serum transferrin levels were persistently abnormal. Therapeutic attempts, including systemic administration of griseofulvin, amphotericin B, clotrimazole, and transfer factor failed. The patient died 5 years after onset of systemic disease.

▶ [This is a very unusual report of a fatal disseminated *T. mentagrophytes* infection in a patient with an abnormal, unspecified immunologic response. Normally, in naturally-induced human infections as well as in experimentally-induced *T. mentagrophytes* infections in animals, a delayed hypersensitivity reaction occurs which parallels inhibition of fungal growth. It is conceivable that chronic antigen excess in this patient might have overwhelmed his immunologic responsiveness, allowing the fungus to grow unchecked. This must be a very rare occurrence with this species of dermatophytes.—E.G.] ◀

(9–1) Arch. Dermatol. 119:482–490, June 1983.

9–2 **Epidemic of Infection With *Trichophyton tonsurans* Revealed in a 20-Year Survey of Fungal Infections in Chicago** is reported by Darryl M. Bronson, Dina R. Desai, Sidney Barsky, and Shirley McMillen Foley (Cook County Hosp., Chicago). *Trichophyton tonsurans* has long been recognized as an important, though previously uncommon, cause of tinea capitis in the United States. It was introduced into the Southwest from Mexico in the 1950s and has replaced *Microsporum audouini* as the causative agent in current epidemics of tinea capitis in many parts of the United States. Infection of the glabrous skin by *T. tonsurans* is less well known. The authors have noticed an increase in the number of cases of tinea corporis due to this fungus in Chicago in recent years. *T. tonsurans* was associated with an increasing proportion of cases of both tinea capitis and tinea corporis in the past 2 decades (table). The incidences of both types of infection have increased dramatically since 1977.

From 1978 to 1980, *T. tonsurans* was isolated from 96% of cases of tinea capitis and 75% of cases of tinea corporis at the authors' hospital. Six patients had concomitant infection of the scalp and glabrous skin. Only 11 of the 207 cases of tinea capitis occurred in adults. More than half the cases were clinically inflammatory, in the forms of kerion and folliculitis. Most cases of tinea corporis occurred in adults, and women predominated heavily. Many of the lesions showed marked inflammation, resembling infection caused by zoophilic species such as *Microsporum canis*. Infection of the hands, feet, groin, and nails by *T. tonsurans* resembled that caused by other species of *Trichophyton*.

Attempts should be made to identify a scalp source whenever tinea corporis caused by *T. tonsurans* is discovered. Persistent infection remains a possibility until the last focus of infection in a school or household has been treated.

▶ [Some epidemiologic facts may account for this phenomenon. Whereas 30 years ago the predominant cause of tinea capitis in children was the genus *Microsporum*, in recent years *T. tonsurans* accounts for more than 90% of all hair infections (*Pediatrics* 72:625, 1983). *Microsporum* infections were easily detectable by the organisms' fluorescence with Wood's lamp and were characterized by spontaneous resolution at puberty. On the other hand, *T. tonsurans* can have protean clinical presentations, do not fluoresce, and induce chronic infection which can continue past adolescence.

	Percentage (Number) of Cases Due to *T. tonsurans*			
Type of infection	**1961-1965**	**1966-1970**	**1971-1975**	**1976-1980**
Tinea capitis	45% (39)	59% (39)	81% (68)	96% (260)
Tinea corporis	15% (8)	32% (11)	74% (23)	76% (117)
Tinea cruris	(0)	(0)	(0)	6% (4)
Tinea manus	(0)	(0)	75% (3)	33% (5)
Tinea pedis	(0)	2% (1)	2% (1)	12% (12)
Tinea unguium	(0)	(0)	(0)	14% (6)

(Courtesy of Bronson, D.M., et al.: J. Am. Acad. Dermatol. 8:322–330, March 1983.)

(9–2) J. Am. Acad. Dermatol. 8:322–330, March 1983.

Hence, infectivity is much higher, causing frequent epidemics of *T. tonsurans* infection of the scalp in school children. Furthermore, according to this epidemiologic study, this fungus has also become the predominant causative agent for tinea corporis in Chicago, especially in adult females, suggesting that the source is the hair of infected children.

Allen et al. (*Pediatrics* 69:81, 1982) demonstrated that the use of selenium sulfide lotion 2.5% as an adjunctive therapy for tinea capitis produced by *T. tonsurans* decreased the duration of positive fungal cultures and reduced infectivity. If selenium sulfide proves to be safe and effective, it might turn around this increasing public health problem.—E.G.] ◀

9–3 **Tinea Capitis in Brooklyn.** Teresita A. Laude, Binita R. Shah, and Yelva Lynfield (Kings County Hosp., Brooklyn, New York) studied data on 144 clinically diagnosed cases of tinea capitis (a disease of children occurring throughout the United States) within a 12-month period. Subjects were divided into 5 groups according to the kind of tinea capitis and the type of treatment: (1) inflammatory, treated with griseofulvin alone; (2) inflammatory, treated with griseofulvin and erythromycin; (3) noninflammatory, treated with griseofulvin alone; (4) noninflammatory, treated with griseofulvin and topical antifungal agents; and (5) inflammatory, treated with griseofulvin and prednisone.

Ninety-six (67%) of the children had positive fungal cultures. In 91 the cultures were positive on the first attempt. In 85 patients the disease was caused by *Trichophyton tonsurans,* and in 11 the cause was *Microsporum* organisms. Twenty-two of 49 bacterial cultures were positive; 15 were positive for *Staphylococcus aureus*. Forty-nine (51%) of the patients with positive cultures were boys, and 47 (49%) were girls; 95 of the 96 children were black and 1 was Hispanic. Peak incidence was at age 4 to 5 years. Seventeen children had 1 affected sibling also enrolled in the study. Animal exposure was also reported. Of the 96 culture-proved cases, 38 (40%) were clinically inflammatory (kerions) and 58 (60%) were not. Marked cervical lymphadenopathic conditions were seen in 53 cases.

Mycologic and clinical cure was obtained after a mean of 4.7 weeks of griseofulvin therapy. Neither systemic erythromycin, topical antifungal agents, nor systemic prednisone resulted in earlier eradication. Prednisone did cause the inflammation of the kerions to subside dramatically. Use of topical antifungal agents may be indicated, however, to prevent spread of the infection to others.

▶ [This article stresses the predominance of *T. tonsurans* as the major etiologic agent in tinea capitis and the responsiveness of the disease to oral griseofulvin. Adjunctive topical agents with haloprogin and tolnaftate were not effective in reducing duration of systemic treatment. Allen et al. (*Pediatrics* 69:81, 1982), however, showed that selenium sulfide lotion 2.5% was a good adjunctive agent to reduce infectivity with *T. tonsurans*.—E.G.] ◀

9–4 **Class-Specific Antibodies in Young and Aged Humans Against Organisms Producing Superficial Fungal Infections.** P. G. Sohnle, C. Collins-Lech, and K. E. Huhta (Milwaukee) measured

(9–3) Am. J. Dis. Child. 136:1047–1050, December 1982.
(9–4) Br. J. Dermatol. 108:69–76, January 1983.

class-specific antibodies (IgG, IgA, and IgM) to *Candida albicans, Pityrosporum orbiculare,* and *Trichophyton rubrum* in 21 young persons (aged 23–44) and 20 elderly persons (aged 70–88) who did not have a history of significant superficial fungal infections.

Antibody to all 3 organisms was present in all individuals in both groups. Except for a reduced level of IgM antibody to *P. orbiculare,* humoral responses in the elderly were similar to those in the younger group. Further, IgA antibody to *C. albicans* was present in higher amounts than IgA antibody to *P. orbiculare* or *T. rubrum* in both groups, and the proportion of IgM antibody to *T. rubrum* was higher than that to the other 2 organisms.

The findings demonstrate that normal persons, both elderly and young, have detectable antibody to 3 organisms that produce superficial fungal infections. The mechanism by which normal individuals become sensitized to these 3 organisms is unclear. These findings suggest that the ecology of these 3 organisms with respect to the normal human host may be reflected in the serologic responses to them.

▶ [This study should have included determination of class-specific antibodies to a zoophilic fungus such as *Microsporum canis,* since subclinical infections with the anthrophilic *T. rubrum* are common and the antibody levels might reflect such an infection. Zoophilic fungal infections, on the other hand, usually produce a brisk and noticeable inflammatory reaction the occurrence of which the patient usually remembers.—E.G.] ◀

9–5 **Antifungal Activity of *Pseudomonas aeruginosa* in Gram-Negative Athlete's Foot.** "Gram-negative athlete's foot," characterized by the presence of *Pseudomonas aeruginosa* and the absence of dermatophytes, has been described as the most severe form of intertriginous infection. The lesions are painful and disabling. It has been suggested that fungi are absent because of the production of an inhibitory substance by *P. aeruginosa.* Carl Abramson and Richard Steinmetz (Pennsylvania College of Podiatric Medicine, Philadelphia) obtained in vitro evidence of a partially purified extracellular diffusible product of *P. aeruginosa* that selectively inhibits dermatophytes, specifically *Trichophyton rubrum.* The factor was purified by ammonium sulfate salt fractionation and column chromatography from the supernatant of a broth culture of *P. aeruginosa* isolated from a patient with severely symptomatic athlete's foot. Diffusion of the antifungal factor in agar gel resulted in large zones of inhibition of *Trichophyton rubrum.*

The antifungal factor produced by *P. aeruginosa* may explain why the recovery of fungi decreases as the infection that is secondary to classic tinea pedis progresses and the fungal flora is replaced by gram-negative bacilli. The factor isolated also inhibits the growth of *Trichophyton mentagrophytes, Microsporum gypseum,* and *Microsporum audouini.* The patient receives a clinical diagnosis of tinea pedis, but laboratory culture and potassium hydroxide studies show no fungus.

▶ [This competitive inhibition has also been demonstrated between diphtheroids like

(9–5) J. Am. Podiatry Assoc. 73:227–234, May 1983.

Brevibacterium species and dermatophytes where the diphtheroid produces a gas, methane-thiol, which is toxic for superficial fungi. This phenomenon explains why obtaining positive KOH mounts and cultures from superinfected tinea pedis is so difficult until antibiotic therapy eradicates the concomitant bacterial infection.—E.G.] ◀

9–6 **Ketoconazole Compared With Griseofulvin in Dermatophytoses: Randomized, Double-Blind Trial.** The imidazoles have made a large contribution to the treatment of superficial and deep mycoses. Ketoconazole is an orally effective agent against both systemic mycoses and chronic, treatment-resistant superficial mycoses. I. Stratigos, N. P. Zissis, A. Katsambas, E. Koumentaki, M. Michalopoulos, and A. Flemetakis (Univ. of Athens) compared the effects of ketoconazole with those of griseofulvin in a double-blind, prospective trial in 50 patients with symptomatic dermatophytosis who either had failed to respond to previous treatment or had extensive lesions unsuitable for local treatment. Patients were given either 200 mg of ketoconazole or 500 mg of griseofulvin daily. Twenty-six patients of both sexes with a mean age of 31 years received ketoconazole, and 24 with a mean age of 32.5 years received griseofulvin. Women of childbearing age without adequate contraception and patients with onychomycosis were excluded from the study. Treatment was continued for 6 weeks or until cultures were negative.

All ketoconazole-treated patients were cured after a median of 2½ weeks, as were 92% of the griseofulvin-treated patients. At 3 weeks, 88.5% of the ketoconazole group and 67% of the griseofulvin group had negative cultures. Differences in therapeutic efficacy between the two drugs were not significant at any interval. One patient in each group returned within 3 months of the end of treatment with symptoms of dermatophytosis and positive cultures. No adverse effects of treatment occurred in either group.

Ketoconazole was at least as effective as griseofulvin in these patients with extensive or treatment-resistant dermatophytoses, and its effects were achieved more rapidly. Ketoconazole has been reported to be effective in patients with severe, extensive *Trichophyton rubrum* infection and in griseofulvin-resistant patients.

▶ [Griseofulvin continues to be the oral treatment of choice for uncomplicated, extensive dermatophyte infections not responsive to topical antifungal agents. The development of griseofulvin-resistant strains has been reported recently, but these cases are rare and, unless identified, do not justify the use of ketoconazole as the first line of therapy. Furthermore, dermatophytosis is still not considered an indication for the use of ketoconazole according to the package insert.—E.G.] ◀

9–7 **Extracutaneous Sporotrichosis** has been reported in only 0.02% of patients infected with *Sporothrix schenckii.* Stephen J. Friedman and John A. Doyle (Mayo Clinic and Found.) reviewed the records of 58 patients with sporotrichosis, a fungal disease most commonly characterized by superficial cutaneous nodules along the lines of lymphatic drainage of limbs. Eleven of these patients had extracutaneous

---

(9–6) Dermatologica 166:161–164, 1983.
(9–7) Int. J. Dermatol. 22:171–176, April 1983.

involvement. This higher incidence is explained by the fact that the Mayo Clinic is a referral center.

Chronic pain and swelling of the knee, ankle, wrist, and elbow was common. Cultures of synovial fluid and tissue were positive for sporotrichosis in most joints tested. The erythrocyte sedimentation rate was elevated in all patients, averaging 60 mm in 1 hour. Chronic granulomatous synovitis was present in 8 patients with arthritis. One patient with multifocal systemic sporotrichosis had organisms in nasal and skin lesions identified by periodic acid–Schiff (PAS)-diastase preparation (Figs 9–1 and 9–2).

Extracutaneous sporotrichosis is seen predominantly in men aged 50 years or older and may be related to outdoor occupations. It rarely follows cutaneous inoculation but is acquired by inhalation with subsequent hematogenous dissemination.

Woman, 54, had a nonproductive cough. A chest x-ray film revealed an interstitial infiltrate in both lower lung fields. No skin lesions were present. Later, granulomatous lesions developed on the skin, nasal septum, and subglottic area that were culture-positive for *S. schenckii.*

The 11 patients initially had many different clinical manifestations that mimicked other serious diseases. This variability contributed to the average time of 17 months from onset of symptoms to diagnosis. Culture of the fungus is necessary for confirmation of the diagnosis. The agglutination and precipitation tests are useful, and no false-positive tests occurred in this study.

Systemic sporotrichosis has been observed in patients with a com-

Fig 9–1 (left).—Giant cell in dermis filled with *S. schenckii (arrow)*. PAS-diastase; original magnification ×100.

Fig 9–2 (right).—Cigar-shaped bodies *(arrow)* and budding organisms *(arrow)*. PAS-diastase; original magnification ×250.

(Courtesy of Friedman, S.J., and Doyle, J.A.: Int. J. Dermatol. 22:171–176, April 1983.)

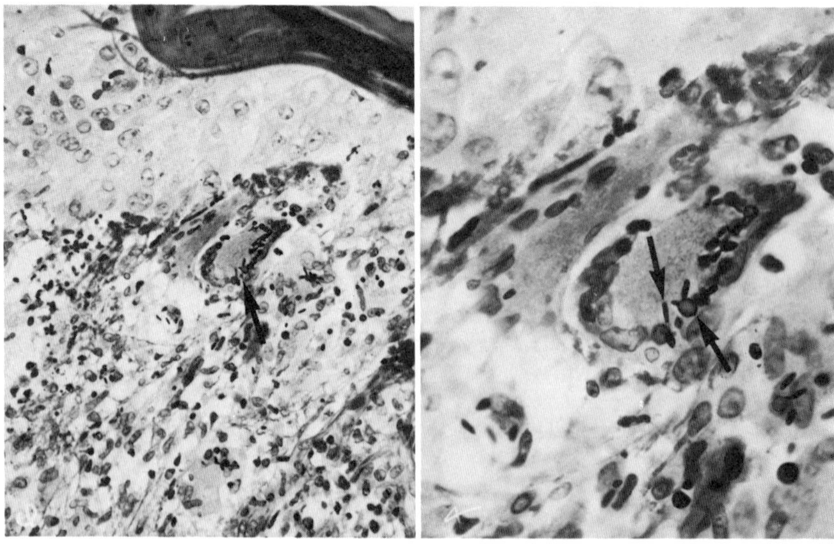

promised immune system, specifically as a result of lymphoreticular disease, corticosteroid therapy, carcinoma, or diabetes. Patients with cutaneous sporotrichosis have had normal cell-mediated immunity, whereas patients with systemic disease have had significant abnormalities.

Iodide therapy, effective in cutaneous sporotrichosis, is seldom successful in extracutaneous sporotrichosis, although results have been better when iodide therapy was accompanied by surgical debridement of a joint. Amphotericin B is the most effective drug for disseminated sporotrichosis, a systemic infection with life-threatening consequences.

▶ [The authors stress some important features of extracutaneous sporotrichosis that should be remembered. The source of the infection in some of these cases was respiratory, which is considered very rare. Most of the cases of dissemination occur from the skin or nodes via hematogenous spread. Even in the famous "epidemic" reported in 1947 in which 3,000 men were infected with contaminated timbers in gold mines near Johannesburg, no evidence of respiratory infections was demonstrated. The second feature is the protean manifestations that make diagnosis so difficult. Third is the reliance on serologic tests rather than cultures to establish a definite diagnosis, and fourth is the lack of response to a supersaturated solution of potassium iodide. The effectiveness of ketoconazole on this form of sporotrichosis remains to be determined, but preliminary studies don't show any advantage over amphotericin B.—E.G.] ◀

9–8 **Sporotrichosis Acquired From a Cat** is reported by Bernard P. Nusbaum, Nita Gulbas, and Stephen N. Horwitz. Two veterinary assistants who handled the same infected cat developed cutaneous sporotrichosis. The cat had ulcerated, draining cutaneous abscesses on the extremities, tail base, and head. Methylene blue staining of exudate from an abscess showed macrophages containing round, yeast-like organisms resembling *Histoplasma capsulatum,* and a culture grew colonies of *Sporothrix schenckii.* The cat was unresponsive to orally adminsitered sodium iodide and was killed. Biopsy specimens from skin lesions and lymph nodes identified the organisms as *S. schenckii.*

One week after being scratched by the cat, 1 veterinary assistant developed painful redness and swelling of the left hand that spread to the arm, and several nodules developed. Three weeks later, there was a red, scaly plaque, 1.5 cm in diameter, on the thumb, with an overlying yellowish crust. Red, pea-sized nodules were present in a linear arrangement from wrist to axilla. Microscopic examination of a punch biopsy specimen from the plaque revealed branched hyphae with conidia in a rosette arrangement characteristic of *S. schenckii.* Treatment with a solution of potassium iodide (90 drops per day) resulted in healing of the lesions within 3 months.

The second assistant had held the same cat without gloves several times against her clothed abdomen and 2 weeks later developed an abdominal papule that had grown into a 5-cm, ulcerated plaque a month later. Fungal culture of the ulcerated exudate grew colonies of *S. schenckii.* Oral potassium iodide therapy (120 drops per day) resulted in resolution of lesions within 3½ months.

(9–8) J. Am. Acad. Dermatol. 8:386–391, March 1983.

Cutaneous sporotrichosis has occurred as an occupational infection in gardeners, miners, and brickyard workers, and infections have followed bites from birds, horses, and rats. Whether intact skin can be infected by direct contact with an animal's draining lesions is not established, although person-to-person transmission has been reported to follow handling of infected dressings. In areas where sporotrichosis is common, even animals that are healthy should be handled with caution.

▶ [This is another report of feline sporotrichosis transmitted to humans. Interestingly, in both reports some of the subjects that developed sporotrichosis didn't remember receiving trauma from the infected cats, suggesting that exposure to exudates might be sufficient for transmission. Fortunately, the feline sporotrichosis has a biologic behavior that is similar to its human counterpart and seems to be localized to the skin and lymph nodes and is responsive to potassium iodide.—E.G.] ◀

9–9 **Primary Cutaneous (Inoculation) Blastomycosis: An Occupational Hazard to Pathologists.** Most skin lesions of blastomycosis are complications of systemic disease; primary cutaneous lesions are rare. Donald M. Larson, Mark R. Eckman, Ronald L. Alber, and Volker G. Goldschmidt (Univ. of Minnesota, Duluth) report two cases of primary inoculation blastomycosis occurring in pathologists.

Case 1.—Man, 31, cut his distal second finger while sectioning a lung that proved to be infected by *Blastomyces dermatitidis*. The wound healed after being washed with benzalkonium chloride, but a tender, red-purple nodule developed 3 weeks later, and a smear of the pus yielded yeast forms typical of *Blastomyces*. No systemic symptoms developed. The skin lesion healed slowly with no treatment other than detergent soaks, and the patient has been well for 11 years.

Case 2.—Man, 59, cut his finger during an autopsy on a patient with pulmonary blastomycosis. A nodule was noted 5 weeks later, and subsequently a large nodule developed in the upper arm. Microabscesses containing yeast forms typical of *Blastomyces* were found in the epidermis at both sites, and cultures yielded *B. dermatitidis*. The lesions resolved after treatment with amphotericin B for 5 days, and the patient has been well for 18 months.

Nine similar cases have been described. No patient had evidence of systemic infection. Five patients received minor lacerations when performing autopsies on patients with blastomycosis. Four infections occurred in the laboratory from accidental inoculation with the organism from *Blastomyces* cultures. All patients recovered, despite the occurrence of lymphangitis and lymphadenitis in several cases. Systemic treatment is not indicated for primary cutaneous blastomycosis in an otherwise normal subject. Special care should be taken when performing autopsies on patients suspected of having systemic blastomycosis. Since the disease is common in dogs, the risk of contracting cutaneous blastomycosis may be increased in those who practice veterinary medicine.

▶ [This rare form of primary chancriform syndrome produced by *Blastomyces* is self-limited and requires no systemic therapy unless the patient is immunocompromised.—E.G.] ◀

(9–9) Am. J. Clin. Pathol. 79:253–255, February 1983.

9–10 **Treatment of Systemic Mycoses With Ketoconazole: Emphasis on Toxicity and Clinical Response in 52 Patients.** Phase-II studies on the in vitro mycologic activity, pharmacologic aspects, toxicity, and efficacy of ketoconazole, an oral imidazole antifungal agent, were begun by the National Institute for Allergy and Infectious Diseases Mycoses Study Group in 1979. William E. Dismukes, Alan M. Stamm, John R. Graybill, Philip C. Craven, David A. Stevens, Robert L. Stiller, George A. Sarosi, Gerald Medoff, Clark R. Gregg, Harry A. Gallis, Branch T. Fields, Jr., Robert L. Marier, Thomas A. Kerkering, Lisa G. Kaplowitz, Gretchen Cloud, Cyndi Bowles, and Smith Shadomy report on the toxic effects of and clinical response to ketoconazole in 52 patients with systemic mycoses treated at 11 different centers.

Of the 52 patients, 16 had blastomycosis, 13 had nonmeningeal coccidioidomycosis, 7 had nonmeningeal cryptococcosis, 8 had histoplasmosis, 7 had sporotrichosis, and 1 patient had both blastomycosis and nonmeningeal coccidioidomycosis. Twenty patients had pulmonary fungal disease, 9 had bone or joint involvement, 16 had skin or soft-tissue involvement, and 7 had multiple organ involvement. The mean age of the patients was 44 years (range, 3–86 years). Maximal daily doses of ketoconazole were as follows: 100 mg in a 3-year-old patient, 200 mg in 23 patients, 400 mg in 12 patients, and 600 mg in 16 patients. The duration of therapy ranged from less than 1 month to 6 months in 52% of the patients, 7 to 12 months in 35%, and 12 to 22 months in 13%. No adverse effects or signs of toxicosis were observed in 35 (67%) patients. In the remaining patients, nausea, vomiting, or anorexia were the most common side effects, occurring in 11 (21%) patients. Miscellaneous side effects included epigastric pain, bilateral hand paresthesias, gingival bleeding, gynecomastia, and photophobia. Three patients had to discontinue use of ketoconazole because of possible adverse reactions consisting of moderate thrombocytopenia, development of pruritic rash, and progressively elevated serum levels of alkaline phosphatase and aspartate transaminase. An increase in serum triglyceride values of more than 50 mg/dl over pretreatment values occurred in 12% of patients who were receiving 200 mg/day, in 33% of those receiving 400 mg/day, and in 56% of patients receiving 600 mg/day. Of the 52 patients, 27 (52%) were cured or showed marked improvement. The primary course of treatment failed in 14 patients (27%), as was evidenced by persistently positive cultures during therapy, and 11 patients (21%) had a relapse after ketoconazole was discontinued. The susceptibility of a pretreatment isolate to ketoconazole was not predictive of the clinical response.

It appears that ketoconazole is a well-tolerated antifungal drug with minimum toxicity. Although clear-cut clinical response data were not obtained in this study series, the results indicate that ketoconazole, in the doses used, was more effective in patients with his-

---

(9–10) Ann. Intern. Med. 98:13–20, January 1983.

toplasmosis and nonmeningeal cryptococcosis than in patients with blastomycosis and nonmeningeal coccidioidomycosis and was least effective in patients with sporotrichosis.

▶ [This collaborative study emphasizes toxicity and clinical response of different systemic fungal infections treated with ketoconazole. Although the authors stress that the drug has minimal toxicity, 33% of the subjects had adverse effects. Except for hepatic dysfunction, thrombocytopenia, gynecomastia, and a dose-related triglyceridemia, the other adverse effects were not serious. Efficacy of the drug in this study was disappointing with 48% of the patients either failing to respond or relapsing after discontinuation of the treatment. Notably unresponsive to the drug were the patients with sporotrichosis among whom 5 of 7 failed to respond or relapsed.—E.G.] ◀

9–11 **Long-Term Therapy of Chronic Mucocutaneous Candidiasis With Ketoconazole: Experience With 21 Patients** (13 males), aged 7–49 years, is reported by Charles R. Horsburgh, Jr., and Charles H. Kirkpatrick (Denver). The *Candida* infections had been present for 3–31 years. Fifteen patients had deficient cellular immunity, 8 had endocrine abnormalities, and 6 had concurrent dermatophytosis or chromomycosis.

In patients weighing less than 40 kg therapy was begun with oral doses of 100 mg of ketoconazole per day, and patients weighing 40 kg or more were given 200 mg per day. The initial dosage had to be increased in 4 patients to obtain satisfactory responses. The drug was given 1½ hours after breakfast for optimal absorption. Potassium hydroxide preparations were made of skin, nail, and mucous membrane scrapings that were cultured on Sabouraud's agar with chloramphenicol and gentamicin. Monitoring for adverse effects of ketoconazole included physical and laboratory examinations.

All patients responded to ketoconazole therapy. Buccal lesions responded in a mean of 7 days, skin lesions in a mean of 23 days, and

Fig 9–2 (left).—Candidiasis of fingernails.
Fig 9–3 (right).—Effects of ketoconazole on nail candidiasis. Improvement was first seen at day 35 and continued until nails were normal.
(Courtesy of Horsburgh, C.R., Jr., and Kirkpatrick, C.H.: Am. J. Med. 75:23–29, Jan. 24, 1983.)

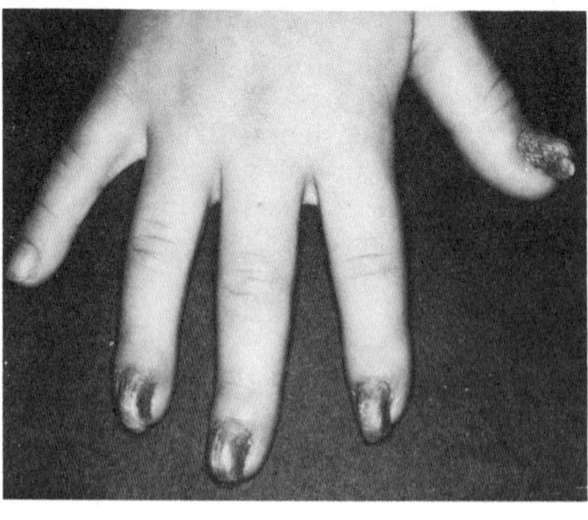
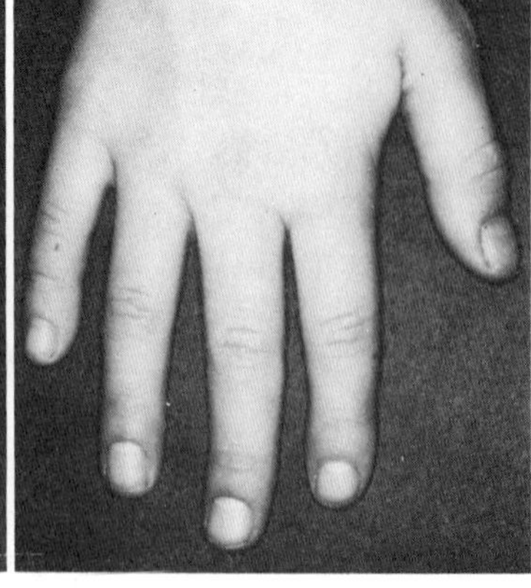

(9–11) Am. J. Med. 75:23–29, Jan. 24, 1983.

nail-bed lesions in a mean of 92 days. One patient with candidal granuloma had to increase the dosage to 200 mg daily before obtaining a satisfactory response. An infection with *Microsporum gypseum* was only controlled at a dose of 400 mg of ketoconazole per day. Figures 9–2 and 9–3 show improvement of nail lesions; by day 103 these nails were essentially normal. Adverse effects were infrequent. One patient had drug-induced hepatitis that resolved on cessation of ketoconazole treatment. Two patients became hypertensive; the relation of hypertension to ketoconazole therapy is unclear. Two patients had relapses when the frequency of dosage was reduced by 50% but responded when the former frequency was reinstituted.

Patients with candidiasis are predisposed to other fungal, acute viral, and bacterial infections; the most persistent and disfiguring lesions are usually due to *Candida* species. Concurrent infection with dermatophytes occurs in 20% of patients with chronic mucocutaneous candidiasis. Therefore, it is important to obtain fungal cultures of involved areas, for ketoconazole is also effective against dermatophytoses, although higher dosage may be required.

Ketoconazole is recommended for treatment of skin, nail-bed, and buccal candidiasis and cutaneous dermatophytosis in the immunocompromised host. Long-term remissions after termination of ketoconazole therapy may require correction of abnormalities of cell-mediated immunity.

▶ [This study confirms previous reports about the efficacy of ketoconazole in mucocutaneous candidiasis. As expected, oral lesions responded faster, whereas paronychia required about 3 months to clear. The possibility that 2 patients who relapsed may have developed a resistant strain is distressing, since no previous reports of resistance to ketoconazole or any of the imidazoles are available; this obviously requires confirmation.—E.G.] ◀

-12 **Clotrimazole and Econazole in Treatment of Vaginal Candidiasis: Single-Blind Comparison.** G. Gabriel and R. N. T. Thin (London) studied the efficacy of 2 antifungal agents, clotrimazole and econazole, in the treatment of vaginal candidiasis in a single-blind trial. Patients included those with a positive culture result for *Candida albicans*. Patients were randomly assigned to receive either one 200-mg clotrimazole pessary or one 150-mg econazole pessary at night for 3 consecutive nights.

The study group included 77 women treated with econazole and 79 given clotrimazole. In the econazole group, 32 were treated with pessaries alone and 45 with pessaries and cream. In the clotrimazole group, 30 were treated with pessaries alone and 49 with pessaries and cream. The drop-out rate was relatively high at the 2-week follow-up in both groups. Of the clotrimazole group, 60 patients were followed for 14 days, and 52 (86.6%) of these had no evidence of fungal infection. In the econazole group there was a slightly higher drop-out rate; 50 patients were followed for 14 days with 45 (90%) of these having no evidence of candidiasis. Of 8 clotrimazole failures, 3 reported observable improvement in symptoms.

(9–12) Br. J. Vener. Dis. 59:56–58, February 1983.

Of the 5 econazole failures, 2 were symptom-free even though *C. albicans* was found on microscopy. All signs of infection resolved in both treatment groups.

The treatments gave similar clinical and mycologic results, both were acceptable to the patients, and neither caused side effects. Thus, the clinician might choose either drug, depending on cost and availability.

▶ [This single-blind controlled study confirms other controlled studies (*Curr. Ther. Res.* 25:590, 1979; *Practitioner* 224:1311, 1980) that show no superiority among the topical imidazoles in the treatment of candidiasis. This also applies to dermatophytosis and tinea versicolor.—E.G.] ◀

9–13 **Treatment of Candidal Diaper Dermatitis: Double-Blind Placebo-Controlled Comparison of Topical Nystatin With Topical Plus Oral Nystatin.** It is currently recommended that candidal diaper dermatitis be treated both orally and topically with nystatin. Diane Munz, Keith R. Powell, and Chik H. Pai (Montreal Children's Hosp.) conducted a prospective double-blind study to evaluate the clinical resolution and recurrence of candidal diaper dermatitis treated with combined oral and topical nystatin therapy or with topical nystatin alone. All 60 patients in the study were treated with cream containing nystatin, 100,000 units/gm. They also received an oral suspension of nystatin, 100,000 units/ml, in a dose of 1 ml by mouth 4 times a day, or a placebo.

Initial skin cultures grew *Candida albicans* in 46 (77%) patients. Forty-eight patients returned at days 10–12 for follow-up; 37 initially had *C. albicans* isolated from the skin; 11 did not. No significant differences between groups were found for medical history or personal habits. All 37 infants whose initial skin cultures grew *C. albicans* had improved in at least 1 of 3 clinical criteria after 10 days of therapy. No differences in clinical course were found between the two treatment groups.

Treatment for longer than 10 days was necessary for 11 (65%) of the combination therapy group and for 9 (43%) of the topical nystatin only group. Recurrence was reported in 10 of 31 patients: 4 (31%) of 13 in the combination therapy group and 6 (33%) of 18 in the topical therapy group. Sixteen of 31 patients had positive skin or stool cultures, or both, for *Candida* species on days 10–12; 5 (31%) of 16 had a recurrence, whereas 4 of 13 (31%) with negative cultures of both skin and stools had recurrences.

The results indicate that topical nystatin alone is as effective as combined oral and topical therapy.

▶ [This study shows convincingly that topical therapy alone is an effective treatment for diaper dermatitis produced by *C. albicans*. The authors stress the fact that many patients required 3 weeks of therapy rather than the customary 10 days of topical nystatin.—E.G.] ◀

(9–13) J. Pediatr. 101:1022–1025, December 1982.

10. Genodermatoses

0–1 **Family Studies in Tuberous Sclerosis: Evaluation of Apparently Unaffected Parents.** Suzanne B. Cassidy, Roberta A. Pagon, Melanie Pepin, and Joel D. Blumhagen (Univ. of Washington) evaluated the apparently unaffected parents of 13 patients with tuberous sclerosis. None of the parents had a personal or family history suggesting this diagnosis. All 26 parents were examined according to a protocol including medical history, physical examination (with Wood's lamp examination of the skin), funduscopic examination through a dilated pupil, roentgenograms of the hands, feet, and skull, renal ultrasound studies, and cranial computed tomography (CT).

In 4 of the 13 families, 1 parent had evidence of tuberous sclerosis. Except for 1 of these, from whom periungual fibromas had been removed, none of the parents who were determined to be affected had previously sought medical care for complications of tuberous sclerosis. Three of the 4 previously unsuspected affected parents were fathers. One parent had no cutaneous findings, and his condition would not have been detected without cranial CT or renal ultrasound examination. Cranial CT findings were abnormal in 3 parents and renal ultrasound findings in 1. In these 4 families, the propositus had no predictable phenotype.

In this study 31% of unaffected parents of propositi demonstrated tuberous sclerosis. The results indicate that a substantial proportion of seemingly normal parents of children with tuberous sclerosis will be heterozygous for this gene. The phenotypes of parents of such patients should be evaluated with a prioritized protocol, including examination for typical skin lesions, cranial CT, renal ultrasound examination or excretory urogram, and dilated eye examination, before recurrence-risk counseling is given.

▶ [This excellent clinical study makes the point that a good history and physical examination may not be adequate to exclude tuberous sclerosis (TS) in an apparently unaffected parent of a patient with TS. Of 21 kindreds with TS available for examination in this study, 13 (62%) had no historical evidence of TS in the parents. After extensive examination and laboratory testing, 4 of the 13 (31%) "unaffected" parents were determined to have TS. In this small study, therefore, 57% (12 of 21) of kindreds with TS demonstrated heterozygosity in a parent of an affected proband. Those of us who are involved in family examinations of patients with TS would do well to carefully consider the standard evaluation used by the authors to exclude TS in parents of an affected individual.—A.R.R.] ◀

–2 **Pregnancy Complications in Type IV Ehlers-Danlos Syndrome.** Type IV Ehlers-Danlos syndrome (EDS), unlike other forms

---

(10–1) JAMA 249:1302–1304, Mar. 11, 1983.
(10–2) Lancet 1:50–53, Jan. 1/8, 1983.

of EDS, appears to be associated with a high incidence of pregnancy complications. Noreen L. Rudd, Carl Nimrod, Karen A. Holbrook, and Peter H. Byers reviewed data on a group of 14 families in which 20 women with type IV EDS were identified. Diagnosis was confirmed in at least 1 member of each family by in vitro measurement of type III collagen produced by dermal fibroblasts. All affected subjects produced lower levels of the protein than controls. Pregnancy experiences of 2 patients are described in detail.

CASE 1.—Woman, 33, had thin skin through which venous vasculature was visible. After 20 weeks of her second pregnancy, she presented with a painful hemorrhage in the left calf. Patient was readmitted at 28 weeks' gestation in premature labor. Isoxsuprine infusion was started and labor ceased. Patient complained of epigastric pain 12 hours later. At 32 hours after admission labor was allowed to proceed; 4 hours after isoxsuprine infusion was stopped, the patient became hypertensive and collapsed suddenly. Resuscitation failed. At autopsy, the uterus was found to have an irregular 4-cm tear which extended completely through the myometrium. The fetus appeared normal.

CASE 2.—Woman, 33, in whom a diagnosis of EDS had been considered had had 2 previous uncomplicated pregnancies. The third pregnancy progressed normally into labor. During the third stage contractions stopped abruptly, blood pressure fell, and uterine bleeding began. Emergency cesarean section revealed the fetus had ruptured through the wall of the uterus. All tissues were extremely friable. Hemostasis could not be achieved and the patient died.

Of the 20 women identified as having type IV 10 had been pregnant, and 5 (including the 2 patients described above) had died from pregnancy-related complications. Overall risk of death in each pregnancy in this group was 25%. Complications of pregnancy included rupture of bowel, aorta, vena cava, or uterus; vaginal laceration; and postpartum uterine hemorrhage.

The authors emphasize that type IV EDS is a distinct form of EDS that differs in clinical and biochemical features from all other forms. They suggest that all patients with this disorder be carefully monitored during labor and for several days postpartum so that prompt intervention can be initiated in the event of vessel or uterine rupture.

▶ [This article serves an extremely important function. Type IV EDS is a disease whose inheritance pattern and biochemical defect are known. Therefore, definitive diagnosis may be made in a woman at risk, and appropriate genetic counseling may be offered with particular emphasis on the very significant maternal mortality. In addition, if pregnancy occurs in such a woman, prenatal diagnosis can be made available. As with many other genetic disorders, detailed clinical and biochemical investigation of type IV EDS will allow couples to make rational decisions regarding reproduction.—J.C.A.] ◀

10–3 **Biochemical Characterization of Variants of Ehlers-Danlos Syndrome Type VI.** In patients with Ehlers-Danlos syndrome type VI, hyperextensibility of the skin and hypermobility of the joints are associated with an almost complete absence of hydroxylysine in skin collagen and with only residual lysyl hydroxylase activity in cultured

---

(10–3) Eur. J. Clin. Invest. 13:357–362, August 1983.

fibroblasts. However, the association between the clinical manifestations and the underlying biochemical defects in this disease are not clear-cut. Annegret Ihme, Leila Risteli, Thomas Krieg, Juha Risteli, Ursula Feldmann, Klaus Kruse, and Peter K. Müller described 3 variants of Ehlers-Danlos syndrome type VI discerned in an analysis of 6 patients with a clinical diagnosis of the disease. Besides determination of the hydroxylysine content of skin biopsy specimens, the ability to hydroxylate lysyl residues in collagen was assessed in cultured fibroblasts in vitro, and the activities of 4 intracellular enzymes of collagen biosynthesis were measured in these cells.

Features characteristic of Ehlers-Danlos syndrome type VI (hyperextensibility of the skin, cigarette paper scars, hypermobility of the joints, and skeletal manifestations) were prominent in patients 1, 2, 3, 4, and 6. Scoliosis was not observed in patient 1, but it was severe in patient 2. Ocular symptoms were the most prominent in patient 5; this patient had no scoliosis, and hyperextensibility of the skin was only mild. Three forms of the syndrome could be identified. One form was severe, with skeletal, dermal, and ocular manifestations associated with an absence of hydroxylysine in skin and little lysyl hydroxylase activity in cultured fibroblasts. In the second form, the skeletal, dermal, and ocular manifestations were also severe, but the content of hydroxylysine in skin was nearly normal, though only residual activity of lysyl hydroxylase was observed in cultured dermal fibroblasts. In the third form, the symptoms were predominantly ocular, with almost normal levels of lysyl hydroxylase activity and hydroxylysine in skin. In all cases, the activities of prolyl 4-hydroxylase and the 2 hydroxylysyl glycosyltransferases were normal, and failure to detect lysyl hydroxylase activity could not be attributed to altered solubility characteristics of the enzyme or to the presence of an enzyme inhibitor. However, the collagen produced in cell cultures was hydroxylated to a considerably greater extent than that found in skin. Hydroxylation of lysyl residues in both mutant and control cells was less sensitive to ascorbate deficiency than that of prolyl residues.

The diagnosis of Ehlers-Danlos syndrome type VI should be based on both measurement of the content of hydroxylysine in skin and determination of lysyl hydroxylase activity. The presence of the usual symptoms in patients with an apparently normal content of hydroxylysine in skin suggests a more complex association between the known biochemical defects and the clinical manifestations than was previously thought to exist.

▶ [The data presented in this article may be interpreted in a way that is different from that suggested by the authors. The patient with pure ocular involvement and normal levels of lysyl hydroxylase and skin hydroxylysine does not have Ehlers-Danlos syndrome type VI. The molecular definition of a genetic disease is the production of an abnormal gene product, in this case, lysyl hydroxylase. Since the enzyme and its finished product are both normal in the patient in question, another form of the syndrome must be present.

The second group reported (normal skin hydroxylysine content but very low in vitro levels of lysyl hydroxylase) may also not have the type VI disease. In this group, the enzyme may have a genetic defect that interferes with in vitro measurement but not with enzyme function. In that case, there could very well be some other enzyme abnormality accounting for the clinical findings, with the lysyl hydroxylase abnormality being a fortuitous finding.

One must interpret biochemical data associated with a constellation of clinical findings very cautiously before assigning a specific inheritance pattern.—J.C.A.] ◀

10–4 **Familial Sea-Blue Histiocytosis With Cutaneous Involvement: Case Report With Ultrastructural Findings.** Sea-blue histiocytes (SBH) are large macrophages with cytoplasmic granules that become blue or blue-green with Giemsa stain and are found primarily in patients with the inherited disorder SBH syndrome. The disorder is characterized by infiltration of the marrow, spleen, liver, nodes, and lungs with SBH. The substance stored in the granules appears to be a glycophospholipid, probably a ceroid. A. M. Zina and S. Bundino (Turin Univ., Italy) report a case of familial primary SBH syndrome in a man with cutaneous nodules. Ultrastructural study of SBH in the skin showed a previously unreported type of inclusion.

Man, 25, presented with hepatosplenomegaly, marrow involvement, and

Fig 10–1 (top).—Plaques over the forehead and infiltration of the eyelids.

Fig 10–2 (bottom).—Histiocytes showing the cytoplasm filled with blue stained granules (May-Grünwald/Giemsa; original magnification ×400).

(Courtesy of Zina, A.M., and Bundino, S.: Br. J. Dermatol. 108:355–361, March 1983.)

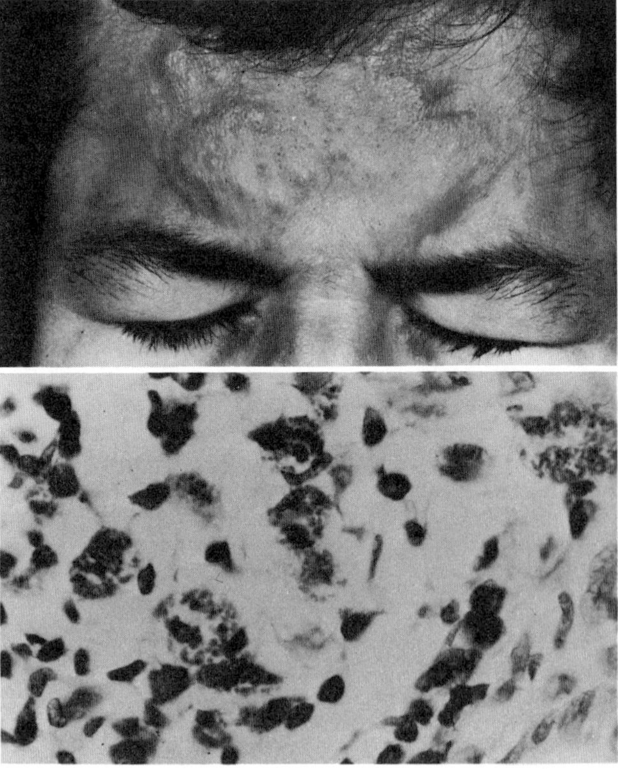

(10–4) Br. J. Dermatol. 108:355–361, March 1983.

diffuse pulmonary micronodules. The initial cutaneous lesions were limited to the eyelids; later, nodular lesions developed on the forehead and chin (Fig 10–1). A biopsy showed a multifocal histiocytic nodular infiltrate in the mid-dermis and deep dermis and a few sarcoid-like granulomas. The stroma exhibited a fibrous reaction. The cells were shown histochemically to be typical SBH (Fig 10–2). Further testing excluded sarcoidosis. Ultrastructural study of a nodular lesion of the face showed the cytoplasm of SBH to be filled with several types of inclusions. All SBH contained pleomorphic large phagolysosomes with whorls of lamellated and membranous structures and microfilaments mixed with dense osmophilic, round, polycyclic, or irregular inclusions. Oval or round inclusions with a dense, amorphous matrix and dense rod-like formations also were observed.

A sister of this patient, aged 17 years, also had SBH syndrome, with involvement of muscles and subcutaneous tissue as well as hepatosplenomegaly and pulmonary infiltrates. The skin was slightly indurated, but no nodules were present. It has been suggested that the stored material in SBH syndrome is a result of an enzyme deficiency that leads to disordered lipid metabolism and the storage of a ceroid substance. It is possible that SBH syndrome is not a unique disease, but that heterogeneous enzyme defects can result in the same clinical picture.

▶ [This interesting report of 2 family members with primary cutaneous nodular infiltrates of sea-blue histiocytes could potentially lead to very interesting biochemical findings. Once the primary gene defect is determined (probably an altered or absent enzyme), it could be compared with the defect in secondary or systemic sea-blue histiocytosis. Important information regarding the propensity for cells to migrate to various tissues could be provided. Alterations in cell surface antigens, abnormal cell membrane structure, or alteration in histiocytic migration factors are several possible effects of the abnormal gene.—J.C.A.] ◀

10–5 **X-Linked Recessive Ichthyosis Vulgaris: Rapid Identification by Lipoprotein Electrophoresis** is described by Heiko Traupe, Peter Michael Kövary, and Hilko Schriewer (Univ. of Münster, Germany). Ichthyoses are a heterogeneous group of hereditary disorders of keratinization. X-linked recessive ichthyosis vulgaris (XRI) is due to a deficiency of steroid sulfatase, which also may lead to birth complications and cryptorchidism. Increased electromobility of low-density lipoprotein particles has been noted in this syndrome, presumably in relation to the accumulation of cholesterol sulfate. Lipoprotein electrophoresis proved diagnostically useful when carried out in 8 cases of XRI and in 2 obligate heterozygous conductors. Four patients with autosomal dominant ichthyosis vulgaris and 1 with atypical ichthyosis vulgaris associated with hypogenitalism also were examined. A marked increase in the mobility of β-lipoproteins and pre-β-lipoproteins was evident in patients with XRI (Fig 10–3). The mobility of these fractions was normal in the heterozygotes and in the patients with other forms of ichthyosis vulgaris. No significant abnormalities in serum triglyceride, cholesterol, high-density lipoprotein cholesterol, or apolipoprotein levels were noted in the patients with XRI.

(10–5) Arch. Dermatol. Res. 275:63–65, February 1983.

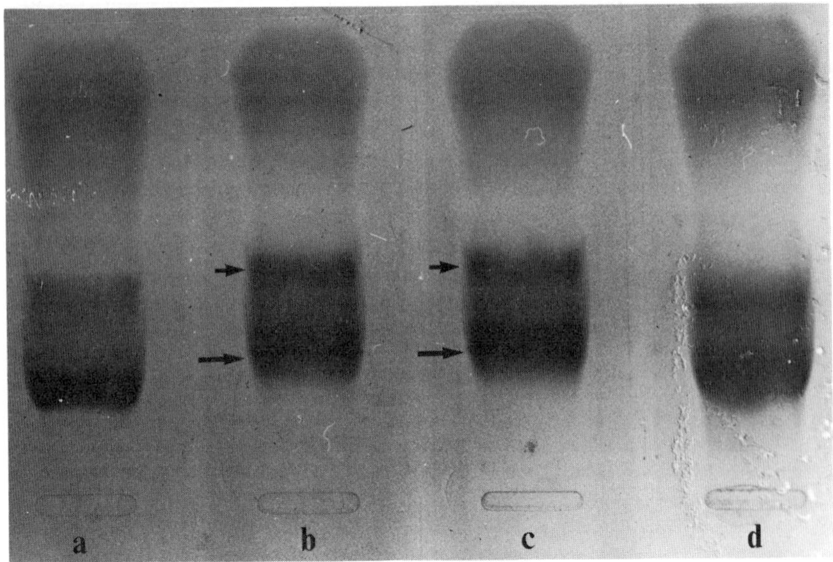

Fig 10–3.—Anode of lipoprotein electrophoresis in 1 heterozygous conductor *(a)*, 2 patients with XRI (*b* and *c*), and 1 patient with autosomal dominant ichthyosis vulgaris *(d)*. Long arrows indicate increased electromobility of β-lipoproteins; short arrows, increased electromobility of pre-β-lipoproteins. (Courtesy of Traupe, H., et al.: Arch. Dermatol. Res. 275:63–65, February 1983.)

Lipoprotein electrophoresis is useful in diagnosing XRI in affected male patients. The pre-β-lipoproteins, as well as the β-lipoproteins, are altered in XRI. The findings of abnormally anionized β-lipoproteins and pre-β-lipoproteins may indicate an increased risk of atherogenesis. Low-density lipoprotein with enhanced negative charge is internalized by vascular macrophages, and massive cholesterol deposition in these cells could result.

▶ [Lipoprotein electrophoresis is a simple screening test to detect X-linked ichthyosis. In this disorder there is a deficiency of steroid sulfatase, thereby causing an accumulation of negatively charged cholesterol sulfate. Therefore those affected show an increased electromobility of low-density lipoprotein particles (β-lipoprotein). It is important that this test be run with a normal control because it is the abnormal mobility—not the quantity—of lipoprotein that must be demonstrated.—R.R.] ◀

10–6 **Treatment of the Ichthyosis of Sjögren-Larsson Syndrome With Etretinate (Tigason).** Sjögren-Larsson syndrome (SLS) is rare. Inheritance is as an autosomal recessive trait. The syndrome consists of mental retardation, spastic diplegia or quadriplegia, and ichthyosis. The ichthyosis is regarded as a variant of lamellar ichthyosis. Sten Jagell and Sture Lidén (Univ. of Umeå, Sweden) evaluated the effect of etretinate, an aromatic retinoid, on the ichthyosis of SLS in 7 patients. Etretinate was administered for 6 months, beginning with a daily dose of 1 mg/kg body weight during the first 2 weeks. Dosage was then reduced to about 0.5 mg/kg/day during the next 4 weeks.

(10–6) Acta Derm. Venereol. (Stockh) 63:89–91, 1983.

During week 7, a further reduction was attempted; if the ichthyosis worsened, dosage was adjusted until a maintenance level was achieved.

During the second week of treatment, desquamation of ichthyotic skin increased, reaching a maximum during week 3. All patients had an increase in pruritus, which often lead to excoriations. The pruritus disappeared with a reduction in dosage. After 4 weeks, all patients showed an excellent treatment result. Attempts to reduce the dosage further resulted in a gradual increase in ichthyosis. Therefore the dosage was successively increased to a maintenance level at which substantial improvement in the ichthyosis was achieved. After treatment all patients required less carbamide cream to relieve dryness and fewer baths. In general, care of the skin became less time consuming. There were no abnormal laboratory findings. Except for pruritus in all patients and cheilitis in 1 patient during the initial phase of the study, there were no significant side effects.

It appears that the usefulness of etretinate for long-term treatment of SLS will depend on its toxicity. The possible adverse effect on blood lipids seems to be the most serious known risk.

▶ [It is not surprising that the lamellar-like ichthyosis of Sjögren-Larsson syndrome responds to treatment with etretinate. Since this ichthyosis dermatosis is usually described as a *mild* lamellar form, one wonders about the indication for chronic retinoid use in this rare genetic disease.—R.R.] ◀

10–7 **Epidermolytic Hyperkeratosis: Ultrastructure and Biochemistry of Skin and Amniotic Fluid Cells From Two Affected Fetuses and a Newborn Infant.** Epidermolytic hyperkeratosis, or congenital bullous ichthyosiform erythroderma, is an autosomal dominant disorder of keratinization characterized by hyperkeratosis, intraepidermal bullae, and condensed keratin bundles in the spinous and granular cells. Amounts of fibrous proteins are decreased in the epidermis, and one of the keratin polypeptides is absent. Karen A. Holbrook, Beverly A. Dale, Virginia P. Sybert, and Richard W. Sagebiel examined skin biopsy and amniotic fluid specimens from two fetuses of the same family at risk of epidermolytic hyperkeratosis. Both fetuses were affected. One was carried to term, and epidermal extracts were prepared from blisters of the newborn infant for analysis of keratin and filaggrin proteins.

The cytoplasm of epidermal cells from both fetuses was poorly preserved, and most cells contained highly condensed bundles of tonofilaments. The cells of the basal and periderm layers were unaffected. A significant proportion of amniotic fluid cells contained filament aggregates. Biochemical studies showed abnormalities in both keratin and filaggrin proteins in blister epidermis and cornified scales from the newborn infant.

Prenatal diagnosis of epidermolytic hyperkeratosis should be possible using cells obtained by amniocentesis, precluding the need for fetal skin biopsy. The structural alterations in tissues of affected fe-

---

(10–7) J. Invest. Dermatol. 80:222–227, April 1983.

tuses and infants may result from a disordered interaction between the abnormal epidermal proteins. Abnormalities in both keratin polypeptides and filaggrin could contribute to abnormal filament aggregation in this disorder.

▶ [Clumps of keratin filaments were not only identified ultrastructurally in the prekeratinized fetal epidermis but were also present in cells obtained from amniotic fluid. Thus, prenatal diagnosis should be possible by amniocentesis alone, avoiding the risk and cost of fetal skin biopsies.

Keratin and filaggrin proteins were assayed from blister fluid of the affected newborn. High-molecular-weight keratins (67,000 and 64,000) were absent and replaced by proteins with molecular weights of 62,000 and 60,000. There was an increase in filaggrin with a molecular weight of 35,000 and additional bands of filaggrin immunoreactive protein not present in normal epidermal extracts. Regarding the pathogenesis of this disorder, the authors correctly conclude that the structural changes may be due to the altered interaction of abnormal keratin and filaggrin proteins.—R.R.] ◀

11. Hair and Nails

11–1 **Evidence for the Importance of Peripheral Tissue Events in the Development of Hirsutism in Polycystic Ovary Syndrome.** Hirsutism can occur in the presence of normal or near-normal serum androgen concentrations, but the serum androstanediol glucuronide (3α-diol G) concentration is markedly increased in idiopathic hirsutism and is an excellent marker of peripheral androgen metabolism and action. Rogerio A. Lobo, Uwe Goebelsmann, and Richard Horton (Univ. of Southern California) assessed in vivo peripheral androgen production and activity, using 3α-diol G as a marker, in 12 hirsute and 12 nonhirsute women, aged 18–26 years, with a diagnosis of polycystic ovary syndrome (PCO). Thirteen age- and weight-matched controls were also studied. All the PCO patients were slightly to moderately obese and had inappropriate gonadotropin secretion.

Serum concentrations of unbound estradiol and LH-FSH ratios were higher in both patient groups than in controls. Concentrations of testosterone, unbound testosterone, and androstenedione were also similar in hirsute and nonhirsute patients and higher than in controls. Hirsute patients had slightly higher dehydroepiandrosterone sulfate and Δ5-androstenediol values than nonhirsute patients. Concentrations of 3α-diol G were above normal in both groups of patients with PCO, but were higher in the hirsute group. The serum 3α-diol G concentration was elevated about 10-fold in hirsute patients, but it was normal in nonhirsute PCO patients. The ratio of serum 3α-diol G to free testosterone was elevated significantly only in the hirsute group.

Women with PCO have increased serum androgen concentrations, regardless of whether hirsutism is present or absent. Hirsutism in these patients is not only a function of the circulating androgen concentrations, but may also be determined by metabolic events in peripheral tissues. There may be greater androgen production in peripheral tissues for a given amount of substrate, but it is unclear whether this occurs through increased 5α or 3α reduction, or both. The 3α-diol G concentration does not reflect a cause of hirsutism but merely serves as a marker of increased androgen formation at the level of the pilosebaceous unit.

▶ [These investigators had presented evidence in a previous publication (*J. Clin. Invest.* 69:1203, 1982) that glucuronidation of the 3α-diol metabolite of dihydrotestosterone is a target cell event and that the measurement of this 3α-diol-glucuronide in the blood can serve as a marker of peripheral androgen action.

In the present study, hirsute and nonhirsute women with polycystic ovaries were

---

(11–1) J. Clin. Endocrinol. Metab. 57:393–397, August 1983.

found to have similarly increased levels of androgens in their peripheral blood, as compared to normal subjects. But the hirsute group had blood levels of the 3α-diol glucuronide 10 times higher than those in the nonhirsute group, thus affording further evidence that the measurement of this end-stage cellular metabolite in the blood reflects the capacity of intracellular androgen transformation. In unpublished studies, the authors have also found increased levels of the 3α-diol glucuronide in patients with acne.—P.E.P.] ◀

11–2 **Adrenal Abnormalities in Idiopathic Hirsutism.** Androgen production is consistently elevated in women with idiopathic hirsutism, but it remains unclear whether the adrenal gland or ovary is the usual source of androgen excess. Aideen Moore, Fergal Magee, Sean Cunningham, Marie Culliton, and T. Joseph McKenna (Univ. College, Dublin) examined the contribution of the adrenal glands to androgen excess in these patients by determining basal androgen concentrations and their responses to exogenous and endogenous adrenal stimulation and adrenal suppression. Thirty-four women with idiopathic hirsutism and regular ovulatory menses participated in the study. Thirty-five normal women also were included. Dynamic studies with ACTH and metyrapone were done in 22 hirsute and 16 normal women.

Basal hormone levels in the 2 groups of women and values after

STEROIDS IN PLASMA (NMOLE/L; MEAN ± SD), IN NORMAL WOMEN (BASAL), AND IN HIRSUTE WOMEN (BASAL AND AFTER ADMINISTRATION OF DEXAMETHASONE)

	Normal women (a)	Hirsute women (b)	a compared with b *P* value	Hirsute women on dexamethasone (c)	b compared with c *P* value	a compared with c *P* value
Testosterone	1·16 ±0·33	1·48 ±0·6	$P<0·05$	0·84 ±0·59	$P<0·001$	$P<0·05$
SHBG	43·9 ±12·7	35·3 ±14·8	$P<0·02$	45·7 ±17·4	$P<0·02$	NS
Testosterone/SHBG	2·84 ±1·05	4·93 ±2·98	$P<0·001$	2·4 ±3·0	$P<0·01$	NS
Dihydrotestosterone	0·59 ±0·19	0·70 ±0·25	$P<0·05$	0·41 ±0·22	$P<0·001$	$P<0·005$
Androstenedione	5·87 ±1·79	7·06 ±2·77	$P<0·05$	5·54 ±2·75	$P<0·05$	NS
DHA	42·8 ±21·5	40·3 ±28·7	NS*	16·34 ±22·66	$P<0·005$	$P<0·001$
DHA-S (μmol/l)	7·14 ±1·86	8·55 ±4·63	NS	2·64 ±2·17	$P<0·001$	$P<0·001$
17-OH-progesterone	2·43 ±0·84	3·01 ±1·23	$P<0·05$	2·48 ±1·63	NS	NS
11-Deoxycortisol	1·44 ±0·96	1·23 ±1·05	NS	1·14 ±1·21	NS	NS
Cortisol	510 ±114	502 ±306	NS	198·9 ±221·3	$P<0·001$	$P<0·001$

*NS, not significant.
(Courtesy of Moore, A., et al.: Clin. Endocrinol. (Oxf.) 18:391–399, April 1983.)

(11–2) Clin. Endocrinol. (Oxf.) 18:391–399, April 1983.

administration of dexamethasone in the hirsute women are given in the table. Basal levels of testosterone and other androgens were significantly elevated in the hirsute women, and levels of sex hormone–binding globulin (SHBG) were significantly suppressed. Increments in plasma levels of dehydroepiandrosterone, androstenedione, cortisol, and 17-hydroxyprogesterone were greater in the hirsute women than in normal subjects after ACTH administration. With metyrapone, only the testosterone response was significantly greater in the patient group. In hirsute women given dexamethasone, plasma androgen responses to ACTH resembled those seen in normal subjects without dexamethasone, but the exaggerated cortisol response was unaltered. The testosterone response to metyrapone was suppressed in dexamethasone-treated patients. More than 50% of the patients responded clinically to 3 months of dexamethasone therapy in a daily dose of 0.5 mg. A more normal body-hair pattern was apparent in responsive patients. Hormone studies were not predictive of the response to dexamethasone therapy.

The dissociation of adrenal androgen and cortisol responsiveness after administration of dexamethasone in women with idiopathic hirsutism suggests that excessive adrenal androgen production, stimulated by a dexamethasone-suppressible factor other than ACTH, may be the primary disorder. Findings of ovarian androgen excess in hirsute patients may represent secondary events.

▶ [The results of this study are similar to those of reports previously published by others that show evidence of mild non-hydroxylase-deficient adrenocortical hyperandrogenism in women with idiopathic hirsutism. The argument about whether the ovary or the adrenal gland is the source of the androgen-induced hirsute state is not really settled, since there is much evidence in the literature to indicate the participation of both the pituitary-adrenal and pituitary-ovarian pathways in idiopathic hirsutism. There is also evidence for the participation of both pathways in other hyperandrogenic disorders, including the polycystic ovarian syndrome. In any event, the common denominator in all patients with "idiopathic" hirsutism is an increase in the production rate of testosterone.

One finding of particular interest in this study was that dexamethasone treatment, 0.5 mg at bedtime, suppressed adrenal androgens but without obtunding cortisol responsiveness to metyrapone administration. Two implications follow from this observation: *(1)* this dosage can be used to suppress adrenocortical androgens without the overriding concern that the adrenal cortex would not be able to respond to stress; and *(2)* it suggests the long-postulated existence of a non-ACTH pituitary peptide responsible for the stimulation of adrenocortical androgen elaboration and the onset of adrenarche in late childhood. A recent report appears to support the presence of such a pituitary-tropic hormone (*Endocrinology* 113:2092, 1983).—P.E.P.] ◀

1–3 **Acquired Hypertrichosis Lanuginosa** is rare. It is usually associated with malignancies. Wannasri Sindhuphak and Amnuay Vibhagool (Chulalongkorn Univ., Bangkok, Thailand) report on the first case discovered in Thailand.

Woman, 32, had rapid onset of generalized hypertrichosis and painful tongue. There was fine white lanugo hair on face and body. Follicular orifices on the trunk and extremities were accentuated. Multiple, hyperpigmented, lichenified, follicular papules were seen on the buttocks and extremities. The

---

(11–3) Int. J. Dermatol. 21:599–601, December 1982.

tongue was markedly erythematous, with multiple, deep furrows. The liver was enlarged to 3 cm below the right costal margin. Routine laboratory tests, x-ray studies, and sigmoidoscopy yielded normal findings. A liver scan showed a space-occupying lesion in the posterior portion of the right upper lobe. Biopsy of the hepatic lesion revealed metastatic adenocarcinoma. The serum carcinoembryonic antigen concentration was 7.7 ng/ml (normal, 0–2.5 ng/ml). No primary cancer was found. During initial hospitalization, discomfort developed in the right upper abdomen, with further enlargement of the liver. The patient was treated with 5-fluorouracil and was doing well 1 year after initial examination.

Of the 24 reported cases of acquired hypertrichosis lanuginosa, 22 have been associated with proved malignancies and 14 occurred in females. The pathophysiologic factors of hypertrichosis are unknown; it may be the result of secretion of a humoral substance by the tumor. Appearance of the disease in a patient is almost always a sign of occult malignancy.

▶ [A timely reminder of the association of this phenomenon with underlying malignancy. In the previously reported cases reviewed by the authors, the associated malignancies occurred in the following organs: 5 in the lung, 7 in the colon or rectum, 2 in the breast, 2 in the bladder, 2 in the uterus, and 1 each in the ovary, gallbladder, mediastinum, and pancreas. The mechanism is not clear, though hormonal factors produced by the tumor are suspected.—R.M.] ◀

11–4 **Photochemotherapy and Alopecia Areata.** A variety of therapeutic agents has been advocated for treating alopecia areata. Mohamed A. Amer and Ahmed El Garf (Zagazig Univ., Zagazig, Egypt) evaluated the effect of photochemotherapy in treating 3 types of alopecia areata in 10 patients (6 male, 4 female) aged 10–50 years.

Patients received 8-methoxypsoralen in an oral dose of 0.6 mg/kg of body weight 2 hours before irradiation for 5 treatments. For the next 5 treatments, topical applications of 0.15% solution of 8-methoxypsoralen applied 1 hour before irradiation was added to the oral treatment. Patients were treated in a stand-up ultraviolet A light box twice a week with 3 days of rest after each exposure. Initial dose of light, 2 joules/sq cm, was increased by 1 joule/sq cm every 4 exposures.

Of the 5 patients with alopecia totalis, 1 showed a good response after 33 treatments; 2 patients had a poor response. A woman with a large single patch of alopecia areata had a moderate response after 40 treatments and 170 joules/sq cm. Four patients with multiple patches of alopecia showed no response. Four of the total of 10 patients showed some regrowth of hair after treatment with psoralen ultraviolet A (PUVA).

The authors conclude that PUVA therapy may have a place in the treatment of alopecia areata. But, because of long-term side effects this therapy should be reserved for those cases of long duration that are resistant to other modalities.

▶ [The results of PUVA treatment of alopecia areata were somewhat disappointing in this study. In 4 patients with multiple patches of alopecia areata, no response was seen. Access of radiation to the treatment sites may be difficult in these patients;

(11–4) Int. J. Dermatol. 22:245–246, May 1983.

similarly, when some regrowth occurs, the effective radiation dose may be reduced. On the other hand, patients with more extensive disease or with alopecia totalis generally have a more resistant disease to start with. There is some evidence that whole body exposure may improve results (E. Gonzalez, personal communication).—R.W.G.] ◀

11–5 **Diphencyprone in Treatment of Alopecia Areata.** Potent contact allergens have been shown to induce regrowth of hair in all forms of alopecia areata, including alopecia totalis. Rudolf Happle, Björn M. Hausen, and Ludwig Wiesner-Menzel evaluated the ability of topically applied diphencyprone (2,3-diphenylcyclopropenone-1), a new, potent contact sensitizer, to induce regrowth of hair in 27 patients, 11 males and 16 females, aged 15–57 years, with extensive alopecia areata (5 patients) or alopecia totalis (22). Diphencyprone, in concentrations ranging from 2% to 0.0001%, was applied to half the scalp; the other side served as a control region. When a difference in hair growth between the two sides became evident, both sides were treated. Treatment lasted 4–17 months.

After 4–8 months of treatment, 23 of the 27 patients exhibited a significant difference in hair growth between the treated and untreated sides; the other 4 showed no therapeutic effect. Hair regrowth occurred either exclusively on the treated side or was faster and more dense on this side (Figs 11–1 and 11–2). In most patients the unilateral response was observed within 3 months, though regrowth was observed as early as 3 weeks in 1 patient and as late as 10 months in another. Treatment of both sides usually produced a good result (Figs 11–3 and 11–4). However, 5 patients who initially had shown a response failed to maintain a continuous response to subsequent treatment, though an eczematous reaction was still present. Despite this failure, a reduction in the concentration of diphencyprone resulted in a resumption of unilateral hair growth in 4 of the 5 patients.

The side effects were basically the same as those associated with dinitrochlorobenzene (DNCB) or squaric acid dibutylester. Initial application of a 2% concentration produced mild irritation of the skin with some itching for 2 or 3 days in 11 patients. On occasion, the eczematous reaction during the eliciting phase was so severe that treatment had to be discontinued for 1 week, after which a lower concentration was chosen. However, no patient discontinued treatment because of adverse effects. None of the laboratory tests performed before and every 3 months during treatment yielded abnormal results.

Diphencyprone is as effective as DNCB and squaric acid dibutylester in the treatment of severe alopecia areata. However, unlike DNCB, it is not mutagenic in the bacterial plate incorporation assay. It is more stable than squaric acid dibutylester, thus being more suitable for storage when dissolved in acetone. The results further support the view that contact allergy, and not merely irritation of the skin, is essential for the successful treatment of alopecia areata.

▶ [Diphencyprone seems to be an effective nonmutagenic contact allergen capable of inducing regrowth of hair in extensive alopecia areata. No patient dropped out of

(11–5) Acta Derm. Venereol. (Stockh.) 63:49–52, 1983.

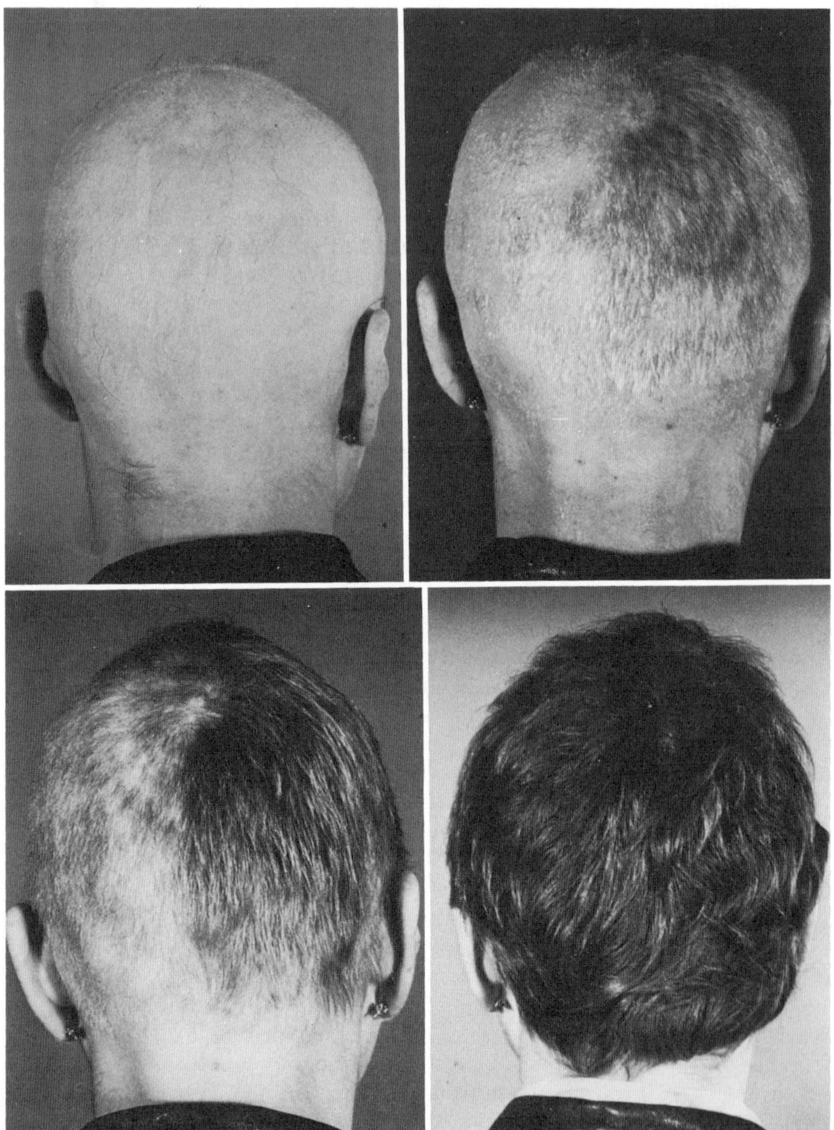

Fig 11–1 (top left).—Alopecia areata before treatment.
Fig 11–2 (top right).—After 15 weeks' treatment of right side with diphencyprone.
Fig 11–3 (bottom left).—Subsequent 6 weeks' treatment of both sides.
Fig 11–4 (bottom right).—After 19 weeks' treatment of both sides.
(Courtesy of Happle, R., et al.: Acta Derm. Venereol. [Stockh.] 63:49–52, 1983.)

the study because of severe side effects of the allergen. The authors state that a "lasting" response was present in the majority of patients—but no follow-up time was actually stated in the article. Further studies are warranted before giving the final word on this therapy.—R.R.] ◀

11–6 **Topical Minoxidil in Treatment of Alopecia Areata.** Minoxidil is a potent, orally active vasodilator that acts directly on vascular smooth muscle. Given systemically, it appears capable of converting vellus to terminal hair. Hypertrichosis is a regular feature in minoxidil-treated patients. David A. Fenton and John D. Wilkinson (High Wycombe, Bucks, England) undertook a modified double-blind crossover trial of topical minoxidil in 17 males and 13 females, with a median age of 43 years, whose median duration of alopecia areata was 5 years. Most had extensive patchy alopecia areata, and 9 had alopecia totalis. Both minoxidil and placebo were administered in ointment and lotion forms. Both active preparations contained 1% minoxidil. The maximum amount applied was based on a minimal oral dose of 5 mg twice daily. Nonresponders were crossed over after 12 weeks.

Active treatment produced a highly significant incidence of regrowth of hair, and 16 patients had cosmetically acceptable responses. There was no significant difference in responses to the ointment and the lotion. Most patients had regrowth of hair within 6 weeks of starting active treatment. Patients with more extensive alopecia had a poor prognosis, but those with an ophiasis pattern of hair loss responded better than expected. Responses could not be related to atopy, a family history of alopecia areata, or duration of disease. Three patients had regrowth of eyelashes and eyebrows, although only the scalp was treated with the active formulation.

Topical minoxidil apparently can induce new hair growth in patients with alopecia areata, but it remains unclear whether treatment can influence the eventual outcome. The few posttreatment biopsies performed suggest that the disease remains active despite regrowth of hair. Minoxidil therapy may at least be a useful stopgap measure, maintaining patients until spontaneous resolution takes place. The treatment seems to be relatively safe. No topical or systemic side effects occurred in the present study.

▶ [Topical minoxidil seems to be a somewhat effective treatment of alopecia areata in approximately 30%–50% of cases. The more extensive the alopecia, the less chance of regrowth. Unfortunately the effects of minoxidil are probably temporary, which will necessitate continual use of the medication. The results of topical minoxidil for male-pattern alopecia are less exciting—rates of cosmetically acceptable hair growth vary from 0 to 30%—R.R.] ◀

11–7 **The Flag Sign of Chemotherapy.** A variety of pigmentary changes have been associated with the use of several chemotherapeutic agents. Ronald G. Wheeland, Walter H. C. Burgdorf, and G. Bennett Humphrey (Univ. of Oklahoma) report a unique case of horizontal hyperpigmented bands appearing in the hair of a patient receiving chemotherapy.

Boy, 4, received a diagnosis of acute lymphoblastic leukemia of the null type at age 2 years. After complete remission with prednisone and vincristine therapy, consolidation therapy was instituted with L-asparaginase and meth-

---

(11–6) Br. Med. J. 287:1015–1017, Oct. 8, 1983.
(11–7) Cancer 51:1356–1358, Apr. 15, 1983.

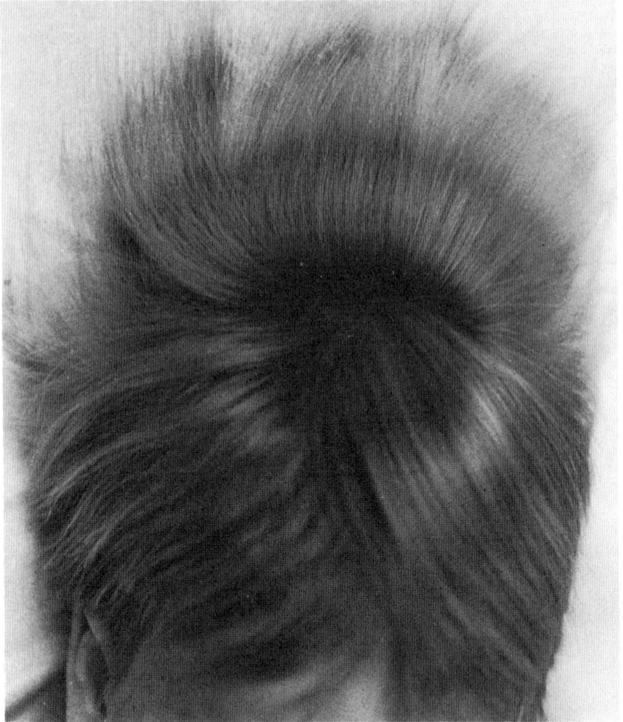

Fig 11–5.—Clinical appearance of pigmented bands within normal blond scalp hair. (Courtesy of Wheeland, R.G., et al.: Cancer 51:1356–1358, Apr. 15, 1983.)

otrexate. Hydrocortisone and arabinosyl cytosine also were used. Maintenance therapy was given with 6-mercaptopurine and oral and intravenous methotrexate with citrovorum rescue. Scalp alopecia developed after induction. As the hair began regrowing, alternating bands of dark pigmentation were noted within the normally blond scalp and eyebrow hair and cilia. Normal blond hair reappeared between high-dose methotrexate treatments, producing a flag-like pattern (Fig 11–5) which has persisted. The length of the normal band of scalp hair corresponds closely with the interval between methotrexate injections. No pigmentary changes developed in the skin or the nails.

Nail hyperpigmentation has been described in association with methotrexate administration. The flag sign seen in this patient has been noted in patients with severe protein-calorie malnutrition, but nutritional deficiency was not a factor in the present case. The hyperpigmentation produced by chemotherapeutic agents appears not to be related to MSH or ACTH activity or to ultraviolet light exposure. A temporary direct effect of the drugs on the activity of hair-bulb melanocytes, leading to increased production of melanosomes and increased distribution to the medullary and cortical cells of the hair shaft, seems to be the most likely explanation.

▶ [The "flag sign" can also occur when dark hair has intermittent *loss* of pigment.

In fact this depigmentation is what occurs in kwashiorkor or in protein-losing disorders such as nephrosis or ulcerative colitis. Also, chloroquine can produce alternating bands of "white" with intermittent therapy. We have not been aware of any disease or treatment, except the one described in this report, that can produce hyperpigmented bands in the hair. The mechanism is not at all clear.—T.B.F.] ◀

12. Leprosy and Other Mycobacterial Diseases

12–1 **Clinical and Immunologic Study of Four Babies of Mothers With Lepromatous Leprosy, Two of Whom Developed Leprosy in Infancy.** Leprosy is infrequent in children aged 4 years and younger, even when household contact occurs. Placental transmission appears to be very rare. M. Elizabeth Duncan, Reidar Melsom, John M. H. Pearson, S. Menzel, and R. St.C. Barnetson (Addis Ababa, Ethiopia) monitored 113 mothers with various types of leprosy through pregnancy and delivery, along with 27 healthy control women. Only 2 of the 36 women with borderline tuberculoid or tuberculoid leprosy had solid-staining bacilli in biopsy specimens or skin smears. Forty of 76 women with lepromatous leprosy showed clinical deterioration during pregnancy or soon afterward, and 28 had frank relapses. Solid-staining bacilli were present in skin smears or biopsies in 38 cases. All 9 milk specimens from mothers with highly bacilliferous leprosy were negative for acid-fast bacilli. Routine examinations of placental sections failed to demonstrate acid-fast bacilli.

In 4 infants, aged 9–17 months, hypopigmented lesions developed that were suspected of being due to leprosy. All of their mothers had active lepromatous leprosy. Two of the infants showed strong clinical evidence of leprosy. Both displayed histologic abnormalities of dermal nerves. On follow-up examination 2–3 years later, the lesions had nearly completely resolved without antileprosy treatment. In the 3 infants studied, no rise in titers of antibody to *Mycobacterium leprae* antigen 7 was noted when the suspicious skin lesions developed. Both infants with clinical evidence of leprosy had a marked rise in levels of IgA and IgM antibodies to *M. leprae.*

Two infants in this series were diagnosed as having leprosy on clinical and histologic grounds, and a third could well have had leprosy. Both infants with proved leprosy had significant increases in serum levels of IgA and, in particular, IgM antibodies to *M. leprae,* and 1 of them had a fall in IgG activity after healing of the lesions.

▶ [Leprosy is purported to have a long incubation period. This case report and the one to follow demonstrate the development of leprosy in four infants as young as 9 months and none older than 18 months. Taken together these 2 reports suggest that incubation periods shorter than 2 years can occur during infancy and that the diagnosis of leprosy should not be excluded from consideration in children younger than 2 years of age who have appropriate contact with affected relatives.—A.J.S.] ◀

(12–1) Int. J. Lepr. 51:7–17, March 1983.

12–2 **Leprosy in 18-Month-Old Children, Bichena District, Gojjam Administrative Region, Ethiopia.** Elisabeth Fekete and Tadele Tedla (Addis Ababa, Ethiopia) undertook a leprosy case-detection survey in an area of Ethiopia with a total population estimated at nearly a quarter of a million. They found 814 new cases of leprosy, 168 of them involving patients aged 5–14 years, and 12 (1.5%) involving children aged 1–4 years. Two patients, aged 18 months, were found to have borderline tuberculoid leprosy. The mother of one of these children had received a diagnosis 7 months before of borderline leprosy, which was treated with dapsone. The father of the other had lepromatous leprosy and had been receiving dapsone therapy for 10 years. A sibling of this child, aged 10 years, was found to have tuberculoid leprosy. The child's mother did not have leprosy.

Although incubation periods of less than 2 years are generally considered to be rare, children younger than age 2 years should not be excluded from leprosy surveys in endemic regions.

12–3 **T-cell-Conditioned Media Reverse T-cell Unresponsiveness in Lepromatous Leprosy.** Patients with disseminated, or lepromatous, leprosy play a major role in transmission of the disease and exhibit deficient T-cell responses to *Mycobacterium leprae* both in vitro and in vivo, but not to other antigens. Abebe Haregewoin, Tore Godal, Abu Salim Mustafa, Ayele Belehu, and Tabebe Yemaneberhan examined the effects of T-cell-conditioned medium rich in interleukin 2 (IL-2) on peripheral blood mononuclear cells from lepromatous patients. It is known that T cells with functional capacity after initial triggering by antigen can be kept in a continuously proliferative state in vitro when cultured in medium containing IL-2. Cells were obtained from 4 patients with borderline leprosy and 13 with lepromatous leprosy.

Blood mononuclear cells from both types of patients responded poorly to exposure to *M. leprae* in culture, but responded well to purified protein derivative. Background tritiated-thymidine incorporation was very high in some cases. Although the cells from lepromatous patients failed to produce IL-2 in response to *M. leprae,* they responded by proliferation to *M. leprae* in the presence of T-cell-conditioned medium. Indirect fluorescence staining showed that most of the proliferating cells present on the fifth day had $OKT4^+$ features. These are inducer-helper cells.

The proliferative defect of lepromatous T cells exposed to *M. leprae* appears to be commonly due to a deficiency in the events leading to antigen-nonspecific factor production. The factor most likely to be involved in the restorative effect is IL-2. Deficient T-cell factor production may be related to the presence of suppressor cells. The findings that helper-inducer T cells proliferate when exposed to *M. leprae* in the presence of T-cell-conditioned medium holds promise for the eventual restoration of immunologic competence in these patients.

(12–2) Lepr. Rev. 54:61–63, March 1983.
(12–3) Nature 303:342–344, May 1983.

▶ [On the basis of in vitro studies, this article suggests that the unresponsiveness in lepromatous leprosy results not from a lack of *M. leprae*–reactive cells but possibly from a deficiency in the production of IL-2. If this is so, one wonders whether future therapy with IL-2 will be feasible, practical, and effective.—S.L.M.] ◀

12–4 **Cutaneous Infiltrates of Leprosy: Cellular Characteristics and the Predominant T-Cell Phenotypes.** It is generally thought that the rapid progression of lepromatous leprosy lesions and their extensive bacillary loads result from a failure of cell-mediated im-

Percentage of Cells Reactive With Monoclonal Antibodies in Cutaneous Infiltrates and Blood of 21 Patients With Leprosy

Patient No.	Diagnosis		Percentage of Infiltrate Cells Positive *			Phenotype of T Cells (Percentage of Total T Cells Positive) †			
						Cutaneous Infiltrates		Blood	
	Clinical ‡	Histologic §	Anti-HLA-DR	Anti-Monocyte	Anti-T Cell	(OKT4/Leu 3a)	(OKT8/Leu 2a)	(OKT4/Leu 3a)	(OKT8/Leu 2a)
1	L	LL	>80	65	20	<5	>90	NT ¶	NT
2	L	LL	>80	60	15	<5	>90	NT	NT
3	L	LL	>80	60	20	<5	>90	60	40
4	L	LL	>80	55	30	<5	>90	61	39
5	L	LL	>80	60	15	<5	>90	NT	NT
6	L	LL	>80	75	15	15	85	NT	NT
7	L	LL	>80	70	30	<5	>90	NT	NT
8	L	BL	>80	50	30	40	60	NT	NT
9	L	BL	>80	70	15	<5	>90	NT	NT
10	B	BL	>80	70	10	<10	>90	NT	NT
11	B	BL	>80	50	20	25	75	69	31
12	B	BL	>80	60	20	35	65	76	24
13	B	BB	>80	30	50	50	50	NT	NT
14	B	BB	>80	50	30	50	50	78	22
15	T	D	>80	35	50	80	20	58	42
16	T	BT	>80	60	25	85	15	76	24
17	T	BT	>80	30	55	85	15	NT	NT
18	T	TT	>80	35	55	90	10	NT	NT
19	L	R	>80	>80	<2	—	—	59	41
20	T	R	>80	>80	<2	—	—	NT	NT
21	T	R	>80	>80	<2	—	—	76	24

*The number of positive infiltrate cells was calculated as follows: (positive cells/total number of cells in infiltrate) × 100. Antibody to HLA-DR was positive with OKIa, antimonocyte antibody with 61D3 or 63D3, and T-cell antibody with Leu 1 or with OKT4 plus OKT8.

†The percentage of positive OKT4 (Leu 3a) or OKT8 (Leu 2a) T cells was calculated as follows: (percentage positive/[percentage OKT8 + percentage OKT4]) × 100 or (percentage positive/percentage Leu 1) × 100. Similar percentages were found for 12 specimens examined by both methods. A dash denotes an insufficient number of T cells for analysis.

‡L denotes lepromatous leprosy; B, borderline; and T, tuberculoid.

§The histologic diagnosis was made according to the Ridley-Jopling scale. LL denotes lepromatous leprosy; BL borderline lepromatous; BB, borderline; BT borderline tuberculoid; TT tuberculoid; D nonspecific dermatitis consistent with resolving Hansen's disease; and R, resolved disease with few or no infiltrates seen.

¶NT denotes "not tested."

(Courtesy of Van Voorhis, W.C., et al.: N. Engl. J. Med. 307:1593–1597, Dec. 23, 1982; reprinted by permission of The New England Journal of Medicine.)

(12–4) N. Engl. J. Med. 307:1593–1597, Dec. 23, 1982.

munity, whereas immunity effectively controls bacillary growth in tuberculoid lesions. Wesley C. Van Voorhis, Gilla Kaplan, Euzenir Nunes Sarno, Marcus A. Horwitz, Ralph M. Steinman, William R. Levis, Nadia Nogueira, Laura S. Hair, Cerli Rocha Gattass, Bradley A. Arrick, and Zanvil A. Cohn (Rockefeller Univ.; Univ. of Tromsø, Norway; and Rio de Janeiro, Brazil) studied the types of cells present in skin lesions of 21 patients with leprosy by applying monoclonal antibodies to tissue sections. A sensitive biotin-avidin system was used to detect cells in frozen sections with the use of monoclonal antibodies. Patients with active lepromatous disease had large, poorly organized infiltrates with many macrophages, and many acid-fast bacilli were present in untreated patients and those in relapse. Patients with tuberculoid lesions had tightly packed, highly organized granulomas with numerous lymphocytes.

The proportions of cells reacting with monoclonal antibodies are given in the table. Many of the lepromatous infiltrates had consisted almost exclusively of suppressor T cells and were devoid of helper cells. The tuberculoid infiltrates, in contrast, contained predominantly helper T cells. The T cells and macrophages expressed HLA-DR antigen in both the lepromatous and tuberculoid infiltrates. No marked alterations in the distribution of blood T-cell phenotypes were observed.

Marked differences are found between the T-cell subsets in infiltrates of lepromatous and tuberculoid leprosy lesions, and they may be related to differences in the microbicidal activity of macrophages in these lesions. The T-cell phenotype in leprosy infiltrates also may be diagnostically useful, particularly for distinguishing various reactive states such as erythema nodosum leprosum from upgrading or borderline reactions. This approach holds potential value for assessing the prognosis of indeterminate leprosy and the effects of chemotherapy and immunotherapy.

▶ [The article supports the suspected immunopathology. Unfortunately a practical in vivo or in vitro test for prognosticating and directing therapy is not available. The lepromin skin test, which could be helpful, is not available.—S.L.M.] ◀

12–5 **Immunotherapy With a Mixture of *Mycobacterium leprae* and BCG in Different Forms of Leprosy and in Mitsuda-Negative Contacts.** The treatment of low-resistance forms of leprosy has been difficult, partly because the host is incapable of mounting an adequate immunologic response to the organism. Lepromatous patients and Mitsuda-negative contacts are unable to eliminate heat-killed *M. leprae* from skin sites, but the injection of both heat-killed *M. leprae* and bacillus Calmette-Guerin (BCG) is followed by the elimination of both mycobacteria. Jacinto Convit, Nacarid Aranzazu, Marian Ulrich, Maria E. Pinardi, Oscar Reyes, and Jorge Alvarado (Caracas, Venezuela) evaluated immunotherapy with a mixture of heat-killed *M. leprae* and viable BCG in 529 patients. They included 25 contacts of lepromatous patients who did not react to Mit-

(12–5) Int. J. Lepr. 50:415–424, December 1982.

suda antigen, 41 patients with indeterminate leprosy who also were Mitsuda negative, 109 patients with borderline lepromatous (BL) or lepromatous (LL) leprosy who were bacteriologically negative after prolonged sulfone therapy, and 354 patients with active BL and LL. Injections were made intradermally at three sites. Standard treatment was continued in most patients with active BL and LL.

Clinical improvement, including sharper definition of lesion borders and progressive flattening and regression of lesions, was seen in 57% of active LL cases and 76% of active BL cases. The lesions were infiltrated by mononuclear cells and exhibited epithelioid differentiation and fragmentation of the organisms. Delayed skin tests with soluble antigen from purified *M. leprae* became positive in significant numbers of patients in all groups. All the Mitsuda-negative contacts developed positive reactions to soluble antigen, but fewer than half the patients with inactive disease became immunologically reactive. Lesions of erythema nodosum leprosum disappeared in some patients and in others were replaced by papular lesions with extensive lymphoid-cell infiltration. A few patients with active disease developed new lesions that later were transformed into structures resembling tuberculoid granulomas.

The findings call into question the assumption that lepromatous leprosy is incurable because bacilli persist after many years of treatment. The development of lymphocytes sensitized to *M. leprae* has been closely associated with lymphocytic infiltration of the lesions, which acquired tuberculoid features, and with the development of positive results in delayed hypersensitivity skin tests. Several vaccinations may be necessary in advanced cases. Combined immunotherapy may be prophylactically useful as well as being of value in treatment of low-resistance forms of leprosy.

▶ [The suppression or congenital absence of cell-mediated response to *M. leprae* in patients with certain types of leprosy is unexplainable. With the current problem of persistent bacilli and resistance to dapsone, there has been a big push to try vaccines for the primary prevention of the disease.

There are 4 vaccines available for trial (Job K. C.: *Leprosy in India* 55:1–7, 1983)

1. The above mixture of *M. leprae* and BCG of Convit et al.
2. Killed and purified *M. laprae* in saline suspension (Mehra, V., Bloom, B. R.: *Infect. Immun.* 23:787, 1979)
3. IRC bacilli killed by γ irradiation (Deo, M. S.: *Science* 216:117, 1982)
4. Mycobacterium W vaccine (Talwar, G. P.: *Leprosy in India* 50:492, 1978.)—S.L.M.] ◀

12–6 **Immunopathology of Erythema Nodosum Leprosum: Role of Extravascular Complexes.** Erythema nodosum leprosum (ENL) is a reactional episode of lepromatous leprosy characterized by large amounts of mycobacterial antigen and corresponding antibodies. The deposit of immunoglobulins and C3 in glomeruli and C1q binding activity in serum support an immune complex cause for ENL. Marian J. Ridley and D. S. Ridley (London) used the immunoperoxidase technique to evaluate 20 patients with ENL. Control biopsy specimens were obtained from 10 patients with nonreacting

---

(12–6) Lepr. Rev. 54:95–107, June 1983.

lepromatous leprosy, 6 of whom had active, untreated disease.

Disintegration of macrophages and release of bacterial antigen in the form of cell walls and particulate components of *Mycobacterium leprae* were consistent findings at the centers of ENL lesions. Various forms of antigenic debris were observed on cell membranes, within vacuoles, and in the intercellular space. The material combined first with IgM and later with IgG. Components of the classic complement pathway were present at the same sites. Both C-reactive protein and β-lipoprotein were present in varying amounts and associated in part with connective tissue. Immunoglobulins and complement components were present in vessel walls later in the course. Granular bacilli and acid-fast debris in nerve bundles were coated with IgM and complement. Lysozyme and IgG were present in the interaxonal spaces. No immunoglobulin was bound to bacilli in control specimens of lesions at a comparable stage of activity. All immunologic components except C-reactive protein were present in smaller amounts than in reacting lesions. Inflammatory cells were scanty in control biopsy specimens.

The findings support the view that ENL is an immune complex disorder, possibly self-perpetuating, that occurs at the site of breakdown of small lepromatous granulomas. The immune complexes are extravascular, in contrast to classic "serum sickness." The occurrence of ENL may be conditional on the slow degradation of large amounts of antigen of low immunogenicity, which would explain why no exact counterpart in other disorders is recognized.

▶ [Two phenomena have been described that may be relevant in the immunopathogenesis of ENL. A controversial one advanced by Mshana (*Lepr. Rev.* 53:1, 1982) that the initiating phase of ENL is due to an imbalance of T-cell subsets with a decrease of suppressed T-cells and a secondary perpetuation phase which might involve immune complexes. The other is that distinctive histologic variations of ENL are related to ethnic groups and present different clinical disease patterns, e.g., the Lucio phenomenon in Mexicans and the occurrence of ENL mainly in the leproma subpolar type of lepromatous leprosy among Malaysians (Ridley et al.: *Lepr. Rev.* 42:65, 1981).—S.L.M.] ◀

13. Melanocytic Nevi and Melanoma

13–1 **Dysplastic Melanocytic Nevi in Histologic Association With 234 Primary Cutaneous Melanomas.** A relationship between cutaneous melanoma and melanocytic nevi is established. Arthur R. Rhodes, Terence J. Harrist, Calvin L. Day, Martin C. Mihm, Jr., Thomas B. Fitzpatrick, and Arthur J. Sober (Boston) examined the association between histologically defined dysplastic melanocytic nevi (DMN) and primary cutaneous melanoma in a series of 234 patients with primary melanoma, who were followed up for a mean of 90 months. All were entered in the Harvard Melanoma Registry. The disease was diagnosed on the basis of a proliferation of variably atypical, singly disposed or loosely aggregated melanocytes in or just above the basal unit in elongated and club-shaped epidermal rete ridges. In contiguity, DMN extended for 3 or more consecutive epidermal retia beyond the most lateral margin of the melanoma.

Nine primary melanomas were lentigo maligna lesions. Of the remaining 225 lesions, 49 (22%) were associated with atypical melanocytic hyperplasia in a lentiginous epidermal pattern (AMHL) in the same histologic section as intraepidermal and invasive melanoma, but beyond its most lateral margin. Further, AMHL was directly associated with the presence of a dermal nevocellular nevus in histologic contiguity with melanoma. It was inversely associated with nodular melanoma. Most AMHL was not related to familial melanoma, but there were few familial cases in the series.

The finding of AMHL in 20% of patients with primary cutaneous melanoma in this series supports the view that at least some cutaneous melanomas may have an origin in DMN. Supposedly normal persons with 1 or more DMN may be a source of AMHL-associated "sporadic" melanomas. The absence of AMHL in ordinary nevocellular nevi and solar lentigines supports the suggestion that patients having pigmented cutaneous lesions with AMHL are at increased risk for the development of melanoma.

▶ [Dysplastic nevi (DN) are currently considered the single most important precursor lesion for malignant melanoma. The frequency with which melanoma arises from DN is unknown, but estimates as high as 50% have been made. In the study abstracted above, histopathologic criteria have been defined for DN, and the frequency with which a residual DN was found in 225 cases of cutaneous melanoma was assessed. In this study approximately 1 melanoma in 5 appeared to have a histopathologically associated DN remnant. Confirmatory studies with clear-cut histologic criteria must be made.—A.J.S.] ◀

13–2 **Familial Atypical Multiple Mole-Melanoma (FAMMM) Syndrome: Segregation Analysis.** Previous studies of 4 pedigrees of the

(13–1) J. Am. Acad. Dermatol. 9:563–574, October 1983.
(13–2) J. Med. Genet. 20:342–344, October 1983.

familial atypical multiple mole-melanoma (FAMMM) syndrome indicated phenotypic variability with respect to cutaneous malignant melanoma (CMM) and other cancers in each kindred. Henry T. Lynch, Ramon M. Fusaro, William J. Kimberling, and Jane F. Lynch (Omaha) and B. Shannon Danes (Cornell Univ.) report the preliminary results of genetic analysis of these kindreds in which the FAMMM phenotype has been verified clinically and pathologically for 16 years. There are 80 affected or at risk family members. The segregation ratio of 0.47 is consistent with autosomal dominant inheritance. There were 3 obligate gene carriers who lacked any FAMMM phenotypic manifestations. The calculated rate of penetrance of the FAMMM gene was 0.93. The risk for cancers other than CMM and intraocular malignant melanoma was increased fivefold in gene carriers after adjustment for age, compared with the population expectation. Possible excesses of cancer of the lung, pancreas, and breast were observed, but a larger sample size would be needed to verify these findings.

The FAMMM syndrome, a cancer-associated genodermatosis, appears to be inherited as an autosomal dominant trait with variable expressivity and reduced penetrance. Unusually long survival with multiple primary CMMs is a feature of these kindreds. The findings suggest a possibly unique host factor mechanism of cancer expression. The variable expressivity of the phenotype poses diagnostic difficulties, particularly when an isolated patient with incomplete expression of the FAMMM phenotype is encountered. Studies of other FAMMM kindreds would be worthwhile.

▶ [Lynch et al. have provided important information for practitioners who care for patients with dysplastic melanocytic nevi (DMN) or cutaneous melanoma or both. From a detailed analysis of 80 "at risk" members of 4 selected kindreds with hereditary melanoma and DMN, 34 (49%) of 72 scorable family members had either cutaneous melanoma or histologically confirmed DMN. More important, 3 members of the kindred were obligate gene carriers on the basis of pedigree analysis (i.e., they had affected parents and children), but did not themselves show manifestations of the disorder. Complicating these studies is the observation that DMN may appear some time later in life and may not be apparent when an individual is studied. Thus, first-degree relatives of persons with cutaneous melanoma need to be seen intermittently in order to exclude the development of DMN or melanoma or both. The increased risk for other cancers in these 4 kindreds is intriguing. However, one wonders about ascertainment bias for families followed so closely for 16 years and about the validity of comparing their cumulative risk of nonmelanoma cancer to age-adjusted incidence data obtained from the Third National Cancer Survey. Clearly, the issues of other cancers in these kindreds requires carefully controlled epidemiologic studies.—A.R.R.] ◀

13–3 **Phenotypic Variation in Familial Atypical Multiple Mole-Melanoma Syndrome (FAMMM).** The FAMMM syndrome is characterized by susceptibility to multiple atypical moles which have varied coloration, structure, and number and are located chiefly on nonexposed areas of skin. Dysplastic changes are found in the melanocytes, with fibroplasia and chronic inflammatory cell infiltration. The lesions can transform to cutaneous malignant melanomas. Henry T.

(13–3) J. Med. Genet. 20:25–29, February 1983.

Lynch, Ramon M. Fusaro, William A. Albano, Judith Pester, William J. Kimberling, and Jane F. Lynch (Omaha) have found that the hereditary form of malignant melanoma as seen in the FAMMM syndrome is more complex than was previously thought. A kindred with a wide-ranging cutaneous and tumor phenotype was studied.

The proband was a woman, 29, who had a cutaneous nodular malignant melanoma that was excised from the forearm. A single papular nevus was present, but no atypical moles were seen. The father had had multiple moles removed from the shoulder and back at age 28 and had also had a nodular malignant melanoma. Examination when he was aged 60 showed several atypical nevi without the histologic features characteristic of fully developed FAMMM moles. None of the proband's 3 children had clinical evidence of atypical moles consistent with the FAMMM syndrome. Three relatives in all had variable clinical and histologic manifestations of the FAMMM syndrome. The proband had a squamous cell cancer of the oral cavity besides the cutaneous melanoma.

Striking phenotypic variation in the FAMMM syndrome is apparent in this relatively small kindred. Studies of FAMMM families have shown variations in the histologic composition of the compound nevi, which may even occur in different regions of the same patient. Preliminary genetic analysis of the present kindred and three others strongly supports autosomal dominant inheritance of the syndrome. The estimated rate of penetrance is 0.86. Sporadic occurrences of the FAMMM syndrome have been described, but it is premature to distinguish familial and sporadic subtypes of the syndrome. Patients must be told of the risk that extracutaneous cancers may develop. It is possible that malignant melanomas can arise without preexistent atypical moles in these patients.

▶ [Lynch et al. point out a problem facing physicians caring for melanoma-prone families. Only one dysplastic melanocytic nevus (DMN) is necessary to give rise to melanoma. Any given melanoma may have arisen in a single DMN, and there need not be other DMN in the same individual. Furthermore, a given individual with DMN or melanoma need not be aware of a family history of melanoma or DMN or both; blood relatives may be at increased risk for melanoma by virtue of carrying potential melanoma precursors but may be unaware of their existence. Until this business is sorted out, it behooves the physician to examine first-degree relatives of individuals with melanoma or DMN, seeking the presence of similar lesions to establish early diagnosis. Also, the absence of DMN in prepubertal individuals does not exclude the diagnosis; DMN may not be apparent until puberty. Pathologists are not yet in complete agreement with respect to the microscopic definitions of DMN or melanocytic dysplasia or both, which only compounds problems for the unwary physician.—A.R.R.] ◀

13–4 **Multiple Melanoma and Atypical Melanocytic Nevi: Evidence of an Activated and Expanded Melanocytic System.** The association between acquired melanocytic nevi and primary malignant melanoma is unclear. Rona M. MacKie (Glasgow) describes 7 patients with malignant melanoma associated with acquired melanocytic nevi and 5 with multiple atypical nevi alone. Mean age at presentation

---

(13–4) Br. J. Dermatol. 107:621–629, December 1982.

with melanoma was 33 years. Three of these patients had a family history of malignant melanoma. Nine of the 12 patients had had excessive solar exposure. Only 2 patients had type I, or "Celtic," skin. All patients have been advised to avoid long-term solar exposure and to use a sunscreen topically if exposure is unavoidable.

All the melanomas had developed on skin regularly exposed to sunlight. The lesions were 0.2–1.9 mm thick. Only 1 patient had had secondary spread on follow-up for 2–12 years. In only 2 of 21 primary tumors was there histologic evidence of a preexistent melanocytic nevus. All the melanomas were of the superficial, spreading type. No primary tumors have developed on a mucosal surface, in the nail bed region, or in the eye. The numbers of melanocytic nevi exceeded those in control subjects in all instances, and many moles were more than 2 cm in diameter and had irregular margins. Lesions in patients without melanoma exhibited changes of compound melanocytic nevus but with increased numbers of large melanocytes at the dermoepidermal junction. The ratio of melanocytes to basal keratinocytes adjacent to lesions was relatively high in all patients; the ratio in distant sites was lower.

Some patients with large numbers of irregularly shaped melanocytic nevi have a tendency to develop malignant melanoma, sometimes in multiple primary sites. The term "activated and expanded melanocyte syndrome" is proposed. The syndrome, whether sporadic or familial, appears to be relatively rare in Britain.

▶ [The author emphasizes three points based on a selected group of patients: *(1)* preexisting melanocytic nevi were detected histologically in contiguity with 2 of 21 primary melanomas (compared to about a quarter of melanomas in other studies); *(2)* numbers of nevi were increased in 13 individuals with melanoma (but lacking a family history of melanoma) compared with 24 "matched" controls; and *(3)* many of the atypical nevi had features that are part of the classic description of dysplastic melanocytic nevi. The author also contends that the number of melanocytes surrounding atypical nevi is increased (based on melanocyte counts in routine sections), that sun exposure has an important role in the evolution of the nevi, and that melanoma may develop on normal skin even in patients with atypical nevi. The author suggests a new term, "activated and expanded melanocyte system." Further studies are required to confirm the latter three observations.—A.R.R.] ◀

13–5 **Dysplastic Nevi on Scalp of Prepubertal Children From Melanoma-Prone Families.** Dysplastic nevi are important in the histogenesis of sporadic cutaneous malignant melanoma and represent a marker for susceptibility to melanoma in affected families. Margaret A. Tucker, Mark H. Greene, Wallace H. Clark, Jr., Kenneth H. Kraemer, Mary C. Fraser, and David E. Elder examined members of 14 families participating in a National Cancer Institute study of hereditary melanoma. They observed dysplastic nevi on the scalp in 4 prepubertal melanoma-prone family members, 3 of whom had normal glabrous skin. The scalp is an uncommon site of ordinary moles. Dysplastic nevi were sought in 400 members of 14 melanoma-prone families, each of which had at least 2 members with documented melanoma.

(13–5) J. Pediatr. 103:65–69, July 1983.

Sixty-seven family members had at least 1 cutaneous malignant melanoma, and in 7 the first melanoma developed before age 20 years. Six of the 67 patients had primary cutaneous melanoma of the scalp, and 5 died of metastatic disease. Scalp melanomas arose in dysplastic nevi in all 6 patients. The initial abnormality in young family members generally was an increased number of morphologically normal nevi, often found at ages 5–9 years. The features of dysplastic nevi appeared at onset of puberty. Scalp nevi were present in 42% of 19 patients under age 20 with dysplastic nevus syndrome (DNS). Scalp nevi in preadolescent and periadolescent children were likely to be dysplastic. The proportion of scalp nevi in patients with dysplastic nevi tended to decline with advancing age.

Dysplastic nevi appear to form the substrate on which nearly all hereditary melanomas occur. The proper management of DNS remains under study, but it seems best to excise dysplastic nevi on the scalp in children. There may be problems in following adolescents regularly, and it is difficult to monitor suspicious nevi that are covered with hair. Melanomas arising at this site carry a very unfavorable prognosis.

▶ [If benign-appearing nevi can be followed easily, they need not be excised, as long as they are stable. "Hidden" nevi present a dilemma. Dysplastic nevi and melanoma-prone families present a difficult problem if some of the dysplastic nevi are in "hidden" areas, making them difficult or impossible to follow. As a general guideline, all nevi on the scalp in individuals with a personal or family history of melanoma or dysplastic nevi or both should be evaluated for prophylactic excision. What to do about hidden nevi in general is a judgment call. Better off!—A.R.R.] ◀

13–6 **Congenital Nevocellular Nevus: A Review of the Treatment Controversy and a Report of 46 Cases.** Marvin S. Arons and Sidney Hurwitz (Yale–New Haven Med. Center) reviewed their experience with 46 children having congenital nevocellular nevi. Most had been referred primarily to a pediatric dermatologist. Girls predominated, probably reflecting an aesthetic bias by parents and primary physicians. All patients but 1 were white. Once a child is aged 10–14 months, the risk of anesthesia does not outweigh that of malignant melanoma developing in the nevus. The excision must include the deep fascia, but only 2 patients had two-stage excisions. Twenty-three patients underwent closure with split- or full-thickness skin grafts. Primary suture closure was feasible in 14 patients.

Malignant changes in congenital nevi often are difficult to recognize, and stage II disease may be present at the time of clinical diagnosis. As the overall prognosis for such patients is unfavorable, these nevi should no longer be considered a primarily cosmetic problem. Malignant melanoma can arise even in small congenital nevocellular nevi. It seems best to excise totally all pigmented congenital nevi as early as is technically possible. All satellite lesions should be removed. Small nevi should be removed even from newborn infants if there are such signs as irregular borders or notable variation in color, or if dark pigmentation or lobulation would make future changes dif-

---

(13–6) Plast. Reconstr. Surg. 72:355–365, September 1983.

ficult to interpret. A cutaneous punch biopsy can be performed when the diagnosis is in question or neoplastic change is a possibility.

About three fourths of these patients had congenital compound nevi, and the rest had dermal nevi. All 38 lesions studied contained mature nevus cells. Both recurrences were in patients who had nevi below the midreticular dermis.

▶ [This article reviews the current treatment controversies surrounding small, large, and giant congenital nevomelanocytic nevi. The series of 46 patients in this report provides no "new" information regarding the malignant potential of small congenital nevomelanocytic nevi. The authors' inclination, based on available information, is to recommend excision of all congenital nevi (where feasible).—A.R.R.] ◀

13–7 **Patterns of Congenital Nevocellular Nevi: Histologic Study of 38 Cases.** Congenital nevocellular nevi are considered to be premalignant lesions, but the actual incidence of malignant change is widely disputed. K. S. Stenn, M. Arons, and S. Hurwitz (Yale Univ.) reviewed the findings in 38 cases of nevocellular nevus diagnosed at birth. All lesions were excised to subcutaneous fat in one step and the defects skin grafted. There were 2 recurrences. Microscopic examination showed either diffuse or patchy infiltration of the upper dermis alone or diffuse or patchy infiltration of the upper and deep dermis with nevoid cells in or below the lower third of the reticular dermis. In 37% of cases, nevoid cells extended into the deepest reticular dermis. The histologic patterns exhibited no correlation with age, sex, lesion site, or size. The 2 patients with recurrent nevi in the surgical site had diffuse upper and deep dermal nevoid cell infiltration. No malignant change was observed in this series.

Several distinct histologic patterns of congenital nevocellular nevus are apparent. The nevoid cells do not necessarily extend into the deep dermis, and the deepest reticular dermis was involved in only just over a third of cases in this study. Both recurrences in this series are attributed to incomplete excision of the primary lesion in the presence of nevoid cells in the deep dermis. Nevi with a diffuse, deep distribution of nevoid cells require more aggressive excision to prevent recurrences. Whether there is any relation between the various histologic patterns and the risk of malignant change remains to be determined.

▶ [The most important observation made in this article is that only 14 (37%) of 38 nevomelanocytic nevi (NMN) known to be congenital by parenteral history had nevus cell involvement of the lower third of the reticular dermis or deeper. For the remaining 24 patients, nevus cells were not found in the lower third of the reticular dermis. For comparison, nevus cells were present in the lower two thirds of the reticular dermis in 59 of 60 congenital NMN studied by Mark et al. (*Hum. Pathol.* 4:395–418, 1973). It is difficult to compare results in the two studies. Walton et al. (*Br. J. Dermatol.* 95:389, 1976) reported that only 2 of 11 NMN excised in the first 72 hours of life had features of congenital NMN described by Mark et al. These issues are vital to the determination of the *sensitivity* of microscopic findings in predicting age at onset of a given nevus (whether in isolation or in contiguity with melanoma) based on histologic features alone. The presence of nevus cells in the deep dermis is sufficient (but not absolutely necessary) to suggest that a given nevus is indeed congenital. The specificity of this finding was not examined by Stenn et al.—A.R.R.] ◀

(13–7) J. Am. Acad. Dermatol. 9:388–393, September 1983.

13–8 **Survival From Preinvasive and Invasive Malignant Melanoma in Western Australia.** Preinvasive melanoma (PIM) is widely believed to be an early stage in a progression of melanocytic changes toward aggressive malignancy, and there is epidemiologic evidence of similarity between PIM and invasive malignant melanoma (IMM). W. M. Lemish, P. J. Heenan, C. D. J. Holman, and B. K. Armstrong (Univ. of Western Australia) reviewed 113 cases of PIM and 415 of IMM in patients who were treated in 1975 and 1976, representing 97% of all new cases in Western Australia in this period. Complete follow-up through 1980 was achieved in 96% of cases.

There was essentially no survival disadvantage in patients with the diagnosis of PIM, and no recurrences were found in this group. The 5-year survival rates of men and women with IMM were 85% and 89%, respectively, and the clinical disease-free rates were 80% and 82%. The prognosis was considerably worse for patients with regional node or distant disease at presentation. Invasive malignant melanoma arising in the head and neck region had the poorest prognosis. Survival rates declined significantly with increasingly deeper invasion. Survival is related to tumor thickness in the table. The difference in survival in relation to tumor thickness was highly significant. Invasive malignant melanoma was generally widely excised with skin graft closure. Node dissection was done for clinical involvement in 7% of patients and prophylactically in another 2%. Adjuvant immunotherapy and chemotherapy were used in 5% and 3% of patients, respectively.

Survival with melanoma in Western Australia is better than in other regions. Lesions with a favorable prognosis may be more frequent in high-incidence populations. No patients with PIM or thin IMM have had recurrences, and these designations need not result in undue anxiety if physicians know of the outlook for patients with these diagnoses and if both patients and the general public receive correct information.

▶ [No universal agreement among melanoma pathologists exists on the diagnostic

Crude and Relative 5-Year Survival Rates From IMM in Western Australia, 1975 and 1976, by Tumor Thickness Group

Tumor thickness group		Five-year survival rate (%) Crude			Relative		
		Men	Women	Total	Men	Women	Total
<0.76 mm	(68)*	93	95	94	100	99	100
0.76–1.49 mm	(49)	67	96	83	82	100	93
1.50–2.99 mm	(44)	63	63	63	74	70	72
3.00+ mm	(36)	45	54	49	58	62	60

*Numbers of cases in parentheses.
(Courtesy of Lemish, W.M., et al.: Cancer 52:580–585, Aug. 1, 1983.)

(13–8) Cancer 52:580–585, Aug. 1, 1983.

criteria for preinvasive melanoma. The terms used at various centers to sign out these lesions would vary from melanoma in situ, to severely atypical melanocytic hyperplasia, to dysplastic nevus. There is universal agreement concerning the benign behavior of this lesion when it has been completely excised. These lesions should be excluded when one is considering mortality from melanoma.—A.J.S.] ◀

13–9 **Cutaneous Factors Related to the Risk of Malignant Melanoma.** Malignant melanoma is described as being most frequent in fair-skinned, blue-eyed, red-haired persons who burn rather than tan when exposed to sunlight. Valerie Beral, Susan Evans, Helen Shaw, and G. Milton undertook a case-control study of various cutaneous factors possibly related to melanoma risk in 287 white women with malignant melanoma and 574 age-matched controls. The women with melanoma were aged 18–54 years.

Hair, skin, and eye color were related to the risk of melanoma. Red hair color at age 5 was associated with a relative risk of 3.0 and blond hair with a relative risk of 1.6. Fair skin was associated with an approximate doubling of the risk. Women with melanoma reported tendencies to burn and freckle when exposed to sunlight, with respective relative risk estimates of 1.4 and 1.9. Hair color, particularly red hair, appeared to be the chief independent determinant of melanoma risk, followed by skin color. A history of an above-average number of nevi on the body carried a relative risk of 3.4. A history of psoriasis and one of vitiligo were also more frequent in cases than in controls. Acne, however, appeared to be protective, with a relative risk of 0.4, and chloasma carried a relative risk of 0.6, as did premature graying of the hair. These relations were independent of hair color and skin color.

Red and blond hair were strongly associated with an increased risk of melanoma in this large case-control study of white women. Fair skin and an increased number of nevi on the body were also associated with an increased melanoma risk. The risk was increased in subjects with a history of vitiligo, whereas a history of hyperpigmentation in the form of chloasma was associated with a reduced risk of melanoma. The higher frequency of psoriasis in cases requires further investigation, especially with regard to treatment.

▶ [Since not all melanoma patients have blue eyes, red or blond hair, skin that burns easily and tans poorly, or a history of extensive solar exposure, other studies are now looking at whether recreational behavior, intermittency of solar exposure, and traumatic solar events (bad sunburns) rather than total cumulative solar exposure may be relevant factors. A preliminary study (Lew, R. A., et al., *J. Dermatol. Surg. Oncol.* 12:981–986, 1983) found a significant risk associated with a history of blistering sunburns in childhood or adolescence. The risks associated with psoriasis, vitiligo, acne, and melasma remain to be evaluated in other studies, and for now the evidence is, at best, weak (see also Elwood, J. M., Hislop, T. G.: *Natl. Cancer Inst. Monogr.* 62:167–171, 1982).—A.J.S.] ◀

13–10 **Incidence and Reporting of Cutaneous Melanoma in Queensland.** Green (Univ. of Queensland, Brisbane, Australia) studied pathology records to ascertain new reports of primary cutaneous mela-

---

(13–9) Br. J. Dermatol. 109:165–172, August 1983.
(13–10) Aust. J. Dermatol. 23:105–109, December 1982.

noma occurring in Queensland during a 12-month period. Records showed 871 incident patients who were residents of Queensland at the time of histologic diagnosis. Three major histologic types were analyzed: superficial spreading melanoma (SSM), lentigo maligna (melanoma) (LM[M]), and melanoma showing no in situ component (nodular).

Between July 1, 1979, and June 30, 1980, of the 871 patients in whom the disease was diagnosed, SSM occurred most frequently overall (57% of the total) and was slightly more common in women; 81% of these tumors were invasive. The LM and LM(M) types constituted 23% of melanomas reported, and 25% of these were invasive at diagnosis. The remainder (15%) were classified as nodular. In women, SSM occurred predominantly in younger age groups, mostly on the trunk and lower limbs, whereas nodular melanoma showed increasing proportions with increasing age, with the lower limbs the major site. Men showed a similar age pattern for nodular melanomas, whereas SSM showed no particular age pattern; the trunk was the major site for both types. The tumor type LM(M) varied least between the sexes, increasing to a peak in those aged 60–69, the head and neck being the predominant sites. With regard to tumor thickness, most SSM and LM(M) tumors were thin in contrast to nodular tumors. Also, 75% of nodular melanomas and about 50% of SSM and LM(M) lesions were noticed by patients. Significantly more women than men noticed their own lesions.

It is likely that education campaigns in Queensland have contributed to public awareness of melanoma and other such lesions. However, it is difficult to distinguish between a true increase in incidence of disease and an increase resulting from early reporting in a community that is aware of the disease. Longitudinal studies are necessary to clarify this issue.

▶ [Australia continues to be on top when incidence figures for melanoma are considered. When comparing these figures to non-Australian data, one must subtract the level I (noninvasive) tumors that are included in the figures. As also seen in other centers around the world, there has been, so far, no leveling off of the rise in incidence. Lifetime risk for melanoma in the United States for whites is between 1/200 and 1/300. The risk in Queensland would be higher. Also of note is the figure of 4%–8% for lentigo maligna melanoma, a clearly solar related tumor which is very similar to that found in less sunny New England. One would expect a greater proportion of lentigo maligna melanomas in areas of more intense solar flux (see abstract below).—A.J.S.] ◀

-11 **Melanoma of the Head and Neck in Queensland.** Trevor J. Harris and Del M. Hinckley (Royal Brisbane Hosp., Queensland, Australia) report that the incidence of melanoma in Queensland is 40 per 100,000 population, the highest rate in the world. Of the 740 melanomas treated between 1974 and 1980, 161 (22%) were located on the head and neck. The peak incidence of head and neck melanoma was in persons aged 50–80 years. The sex ratio was 1.33 males to 1 female. Most lesions occurred on the skin of the cheek, temple, and

---

(13–11) Head Neck Surg. 5:197–203, Jan.–Feb., 1983.

neck, with melanomas of the scalp and lower lip being relatively uncommon.

Geographically, the highest risk area for skin cancer is Queensland, centered on the Tropic of Capricorn. The cumulative effect of this exposure to sunlight produces typical "Queensland skin," an admixture of solar keratoses, basal cell carcinomas, squamous cell carcinomas, and Hutchinson's melanotic freckle. In this series, 46.5% of melanomas of the head and neck were Hutchinson's melanotic freckle melanoma, and two thirds of these were superficial lesions. Further, 54.8% of head and neck melanomas were treated at the superficial levels I and II, another 20% at level III (varying in thickness from 0.65 mm to 1.5 mm), and 25% at levels IV and V (more than 1.5 mm thick). Superficial melanoma required a histologically adequate excision with a small margin (1 cm). Flap cover rather than a graft is used in early lesions, because they are unlikely to recur locally, a good cosmetic result is desirable, and the repair is definitive. Anatomical variations in areas as the ear, nose, eyelid, and scalp influenced the patterns of spread and necessitated different treatments at each site.

Melanoma level and thickness can be used as a guide to the extent of surgery necessary in the treatment of primary tumors and affected notes. The treatment undertaken is based on frozen section determination of depth of invasion. A public awareness program continues in Queensland, because early detection combined with adequate initial surgical treatment appears to lead to a successful outcome in most patients.

▶ [Queensland, Australia, and Tucson, Arizona, are "head and shoulders" above other areas of Australia and the United States in melanoma incidence. In this series of head and neck melanomas from Queensland, nearly half were of the lentigo maligna melanoma type, the one type clearly related to chronic solar exposure. Some caution must be exercised in comparing these incidence figures with United States data, as mentioned in the preceding abstract, because the Australians include level I (in situ) lesions in their rates, whereas figures from the United States do not.—A.J.S.] ◀

13–12 **Geographic Distribution of Cutaneous Melanoma in Queensland.** Adele Green and Victor Siskind (Herston, Queensland) examined the geographic distribution of melanoma in Queensland in light of the large increase in incidence (doubling from 16.4 cases per 100,000 population in 1965 to 32.7 per 100,000 in 1977), and to reassess whether the observed distribution provides support for the solar radiation hypothesis. They considered all cases of first primary cutaneous melanomas that appeared in the records of the 24 Queensland pathology laboratories from July 1, 1979, to June 30, 1980. Patients with Hutchinson's melanotic freckle (HMF) or Hutchinson's melanotic freckle melanoma (HMFM) were separated from the others. For comparison, Queensland was partitioned into 4 regions—tropical and subtropical, divided by the Tropic of Capricorn, and inland and coastal, divided by the Great Dividing Range. Regional incidence

---

(13–12) Med. J. Aust. 1:407–410, Apr. 30, 1983.

MORTALITY AND INCIDENCE RATES OF MELANOMA*
IN QUEENSLAND

Region	Mortality rate†	Incidence rate‡
Subtropical	4.7	35.8
Tropical	4.9	34.9
Coastal	5.0	37.0
Inland	4.2	25.3

*Excluding Hutchinson's melanotic freckle and Hutchinson's melanotic freckle melanoma.

†Deaths per 100,000 population, calculated from 1974–1979 data of the Australian Bureau of Statistics and indirectly standardized to the age distribution of Queensland in 1976.

‡Incidence per 100,000 population indirectly standardized to the age distribution of Queensland in 1976.

(Courtesy of Green, A., and Siskind, V.: Med. J. Aust. 1:407–410, Apr. 30, 1983.)

rates for melanoma, excluding HMFM, were standardized directly to the age distribution of the Queensland population.

In all, 871 patients had first primary cutaneous melanomas diagnosed in Queensland during the study period. This represents an overall crude incidence rate of 39.6 cases per 100,000 population, or 45.1 per 100,000 when standardized to the age distribution of the standard European population. There were 201 patients reported as having an in situ component of HMF. The differences between the 4 broad regions for age-standardized rates were statistically significant, with the source of significance being between inland and coastal regions. Indirectly age-standardized mortality and incidence rates in broad geographic areas are presented in the table. The main difference in mortality occurred between coastal and inland areas rather than between tropical and subtropical areas.

The findings indicate that even after the sharp increase in incidence in cutaneous melanoma, the place of residence of melanoma patients in Queensland bears no consistent relation to latitude. The only statistically significant geographic difference in the incidence of melanoma is the higher rate in the coastal strip compared with inland areas, despite the greater summer erythemal ultraviolet doses in the latter regions. Many local factors, including altitude, atmospheric ozone levels, and variations in cloud cover, may modify the linear dependence of ultraviolet dose on latitude, which may yet explain the variation in actual exposure to ultraviolet radiation received by the population.

▶ [The relationship of solar exposure to melanoma incidence is not a clear-cut one. Latitude gradients seem to operate within countries but not within small regions of the country or between countries. Other factors clearly are operating, and the effects of microenvironment, behavior, and precursor lesions must be evaluated (see the two preceding abstracts).—A.J.S.] ◀

-13 **Cutaneous Malignant Melanoma in Hawaii: An Update** is pre-

(13–13) West. J. Med. 138:50–54, January 1983.

sented by M. Ward Hinds and Laurence N. Kolonel (Univ. of Honolulu). The incidence of cutaneous malignant melanoma has been increasing in white populations for at least 3 decades and possibly for longer; many believe that increasing exposure to solar radiation is the chief cause. A previous review indicated a tripling of the age-adjusted incidence of cutaneous melanoma in whites of both sexes in Hawaii between 1960 and 1977, and an even greater increase has occurred subsequently. Eighty percent of cases of invasive melanoma were diagnosed in whites between 1960 and 1980, whereas whites constituted only 34% of the population in 1970. The frequency of melanoma in whites rose steadily over the review period (Fig 13–1) and included all age groups. A large proportion of the diagnoses were made in persons younger than 40 years of age in both sexes. The only decline was in cutaneous melanoma of the lower extremity in men. The many other ethnic groups in Hawaii all exhibit a tenth or less of the risk of malignant cutaneous melanoma apparent in whites. The risk also is relatively low in the small proportion of whites of Portuguese ancestry.

The incidence of cutaneous malignant melanoma continues to in-

Fig 13–1.—Incidence of invasive cutaneous malignant melanoma in whites and nonwhites in Hawaii shown by sex and year of diagnosis, 1960–1980. (Courtesy of Hinds, M.W., and Kolonel, L.N.: West. J. Med. 138:50–54, January 1983.)

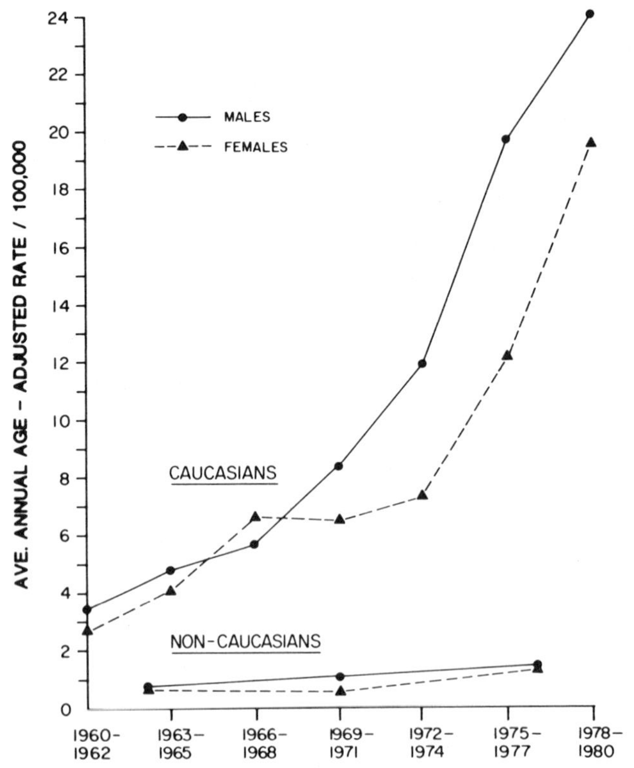

crease rapidly in whites in Hawaii, as in many other parts of the world. However, there is little evidence of an increasing incidence in nonwhites in Hawaii. The findings are consistent with a predominant role for solar ultraviolet radiation in cutaneous malignant melanoma. Recognition of this probable causal association is essential if the increase is to be stemmed. The risk appears to be increased by intermittent leisure-time exposure to solar radiation, but a contribution by nonsolar factors must not be ignored. These may include genetic predisposition, dietary factors (e.g., use of retinoids), trauma, hormonal factors, viruses, and certain drugs. The best current means of reducing the risk, however, is to modify solar exposure patterns.

▶ [Whites in Hawaii appear to share the increasing incidence of cutaneous melanoma that has been observed for whites elsewhere, whereas nonwhites in Hawaii have maintained relatively flat rates. These data once again support the apparent association of high cutaneous melanization and lower risk for development of melanoma.—A.J.S.] ◀

–14 **Epidemiology of Malignant Melanoma in the German Democratic Republic and the Federal Republic of Germany.** Heinz-Dieter Jung reports data on the incidence of malignant melanoma in the German Democratic Republic. Although malignant melanoma is rare, it is a severe form of skin tumor. In 1964 in the German Democratic Republic, the incidence was less than 1% of all malignant tumors and less than 6% of malignant neoplasms of the skin. The incidence is low but increases considerably during puberty.

Melanoma as a percentage of all neoplasms occurring in one age group is highest between ages 15 and 20, in which more than 8% of all malignant tumors were melanomas. In the age group of 20–25 years, the number rose from 0.45 per 100,000 (1968) to 0.88 per 100,000 (1975) in men, and 0.69 per 100,000 (1968) to 0.94 per 100,000 (1975) in women (age-standardized values). The incidence of malignant melanoma steadily increased from 1955 to 1975, i.e., from 1.55 per 100,000 in men and 1.80 per 100,000 in women to 3.1 per 100,000 in men and 4.3 per 100,000 in women. A genuine increase in incidence is seen when age-specific rates from 1968 to 1975 are compared. Between 1955 and 1975 the incidence in men and women doubled in the German Democratic Republic. An increase in the incidence in both sexes can be observed worldwide.

Ultraviolet radiation and chemical carcinogens influence the incidence of malignant melanoma in the German Democratic Republic, although the contribution of chemical carcinogens has not been thoroughly examined. However, in the northern areas (Karl-Marx-Stadt, East Berlin, and Kohle) this causative factor is evident; these regions are concentrated areas of industry.

The death rate from malignant melanomas is almost stationary. The survival rate in men is about 50%; in women it is higher. In the Federal Republic of Germany there were about 1,674 cases of malignant melanoma in 1969 and about 1,825 in 1974; and more than 2,000 in 1975 were to be expected.

(13–14) Hautarzt 33:636–639, December 1982.

There are many unsolved problems. Epidemiologic studies with a greater range of data over a longer period will enable modern methods of diagnosis and analysis to evaluate the incidence of malignant melanoma.

▶ [From this report incidence rates for melanoma in Germany appear lower than those for the United States. Putative association of chemical carcinogens and melanoma remains to be established. Survival rates for men also appear lower than United States rates.—A.J.S.] ◀

13–15 **A Comparison of Prognostic Factors and Surgical Results in 1,786 Patients With Localized (Stage I) Melanoma Treated in Alabama, USA, and New South Wales, Australia.** Charles M. Balch, Seng-Jaw Soong, Gerald W. Milton, Helen M. Shaw, Vincent J. McGovern, Tariq M. Murad, William H. McCarthy, and William A. Maddox compared 12 clinical and pathologic variables in two series of patients with stage I melanoma who were treated at the University of Alabama in Birmingham (676 patients) and at the University of Sydney in New South Wales, Australia (1,110 patients).

Actuarial survival rates were virtually the same at the two institutions over a 25-year follow-up period. The incidence of thin melanomas (less than 0.76 mm thick) was also similiar at both geographic locations (25% vs. 26%). Other similarities between these two patient populations included tumor thickness, level of invasion, surgical results, sex distribution, and age distribution. The greatest differences between the populations consisted in the anatomic distribution and growth pattern of the melanomas and the incidence of ulceration. The trunk was the most common site of melanoma, and tumors occurred there more frequently in Australian patients (37% vs. 28%).

A multifactorial analysis that included comparison of the two institutions as a variable showed the dominant prognostic factors ($P <$ .0001) to be *(1)* ulceration, *(2)* tumor thickness, *(3)* initial surgical management (wide excision with or without node dissection), *(4)* anatomical location, *(5)* pathologic stage (i.e., I vs. II), and *(6)* level of invasion. The benefit of elective lymph node dissection was demonstrated in both series for patients with intermediate-thickness melanoma (0.76–3.99 mm). For melanomas ranging from 0.76 to 1.5 mm in thickness, the benefit of node dissection was demonstrated primarily in male patients. Survival rates for melanoma at the two institutions were not significantly different from each other in the multifactorial analysis.

The authors conclude that the biologic behavior of melanoma in these two different parts of the world was virtually the same, with only minor differences that did not significantly influence survival rates. They stress that long-term follow-up exceeding 8–10 years is critical in the interpretation of these prognostic factors and surgical results, since some patients are at risk for clinically evident metastatic disease for 10 years or longer after the initial treatment.

▶ [Melanoma in whites appears to behave in a remarkably similar manner from con-

(13–15) Ann. Surg. 196:677–684, December 1982.

tinent to continent if similar patient stages are studied. Drs. Balch and Milton are preparing a monograph comparing data from 17 centers worldwide. The results should be most informative. The value of elective regional lymph nodal dissection is still disputed. A randomized prospective multicenter trial is now underway in the United States.—A.J.S.] ◀

13–16 **Uveal Findings in Patients With Cutaneous Melanoma.** Daniel M. Albert, Steven S. Searl, Bernadette Forget, Philip T. Lavin, John Kirkwood, and James J. Nordlund studied findings in the uveal tracts of 197 white patients with known cutaneous melanomas and compared them with findings in controls. All of the patients had a proved cutaneous melanoma that had been surgically excised. An iris nevus (Fig 13–2) was defined as a raised, discrete, pigmented mass or nodule located within the anterior iris stroma obscuring the normal iris architecture. A choroidal nevus (Fig 13–3) was defined as a flat or slightly raised, blue to slate-gray, oval to round lesion with well-defined but not sharp margins.

Patients with cutaneous melanoma had a significantly higher frequency of iris nevi (101 [51%] of 197 patients) than controls (58 [39%] of 147). Also, the frequency of choroidal nevi was higher in the group with cutaneous melanoma, but the number (8 of 197 patients vs. 2 of 147 controls) was too small to have statistical significance. Patients with cutaneous melanoma, especially women, had more skin nevi than controls had.

These findings suggest that the frequency of iris, and possibly of cutaneous, nevi is increased in patients with cutaneous melanoma.

▶ [Patients with vitiligo, melanoma, and melanoma with hypomelanosis should have ophthalmologic examinations. In each of these groups of patients a substantial proportion appear to have evidence of inflammatory disorders of the choroid, raising the

Fig 13–2 (left).—Discrete pigmented masses are seen to obscure the underlying iris stroma in this example of an iris nevus.

Fig 13–3 (right).—A choroidal nevus has a flat appearance with pigmented feathery borders.

(Courtesy of Albert, D.M., et al.: Am. J. Ophthalmol. 95:474–479, April 1983. Copyright 1983 by the Ophthalmic Publishing Company; reprinted by permission.)

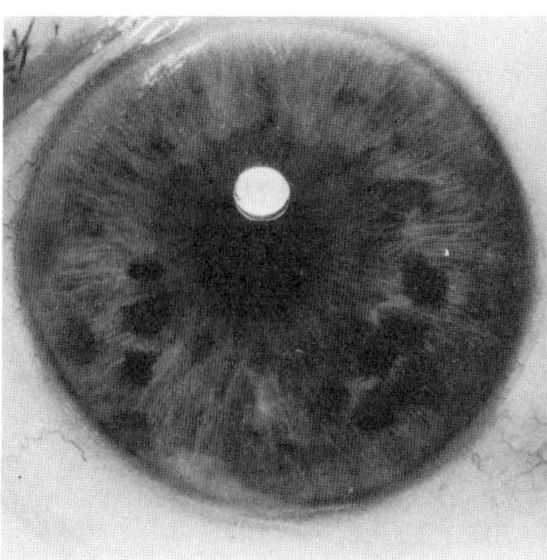

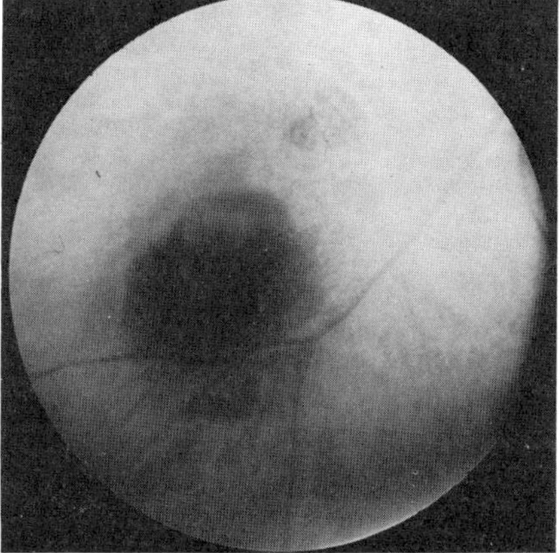

(13–16) Am. J. Ophthalmol. 95:474–479, April 1983.

speculation that reactivity directed against cutaneous melanocytes (vitiligo) or malignant melanocytes (melanoma) or both (melanoma with hypomelanosis) may have reactivity directed against choroidal melanocytes as well. (see Koh, H., et al.: *J. Am. Acad. Dermatol.* 9:696–708, 1983; and Albert, D. M., et al.: *Ophthalmology* 86:1145–1158, 1978).—A.J.S.] ◀

13–17 **Acral Lentiginous Melanoma: Clinicopathologic Study of 36 Patients.** Acral lentiginous melanoma (ALM) is a distinct variant of malignant melanoma with a predilection for the soles, palms, and nail beds. Rao R Paladugu, Carl D. Winberg, and Robert H. Yonemoto (City of Hope Natl. Med. Center, Duarte, Calif.) reviewed 36 histologically confirmed cases of ALM seen in 1955–1979. All patients were followed for 2 years or until death. Cases of ALM constituted 7% of all melanomas seen at the authors' center in this period. Most of the 53 patients with volar-subungual melanoma had ALM. A majority of patients had plantar lesions. The age distribution is shown in Figure 13–4. Several polypoid plantar-palmar lesions were ulcerated and bleeding. Some plantar lesions contained areas of necrosis and were fungating. Two patients had amelanotic lesions. Microscopic examination showed evidence of regression in 39% of cases.

Most plantar-palmar lesions were excised widely with regional node dissection. Only 3 of these patients had amputations, but all those with subungual lesions had amputation of the digit followed by node dissection. Patients in both groups received combination chemotherapy, and some received immunotherapy as well, usually with

Fig 13–4.—Age distribution of patients. (Courtesy of Paladugu, R.R., et al.: Cancer 52:161–168, July 1, 1983.)

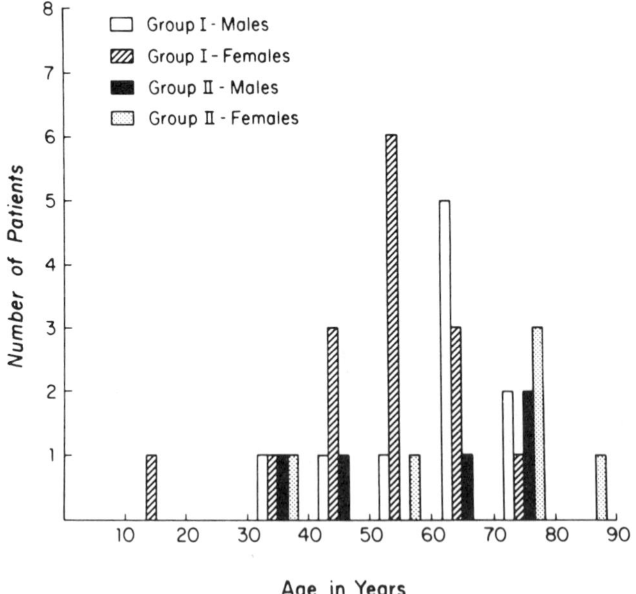

(13–17) Cancer 52:161–168, July 1, 1983.

bacillus Calmette-Guerin. Fifteen of the 25 patients with plantar-palmar melanomas died, 1 without evidence of disease. Ten were well at the time of follow-up examinations after 26–181 months. All but 1 of the patients who died had extensive disease terminally. Five of the 11 patients with subungual melanomas died; the other 6 were without disease after 26–288 months. One patient died without evidence of melanoma. Overall median survival was 73.5 months. Possible correlations were found between survival time and both the level and the thickness of melanocytic proliferation.

Acral lentiginous melanoma has been the most common type of volar-subungual melanoma. Subungual lesions more than 1 mm deep and those showing severe regression should be widely excised, and node dissection should be performed. Volar lesions less than 1 mm deep and those showing radial growth with minimal invasion require only wide local excision. Subungual melanomas in the vertical growth phase are managed by digital amputation and node dissection.

▶ [Acral lentiginous melanoma appears to be a distinct form of melanoma and is a type of melanoma that occurs commonly in blacks and Orientals. The mean age is at least a decade older for ALM than for superficial spreading melanoma. Thin lesions appear to be associated with relatively good outcome, but, as a group, patients with thick lesions do poorly. Early biopsy is recommended.—A.J.S.] ◀

3–18 **Amelanotic Lentigo Maligna Melanoma Manifesting as a Dermatitis-Like Plaque.** Steven P. Borkovic and Robert Allen Schwartz (San Francisco) describe a patient in whom a second primary tumor resembled a dermatitis. Review of the patient's medical record suggested that what had been recorded as the first primary tumor might also have been dermatitis-like.

Man, 73, was seen in 1981 because of a 5-year history of an erythematous lesion over the right deltoid area that had gradually increased in size. Ten years prior to examination he had a dermatitic lesion excised from his left forearm; the lesion had been described by the dermatologist as an erythematous scaly patch. Histopathologic examination revealed atypical melanocytes invading the dermis and epidermis with no melanin pigmentation on hematoxylin-eosin and Fontana's staining. No metastases had been found, but this previous tumor was highly suggestive of a primary amelanotic lentigo maligna melanoma.

On examination in 1981, the patch overlying the right deltoid area appeared slightly erythematous and amelanotic. Results of chest roentgenogram and tomograms and blood chemistry tests were normal. A biopsy specimen from the raised portion of the lesion showed proliferation of moderately atypical melanocytes in the basal cell layer and in the overlying stratum granulosum. The tumor cells had oval to irregularly shaped dense chromatin surrounded by an indistinct faint rim of basophilic cytoplasm. There was a high nuclear-to-cytoplasmic ratio and an unusually high incidence of mitoses. Abnormal melanocytes were present in the upper papillary dermis. Biopsy findings were consistent with a diagnosis of amelanotic lentigo maligna melanoma. Histologic examination confirmed this diagnosis. The patient was free of recurrence or metastases 6 months after excision of the lesion. Since there

---

(13–18) Arch. Dermatol. 119:423–425, May 1983.

were no palpable lymph nodes, lymph node dissection was deemed unnecessary.

▶ [There have been several reports of amelanotic lentigo maligna melanoma in recent years (Paver, K., et al.: *Aust. J. Dermatol.* 22:106–108, 1981), suggesting that this lesion may be relatively underdiagnosed. In their less differentiated variants, they may be difficult to distinguish from certain tumors of neural origin. Biopsy is the only means for the diagnosis of this lesion.—A.J.S.] ◀

13–19 **Skin Markings in Malignant Melanoma.** Edward E. Bondi, David E. Elder, Dupont Guerry IV, and Wallace H. Clark, Jr. (Univ. of Pennsylvania) studied, via photographic analysis, the skin markings in 89 patients with 66 superficial spreading melanomas (SSM), 7 nodular melanomas (NM), 12 acral lentiginous melanomas (ALM), and 7 lentigo maligna melanomas (LMM). Clinical evidence of vertical growth phase disease was noted in 30 SSMs, the 7 NMs, 8 ALMs, and 3 LMMs. In every case, vertical growth phase disease was associated with focal loss of skin markings, and in 6 of these, ulceration was noted. Clinical regression was observed in 33 SMMs, 4 ALMs, and 3 LMMs. In 21 of these, skin markings were totally eliminated, and in 7 instances they were partially eradicated. In 66 SSMs, 12 ALMs, and the 7 LMMs, radial growth phase was observed; in all but 2 of these, skin markings were preserved. There were 23 SSMs in which skin markings were preserved throughout the entire lesion. Mean thickness of these 23 lesions was significantly less than that of SSMs having areas with loss of skin markings. Similar results were obtained from thickness measurements of LMMs and ALMs.

These findings indicate the value of obtaining photographs of all lesions suspected of being melanoma. Photographic analysis facilitates the assessment of fine morphological criteria such as skin markings. The radial growth phase of malignant melanoma is not characterized by loss of skin markings. If obliteration of these furrows is used as a key for diagnosing malignant melanoma, many early, curable melanomas will not be recognized. Rather, careful attention should be focused on variations in color, size, and shape as reliable early signs of malignancy in pigmented lesions.

▶ [Effacement of skin markings has been offered as a sign that should raise suspicions of malignancy. Patients with *vertical growth* usually lose skin markings in that area of the tumor, whereas skin markings are usually maintained in the radial growth phase. In contrast with the findings in this study, we have seen cases of regressing lesions in which skin markings are maintained. Increase in prominence of skin markings as an early sign needs confirmation by others before widespread acceptance is recommended.—A.J.S.] ◀

13–20 **Proposal for Staging Malignant Melanoma.** Posttherapeutic T categories in the TNM classification of the International Union against Cancer for malignant melanoma, as defined by tumor thickness, correspond to the same classes defined by level of invasion in a few cases. Ch. Kuehln-Petzold, H. Wiebelt, H. Berger, and G. Wagner sought a better TNM classification by analyzing 1,310 clinical stage I melanoma cases, followed for at least 8 years in the prospective Ger-

---

(13–19) JAMA 250:503–505, July 22–29, 1983.
(13–20) Arch. Dermatol. Res. 275:255–256, August 1983.

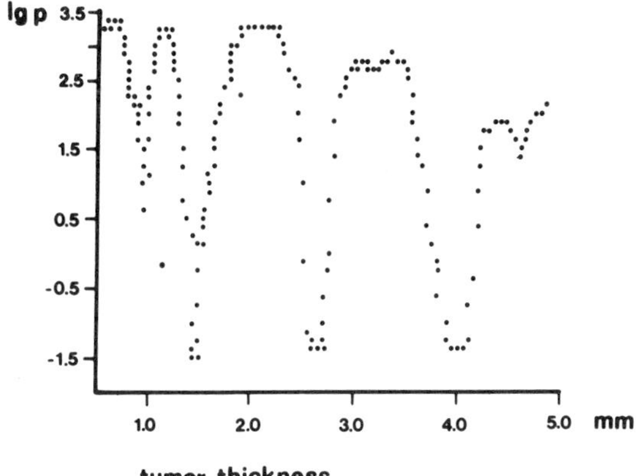

Fig 13–5.—Definition of prognostic subgroups according to thickness of melanoma. There are periodic depressions for *P* values between adjacent curves. They form negative peaks at melanoma thicknesses of 1.0, 1.5, 2.75, and 4.0 mm. (Courtesy of Kuehnl-Petzold, C., et al.: Arch. Dermatol. Res. 275:255–256, August 1983; Berlin-Heidelberg-New York: Springer.)

man Melanoma Group. Most tumors were excised with a 2-cm margin. The level of invasion was determined by Clark's method and the tumor thickness by Breslow's method.

The prognosis did not decrease linearly with increasing tumor thickness when calculated as significant difference between two adjacent survival curves of melanomas differing in thickness by only 0.2 mm (Fig 13–5). Three prognostic classes were defined by tumor thicknesses of less than 1.5 mm, 1.5–4.0 mm; and greater than 4.0 mm. These classes were reproducible in both sexes, although females in all categories had a significantly better prognosis than males. Exophytic growth of tumors above the skin surface correlated closely with their thickness, and classes of exophytic growth of less than 1.5 mm, 1.5–3.0 mm, and greater than 3.0 mm were distinguished. In 76% of cases these classes corresponded to the posttreatment categories defined by tumor thickness.

These prognostic classes for clinical stage I melanoma appear to be more practical than existing systems. They take into account the fact that survival may not decline linearly with increasing tumor thickness. Further, overestimation of minor differences in melanoma thickness is avoided.

▶ [In agreement with this article, we feel that melanoma survival does not vary in a continuously linear manner with increasing thickness, but that there appear to be certain thicknesses at which noticeable step-ups in risk are observed. These step-ups in risk may correlate in some manner with biologic changes taking place in the tumor as it evolves along its natural course. Similar to the groups defined by Figure 13–5 with peaks at 1.0, 1.5, 2.75, and 4.0 mm, our group found divisions at 0.85, 1.70, and 3.6 mm (Day, C. L. Jr., et al.: *N. Engl. J. Med.* 305:1155, 1981). It is to be hoped that a consensus will soon be reached for optimal values that will be applicable to all melanoma patients. The groups are not far apart at present. Also of note is the male-female ratio of melanoma incidence of 0.5 in the German series, whereas that for most series in the United States and Australia is 1.0. I know of no explanation for this difference.—A.J.S.] ◀

13–21 **Effect of Anatomical Location on Prognosis in Patients With Clinical Stage I Melanoma.** Gary S. Rogers, Alfred W. Kopf, Darrell S. Rigel, Robert J. Friedman, Jeffrey L. Levine, Marcia Levenstein, Robert S. Bart, and Medwin M. Mintzis (New York Univ.) attempted to identify tumor-involved subsites of the body surface at which the recurrence rate for stage I melanoma was substantially different from the overall recurrence rate and thus to identify subsets of anatomical sites that would be predictive of disease-free survival. The series included 1,090 patients with primary cutaneous malignant melanoma. There were 971 patients with clinical stage I disease, in 194 of whom recurrence developed during the mean follow-up period of 39 months.

High-risk locations (recurrence rates of more than 35%) included the scalp, mandibular area, anterior and posterior midline of the trunk, hands, feet, popliteal fossae, and external genitalia. Low-risk sites (recurrence rates of less than 10%) were the forearms and thighs. Intermediate-risk locations (recurrence rates between 10% and 35%) comprised all other cutaneous sites (Fig 13–6). Of 971 patients with clinical stage I disease, 154 (15%) had primary lesions in high-risk areas, 150 (15%) in low-risk areas, and 667 (70%) in intermediate-risk areas. Overall cumulative 5-year disease-free survival

Fig 13–6.—Relative risk of melanoma metastasis or recurrence according to location of primary lesion. High-risk locations are indicated by black, intermediate-risk areas by stripes, and low-risk areas by white. (Courtesy of Rogers, G.S., et al.: Arch. Dermatol. 119:644–649, August 1983; copyright 1983, American Medical Association.)

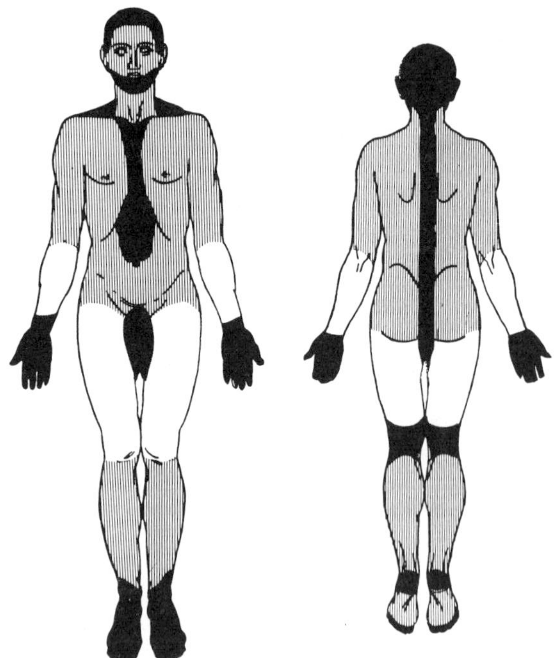

(13–21) Arch. Dermatol. 119:644–649, August 1983.

for the 971 patients with 80.6%. Patients with lesions in high-risk areas had a 5-year survival of 54.3%, and those with lesions in intermediate-risk sites, 79.3%; survival in those with lesions in low-risk areas was 93.4%. These differences were statistically significant. Melanomas occurred more frequently in high-risk areas in male patients than in female patients. Age was not a factor in these results. Differences in lesion thickness among the 3 risk groups were statistically significant with lesions in high-risk areas being significantly thicker than those in the other 2 groups. There was a statistically significant difference in distribution of histologic types of melanoma among the 3 risk groups with more nodular melanomas in the high-risk areas. Melanomas in high-risk sites generally had less host lymphocyte response than did those in the other 2 groups. Cox proportional hazards analysis demonstrated that grouping the lesions by their anatomical risk location had prognostic value that was significant in a model of 8 other known predictive variables (lesion thickness, sex and age of patient, lesion type, level of invasion, mitotic index, ulceration, and pressure of prexistent nevus). These findings underscore the importance of the anatomical location of the tumor in assessing the prognosis of patients with clinical state I malignant melanoma of the skin.

▶ [Several studies have been published in the last few years that suggest that for a given tumor thickness the prognosis of tumors at certain sites will be better than for tumors at other sites. It remains to be established exactly where these preferred anatomical locations are through the comparative studies of several large series of clinical stage I (no clinically evident disease other than the primary tumor) patients. This editor predicts that scalp, hands, and feet will prove to be unfavorable locations after adjustments are made for thickness and that the remainder of the extremities will prove to be of relatively lower risk than the general risk for the body overall. (Day, C., Jr., et al.: *CA* 32:113–122, 1982).—A.J.S.] ◀

13-22 **Metastases of Thin Melanomas.** Although melanomas less than 0.76 mm thick generally carry a very good prognosis, histologic signs of regression in such lesions have been associated with an increased tendency to metastasize. Henri Trau, Darrell S. Rigel, Matthew N. Harris, Alfred W. Kopf, Robert J. Friedman, Stephen L. Gumport, Robert S. Bart, and W. Robson N. Grier (New York Univ.) attempted to confirm this association in a serial study of 116 step-sectioned cases of malignant melanoma seen between 1972 and 1980 that were less than 0.76 mm thick. None of the patients had clinical or histologic evidence of regional or distant metastasis. In situ melanomas were excluded. Histologic evidence of partial regression was present in 41 cases, which were followed up for a mean period of 43 months. Only 1 of these patients had metastatic disease. He died of brain metastasis despite wide excision of the primary lesion. The patients without evidence of regression were followed up for a mean period of 35 months. The two groups did not differ significantly with regard to age, sex, duration of melanoma, type of melanoma, thickness, or greatest and smallest tumor diameters.

(13–22) Cancer 51:553–556, Feb. 1, 1983.

These findings fail to support the suggested association of metastasis with partial regression of thin melanomas. Metastasis was an exceptional event in these cases of thin melanoma that were step-sectioned, even in the presence of partial regression. Other researchers may have failed to include only step-sectioned specimens of primary melanomas in their material. Alternatively, geographic differences in the biologic behavior of this neoplasms may be of importance.

▶ [Like the authors of this article from New York University, we have only seen a few cases of metastases from melanomas less than 0.75 mm thick. However, taken together with reports in the literature it is reasonably well established that not all melanomas less than 0.75 mm thick are cured. Even though the likelihood of cure from a melanoma less than 0.75 mm thick is probably close to 100% (98%–99% 5-year disease-free survival at our institution), it seems desirable to inform the patient with thin melanomas that there is a risk of recurrence, but that this risk is very slight.—A.J.S.] ◀

13–23 **Metastasis and Death in Patients With Thin Melanomas (Less Than 0.76 mm).** Athough thickness is an accepted prognostic indicator in melanoma, fatal metastatic disease may develop in occasional patients with lesions less than 0.76 mm in thickness. John E. Woods, Edward H. Soule, and Edward T. Creagan (Mayo Clin. and Found.) reviewed findings in 1,370 patients with malignant melanoma seen from 1970 to 1979; about 30% of the melanomas were thin. Of 20 patients who appeared to have metastases from thin lesions, metastases were documented in 12, 9 men and 3 women aged 30–69. Ten patients had superficial spreading melanomas and 2 had nodular melanomas. The lesions ranged from 0.3 to 0.75 mm in thickness, most being more than 0.5 mm thick. The level of penetration did not correlate closely with lesion thickness. Four patients had lesions on the upper back, upper posterior arms, posterior neck, or posterior scalp, which constitute a recognized danger zone. All but 1 of the 12 patients died of melanoma; the exception was alive without disease 10 years after groin dissection for inguinal metastases.

These findings indicate that malignant melanomas less than 0.76 mm thick can metastasize and must be watched carefully. There was no evidence of a prior undetected disappearing melanoma or a second, unsuspected primary melanoma in any of the present series. It appears that most patients with thin, metastatic melanomas die of the disease.

13–24 **Biologic Behavior of Thin Malignant Melanomas With Regressive Changes.** Rao R. Paladugu and Robert H. Yonemoto (City of Hope Natl. Med. Center, Duarte, Calif.) reviewed data on all cutaneous melanomas less than 0.76 mm in thickness observed and treated at this center, and they evaluated the biologic behavior of lesions associated with regressive changes. Satisfactory information concerning primary lesions was obtained from 219 patients; 132 were studied retrospectively, and 87 were studied prospectively.

(13–23) Ann. Surg. 198:63–64, July 1983.
(13–24) Arch. Surg. 118:41–44, January 1983.

Among these 219 patients with cutaneous malignant melanoma, 36 had primary lesions measuring less than 0.76 mm (21 women, 15 men). Thirty-one of the 36 lesions were classified as superficial spreading. Eleven of the 36 showed regressive changes; 8 (22.2%) of the 36 had metastasized. In 2 patients micrometastases were found in the prophylactically dissected lymph nodes. In the remaining 6, distant metastases were found in lymph nodes, lungs, liver, bones, and brain within 2 months to 10 years. Six of these lesions were level II; 2 were superficial level III. Of the 11 lesions showing regression, 5 (45.5%) metastasized. Of 25 thin melanomas without regressive changes, only 3 (12%) metastasized. The difference is statistically significant. None of the patients had clinically palpable lymph nodes at the initial appearance. No statistically significant differences in either mean age at primary diagnosis or mean time to relapse among patient groups with and without regressive changes were found. Four patients died 12–182 months from date of diagnosis.

The findings indicate that *(1)* melanomas with regressive changes, active or quiescent, merit separate classification and cautious treatment; *(2)* thinness of these regressing lesions should not influence the clinician to use the usual guidelines for treatment of usual thin melanomas; *(3)* regressive changes should serve as a warning signal rather than inducing a false sense of security; and *(4)* the entire lesion needs to be examined thoroughly by the pathologist because regression can involve only parts of the tumor in some instances.

▶ [The findings in this article are similar to the experience reported by Gromet et al. (*Cancer* 42:2282–2292, 1978) in which approximately 20% of the patients with regressed melanomas less than 0.76 mm thick developed metastases. The high rate of metastases in melanomas less than 0.76 mm thick of the City of Hope National Medical Center is at variance with our experience in the New York University Medical Center Melanoma Clinical Cooperative Group analyses. It would be of value to know how many of the 8 patients who metastasized had serial tissue block sections available for complete histopathologic evaluation of their primary tumors.—A.J.S.] ◀

3–25 **Favorable Prognosis for Malignant Melanomas Associated With Acquired Melanocytic Nevi.** The level of penetration of cutaneous malignant melanomas into the underlying dermis, subcutaneous tissue, or both, has significant prognostic importance. Prognosis may also be influenced by whether the melanoma is associated with an acquired melanocytic nevus or arose de novo. Robert J. Friedman, Darrell S. Rigel, Alfred W. Kopf, Lawrence Lieblich, Robert Lew, Matthew N. Harris, Daniel F. Roses, Stephen L. Gumport, Anna Ragaz, Elaine Waldo, Jeffrey Levine, Marcia Levenstein, Rhonda Koenig, Robert S. Bart, and Henri Trau prospectively evaluated the incidence of metastatic disease, death, or both in a clinicohistopathologic study of 557 patients with primary cutaneous malignant melanoma examined between 1972 and 1980. Generally accepted, specific histologic characteristics of nevus cells were used to distinguish small melanoma cells from dermal nevus cells (table).

Of the total, 130 patients had a melanocytic nevus, and the other

---

(13–25) Arch. Dermatol. 119:455–462, June 1983.

Histologic Differentiation Between "Small Melanoma Cells" and Dermal Nevus Cells*

Small Melanoma Cells	Dermal Nevus Cells
Melanin pigment commonly present	Melanin pigment generally absent
Generally have a nested pattern, reticulin fibers surround each nest of cells and do not penetrate between each individual cell	Generally lose their nested pattern, with each individual nevus cell separated from its neighboring cell by intercellular eosinophilic material (reticulin)
Continuity of the "small melanoma cells" with the usually diagnostic overlying malignant melanoma	Abrupt transition between nevus cells and atypical melanocytes of the melanoma
Usually significant nuclear pleomorphism and hyperchromatism; mitoses rare; nucleoli prominent	Lack of nuclear atypia; no mitoses

*Adapted from Elder, D.E., Ainsworth, A.M., and Clark, W.H., Jr.: The surgical pathology of cutaneous malignant melanoma, in Clark, W.H., Jr., Goldman, L.I., and Mastrangelo, J.J. (eds.): *Human Malignant Melanoma.* New York, Grune & Stratton, 1979.

(Courtesy of Friedman, R.J., et al.: Arch. Dermatol. 119:455–462, June 1983; copyright 1983, American Medical Association.)

427 had melanoma without histologic evidence of a nevus (de novo). Mean follow-ups were 44.6 months for those with nevus-associated lesions and 40.4 months for the de novo group. Evidence of metastatic disease, death from melanoma, or both occurred in only 10 (7.7%) of the patients with nevus-associated melanoma, but in 78 (18.2%) of those with malignant melanoma arising de novo. The 5-year disease-free survival rates were 91% for patients with nevus-associated melanoma and 78% for those with de novo melanomas ($P = .02$). The mean thickness of the malignant melanomas associated with an acquired melanocytic nevus was 1.34 mm, compared with 1.89 mm for the de novo melanomas ($P = .002$). Adjustment for this difference using a stratified life-table analysis and log-rank test for survival confirmed the significance of the difference in 5-year disease-free survival between the two groups ($P = .02$).

The overall favorable outcome observed in patients with malignant cutaneous melanomas associated with acquired melanocytic nevi was independent of lesion thickness and six other clinical and histologic variables reportedly related to the biologic behavior of malignant melanoma. Accordingly, the presence of nevus cells in a malignant melanoma indicates a better prognosis and may have important implications in the understanding of the pathobiologic nature of this neoplasm.

▶ [One of the criticisms of this study and other similar ones is that the more invasive melanomas (worse prognosis) may have destroyed any evidence of a preexistent nevus as they have evolved, leading to the apparent worse prognosis in the absence of a nevus. The frequency with which one finds a nevus is a direct function of the number of blocks examined from each specimen (Rhodes, A. R., et al.: *J. Am. Acad. Dermatol.* 6:230–241, 1983). The distinction between nevus and small cell melanoma cells is sometimes obscure.—A.J.S.] ◀

13–26 **Major Histocompatibility Antigens and Mononuclear Inflammatory Infiltrate in Benign Nevomelanocytic Proliferations and Malignant Melanoma.** Histocompatibility antigens play a major role in the recognition of foreign antigens by T lymphocytes, and it has been suggested that their presence on tumor cells is important in the generation of a host response. Dirk J. Ruiter, Atul K. Bhan, Terence J. Harrist, Arthur J. Sober, and Martin C. Mihm, Jr. (Harvard Med. School), undertook an immunohistochemical study using monoclonal antibodies and an immunoperoxidase method to assess the distribution of major histocompatibility antigens in nevomelanocytes and the nature of the associated inflammatory infiltrate in malignant melanoma and various benign nevomelanocytic lesions. Twelve surgical specimens of malignant melanoma, 11 of nevomelanocytic dysplasia, 10 of nevomelanocytic hyperplasia or nevocellular nevus, and 1 of halo nevus were evaluated. The specimens were examined using a series of monoclonal antibodies reactive with thymocyte antigens, peripheral T lymphocyte surface antigens, or both.

The HLA-A, B, and C antigens and β_2-microglobulin were found on malignant melanocytes in primary cutaneous and metastatic melanomas. The HLA antigens were not found on nevomelanocytes in benign hyperplasia or nevocellular nevi, but faint staining for β_2-microglobulin was present in some cases. Staining for both HLA antigens and β_2-microglobulin was variable in cases of nevomelanocytic dysplasia. Most of the inflammatory cells were T cells, and a majority of these were of the helper-inducer phenotype.

Expression of the HLA antigens may be involved in triggering or eliciting a cellular immune response against dysplastic or malignant nevomelanocytes. Antigenic modulation may occur in the process of malignant transformation, resulting in the appearance of tumor-associated antigens. Both helper-inducer T cells and cytotoxic-suppressor T cells appear to be involved in the tumor-directed immune response. The expression of HLA antigens and β_2-microglobulin antigen may be involved in eliciting an inflammatory cellular response in cases of nevomelanocytic dysplasia, halo nevus, and malignant melanoma.

▶ [In light microscopic studies, the absence of an inflammatory host response below the vertical growth phase of cutaneous melanoma is a sign of poor prognosis. Conversely, most melanomas in their radial growth phases have a distinctly prominent host response below the invasive portions of the tumor. These observations have raised questions about whether there is a change in surface tumor antigenicity associated with deep invasion such that the "new" surface antigens are less well recognized by the host (Brocker, E.-B.: *J. Invest. Dermatol.* 82:244–247, 1984).—A.J.S.] ◀

(13–26) J. Immunol. 129:2808–2815, December 1982.

13–27 **Presence of Fibroblast-Type Intermediate Filaments (Vimentin) and Absence of Neurofilaments in Pigmented Nevi and Malignant Melanomas.** All nucleated cells of adults have a cytoplasmic network of 10-nm filaments, or "intermediate filaments," that form part of the cytoskeleton. These are classified into five types that have characteristic cell-type specificities. M. Miettinen, V.-P. Lehto, and I. Virtanen (Univ. of Helsinki) assessed the intermediate filaments in 9 cases each of pigmented nevus and malignant melanoma, using monospecific antibodies to intermediate-filament proteins and immunofluorescence microscopy. Frozen sections were available from 9 pigmented nevi, 3 malignant melanomas of the skin, and 1 metastatic cutaneous melanoma from the mesentery. Five other malignant melanomas were assessed from paraffin-embedded material, as were 3 cases of cellular blue nevi.

All of the pigmented nevi showed positive cytoplasmic staining in the nevus cells with anti-vimentin. The same pattern was seen in the cellular blue nevi. All 9 melanomas stained strongly with anti-vimentin. None of the lesions stained with antineurofilament, anti-keratin, anti-desmin, or anti-glial fibrillary acidic protein antibodies.

Pigmented nevi and malignant melanomas express only the intermediate filaments of fibroblast-type, or vimentin. In this respect they resemble mesenchymal tumors of nonmuscular origin and differ from neural cells, which express neurofilaments. Most carcinomas express keratin but not vimentin, making this a method of value in differential diagnosis. The differentiation between pleomorphic melanomas and pleomorphic rhabdomyosarcomas is aided by the presence of desmin in rhabdomyosarcomas. Further studies are needed to obtain a comprehensive picture of the cytoskeleton of melanomas and related tumors.

▶ [Although the total number of tumors assessed was small. Miettinen et al., using monospecific antibodies against intermediate filament proteins and immunofluorescence microscopy, show quite definitely that melanomas and pigmented nevomelanocytic nevi have intermediate filaments of the vimentin-type, but not keratin, neurofilaments, desmin, or glial fibrillary acidic protein. This method may be useful in the practical differentiation of melanomas from neuroectodermal tumors.—A.R.R.] ◀

13–28 **Predictors of Late Deaths Among Patients With Clinical Stage I Melanoma Who Have Not Had Bony or Visceral Metastases Within the First 5 Years After Diagnosis.** Calvin L. Day, Jr., Martin C. Mihm, Jr., Arthur J. Sober, Matthew N. Harris, Alfred W. Kopf, Thomas B. Fitzpatrick, Robert A. Lew, Terence J. Harrist, Frederick M. Golomb, Allen Postel, Patrick Hennessey, Stephen L. Gumport, John W. Raker, Ronald A. Malt, A. Benedict Cosimi, William C. Wood, Daniel F. Roses, Fred Gorstein, Darrell Rigel, Robert J. Friedman, and Medwin M. Mintzis studied 14 prognostic factors in 340 patients with clinical stage I malignant melanoma who were free of bony or visceral metastases 60 months after diagnosis.

Malignant melanoma survival rate (MMSR) was 95% for these pa-

---

(13–27) J. Cutan. Pathol. 10:188–192, June 1983.
(13–28) J. Am. Acad. Dermatol. 8:864–868, June 1983.

tients during the ensuing 40 months (100 months after diagnosis). Deaths from malignant melanoma occurred exclusively in patients with primary lesions 1.70–3.64 mm thick. The 74 patients in this thickness group who were free of bony or visceral metastases at 60 months had a 100-month MMSR of 73%. Patients in other thickness groups, including 19 with melanomas more than 3.64 mm thick, had a 100-month MMSR of 100% (if bony or visceral metastases had not occurred in the first 60 months after diagnosis). Within the 1.70–3.64-mm thickness group, statistical analysis showed no other significant prognostic factors among the remaining 13 variables. As a result of continuing deaths after 60 months in the 1.70–3.64 mm thickness group, these patients had a cumulative 100-month MMSR that was only 17% higher than that for the thicker (greater than 3.65 mm) group.

These data, when combined with 1–60-month results, suggest that most melanomas do not become lethal until a critical volume is reached. The thickness measurement parallels the metastatic tumor burden. Thickness is an index not only of the lethal potential but also of survival interval after surgical removal of the tumor.

▶ [It is now apparent that a 5-year disease-free interval is not sufficient to consider a patient with melanoma cured of his disease. This situation is analagous to that seen with breast cancer. The essential point of this article is the necessity of continued follow-up of these patients for at least 10 years. Recent reports of recurrence after 10 years are also of note (Briele, H. A., et al.: *Arch. Surg.* 118:800–803, 1983; and Koh, H. K., et al.: *JAMA* [in press]). For predictors of survival at 2 years and 5 years see Sober, A. J., et al.: *J. Invest. Dermatol.* 80:50s–52s, 1983; and 80:53s–55s, 1983.—A.J.S.] ◀

13–29 **Late Recurrence of Cutaneous Melanoma.** Henry A. Briele, Craig W. Beattie, Salve G. Ronan, Prabir K. Chaudhuri, and Tapas K. Das Gupta (Chicago) studied 7 patients exhibiting late local or regional recurrences of cutaneous melanoma. They were among 105 patients with clinical stage-I melanoma who were followed up for 10 years or until death. The clinical findings are given in the table. Six patients were women aged 50 years and younger who were premenopausal at the time of primary diagnosis. All 3 of the primary tumors assessed were Clark's level III nodular lesions, ranging in thickness from 1.45 to 2.5 mm. Two of them were ulcerated. Four patients were first seen with lymph node metastasis alone; 3 were alive without disease 42–68 months after adenectomy, but 1 died of systemic disease after 37 months. Both patients who were first seen with node metastasis and either local recurrence or in-transit metastasis died of systemic disease. A patient who was treated for local recurrence alone is currently being treated for regional and systemic disease. Recurrences developed in 78% of the entire study group, but were noted in the 7 selected patients more than 10 years after primary diagnosis.

Thus about 7% of this group of patients with primary stage I cutaneous melanoma had recurrent disease more than 10 years after initial diagnosis. Premenopausal women predominated; hence the dis-

(13–29) Arch. Surg. 118:800–803, July 1983.

PATIENTS WITH FIRST CLINICAL EVIDENCE OF RECURRENT MELANOMA MORE THAN 10 YEARS AFTER PRIMARY DIAGNOSIS*

Patient No./ Sex/Age at Primary Diagnosis, yr (Date)	Location of Primary Tumor	Histologic Findings or Primary	Age at Recurrence, yr (Date)	Disease-Free Interval, yr	Location of Recurrence	Outcome
1/F/39 (7/53)	L leg	Slides unavailable	55 (5/69)	16	L femoral nodes	Died 6/72
2/F/39 (6/54)	L leg	2.5 mm, level III, nodular, ulcerated	61 (2/77)	23	L femoral nodes and in-transit metastases	Died 9/79
3/F/24 (6/57)	R leg	1.77 mm, level III, nodular, ulcerated, diagnosed when pregnant	45 (11/77)	21	R femoral nodes	NED* 8/82
4/F/22 (6/58)	L forearm	Slides unavailable; pathologic report: melanoma, superficial dermis involved	43 (1/79)	20	L axillary nodes	NED 8/82
5/M/44 (5/62)	L thigh	Slides unavailable	55 (8/73)	11	L femoral nodes and local recurrence	Died 5/78
6/F/24 (11/62)	L scapula	Slides unavailable; pathologic report: cellular compound nevus diagnosed when pregnant	38 (12/76)	14	L axillary nodes	NED 8/82
7/F/38 (11/67)	R leg	1.45 mm, level III, nodular	49 (8/78)	11	Local recurrence	Alive with systemic and regional disease 8/82

*NED indicates no evidence of disease.

(Courtesy of Briele, H.A., et al.: Arch. Surg. 118:800–803, July 1983; copyright 1983, American Medical Association.)

ease-free interval before recurrence may be very long in these patients. An endocrine source is possible, but prolonged disease-free intervals may also reflect host resistance on an immunologic basis. These cases emphasize the need for continued long-term follow-up of patients treated for invasive cutaneous melanoma, especially those not undergoing node dissection as part of their primary treatment. Women who are premenopausal at the time of primary diagnosis particularly require prolonged follow-up.

▶ [Melanoma, like cancer of the breast, cannot be considered cured, even if the patient is disease-free at 5 years after removal of the primary tumor. There appears to be an inverse relationship between primary tumor thickness and time to recurrence; thick tumors tend to recur earlier. In the recent paper by Day et al. (*J. Am. Acad. Dermatol.* 8:864–868, 1983) the recurrences after 5 years were noted in patients with tumors 1.70–3.64 mm thick. Koh et al. (*JAMA* [in press]) have reported on two patients who first had recurrences more than 10 years after removal of the primary tumor; an observation similar to that reported in this article. Both of these patients had primary tumors in the range of 0.85–1.69 mm thick. In the study by Briele et al. 3 patients have primary tumor thickness reported: 1.45 mm, 1.77 mm, and 2.5 mm. All 3 of these patients fall into the intermediate risk categories for melanoma.—A.J.S.] ◀

13–30 **Local and In-Transit Metastases Following Definitive Excision for Primary Cutaneous Malignant Melanoma.** Daniel F. Roses, Matthew N. Harris, Darrell Rigel, Zev Carrey, Robert Friedman, and Alfred W. Kopf (New York Univ.) managed 672 consecutive patients with clinical stage I and stage II primary cutaneous malignant melanoma by excising 3–5 cm of surrounding skin down to and including the fascia when the lesion was more than 0.5 mm in thickness. Thinner lesions and those in cosmetically and functionally crit-

(13–30) Ann. Surg. 198:65–69, July 1983.

TIME FROM DEVELOPMENT OF LOCAL AND IN-TRANSIT METASTASES TO CLINICALLY DEFINED SYSTEMIC METASTASES IN 25 PATIENTS

Classification	n	No. (%) Who Developed Systemic Disease n (%)	Time Range until Systemic Disease (Months)	Average Time until Systemic Disease (Months)
Stage I with local metastases	7	6 (85.7)	0–23	9.7
Stage I with in-transit metastases	15	10 (66.7)	0–18	4.7
Stage II with local and/or in-transit metastases	3	3 (100)	0–10	3.3

(Courtesy of Roses, D.F., et al.: Ann. Surg. 198:65–69, July 1983.)

ical sites were excised with smaller margins. Only 14 patients in the series had stage II disease. The overall mean follow-up was 45 months. Elliptical excisions were generally carried out to achieve primary closure where possible. Skin grafts were necessary in two thirds of the 365 patients with lesions 1 mm or more thick. Elective regional node dissections were done in 49.5% of stage I cases.

Local metastasis developed in 1.1% of patients with clinical stage I disease. The life table–adjusted local recurrence rate at 5 years was 1.8%. In-transit metastasis developed in 2.3% of patients. No patient with a primary lesion less than 1 mm thick developed local metastasis, although 1 had in-transit metastasis. Three of the 14 patients with clinical stage II disease had local metastasis, and 2 of them also had in-transit metastasis. Disseminated systemic melanoma developed in 6 of the 7 stage I patients with local metastasis and in 12 of the 17 patients with in-transit metastasis (table).

These results warrant a policy of treatment based on accurate histologic evaluation of the primary tumor, excision with conservative margins for thin lesions, and excision with more extensive margins for thicker lesions, an approach to be modified by cosmetic and functional considerations where appropriate. Local and in-transit metastases that follow definitive excision are a significant marker of disseminated systemic melanoma.

▶ [The data in this paper can be interpreted to show the relative rarity of local recurrence developing with thin melanoma even when excisions of less than 3-cm free margins are employed. Of the 7 clinical stage I patients with local recurrence 6 had primary tumors more than 2.50 mm thick. Only 1 local recurrence developed in 533 patients with primary tumors less than 2.50 mm. Conversely, patients with advanced disease (clinical stage II, i.e., palpable nodes suspicious for tumor) are highly likely to have intracutaneous local metastases, satellitosis, and in-transit metastases in addition to lymph nodal metastases, since the former 3 events can occur prior to tumor reaching the regional nodes.—A.J.S.] ◀

13–31 **Prognostic Parameters in Recurrent Malignant Melanoma.** C. P. Karakousis, D. F. Temple, R. Moore, and J. L. Ambrus (Roswell Park Meml. Inst., Buffalo) reviewed data on 361 patients with recurrent malignant melanoma, who were seen between 1965 and 1975, to identify factors related to survival. All patients were initially seen

(13–31) Cancer 52:575–579, Aug. 1, 1983.

with stage I disease. Nearly two thirds of patients were men. Mean age was 48 years. Regional or distant lymph nodes were involved at the time of first recurrence in 56% of cases. The lungs were involved in 10.5% of cases, the liver in 7%, and the skin or subcutaneous tissue in 6%. About one fifth of patients had multiple sites of involvement at the first recurrence. Operation was performed on 201 patients, mainly with stage II or stage III involvement.

Nineteen percent of patients were without disease 5 years or longer after recurrence. Another 2% have disease, and 2% died without disease. Clinical stage was the strongest determinant of survival. The number of distinct initial lesions was an important factor in stage IV cases. In patients with regional node disease, the disease-free interval from excision of the primary melanoma to recurrence correlated with subsequent survival. Patients free from disease for less than a year had a median survival of 16 months, and 16% were alive at 5 years. Those with a longer disease-free interval had a median survival of 2 years, and 30% were alive at 5 years. In patients with stage IV disease, the disease-free interval was a significant factor only when it exceeded 2 years. Twelve patients with stage IV disease had a median survival of 2 years after excision of metastatic disease, and 4 of them were without disease at 5 years.

Clinical stage appears to be the chief determinant of survival in patients with recurrent melanoma. The disease-free interval after primary treatment and the number of recurrent lesions are also prognostic factors.

▶ [Patterns and time of recurrence in patients with clinical stage I disease are highly dependent on the initial definitive surgery. In centers where elective regional lymph node dissections (ERNDs) are performed, lymph node recurrences are rare and visceral recurrences predominate. Where ERNDs are not performed, the lymph nodes are often the first area for recurrence. In general, lymph node recurrences develop sooner than visceral presentation. This study emphasizes the high risk associated with recurrent disease (19% 5-year disease-free survival).—A.J.S.] ◀

13–32 **Metastatic Malignant Melanoma With an Unknown Primary.** Malignant melanoma accounts for 11% of all instances of spontaneous remission of cancer. D. S. Reintgen, K. S. McCarty, Brett Woodard, Edwin Cox, and H. F. Seigler (Duke Univ.) conducted a retrospective computer-aided review of the literature concerning diagnosis, treatment, and prognosis of patients with melanoma with an unknown primary. The study population comprised 124 patients. Caucasian to black ratio was 42:1. Average age at diagnosis was 47.9 years. The most common site of secondary presentation for primary melanoma is regional lymph node disease, stage II, with 64% of patients falling in this category. Several control groups were compared with patients with unknown primaries.

Of the 124 patients with unknown primary melanoma, 62% eventually had a recurrence after a mean follow-up of 5 years. Of the 73 patients who presented with metastatic melanoma in lymph node sites, 45% continued to be disease free during the observation period.

(13–32) Surg. Gynecol. Obstet. 156:335–340, March 1983.

Forty-four percent of the recurrences occurred within 6 months after documentation of initial metastatic disease, and 88% took place within 2 years. Median survival for stage I, II, and III patients was 28.3 months, 31.4 months, and 7.3 months, respectively. When those with stage I and III disease with blood-borne metastases were compared with those with stage II disease with lymphatic metastasis, patients with unknown primary melanoma who had nodal disease at diagnosis had a significant increase in survival time. In those with stage I disease median survival time for the unknown group was 28.3 months and for the known group, 80.9 months.

If the minority of patients with subcutaneous metastatic disease is eliminated from the analysis, the actuarial survival times of comparable groups of patients with known and unknown primary melanoma are virtually indistinguishable. Although it is likely that the body's own defense destroyed the primary lesion, this does not lead to increased protection against subsequent metastatic spread or increase in survival time.

▶ [Not all patients with metastatic melanoma will die from the disease even if the primary tumor eludes detection. In this series, 38% of patients were disease free after 5 years. From the several studies that have been reported recently, survival of patients with unknown primary tumors seems comparable to similar patients in whom a primary tumor has been surgically eliminated (Giuliano, A., et al.: *Ann. Surg.* 191:98–104, 1980).—A.J.S.] ◀

13–33 **Imaging of Melanoma With ^{131}I-Labeled Monoclonal Antibodies.** Steven M. Larson, Joseph P. Brown, Peter W. Wright, Jorge A. Carrasquillo, Ingegerd Hellström, and Karl Erik Hellström (Seattle) used mouse monoclonal antibodies and Fab fragments specific for the melanoma-associated antigen p97 to image metastatic human melanomas. Two antibody preparations specific for p97 and three control immunoglobulin preparations were evaluated in athymic mice and in toxicity tests in rabbits. The antibodies were purified from ascites fluid of mice bearing hybridoma ascites tumors. The patients studied had widespread inoperable melanoma and significant amounts of p97 on their tumors. Most had failed to respond to all conventional treatment measures. Thyroid uptake was blocked with potassium iodide before labeled antibody was injected. Images were obtained 48 hours after nuclide injection, using a blood-pool subtraction method without injection of pertechnetate.

Studies in mice showed antigen-specific uptake in melanoma xenografts. Toxicity tests in rabbits that received as much as 100 times the amount of antibody used in patients gave no evidence of tissue damage. Six patients received 1 mg of labeled antibody and 1 received 1 mg of labeled Fab without toxic side effects. All patients had positive scans. All but 3 of 25 lesions larger than 1.5 cm were visualized. Greater tumor uptake of p97-specific antibody than of control IgG or Fab was confirmed by biopsy in 2 cases. In three patients who were given 1 mg or more of labeled antibody, antibodies to mouse immunoglobulin developed within several weeks of injection. Calculated ra-

---

(13–33) J. Nucl. Med. 24:123–129, February 1983.

diation doses from ^{131}I-labeled IgG were 4.9 rad/mCi to the liver, 2 rad/mCi to the marrow, and 0.7 rad/mCi to the whole body. Gonadal doses were less than 1 rad/mCi.

Monoclonal mouse antibodies to p97 can safely be given to patients in milligram doses, producing immunologically specific uptake by melanomas. This approach may be useful in diagnosing occult melanoma in selected patients. Development of this technique into a clinically useful procedure will require methods of limiting hepatic uptake and increasing the in vivo targeting of antibody to tumor.

▶ [This is a pioneer study in the use of monoclonal antibodies for diagnostic and therapeutic purposes. As an experimental model these investigators have shown that by labeling monoclonal antibodies directed against melanoma-associated antigens, melanoma metastases can be discerned. By linking a therapeutic agent to the antibody, selective toxicity to melanoma cells would be possible. With this in mind, one group has attempted to attach diphtheria toxin to melanoma-seeking antibodies as a therapeutic approach. Much needs to be done before this approach will be clinically relevant for the general patient with metastatic melanoma.—A.J.S.] ◀

13–34 **Optimal Resection Margin for Cutaneous Malignant Melanoma.** Wide local excision of cutaneous melanoma often causes significant morbidity and cosmetic deformity, and it has been suggested that wide excision is not always necessary. David E. Elder, DuPont Guerry, IV, Richard M. Heiberger, Donato LaRossa, Leonard I. Goldman, Wallace H. Clark, Jr., C. Jean Thompson, Isabel Matozzo, and Marie Van Horn examined the relationship between the surgical margins and outcome in a prospective study of 105 patients with melanoma. All had histologically confirmed primary malignant melanoma and were followed up for 3 years. The modal patient age was 40–44 years. Forty-four of the 109 primary lesions were intact at initial examination. Most were of the superficial spreading type. The most common procedure was excision with grafting. Prophylactic node dissection was performed in 28 cases, and 5 patients had clinically positive nodes dissected.

Neither survival nor disease-free survival was related to the operative or pathologic width of the excision margin. The disease-free survival rate 3 years later was 78%. Both tumor thickness and level were significant prognostic factors. No patient had locally recurrent disease, but 19 had regional recurrences. All 6 patients with in-transit metastases had minimal operative margins exceeding 30 mm. Satellite tumor deposits were found in 5 wide excision specimens. In 2 cases, the satellite lesions were clinically obvious. Two of these 5 patients were alive without disease 3 years later. All 3 who died had level IV or V primary lesions more than 2.5 mm thick.

Survival of cutaneous melanoma patients in this study series was not related to the width of the surgical margins, and no local recurrences were observed. Satellitosis and in-transit cutaneous metastases indicate that melanomas can recur locally, but these changes were seen only in tumors more than 2 mm thick. These findings sup-

---

(13–34) Plast. Reconstr. Surg. 71:66–72, January 1983.

port the wide excision of "thick" melanomas and more modest local treatment for thin melanomas.

▶ [Optimal resection margins for cutaneous melanoma have not as yet been established with certainty. What is clear, however, is that for most cases of clinical stage I melanoma, margins substantially less than the classic 5-cm margins are adequate to control the disease. Randomized studies are ongoing comparing 1.0-cm with 3.0-cm margins for thin melanoma; the results should be available soon. From results published to date, narrower margins may be associated with a slightly higher local recurrence rate, but survival rates appear comparable for narrower margins compared with wider resections (Day, C. L., Jr., et al.: *N. Engl. J. Med.* 306:479–482, 1982).—A.J.S.] ◀

13–35 **Phase II Study on Postsurgical Management of Stage II Malignant Melanoma With Newcastle Disease Virus Oncolysate.** At present, surgery is the most effective treatment of malignant melanoma with regional node involvement; however, most patients die of the disease. William A. Cassel, Douglas R. Murray, and Helen S. Phillips (Emory Univ.) evaluated a Newcastle disease virus lysate of malignant melanoma cells for use in delaying the progression of stage II melanoma to the disseminated stage in patients having therapeutic lymphadenectomy. Patients were entered consecutively into the study over a 4-year period. A dose of 2.5 ml of the virus oncolysate was

Fig 13–7.—Disseminated disease status of stage II melanoma patients after undergoing regional lymphadenectomy. Percentages are compared between patients remaining disease free after lymphadenectomy alone (controls) and patients who after lymphadenectomy were treated with viral oncolysate. Each treated patient was given viral oncolysate for 160 weeks. (Courtesy of Cassel, W.A., et al.: Cancer 52:856–860, Sept. 1, 1983.)

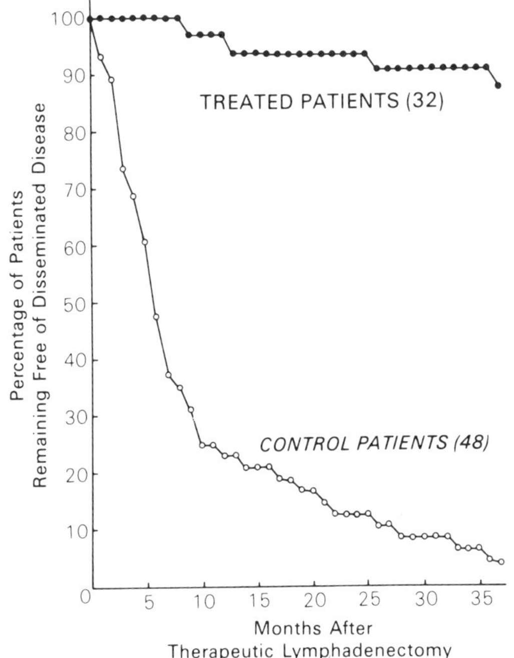

(13–35) Cancer 52:856–860, Sept. 1, 1983.

given subcutaneously, and most patients received allogeneic cell preparations. Initially, oncolysate was given weekly for 1 month; then every 2 weeks until 1 year after surgery, and every 3 weeks for as long as 120 weeks after surgery; thereafter, the preparation was administered every 6 weeks to 160 weeks.

The 32 patients given viral oncolysate did considerably better than 48 retrospectively studied controls (Fig 13–7). Evidence of disseminated disease was present in 6% at 1 year and in 12% after 3 years. All patients were sensitive to skin test antigens.

There is evidence of antigenic cross-reactivity between nearly all human melanomas. It is not clear how tumor-specific the antigens are, but the immunogenicity of human melanomas is accepted. The present findings suggest that a Newcastle disease virus oncolysate can help delay the occurrence of disseminated disease in patients with clinical stage II melanoma after therapeutic lymphadenectomy. A more defined viral oncolysate may be developed when the antigenic composition of human melanomas is better defined. The present preparation is a helpful adjunct to surgery in the management of clinical stage II malignant melanoma.

▶ [This is a preliminary nonrandomized study with small numbers of patients followed for a short period of time. The differences compared with historical controls are striking, but "historically" the use of historical controls has often been misleading. Prospective randomized trials must be done, and since no other obviously promising agent is currently being used, a good trial with this agent seems warranted. Its usefulness is far from being proved at this point.—A.J.S.] ◀

13–36 **Evaluation of Human Lymphoblastoid Interferon in Advanced Malignant Melanoma.** S. Retsas, T. J. Priestman, K. A. Newton, and G. Westbury (London) evaluated the effect of human lymphoblastoid interferon in 17 patients with malignant melanoma (10 men and 7 women with a median age of 50 years). All patients but 1 had previously received chemotherapy for systemic disease and most had received radiotherapy to localized metastases. All patients had advancing tumor at the time of interferon therapy. Three different batches of interferon were used in these patients. Planned treatment consisted of 2.5 megaunits/sq m of body surface, to be given intramuscularly each day for 30 days.

Anorexia and prostration were most troublesome in the first week of treatment. Patients receiving dexamethasone did not become febrile during interferon therapy. A suppressive effect on hematopoiesis was evident. Tumor regression was observed in only 1 patient, who received intramuscular injections of interferon for in-transit cutaneous metastases in one leg. Disease progressed in a patient who had interferon injected directly into the tumor. Disease progressed rapidly in most patients.

These findings suggest that human lymphoblastoid interferon has minimal activity in advanced and previously treated malignant melanoma. Any activity is confined to cutaneous metastases and is not superior to that of existing treatments. The role of interferon as an

---

(13–36) Cancer 51:273–276, Jan. 15, 1983.

adjuvant treatment in patients with earlier stages of disease or in combination with effective cytotoxic chemotherapy in advanced cases, remains to be established.

▶ [Interferon is not an innocuous drug. Most patients experience fever, chills, and malaise when treatment has begun. Associated with high doses have been neurologic consequences of seizures and peripheral neuropathies. In the present study very little evidence for activity was seen; however, 2.5 million units/sq m/day is a relatively low dose. Studies with higher doses, adjuvant studies, or combination therapy studies are anticipated.—A.J.S.] ◀

13–37 **Solitary Pulmonary Metastases in High-Risk Melanoma Patients: Prospective Comparison of Conventional and Computed Tomography.** Removal of melanoma metastases may improve the prognosis, but the best means of detecting pulmonary spread at a relatively early stage is unknown. Dennis K. Heaston, Charles E. Putman, Bruce A. Rodan, Evelyn Nicholson, Carl E. Ravin, Melvyn Korobkin, James T. T. Chen, and Hilliard F. Seigler undertook a prospective comparison of conventional chest roentgenography, conventional tomography, and computed tomography (CT) in 42 patients at high risk of primary relapse of malignant melanoma because of the depth of invasion of the primary lesion or a history of skin or node metastases. Half the patients had had 2 or 3 skin or lymph node recurrences, and only 11 patients had not had recurrent melanoma. Median patient age was 49 years. Initial screening was with high-kilovoltage posteroanterior and lateral roentgenograms. Both 30-degree linear tomograms and contiguous CT scans 1 cm thick were obtained.

Chest roentgenograms showed "definite" pulmonary nodules in 11 patients, conventional tomography in 16, and CT in 20. Both plain roentgenography and conventional tomography yielded normal findings in 3 patients in whom follow-up verified pulmonary metastasis. Computed tomography detected more pulmonary nodules than did conventional tomography in 11 patients and also identified lesions at extrapulmonary sites. Computed tomography alone altered management in only 1 instance, in a patient with normal chest x-ray films who underwent wedge resection of a solitary metastasis initially detected by CT. Nineteen other patients continued immunotherapy or began multidrug chemotherapy on the basis of new CT or conventional tomographic findings or corroboration of the chest roentgenograms.

Chest CT should be done before immunotherapy is started or a presumed solitary pulmonary metastasis of malignant melanoma is removed surgically. Computed tomography and conventional tomography give comparable results once chemotherapy has been started for bulky regional or cutaneous disease.

▶ [Early detection of solitary pulmonary metastases from melanoma is a worthwhile effort, since surgical removal may result in cure of the patient. More often, however, patients with a solitary metastasis will develop multiple metastases within months following the presentation of the solitary nodule. Before pulmonary resection is contemplated, a full metastatic work-up should be done to rule out, to the degree possible, evidence of disease elsewhere.—A.J.S.] ◀

(13–37) AJR 141:169–174, July 1983.

13–38 **0-7-21 Radiotherapy in Nodular Melanoma.** There is increasing evidence that malignant melanoma is not intrinsically radioresistant, and that large-dose-per-fraction radiotherapy produces better responses than conventional 200-rad/day fractions. Curtis R. Johanson, Andrew R. Harwood, Bernard J. Cummings, and Ian Quirt (Princess Margaret Hosp., Toronto) reviewed the results of such treatment in 54 patients seen between 1975 and 1980 with biopsy-proved malignant melanoma who were followed up for 3 months or longer. Fractions of 800 rad were given on days 0, 7, and 21. About half of the patients received 850 mg/sq m of imidazole dicarboxomide (DTIC) 12 hours before the first and third fractions of radiotherapy. Twenty-two patients were treated for microscopic residual melanoma, 9 for gross residual disease after surgery, and 23 for recurrent melanoma. Thirty-two patients received DTIC as well as radiotherapy.

Eighteen of the 22 patients treated for residual microscopic melanoma had no evidence of recurrence within the irradiated volume. Two of the 4 with "in-field" recurrences had a very aggressive form of melanoma. Eight patients without in-field recurrence died of distant metastases, 6 within 15 months of radiotherapy. Five patients treated for gross residual disease achieved complete remission, and 2 others had no progression in the treated volume before they died. Seven of the 23 patients treated for recurrent melanoma had a complete remission, and 2 others had complete remission followed by in-field recurrence. Five patients had partial responses, and 3 experienced stabilization of their disease. Local responses were not influenced by DTIC therapy. Three patients experienced complications of radiotherapy. Although complete responses to radiotherapy were more frequent in patients with smaller lesions, some with massive disease showed complete responses as well.

Large-dose-per-fraction radiotherapy can be effective in the treatment of nodular melanoma. A randomized prospective trial is planned to evaluate adjuvant 0-7-21 radiotherapy in high-risk patients.

▶ [Follow-up reports from this group are a welcome addition to the melanoma literature, since this group is one of the few with any extensive experience with radiotherapy and melanoma. Clearly, useful palliation can be achieved in certain patients with metastases that are unresponsive to chemotherapy. The role of radiation therapy for primary melanoma is much less clear. It should be pointed out that the title of this article is misleading in that the authors' reference to "nodular" melanoma does not mean nodular melanoma according to the Clark classification but refers to the vertical growth phase melanoma nodules that can be seen in any of the types of melanoma.—A.J.S.] ◀

(13–38) Cancer 51:226–232, Jan. 15, 1983.

14. Nonmelanoma Skin Cancer

14–1 **DNA Repair in Cells From Patients With Actinic Keratosis.** Actinic keratosis (AK) is a relatively common disorder associated with both aging and exposure to sunlight, which may progress to carcinoma in situ and then invasive squamous cancer. There is evidence that patients with AK may have a reduced capability of unscheduled DNA repair synthesis. Jerrar M. Abo-Darub, Rona MacKie, and John D. Pitts (Univ. of Glasgow, Scotland) examined the DNA repair capacity of peripheral blood lymphocytes from patients with multiple actinic keratoses requiring surgical treatment and from age-matched controls. Studies were done with methy-^{3}H-thymidine. Deoxyribonucleic repair activity in lymphocytes from AK patients 4 hours after ultraviolet irradiation was only 50% of that in control lymphocytes. At 21 hours the extent of DNA synthesis in cells from AK patients was similar to that in control cells.

Ultraviolet-irradiated peripheral blood lymphocytes from AK patients exhibit an impaired capacity for DNA repair. The repair activity in cells from AK patients ranges from 30% to 60% of that in cells from age-matched controls. The effect is similar to that described by others. Given enough time, AK cells can achieve as much repair synthesis as normal cells, as has been observed in xeroderma pigmentosum cells.

▶ [From animal studies there is evidence that sunlight is not only capable of tumor induction but also may be immunosuppressive. This immune suppression may facilitate tumor growth once induction has occurred. The mechanisms of tumor induction and immune suppression in man are just beginning to be evaluated. The work described in this article and that by Sbano et al. (*Arch. Dermatol. Res.* 262:55–61, 1978) suggests that sunlight can create an acquired xeroderma pigmentosum–like defect in the DNA repair process and that this repair defect may contribute to tumor induction. There is adequate penetration of the ultraviolet A and visible wavelengths of sunlight to irradiate lymphocytes circulating through the dermis.—A.J.S.] ◀

14–2 **Detection of Human Papillomavirus Type 5 DNA in Skin Cancers of an Immunosuppressed Renal Allograft Recipient.** Genome copies of human papillomaviruses (HPV) have been detected in several kinds of human cancer of the skin and mucosa. Until now, the HPV-5 genome has been found only in squamous cell carcinomas of the skin from patients with the rare disease epidermodysplasia verruciformis. Marvin A. Lutzner, Gérard Orth, Viviane Dutronquay, Marie-Françoise Ducasse, Henri Kreis, and Jean Crosnier (Paris) report the results of a search for HPV DNA in the benign and malignant skin lesions of a renal allograft recipient.

(14–1) J. Invest. Dermatol. 80:241–244, April 1983.
(14–2) Lancet 2:422–424, Aug. 20, 1983.

Man, 35, had received a cadaver renal allograft for treatment of renal failure associated with glomerulonephritis. He had undergone immunosuppression for 13 years with azathioprine and corticosteroids and had had multiple in situ and invasive skin cancers of sun-exposed skin during the preceding few years. Examination revealed about 20 macular, scaly lesions on the arms and trunk, which clinically and histologically resembled the pityriasis versicolor–like benign lesions of epidermodysplasia verruciformis. Two more cancers that had developed on the cheek 1 year previously were excised. The scaly lesions disappeared after withdrawal of azathioprine.

Light microscopic examination showed one of the cheek cancers to be a carcinoma in situ and the other to be an early invasive squamous cell carcinoma. Neither the immunoperoxidase method nor electron microscopic examination revealed any evidence of papillomavirus group antigen or papillomavirus-like particles. Viral DNA extracted from the benign warty lesions was analyzed by the Southern blot hybridization technique, with the probes specific for HPV-3, -5, -8, and -9, all of which are associated with epidermodysplasia verruciformis. Autoradiography after hybridization showed heavily labeled bands with the HPV-5 probe and less heavily labeled bands with the HPV-8 probe, an HPV known to have 15% DNA sequence homology with HPV-5. The mobility of the labeled bands corresponded with forms II and III of the HPV-5 DNA prototype isolated from benign lesions of a patient with epidermodysplasia verruciformis. Total DNA extracted from the two skin cancers was cleaved by the restriction endonucleases BamHI and PstI and analyzed by the Southern blot hybridization technique. Bands for both cancers were detected with the HPV-5 probe, which corresponded in mobility with those seen in the benign lesions. Deduction from reconstruction experiments showed the intensity of the bands to correspond with one or two copies of viral DNA per diploid cell DNA content. No bands were observed with the HPV-3 or HPV-9 probes; viral DNA was insufficient for detection with the HPV-8 probe.

The observations that skin cancers in renal allograft recipients and in patients with epidermodysplasia verruciformis occur almost exclusively in sun-exposed skin, and that the frequency of skin cancer in renal allograft recipients is proportional not only to the duration of immunosuppression, but also to the duration of exposure to sunlight, suggest that ultraviolet light may be a cofactor for oncogenesis. The findings in this patient point to a role for HPV-5 in the pathogenesis of skin cancers in renal transplant recipients.

▶ [Evidence favoring a viral causation of squamous cell carcinoma has been proposed for epidermodysplasia verruciformis (Ostrow, R., et al.: *Proc. Natl. Acad. Sci. USA* 79:1634–1638, 1982) and for renal transplant patients. The problem has been to determine whether the presence of wart material is of etiologic significance or whether the wart is merely a saprophyte. Sun-damaged skin seems to be required for the enhanced development of skin cancers in transplant patients. It appears as if the carcinogenesis processes are accelerated; changes that would be expected over 10–20 years occur within a few years of transplantation.—A.J.S.] ◀

14–3 **Lichenoid Solar Keratosis: Prevalence and Immunologic Findings.** Chin Y. Tan and Ronald Marks (Welsh Natl. School of

(14–3) J. Invest. Dermatol. 79:365–367, December 1982.

Medicine, Cardiff, Wales) note that solar keratoses may show basal cell liquefactive degeneration (BLD) that, when extensive, can result in a superficial resemblance to lichen planus. The frequency of these phenomena and immune mechanism involvement were investigated. In all, 212 histologic specimens were examined retrospectively from lesions diagnosed histologically as solar keratoses between 1975 and 1980. The prospective study examined 28 patients with typical solar keratoses. Half of each lesion was submitted to routine histologic testing and hematoxylin and eosin staining. The other half was studied by immunofluorescence.

The prevalence of lichenoid keratosis was 6.1% in 212 solar keratoses examined retrospectively and 10.7% in 28 lesions examined prospectively. Change in BLD (occupying one-third or more of the basal layer available for inspection) occurred in 27.8% of the 212 lesions. When histologic features were scored on analogue scales, their interrelationships showed that BLD could not be correlated with epidermal atypia, acanthosis, acantholysis, or inflammatory cellular infiltrate; a negative correlation occurred with parakeratosis. Immunoglobulins or fibrin and complement were found by immunofluorescence in 78.8% of the 28 specimens examined prospectively. Immunofluorescent findings in 3 lichenoid keratoses were similar to those in ordinary solar keratoses. No circulating antibodies to epidermal structures were detected in patients with solar keratoses.

Thus, no feature of the solar keratoses investigated predisposed to lichenoid change; BLD was a frequent feature in solar keratoses, whereas full development of lichenoid keratoses occurred much less frequently. Immunoprotein deposits were not related to the development of BLD. Clinically, lichenoid keratoses could not be distinguished from ordinary solar keratoses.

▶ [That immunosurveillance is operative in epithelial neoplasms is amply illustrated by the high incidence of invasive squamous cell carcinoma in *(1)* renal allograft patients receiving immunosuppressive medications (corticosteroids and azathioprine) and *(2)* older patients with chronic lymphatic leukemia. We have older patients who have a long history of sun damage who develop chronic lymphatic leukemia and may have 3–5 new invasive epithelial carcinomas in a matter of weeks. These patients must be carefully monitored and managed only with Mohs' surgery for those invasive lesions on certain areas of the face (nasolabial folds and canthi).—T.B.F.] ◀

14–4 **Keratin Polypeptide Composition as a Biochemical Tool for Discrimination of Benign and Malignant Epithelial Lesions in Man.** Fibrous keratin proteins, the constituents of tonofilaments, are a family of 8–12 proteins present in various stratified epithelia besides the epidermis. They are lacking in malignant tumors of cornifying epithelia in rodents, but they are synthesized by benign tumors. Hermelita Winter, Jürgen Schweizer, and Klaus Goerttler (Heidelberg, Federal Republic of Germany) attempted to determine whether this can be observed in human epithelial lesions. Samples of normal human skin at various sites and of benign and malignant skin tumors were subjected to extraction of keratins by a high-salt-buffer proce-

---

(14–4) Arch. Dermatol. Res. 275:27–34, February 1983.

dure. Keratins were analyzed by one-dimensional polyacrylamide gel electrophoresis and two-dimensional gel electrophoresis.

The keratin patterns of benign tumors were similar to those of normal epithelium or stratum corneum. The relative proportion of stratum corneum–associated keratin polypeptides to those characteristic of the living layers corresponded to such morphological features as hyperkeratosis and acanthosis. The epithelial cancers totally lacked high-molecular-weight keratins. The reduced-keratin patterns of morphologically disparate cancers exhibited striking uniformity.

The most abundant differentiation products of the epidermis and other cornifying epithelia are generally identical with respect to molecular-weight range and electric-charge range within mammalian species, including man. An absence of large keratins from epithelial cancers, which was first described in rodents, has been confirmed for human epidermal and vaginal malignant lesions. It is best demonstrated by one-dimensional gel study. The finding could be useful in diagnostic pathology, especially if antibodies related to the keratin polypeptides are used. Specific monoclonal antibodies will be necessary, since antiserums to distinct keratin components may cross-react immunologically with other keratin polypeptides.

▶ [In this study a change in composition of a *specific* epidermal protein is used to distinguish the benign or malignant nature of tumors of epidermal origin. The findings in this study should be considered as preliminary observations, since only a small number of skin cancers were analyzed. The development of objective tests capable of determining malignancy should be encouraged as adjuncts to or replacements for standard light microscopic diagnoses in which a high degree of subjectivity is often involved.—A.J.S.] ◀

14–5 **Recurrent Squamous Cell Carcinoma of the Skin.** Squamous cell carcinoma of the skin is often said to have a very low rate of recurrence and minimal potential for metastasis, but widely divergent observations have been reported. Steven C. Immerman, Edward F. Scanlon, Miriam Christ, and Kerry L. Knox (Northwestern Univ.) encountered several patients with very aggressive recurrences of squamous cell cancer of the skin. Review was made of the data on all patients receiving diagnoses of primary squamous carcinoma of the skin during a 10-year period. Eighty-six of the 1,833 skin cancers removed during this period were invasive squamous cell carcinomas. Forty-seven other patients had in situ lesions, or Bowen's disease.

None of the patients with noninvasive squamous cell carcinoma had recurrent disease during an average follow-up period of 4.3 years. Three underwent reexcision because of positive margins. Two of the patients with invasive lesions were treated with biopsy and primary irradiation and the rest with surgical excision. Fifteen of the 24 patients with tumor at the resection margins underwent wide excision, and another was irradiated. Two untreated patients had recurrences that were controlled by superficial radiation. Local or regional recurrences developed in 17 patients (20%) with invasive squamous cell

(14–5) Cancer 51:1537–1540, Apr. 15, 1983.

cancer, but none had distant disease. Eleven recurrences involved structures deep to the skin or regional nodes or required multiple reexcisions. Ten of the 17 patients with recurrences had initial lesions 1 cm or more in greatest diameter. Patients with moderately or poorly differentiated primary lesions were more likely to have recurrent disease. None of 23 patients with level I, II, or III lesions had recurrent disease.

Squamous cell carcinomas of the skin that penetrate to Clark's level IV or V have the potential to recur and metastasize to regional nodes and should be considered malignant lesions, even if associated with actinic skin changes. One fifth of these patients with invasive squamous cell carcinoma of the skin had recurrences.

▶ [The application of Clark's anatomic levels of invasion to prognosticate squamous cell carcinoma recurrence is a novel one. Penetration into reticular dermis or subcutaneous fat, levels IV and V, respectively, probably reflect both aggressiveness of tumor and increased tumor volume (advanced primary tumor). The 20% recurrence rate seems high and may reflect the more advanced nature of cases that are treated within hospital settings compared with those treated in outpatient offices. With increased use of Mohs' surgical techniques for squamous cell carcinoma, a drop in the local recurrence rates would be anticipated.—A.J.S.] ◀

14–6 **Multivariate Risk Score for Recurrence of Cutaneous Basal Cell Carcinomas.** Neil Dubin and Alfred W. Kopf (New York Univ.) performed a multiple logistic analysis relating prognostic factors to risk of recurrence for 1,417 basal cell carcinomas treated from 1955 to 1969. Of special interest was the delineation of patient and lesion characteristics within each treatment group that would be indicative of an increased risk of recurrence within 5 years after treatment.

A majority (758 of 1,417) of lesions were treated with curettage-electrodesiccation, and 26% recurred within 5 years. Significant associations with recurrence were seen for patient's age at treatment, previous therapy, and lesion diameter. No lesion less than 2 mm in diameter recurred within 5 years; the recurrence rate increased with increasing diameter. Lesions that had been treated previously recurred more frequently than those that had not. Recurrence rates also increased substantially with patient's age at treatment. Of 412 lesions treated by irradiation, 9.7% recurred within 5 years. Only sex was significantly associated with risk of recurrence, men having double the recurrence rate of women. Surgical excision was used to treat 247 lesions, of which 9.3% recurred. The only significant factor in surgically treated patients was previous therapy, with recurrence in 19.4% of those previously treated but in only 7.6% of those not previously treated.

Factors significantly correlated with increased risk of recurrence of carcinoma after each treatment approach were as follows: surgical excision—greater lesion diameter and lesion located on the scalp, ears, eyes, nose, or face; irradiation—greater lesion diameter, lesion located on the nose, and male sex; curettage-electrodesiccation—greater lesion diameter, lesion located on the forehead, ears, eyes,

---

(14–6) Arch. Dermatol. 119:373–377, May 1983.

nose, or face, prior therapy, and older age of patient. Basal cell carcinoma caused no fatality in this series.

▶ [Multivariate (Cox) analyses are valuable in assessing relative importance of risk factors where several factors are considered simultaneously. A 26% recurrence rate for desiccation and curettage seems excessively high for this procedure and much below the 90%–95% cure rates reported. What has become clear is that there are certain areas, such as the scalp, for which recurrence rates with desiccation and curettage are very high. Location and tumor size are major factors that should influence the selection of treatment method.—A.J.S.] ◀

14–7 **Effectiveness of Curettage and Electrodesiccation in Removal of Basal Cell Carcinoma.** The goal of treatment of basal cell cancer is removal of the tumor with the least risk of local recurrence and with minimal cosmetic and functional defects. B. L. Edens, G. A. Bartlow, P. Haghighi, R. W. Astarita, and T. M. Davidson compared the efficacy of curettage and electrodesiccation in removing biopsy-proved basal cell cancers less than 2 cm in diameter from previously untreated patients. Lesions with morpheaform histologic pattern were excluded. Patients either had their tumors curetted and desiccated once or curetted and desiccated 3 times before being excised with a 2-mm margin about the curetted, desiccated crater.

Of the 45 patients having a single curettage-desiccation, 47% had tumor at the surgical margin. Another 2% had tumor in the specimen but not at the margin. Of 40 patients having 3 treatments before excision, 33% had involved surgical margins. One specimen with normal margins contained tumor. Eighty-seven patients in all who had a single treatment, in some of whom only the surgical margins were examined, had a 45% rate of diseased margins, and 87 who had 3 treatments had a 37% rate of diseased margins, tumor in the specimen, or both.

The findings suggest that there are 2 growth patterns of nonmorpheaform basal cell carcinoma. One is a circumscribed pattern that is checked by dermal immune processes and is totally removed by curettage and electrodesiccation. The other growth type is invasive, possibly a result of deficient immunity, and tumor may remain even after 3 curettage-desiccation treatments and excision with a 2-mm margin.

▶ [Previous studies have documented a 95% cure rate following electrodesiccation and curettage for basal cell carcinoma. The finding of residual tumor in one third of patients following this treatment seems inconsistent with the low recurrence rates. An observation that may help resolve this apparent discrepancy is the phenomenon of microscopic residual tumor in clinically clear surgical excision margins. When such patients are followed without reexcision, a substantial proportion do not recur, suggesting that the residual tumor may not be biologically significant (Salasche, S.: *J. Am. Acad. Dermatol.* 8:496–503, 1983).—A.J.S.] ◀

14–8 **Curettage and Electrodesiccation in Treatment of Midfacial Basal Cell Epithelioma.** Stuart J. Salasche (Brooke Army Med. Center) compared the efficacy of curettage and electrodesiccation (C and D) in the treatment of primary, small, uncomplicated basal cell

---

(14–7) J. Am. Acad. Dermatol. 9:383–388, September 1983.
(14–8) Ibid., 8:496–503, April.

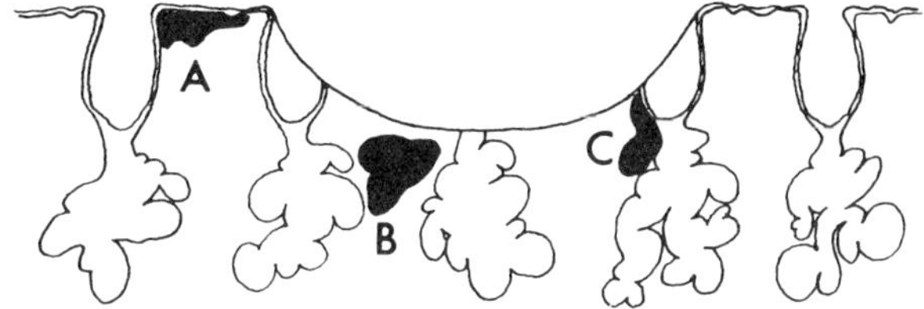

Fig 14–1.—Three patterns of residual tumor: *A*, superficial; *B*, deep, between hair follicles; and *C*, deep, originating from outer root sheath of hair follicle. (Courtesy of Salasche, S.J.: J. Am. Acad. Dermatol. 8:496–503, April 1983.)

epitheliomas (BCEs) on the nose and nasolabial fold (NLF) with that of BCEs elsewhere on the head and neck in 100 patients.

Curettage and electrodesiccation were performed 3 times on each lesion. A one-stage Mohs' chemosurgical procedure was done to ensure adequacy of the C and D. Residual tumor was found in 30% of the nasal and NLF lesions, compared with 12% of those elsewhere on the head and neck (table). Residual tumor was seen in 3 patterns (Figure 14–1). Most deep patterns were on the nose and NLF.

Success of C and D depends on the ability to separate the "soft" tumor from surrounding normal skin with the curette and the presence of normal dermis at the base of the lesion. The mushy, friable, cancerous material is softer than normal skin and is easily dislodged from it. This distinction is lost if the curette "drops" into the subcutaneous fat and an alternative such as excision or Mohs' procedure is required. Progressively smaller curettes must be used, and tiny pockets of cancer cells are destroyed by electrodesiccation. A 3-mm rim of normal tissue must be destroyed if high cure rates are to be achieved. Proper setting of the desiccating current is just beyond that required for hemostasis because increasing the current causes more heat, deeper penetration, excessive tissue destruction, and scarring.

The skin of the nose is composed of numerous sebaceous follicles embedded in dense fibrous stroma and supported by little subcutaneous fat. These follicles may effectively "hide" tumor islands from the curette. Tumor growth from the outer root sheath of hair follicles is also impossible to discern with the curette.

Curettage and electrodesiccation can afford cure rates in excess of

"Chemo-check" After Curettage and Desiccation

	Number	Positive	% positive
Total cases	100	21	21%
Nose and NLF	50	15	30%
Head and neck (non-nose)	50	6	12%
		$p < 0.001$	

(Courtesy of Salasche, S.J.: J. Am. Acad. Dermatol. 8:496–503, April 1983.)

95% in treatment of basal cell epitheliomas. The nose and NLF, however, are high-risk areas to be avoided, since local anatomical peculiarities make eradication of the entire tumor difficult. Recurrences may lead to deformities and functional impairment. Excision and histologic control, Mohs' chemosurgery, or C and D followed by chemocheck is recommended; a "positive" chemo-check is followed by further excisions and repeated until a tumor-free plane is attained.

14–9 **Therapy for Basal Cell Epitheliomas by Curettage Only: Further Study.** William E. McDaniel (Univ. of Kentucky) reports a follow-up of 437 patients having 644 basal cell epitheliomas (BCEs) treated by curettage only. The treatment was started in 1958 because of unsatisfactory cosmetic results from electrocoagulation following curettage. In addition, the long-term cosmetic results of irradiation frequently were unsatisfactory. Curettage only is a simpler, more rapid, and less expensive approach. The procedure is carried out under lidocaine anesthesia. A virtual excision biopsy is performed with a dermal curette 10 × 7 mm in size, proceeding 3–4 mm beyond the tumor margin. The wound is filled with Gelfoam pieces and covered with gentamicin cream. The wound heals within 3 weeks.

Most of the lesions were on the face, and virtually all were at sites of frequent solar exposure. The average reported duration of the lesions was 13 months when 4 estimates of 10 or more years were excluded. The average follow-up was a little less than 4 years. Twenty-eight recurrences developed in 328 treatment sites observed for 5 years or longer. Eight developed in patients with multiple BCEs, a frequency slightly higher than that in the other patients. No second recurrences developed after alternative treatment, although many patients were followed for 2 years or less. None of 28 deaths was related to BCE or to treatment complications. Hypopigmentation at the wound site was the most common sequel of treatment, but the cosmetic results continue to be good to excellent.

A 5-year cure rate of 91.5% was achieved with curettage alone for BCEs on exposed skin surfaces in patients followed up for more than 5 years. The author presently treats virtually all BCEs up to 14–15 mm in size by this method when they are at sites suitable to vigorous curettage. Eyelid and lip lesions are not treated in this way, and only small, superficial lesions on the back and shoulders are curetted. Good to excellent cosmetic results are obtained by curettage only.

14–10 **Metastatic Basal Cell Carcinoma.** Basal cell carcinoma (BCC) is the most common malignant tumor of the skin, accounting for 70%–75% of all skin tumors. It rarely metastasizes; only 113 documented cases of metastasis have been reported, 25 of which were metastases to bone. Erlinda S. McCrea, Donald D. Coker, and Mohammad A. Hafiz (Univ. of Maryland) report another case of BCC that metastasized to bone.

Woman, 63, was well until 1972, when she noticed a posterior scalp mass

---

(14–9) Arch. Dermatol. 119:901–903, November 1983.
(14–10) South. Med. J. 76:686–688, May 1983.

that slowly enlarged and eventually ulcerated. In October 1976, examination showed two ulcerated, infected, indurated posterior scalp lesions with heaped-up margins. The larger one measured 7×6 cm and the other was 4×4 cm. Bilateral multiple posterior cervical adenopathy was observed in the trapezius area. The lesions extended to the periosteum of the skull. The initial impression was of squamous cell carcinoma, but biopsy of the scalp lesions and multiple cervical node excisions disclosed keratinizing BCC of the skin with metastases to the lymph nodes. Some areas showed a hint of sebaceous differentiation. The patient received 6,600 rad to the scalp and 5,275 rad to the posterior cervical nodes bilaterally. A ^{99m}Tc bone scan revealed areas of increased uptake in the cervical and lumbar spine, right sacroiliac joint, left first rib, and distal part of the right femur. A bone survey revealed degenerative changes. No symptoms were referable to the skeleton, and there were no findings specific for metastases. A recurrent skin lesion was found on the left side of the scalp in January 1977. A right preauricular mass was also seen, but it was thought to be due to metastatic lymph node involvement. The skin lesion and the preauricular mass were irradiated. A left posterior scalp biopsy in June 1977 revealed recurrent BCC. Further radiotherapy was given, but a new nodule was found in the left side of the scalp in July 1977. Because of failure of the right preauricular mass to regress, a right superficial parotidectomy was performed in August. This revealed adenocarcinoma of the salivary duct. The recurrent scalp lesion was excised. A ^{99m}Tc bone scan in September demonstrated a progressive increase in activity in the areas previously described, though the bone survey was unchanged. The patient was free from skeletal symptoms until March 1979, when she began to limp and had back pain. A bone scan revealed marked progression, with new areas of increased uptake. A bone survey was consistent with the scan abnormalities, demonstrating osteoblastic and osteolytic lesions in the thoracolumbar spine and pelvis and proximal parts of the humeri. The alkaline phosphatase activity had risen to 263 IU at this time; on heating, the value fell to 22 IU, indicating its bony origin. A liver-spleen scan, upper gastrointestinal tract tests, barium enema, chest roentgenograms, and xeromammograms revealed no abnormalities. Biopsy of the left iliac crest in April 1979 showed metastatic BCC that was histologically similar to the original scalp lesion but had no histologic resemblance to the excised parotid tumor. The patient showed tremendous subjective improvement in response to treatment with *cis*-platinum and bleomycin. This improvement was accompanied by a fall in alkaline phosphatase activity to 198 IU in September 1979. The patient was well until March 1980 when a chest film revealed a solitary nodule in the right lung, with increased sclerosis of the osseous lesions. An iliac crest biopsy revealed continuing metastatic BCC. One course of epipodophyllotoxin (VP-16) therapy resulted in clinical and laboratory improvement, with a fall in alkaline phosphatase activity to 68 IU.

Basal cell carcinoma requires its stromal support for survival, whereas epidermoid carcinomas do not and thus metastasize more readily. The presence of a normal basement membrane may be a good barrier to prevent BCC from metastasizing. Surgical treatment and radiotherapy can cause this barrier to break down and may facilitate spread.

▶ [Each year a few reports of metastasizing basal cell carcinoma appear to remind us that this entity is not always a benign actor. The one case that I personally have seen (unreported) presented with metastases to the pelvic bones. Response to chemotherapy is often poor.—A.J.S.] ◀

14–11 **Early Lesions of Kaposi's Sarcoma in Homosexual Men: Ultrastructural Comparison With Other Vascular Proliferations in Skin.** N. Scott McNutt, Van Fletcher, and Marcus A. Conant (San Francisco) note that an aggressive variant of Kaposi's sarcoma (KS) has appeared in young homosexual men with evidence of systemic immunosuppression. The ultrastructure in biopsy specimens from 8 young homosexual men with KS was compared with that in biopsy

Fig 14–2.—Kaposi's sarcoma in this abnormal dermal vascular channel reduces the lumen **(L)** to a slit, which would probably be undetected by light microscopy. Small, sparse intercellular junctions are seen **(J)**, and the basal lamina is fragmented. Pericyte processes were either absent or greatly reduced in prominence. ×17,900. (Courtesy of McNutt, N.S., et al.: Am. J. Pathol. 111:62–77, April 1983.)

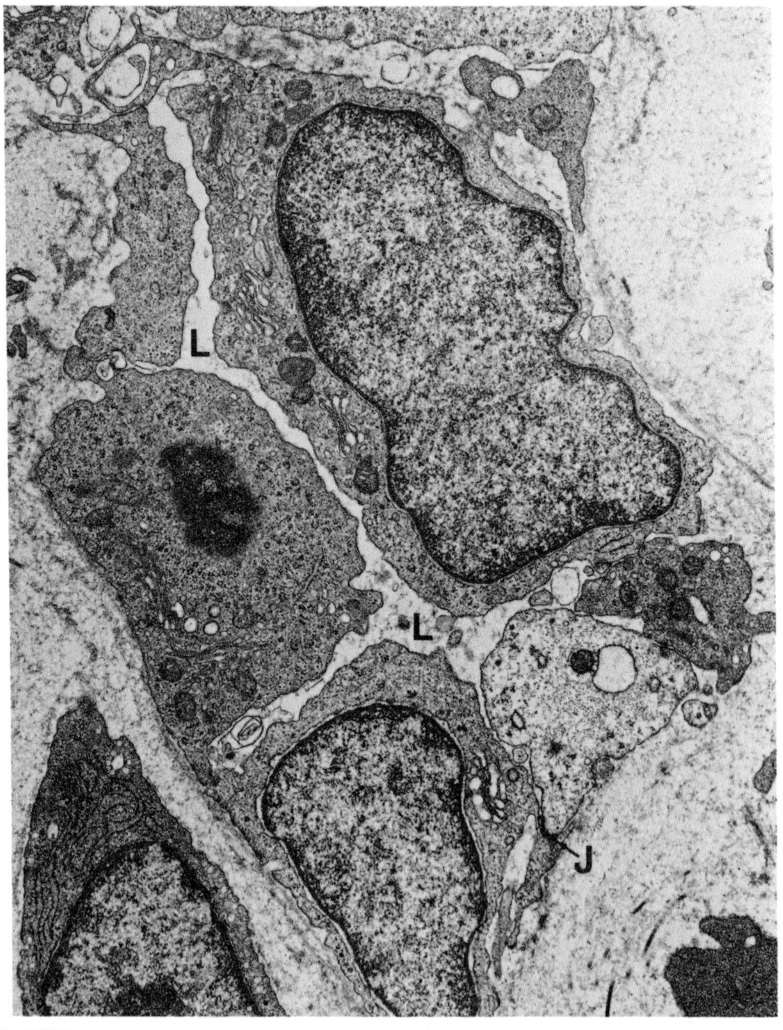

(14–11) Am. J. Pathol 111:62–77, April 1983.

specimens from 4 elderly heterosexuals with KS and from 23 patients having benign vascular disorders of the skin.

In all KS patients, the small blood vessels lacked a prominent investment of pericytes and their processes and had a fragmented and often absent basal lamina, frequent discontinuities in the endothelial lining, and only a few small junctional densities between endothelial cells. In some patients with clinically aggressive KS, there also was necrosis of individual endothelial cells and prominent cytoplasmic processes entrapping individual collagen fibers. The benign disorders lacked these features. These differences in the structure of the small vessels may be of diagnostic value in some patients with early KS. In early or patch-stage lesions of KS in both homosexuals and heterosexuals, electron micrographs confirm the endothelial nature of most of the cells infiltrating the reticular dermis (Fig 14–2). These endothelial cells line cleftlike lumens, which may be either very thin or more dilated. Very few lumens contained erythrocytes. The cellular lining of the clefts was continuous in most areas.

It was not possible to find unequivocal ultrastructural features that correlated with the rapidity of the spread of KS. An inherent problem is that KS skin lesions follow varying rates of progression in both young homosexual and old heterosexual patients and do not allow a simple type of comparison. The loss of dendritic pericytes in blood capillaries in KS may relate to the telangiectasia that is a prominent feature of the early KS lesion.

▶ [Clinically, early lesions of KS in the acquired immune deficiency syndrome may appear quite innocent, and a high index of suspicion is required to perform a biopsy on these lesions. The pathologist is then faced with the problem of distinguishing between KS and other forms of benign or malignant vascular proliferations. This study of relatively small numbers of patients suggests that the electron microscope may be of help in this sometimes difficult differential. Further studies by this and other groups are eagerly awaited.—A.J.S.] ◀

14–12 **Kaposi's Sarcoma and Community-Acquired Immune Deficiency Syndrome: Update With Emphasis on Its Head and Neck Manifestations.** Kaposi's sarcoma (KS) was previously considered to be an indolent sarcomatous disorder of the elderly, which was also seen in immunosuppressed hosts; but now it is associated with acquired immune deficiency syndrome (AIDS). Elliot Abemayor and Thomas C. Calcaterra (Univ. of California, Los Angeles) reviewed the records of 45 patients with AIDS, with or without KS, 18 of whom initially had evidence of involvement of the head and neck region. All patients were men, with an average age of 34 years. Average duration of symptoms was 8 months. Only 6% of patients claimed to be exclusively heterosexual. All reported drinking moderately, and 3 patients were intravenous drug abusers. Twelve patients each reported having had gonorrhea and syphilis in the preceding 5 years, and 6 had had hepatitis B.

The head and neck abnormalities involved the skin in 8 patients, the oropharynx in 7, lymph nodes in 6, and other sites in 4. The skin

---

(14–12) Arch. Otolaryngol. 109:536–542, August 1983.

lesions were painless macules or blue-purple nodules. Biopsies of enlarged posterior cervical nodes showed changes of KS. Four patients had dermal KS lesions in conjunction with oral candidiasis. Eight patients had evidence of KS in the gastrointestinal tract. Five patients developed *Pneumocystis carinii* pneumonia, and 4 of them died. Two other patients had multisystem failure and died. Eleven patients were alive with disease when last seen. One other patient had no lesions.

Many relations exist among KS, the immune system, and viruses. The current outbreak of AIDS is ascribed to an accumulation of risk factors, with possible infectious spread of disease. The defect in immune function appears to involve immune regulation rather than any single portion of the immune system. No effective treatment has been found. The KS seen in patients with AIDS is poorly responsive to chemotherapy. Interferon is under study, but thymosin has not been helpful. The *P. carinii* pneumonia seen in patients with AIDS has also been difficult to treat effectively.

▶ [Head and neck presentation for classic KS would be most unusual. The more widespread presentation in the context of AIDS is becoming well known. This article emphasizes the observation of initial presentation in head and neck sites. A high index of suspicion for KS must be maintained in patients with AIDS.—A.J.S.] ◀

14–13 **Preliminary Observations on Effect of Recombinant Leukocyte A Interferon in Homosexual Men With Kaposi's Sarcoma.** Susan E. Krown, Francisco X. Real, Susanna Cunningham-Rundles, Patricia L. Myskowski, Benjamin Koziner, Seymour Fein, Abraham Mittelman, Herbert F. Oettgen, and Bijan Safai state that preliminary clinical trials have shown that both natural and recombinant-DNA-produced human interferon occasionally inhibit the growth of certain tumors. The effect of administration of recombinant leukocyte A interferon (IFLrA), a purified human interferon produced by recombinant-DNA techniques, on tumor growth and immune function was examined in 13 patients treated during the course of a phase I trial of this agent. The interferon was prepared from *Escherichia coli*. All patients had measurable, biopsy-confirmed Kaposi's sarcoma, and all were homosexual or bisexual men aged 32–50.

Of the 12 evaluable patients, 5 experienced a major objective response (3 had a complete response and 2 a partial response); 3 had a minor response, and 4 had disease progression. A complete response occurred in 1 patient with lesions confined to the skin; in another with involvement of the skin, lymph nodes, oral mucosa, and stomach; and in the third with skin, oral mucosa, and node lesions. Minor responses were observed in 3 patients during the first month of treatment; however, when the dosage schedule was reduced in the second month, new lesions appeared.

Side effects included fever, chills, weakness, fatigue, anorexia, headache, myalgias, and joint pain. Hair loss and paresthesias occurred infrequently. Orthostatic hypotension developed in several pa-

---

(14–13) N. Engl. J. Med. 308:1071–1076, May 5, 1983.

tients. The mean nadir for the white blood cell count was 2,200/cu mm. Major episodes of infection were infrequent during treatment. The percentage of sheep erythrocyte–rosetting lymphocytes was within the normal range for all patients. Eight of 13 patients lacked natural killer-cell activity. Augmentation of natural killer-cell activity in vitro by IFLrA occurred in 5 of 9 patients. The response to phytohemagglutinin increased to normal in 6 patients during treatment. The presence of circulating interferon activity before treatment was not correlated with pretreatment blood counts or measures of immune function. Neutralizing antibody to IFLrA developed in 1 patient.

These findings, although preliminary, suggest that IFLrA may be a useful agent in the treatment of Kaposi's sarcoma in immunosuppressed patients and that it is capable of restoring at least some aspects of cell-mediated immune function. The study provided no evidence in support of or against either a viral origin for the sarcoma or an antiviral mechanism for the antitumor activity of interferon in this disease.

▶ [The failure of Kaposi's sarcoma in patients with acquired immune deficiency syndrome (AIDS) to respond to conventional therapies has lead to a search for new and innovative approaches. Interferon seems to offer some evidence of activity in certain patients with AIDS. From the cases presented, this agent alone would not appear to be the likely cure but may be useful in combination with other forms of treatment. This area is evolving rapidly (see also Volberding, P., et al.: *Am. J. Med.* 74:652–656, 1983).—A.J.S] ◀

4–14 **Kaposi's Sarcoma: A New Staging Classification.** Until recently, Kaposi's sarcoma was considered to be rare in North America and Europe, but an increasing number of homosexual men with an aggressive, often lymphadenopathic form of the disease are being encountered. Robert L. Krigel, Linda J. Laubenstein, and Franco M. Muggia (New York Univ.) propose a new staging system for Kaposi's sarcoma, based on the findings in 49 homosexual men with the disease. The system comprises stage I disease, with the typical locally indolent lesions; stage II, a locally invasive, aggressive form seen mostly in equatorial Africa; stage III, a disseminated, mucocutaneous form, often with node involvement, seen in both African children and North American male homosexuals; and stage IV, a disseminated, mucocutaneous disorder with visceral involvement, seen in the same groups.

Most of the patients were first seen with skin lesions, and adenopathy was also frequent. The skin lesions ranged from pink-red macules or papules to plaques or elevated nodules. Nearly two thirds of patients had innumerable lesions widely distributed over the skin surface. Thirty of the 49 patients had generalized adenopathy at presentation. All 24 node biopsies confirmed Kaposi's sarcoma. Five patients had splenic enlargement. Splenectomies performed in 2 patients confirmed the presence of disease in both, and the 3 liver biopsies in patients with hepatomegaly were also confirmatory. Gas-

---

(14–14) Cancer Treat. Rep. 67:531–534, June 1983.

trointestinal involvement was present in 45% of patients. Pulmonary disease was a cause of death in 3 early cases. Three subsequent patients had fever and reticulonodular pulmonary infiltrates; *Pneumocystis carinii* pneumonia was confirmed in 2, and the third had Kaposi's sarcoma alone. Six patients had stage I disease, 1 had stage II, 29 had stage III, and 13 had stage IV. Seven patients with stage III and 8 with stage IV disease had systemic symptoms.

This staging system resembles that used for lymphoreticular neoplasms. Patients with stage I disease can be managed by local measures such as radiotherapy, whereas single-agent trials are appropriate for those with stage II and stage III disease. Patients with stage IV disease and those with systemic symptoms can be given early, aggressive combination chemotherapy.

▶ [Staging systems are helpful in comparing results from studies of natural history and response to therapy from different institutions. Usually more than one staging system is in use at any particular time so that the definition of each stage as used by the authors must be kept in mind.—A.J.S.] ◀

14–15 **Frequencies of HLA and Gm Immunogenetic Markers in Kaposi's Sarcoma.** There is evidence that HLA-DR5 is associated with homosexuals who have acquired immune deficiency syndrome, and that both the homosexual and classic forms of Kaposi's sarcoma may have a viral cause. M. S. Pollack, B. Safai, P. L. Myskowski, J. W. M. Gold, J. Pandey, and B. Dupont examined the roles of the HLA- and Gm-linked immune response factors in Kaposi's sarcoma in 39 white patients with histologically documented disease. Nineteen had the homosexual form, and the other 20 had classic Kaposi's sarcoma.

A highly significant increase in HLA-DR5 was found in both groups of patients. Both groups showed a decreased frequency of the DR3 antigen. The homosexual group had an increase in the HLA-B antigen Bw35. Both groups had a marked reduction in the frequency of B8 antigen. The increases in DR5 and Bw35 persisted when comparison was made with control populations of Italian, Ashkenazi Jewish, or Hispanic descent. An increase in homozygosity for the Gm haplotype 3;5,13 was observed, but the effect was not statistically significant. Several of the Gm 3;5,13-homozygous patients lacked DR5, and there was no evidence for an interactive effect between these antigens.

The findings suggest that HLA response factors may have a role in the induction of both the homosexual and the classic forms of Kaposi's sarcoma. Immune response factors that are Gm linked may also be involved.

▶ [This study needs confirmation in other series. Sixty-four HLA and HLA-DR antigens were measured. When small sample sizes are involved and large numbers of factors are being examined, it is not difficult to obtain a statistically significant result from one factor by chance alone.—A.J.S.] ◀

14–16 **Clinical Course of Retrovirus-Associated Adult T-Cell Lymphoma in the United States.** Paul A. Bunn, Jr., Geraldine P.

(14–15) Tissue Antigens 21:1–8, January 1983.
(14–16) N. Engl. J. Med. 309:257–264, Aug. 4, 1983.

Schechter, Elaine Jaffe, Douglas Blayney, Robert C. Young, Mary J. Matthews, William Blattner, Samuel Broder, Marjorie Robert-Guroff, and Robert C. Gallo reviewed the clinical findings in 11 patients with adult T-cell lymphoma and natural antibodies to human T-cell lymphoma virus.

Generally, the patients were young (median age, 33 years), black, and male and had been born in the southeastern United States. The disease had an aggressive course with rapid onset of disseminated skin lesions or symptoms associated with hypercalcemia, or other metabolic disturbances, or both. The median interval between onset of symptoms and diagnosis was 2 months (range, 1–12 months). The cutaneous lesions showed considerable variation. Two patients had large, discrete tumor nodules, 3 had smaller nodules, 1 had generalized maculopapular lesions, and 2 had more nonspecific, generalized, erythematous or parapsoriatic rashes. Except for the biopsy in the patient with the parapsoriatic rash, all skin biopsies were diagnostic of lymphoma. Pautrier microabscesses were present in the epidermis in 4 patients. Five of the 6 patients who initially had skin lesions became hypercalcemic within several weeks to months after presentation and before specific treatment for lymphoma. Common abnormalities included rapid enlargement of peripheral, hilar, and retroperitoneal lymph nodes, with sparing of the mediastinum; invasion of the CNS, lungs, or gastrointestinal tract; and opportunistic infections. All patients had a paraneoplastic syndrome characterized by increased bone turnover, abnormal bone scintigraphy, and hypercalcemia. All were treated with combination chemotherapy, which produced prompt, complete clinical remission, though generally of short duration. Third-line chemotherapy was unsuccessful. Survival was short, with a projected median survival of only 11 months by life-table analysis.

The features characterizing these patients are similar to those described in patients in Japan and the West Indies with adult T-cell lymphoma, which is also associated with the human T-cell lymphoma virus. Retrovirus-associated T-cell lymphomas should be strongly suspected in patients with the acute onset of generalized skin lesions or hypercalcemia with metabolic bone abnormalities or both. Detection of antibody to human T-cell lymphoma virus is important in establishing the subtype of T-cell lymphoma. Diagnosis of the syndrome can be confirmed by appropriate serologic and virologic studies. Staging should emphasize CNS, gastrointestinal, and pulmonary lesions.

► [This abstract and the one that follows report on retrovirus-associated T-cell lymphoma and leukemia. The authors of the first study feel that this form of non-Hodgkin's lymphoma belongs in the high-grade category of the National Cancer Institute's disease classification and should be classified separately from other high-grade lymphomas. This form of lymphoma presents a unique paraneoplastic syndrome with increased bone resorption and hypercalcemia, aggressive course, rapid dissemination, infiltration of skin and organs, metabolic abnormalities, opportunistic infections, and brief response to chemotherapy. The case report that follows shows that a vasculitis-arthritis syndrome may be seen in association with these retrovirus-induced disorders.—A.J.S.] ◄

14–17 **Identification of Human T Cell Leukemia Virus in a Japanese Patient With Adult T-Cell Leukemia and Cutaneous Lymphomatous Vasculitis.** Adult T-cell leukemia (ATL) has been found to be endemic to restricted areas of Japan. Recently, human T-cell leukemia virus (HTLV) has been associated with various clinical mature T-cell lymphoproliferative syndromes in various areas of the world. Barton F. Haynes, Sara E. Miller, Thomas J. Palker, Joseph O. Moore, Philip H. Dunn, Dani P. Bolognesi, and Richard S. Metzgar describe in detail a Japanese patient with ATL and unusual clinical manifestations (arthritis and cutaneous lymphomatous vasculitis) in whom a strain of HTLV was isolated from cultures of peripheral blood T cells.

Woman, 49, was seen with swelling of the left index finger, right fourth proximal interphalangeal joint, and right ankle. One week later a nodular rash developed on the neck, chest, back, and right ear lobe. The only laboratory abnormalities were a white blood count of 20,000/cu mm with 54% lymphocytes and an alkaline phosphatase level of 331 units (normal, less than 240 units). One month later the skin lesions had begun to ulcerate and the peripheral white blood cell count was 24,000/cu mm with 90% abnormal-appearing lymphocytes, 91% of which rosetted with sheep erythrocytes. As the patient had been born in Japan and had lived there until age 23 years, Japanese ATL was suspected. After admission, physical examination showed multiple 0.5–3-cm nodular skin lesions, many of which had ulcerated centrally. Laboratory abnormalities included a peripheral white blood cell count of 27,000/cu mm with 85% lymphocytes and a lactate dehydrogenase activity of 426 units. Serum calcium concentration was within the normal range. Histologic examination of the skin lesions revealed marked infiltration of the dermis and subcutaneous tissue with lymphocytes. Numerous foci of lymphocytes were nested in the epidermis. The lymphocytic infiltrate was angiocentric, with foci of malignant-appearing cells around virtually every vessel. Most vessels showed marked perivascular hemorrhage or intravascular thrombosis. Malignant T cells in peripheral blood, skin, and joint fluid before culture in vitro did not express the p19 HTLV-associated antigen. Electron microscopic examination, however, revealed intracellular type C viral particles in skin-infiltrating T cells. After 7 days in culture supplemented with T-cell growth factor, peripheral blood malignant cells expressed the p19 antigen. Electron microscopic examination showed type C virus particles to be budding from malignant T lymphocytes. Treatment of peripheral blood T cells with mitomycin-C induced the transformation of cord blood T cells into HTLV-infected p19$^+$ T cells.

In this patient, the demonstration of HTLV in malignant T cells confirms the association of HTLV with Japanese ATL. The virus may also be associated with a vasculitis-arthritis syndrome.

14–18 **Mycosis Fungoides: Importance of Pulmonary Cytology in Diagnosis of a Case With Systemic Involvement.** Mycosis fungoides, an uncommon but distinct cutaneous T-cell lymphoma that tends to become a disseminated malignant neoplastic disease involving the viscera, predominantly affects middle-aged persons and generally re-

(14–17) Proc. Natl. Acad. Sci. USA 80:2054–2058, April 1983.
(14–18) Acta Cytol. (Baltimore) 27:198–201, March/April 1983.

sults in death 4–5 years after diagnosis. It is characterized by a typical cellular infiltrate, including neoplastic lymphoid cells with indented, infolded, and hyperchromatic nuclei (mycosis cells). Rebecca A. Ludwig and Indra Balachandran (SUNY, Upstate Med. Center) describe a patient with cutaneous myosis fungoides who developed pulmonary lesions while undergoing radiation therapy.

Man, 39, with compensated renal failure, had developed eczematous blistering lesions on the trunk, soles of the feet, and neck 1 year before admission. Two months before admission, new skin eruptions developed on the face, mucous membranes of the oropharynx, trunk, buttocks, extremities, and external genitalia. At admission the disseminated skin lesions appeared as lichenoid, indurated plaques, with central clearing and ulceration of the overlying skin, and were accompanied by moderate pruritus. There was no peripheal lymphadenopathy, and the spleen and liver were not enlarged. The clinical impression of mycosis fungoides was confirmed by skin biopsy. There was no evidence of malignant cells on bone marrow examination. Topical nitrogen mustard therapy was begun but was poorly tolerated, and electron beam therapy was subsequently initiated. Over the next 4 months, the patient completed a course of total skin electron beam therapy, with a good result. However, he had increasing shortness of breath and hemoptysis 1 month later. A chest x-ray film demonstrated new, diffuse, fluffy alveolar and nodular infiltrates in both lungs. Transbronchial biopsy, with pulmonary cytologic examination including bronchial washings and brushings, revealed malignant lymphoma cells resembling those seen on the previous skin biopsy (Fig 14–3). These cells showed hyperchromatic nuclei, with scanty cyanophilic cytoplasm. Some nuclei had clefts or indentations, giving a grooved or folded appearance. For the most part, the chromatin was finely granular and irregularly distributed. Prominent, occasionally multiple, nucleoli were seen in most cells. Open-lung biopsy of the lingula revealed an infiltrate of similar malignant lymphoma cells. Three courses of chemotherapy were begun with cyclophosphamide, doxarubicin, vincristine, prednisone, and bleomycin. A repeat chest film showed improvement of the pulmonary infiltrates. Three months after the development of pulmonary symptoms, the patient had a

Fig 14–3.—Bronchial washing showing hyperchromatic, convoluted lymphoid cells with macronucleoli. Papanicolaou; original magnification, ×800. (Courtesy of Ludwig, R.A., and Balachandran, I.: Acta Cytol. [Baltimore] 27:198–201, March–April 1983.)

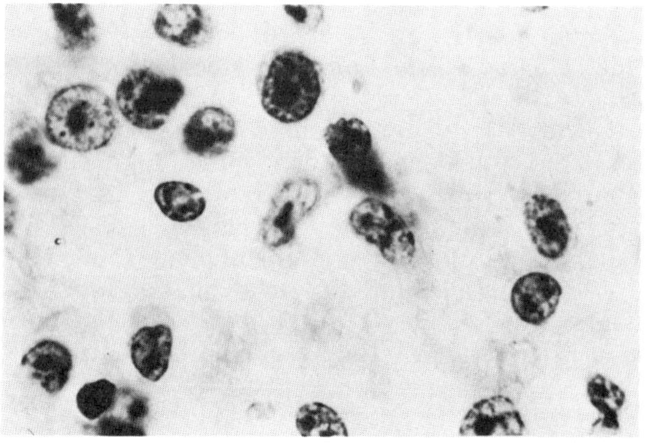

grand mal seizure. A computed tomographic scan of the skull and brain yielded normal findings, but cytologic examination of the cerebrospinal fluid revealed many single, pleomorphic lymphoid cells. Two intrathecal courses of methotrexate were administered, but the patient became lethargic and unresponsive over the next 10 days. Septic shock was diagnosed. Despite vigorous support, the patient died of cardiopulmonary arrest 6 months after the original diagnosis of mycosis fungoides.

In this patient the appearance of characteristic dysplastic lymphoid cells in pulmonary cytology specimens and in open-lung biopsy tissue allowed the diagnosis of a malignant pulmonary lymphomatous process in the presence of known mycosis fungoides and pulmonary infiltrates. The recognition of mycosis fungoides cells was critical in differentiating this disease from other malignant lymphomas and opportunistic pulmonary infection.

14–19 **Cutaneous Lymphomas: Correlation of Histochemical and Immunohistochemical Characteristics and Clinicopathologic Features.** Lymphomatous diseases of the skin include a heterogeneous group of malignant disorders whose classification has caused considerable confusion. Jayashree Krishnan, Chin-Yang Li, and W. P. Daniel Su (Mayo Clinic and Found.) classified 24 cases of cutaneous lymphoma on the basis of histochemical and immunohistochemical features. There were 18 T-cell, 3 B-cell, and 3 true histiocytic lymphomas. Significant clinical and histopathologic differences were evident among these 3 types.

The skin lesions of T-cell lymphoma usually were chronic and pruritic and sometimes were ulcerative. Two of the 18 patients died. The T-cell lymphomas exhibited epidermal infiltration without a grenz zone. Strong focal positivity for acid phosphatase in the Golgi zones was characteristic of these lesions. The lesions of B-cell lymphoma were nonpruritic and nonulcerative. Two of the 3 patients died within 2 years of diagnosis. Histologically, the B-cell lesions showed a grenz zone in the upper dermis and no epidermal involvement. The lesions of true histiocytic lymphoma often were pruritic and ulcerative. Like those of T-cell lymphoma, these lesions exhibited epidermal infiltration and no grenz zone. All 3 patients with true histiocytic lymphoma died within 6 months of diagnosis.

Cutaneous lymphomas can be classified on the basis of their cell origin, by histochemical and immunohistochemical techniques, into B-cell, T-cell, or true histiocytic lymphomas. True histiocytic lymphoma can resemble T-cell lymphoma clinically and histologically on routine assessment, but it has a much worse prognosis.

14–20 **Severe Pruritus Should be a B-Symptom in Hodgkin's Disease.** Pruritus occasionally is noted in Hodgkin's disease, but its clinical and prognostic significance remains unclear. Paolo G. Gobbi, Giuseppe Attardo-Parrinello, Gaetano Lattanzio, Salvatore C. Rizzo, and Edoardo Ascari (Univ. of Pavia, Italy) evaluated the occurrence and significance of pruritus in a study series of 360 patients with Hodg-

---

(14–19) Am. J. Clin. Pathol. 79:157–165, February 1983.
(14–20) Cancer 51:1934–1936, May 15, 1983.

kin's disease, staged or restaged between 1971 and 1979. One fourth of the patients had mild itching when admitted, and 5.8% had severe, generalized pruritus. In all cases, itching was at least partly responsive to antitumoral therapy. The patients with severe pruritus showed a shorter survival than the others, and this difference remained after adjustment for initial characteristics, stage, A or B category, histotype, and treatment. The difference in survival rates between patients with severe pruritus and the others was apparent from the first years of follow-up.

Although severe pruritus seems to be somewhat more frequent in advanced Hodgkin's disease and when other systemic symptoms are present, it is independently related to a relatively unfavorable prognosis. Generalization of pruritus is useful in distinguishing severe from less severe cases. Severe pruritus should be included with the recognized B symptoms: fever higher than 38 C, night sweats, and weight loss greater than 10%. Pruritus could be designated as severe in the presence of multiple excoriations and a generalized distribution and when local and systemic antipruritic measures are ineffective. Severe pruritus may be related to the biologic characteristics of Hodgkin's disease.

▶ [The authors classify pruritus as severe when *(1)* there are multiple excoriations, *(2)* local and systemic antipruritics have proved to be ineffective, and *(3)* it is generalized. In their series, pruritus that was defined as severe by these criteria was associated with a poorer prognosis. They propose that severe pruritus be included in the definition of the B clinical category (as defined at the Ann Arbor meeting of the committee on Hodgkin's disease staging classification).—R.M.] ◀

4–21 **Sézary Syndrome: Transformation to High-Grade T-Cell Lymphoma After Treatment With Cyclosporine.** M. D. Catterall, B. J. Addis, J. L. Smith, and P. E. Coode used cyclosporine to treat a patient with Sézary syndrome. This patient's disease was characterized by intensely pruritic erythroderma, lymphadenopathy, and the presence of abnormal T lymphocytes (Sézary cells) in his affected skin and peripheral blood.

Man, aged 28, had a 3-year history of increasing generalized pruritus. A diagnosis of Sézary syndrome was confirmed by histologic examination of the skin and lymph nodes, and by lymphocyte marker studies. Treatment with cyclosporine began in September 1978 with an oral dose of 25 mg/kg daily for the first week and 12 mg/kg daily for another week. Within a few days of beginning therapy, significant elevations of the serum bilirubin, aspartate aminotransferase, serum creatinine, and blood urea levels occurred and the patient became clinically icteric. During the early posttreatment period, a moderate subjective diminution in degree of pruritus coincided with the gradual emergence of islands of leukoderma. In June 1979, the patient reported rapid weight gain, swelling of the lower limbs and abdomen, and palpitations occurring in a 2-week period. Lymph nodes were massively enlarged and splenomegaly developed. Lymphangiography confirmed massive intra-abdominal lymphadenopathy and lymphoma. The patient received 6 courses of combined chemotherapy with vincristine, adriamycin, methotrexate, and prednisolone between June and September 1979. Substantial tumor regres-

(14–21) Clin. Exp. Dermatol. 8:159–169, March 1983.

sion occurred, but pruritus reemerged as the dominant symptom. Chemotherapy resumed with the combination of cyclophosphamide, vincristine, adriamycin, and prednisolone, which promoted a period of relative stability. The patient died in April 1980 from progressive deterioration.

The first skin biopsy showed a patchy, predominantly perivascular infiltrate in the dermis. The first lymph node biopsy included several slightly enlarged nodes, and the second lymph node biopsy showed a predominance of the large cells with effacement of the normal nodal structure. In this patient, progression to a high-grade lymphoma occurred about 4 years after onset of symptoms and 8 months after a short course of cyclosporine. Surface marker studies and cytochemistry demonstrated that the acute-phase cells were related to the original atypical lymphocytes.

Recent reports suggest a high incidence of malignant lymphomas in transplant patients receiving cyclosporine. Some of these tumors are of B-cell origin, but others have not been fully documented. Findings in the present patient raise the possibility that the drug accelerated or altered the natural history of the disease.

▶ [Cyclosporine is a lymphocytotoxic drug that will probably be more widely used in the future because of its introduction as an immune suppressant in the organ transplant field. In the United States its use has so far been limited to investigational trials. The issue of lymphoma development in patients receiving cyclosporine requires close watching. Other recent innovative approaches to the treatment of Sézary syndrome have included extracorporeal irradiation of blood with psoralen–ultraviolet A and administration of monoclonal antibodies directed against T cells. All of these approaches have produced temporary improvement in some of the treated patients.—A.J.S.] ◀

14–22 **Investigation of 2′-Deoxycoformycin in the Treatment of Cutaneous T-Cell Lymphoma.** Mycosis fungoides is an uncommon malignancy best characterized as a cutaneous T-cell lymphoma. 2′-Deoxycoformycin (DCF), a potent inhibitor of adenosine deaminase, has been investigated in phase I clinical trials as a possible anticancer agent because of its adverse effect on the survival of leukemia T-cell lines. Michael R. Grever, Emil Bisaccia, Dwight A. Scarborough, Earl N. Metz, and James A. Neidhart (Ohio State Univ.) report the results of DCF treatment in 4 patients with advanced mycosis fungoides. A total of 8 courses of DCF was administered. As the study was part of an ongoing phase I clinical trial, each patient was given a fixed dosage (range, 4–10 mg/sq m/day for 3 consecutive days) for 28 days. All 4 patients had a poor prognosis as evidenced by extensive skin plaques, skin tumors, lymphadenopathy, or hepatosplenomegaly.

Lymphadenopathy resolved in all patients after administration of DCF. Two patients achieved complete remission after receiving 1 and 3 courses (8 mg/sq m/day), respectively. These 2 patients have shown no progression of disease since the last course of DCF; durations of remission have been longer than 9 and 7 months, respectively. Both these patients showed a 100% inhibition of adenosine deaminase. The other 2 patients achieved partial remission, with complete resolution

---

(14–22) Blood 61:279–282, February 1983.

of lymphadenopathy and 80%–90% clearing of skin plaques. One of these patients showed a substantial partial remission after 3 courses, followed by a plateau in response. Several more doses of DCF were followed by progression of skin lesions (10% of body area) after 9 months. Adenosine deaminase inhibitions in the 2 patients showing partial remission were 60% and 100%. The patient with 60% adenosine deaminase inhibition had received only 1 course of DCF at a lower dosage (4 mg/sq m/day) than the other patients. This patient showed elevated serum creatinine concentrations after DCF administration that returned to normal with conservative medical management. During this period, he had mild conjunctival inflammation, fever, nausea, and diarrhea, which resolved completely within 2 weeks. The other 3 patients had mild nausea and vomiting but no nephrotoxicity. Two patients developed moderate and 1 developed significant leukopenia.

Effective antitumor activity can be achieved with DCF at dosages that inhibit adenosine deaminase but are not associated with irreversible clinical toxicity. Phase II investigations will provide further information about the value of DCF in the treatment of mycosis fungoides.

▶ [Three years ago, Dr. Michael Wick of the Farber Cancer Research Institute used similar doses of DFC to treat two of my patients with advanced cases of mycosis fungoides. Both patients showed initial impressive responses but developed significant unpredicted renal and central nervous system toxicity which discouraged further experimental use of this potent drug.—S.L.M.] ◀

14–23 **Topical Carmustine (BCNU) for Mycosis Fungoides and Related Disorders: A 10-Year Experience.** Herschel S. Zackheim, Ervin H. Epstein, Jr., N. Scott McNutt, David A. Grekin, and William R. Crain (Univ. of California, San Francisco) reviewed the results of topical carmustine (BCNU) therapy in 91 patients treated since 1971, including 86 with mycosis fungoides (MF), 3 with lymphomatoid papulosis, and 2 with parapsoriasis en plaques. All the diagnoses were confirmed histologically. More than a third of the patients with MF had received specific treatment previously, usually with topical mechlorethamine application. Both a BCNU ointment and an intralesional solution were used. More intensive treatment was used in earlier years. Seventy patients received 116 total-body courses with a mean dose of 607 mg. Most patients also used supplementary local applications of ointment. Twenty-one patients were treated only locally or regionally.

Only 3 patients had hypersensitivity reactions to treatment. Erythema and telangiectasis often spared the lesion site. A lichenified dermatitis sometimes resulted from local treatment; it usually resolved spontaneously in 1–2 months. A benign nevus developed in 1 patient, and in another a linear epidermal nevus became prominent during treatment. Three patients had mild to moderate bone marrow depression. Complete remission of MF was achieved in 84% of pa-

---

(14–23) J. Am. Acad. Dermatol. 9:363–374, September 1983.

tients with less than 10% involvement and in 52% of those with more extensive disease. The respective median response durations were 12 and 23 months. None of these patients died of MF. Local treatment only gave good results in several patients with less than 5% involvement. Five of 7 patients with poikilodermatous MF did well, as did the 3 patients with lymphomatoid papulosis and both patients with parapsoriasis en plaques.

Topical BCNU application is an effective treatment for cutaneous T-cell lymphomas such as MF. Marrow depression has not been a serious problem, and premalignant changes have not been observed in the skin. Hypersensitivity to BCNU is rare. Both pulmonary toxicity and renal toxicity are possibilities with BCNU therapy.

▶ [Although the authors point out that hypersensitivity reactions are rare and although they fail to describe any, one wonders whether contact urticaria and anaphylactoid reaction as induced by topical application of nitrogen mustard (Grunnet, E.: *Br. J. Dermatol.* 94:101, 1976) have been experienced or will be described.—S.L.M.] ◀

14–24 **Treatment of Cutaneous Lymphoma With Etretinate.** A. L. Claudy, B. Rouchouse, S. Boucheron, and J. C. Le Petit (St. Etienne, France) used etretinate to treat 12 patients with parapsoriasis en plaques and various stages of epidermotropic and nonepidermotropic cutaneous lymphoma (NECL). The 7 men and 5 women were aged 47–77 years. Four patients had large plaques or diffuse atrophic parapsoriasis. The 6 with epidermotropic lymphoma included 3 patients with infiltrative erythroderma, 2 with Sézary syndrome, and 1 with mycosis fungoides. Two patients had NECL with low-grade malignant B-cell lymphoma and multiple nonulcerated nodules and plaques. Seven patients had failed to respond to various treatments. Etretinate was given in a dosage of 0.8–1.0 mg/kg daily for 2–14 months. Eight patients received maintenance therapy with 0.5 or 1 mg/kg daily.

The patients with parapsoriasis en plaques or diffuse atrophic parapsoriasis had a poor response to treatment. Those with infiltrative erythroderma had impressive results. The patients with deeply infiltrating tumors were unresponsive to etretinate. Three of 4 patients who discontinued treatment had recurrences after 3–4 months, but 1 remained free from disease. No severe toxic effects of etretinate were seen even with a dosage of 1 mg/kg daily, and there were no changes in serum enzyme activities. Three of 9 patients had a twofold rise in blood triglyceride concentrations during treatment, but these patients were at risk because of preexistent obesity or diabetes.

The short-term results obtained with etretinate in these patients with cutaneous lymphomas appeared to equal those reported with other treatments, which are usually more aggressive and not without severe side effects. Further study is needed to determine whether etretinate influences the survival of patients with cutaneous lymphomas.

(14–24) Br. J. Dermatol. 109:49–56, July 1983.

▶ [Although etretinate is unavailable in the United States, Kessler et al. of the University of Arizona (see abstract below) have demonstrated similar efficacy with 13-*cis*-retinoic acid in cutaneous T-cell lymphoma. One wonders whether the efficacy of psoralen–ultraviolet A would be enhanced by combined therapy with oral retinoids.—S.L.M.] ◀

14–25 **Treatment of Cutaneous T-Cell Lymphoma (Mycosis Fungoides) With 13-*cis*-Retinoic Acid.** Retinoids can inhibit proliferation and lead to differentiation and maturation in malignant disorders, and they have also been found to alter T-lymphocyte maturation. John F. Kessler, Frank L. Meyskens, Jr., Norman Levine, Peter J. Lynch, and Stephen E. Jones (Univ. of Arizona) evaluated 13-*cis*-retinoic acid in 4 patients with refractory cutaneous T-cell lymphoma. All had generalized plaques and erythroderma due to mycosis fungoides. Symptoms of disease had been present for 4–10 years. The drug was given in doses of 1–3 mg/kg daily. Nearly complete clearing of extensive tumors and plaques was seen in 1 case, and the patient remains in partial remission after 15 months. Two other patients had improvement of pruritus and a 50% reduction in plaques after 4 and 6 weeks, respectively. The fourth patient also had improvement of pruritus and clearing of plaques, but dryness and scaling necessitated withdrawal of treatment.

Most patients with cutaneous T-cell lymphoma have an infiltrate of helper T-cells, and reduced levels of natural killer lymphocytes have been reported. Whether retinoids exert an effect on natural killer lymphocyte activity, which may have antitumor effects, is unknown. Retinoids do influence the immune function of epidermal mononuclear cells, and they could conceivably influence tumor activity through their effects on immunity. The present experience supports further clinical studies of retinoids in the treatment of cutaneous T-cell lymphoma.

14–26 **Merkel Cells and Merkel Cell Tumors: Ultrastructure, Immunocytochemistry, and Review of the Literature.** Forty-six cases of monomorphic cellular dermal tumors, termed trabecular carcinomas or Merkel cell tumors, have been reported. Thomas F. C. S. Warner, Hideo Uno, G. Reza Hafez, John Burgess, Craig Bolles, Ricardo V. Lloyd, and Masamichi Oka (Univ. of Wisconsin, Madison) reviewed these cases and report 6 more, including 4 with unique features strongly supporting an origin from the Merkel cell or its precursor. The clinical features of the authors' cases are given in the table. All but 1 of the tumors were examined by electron microscopy and the immunoperoxidase technique.

All but 1 of the Merkel cell tumors involved the dermis and the subcutaneous adipose tissue. Lymphocytic and plasma cell infiltration was present and in 1 case was prominent (Figs 14–4, 14–5, 14–6). The tumor borders were infiltrative in 2 instances. Sheets of cells predominated, but focal trabecular patterns were evident in all cases. Pseudorosettes were unusual. Mitoses were

---

(14–25) Lancet 1:1345–1347, June 18, 1983.
(14–26) Cancer 52:238–245, July 15, 1983.

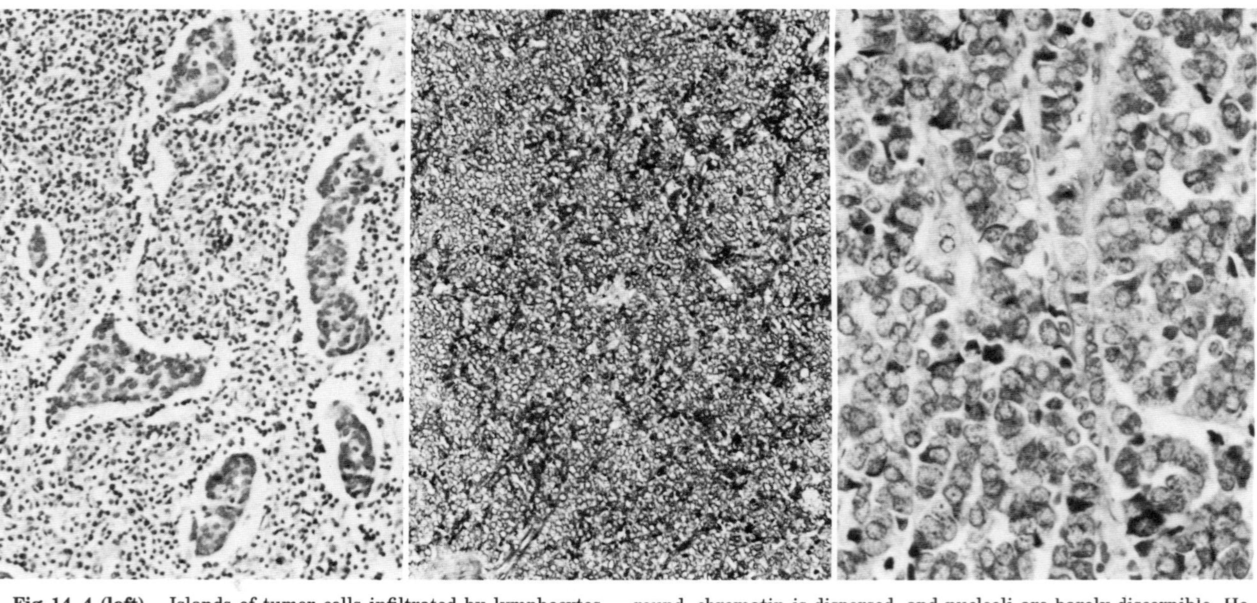

Fig 14–4 (left).—Islands of tumor cells infiltrated by lymphocytes. Hematoxylin-eosin; original magnification, ×125.

Fig 14–5 (center).—Sheets of tumor cells containing vesicular nuclei. Hematoxylin-eosin; original magnification, ×125.

Fig 14–6 (right).—Tumor cells in trabecular array. Nuclei are round, chromatin is dispersed, and nucleoli are barely discernible. Hematoxylin-eosin; original magnification, ×300.

(Courtesy of Warner, T.F.C.S., et al.: Cancer 52:238–245, July 15, 1983.)

CLINICAL FEATURES OF MERKEL'S CELL TUMORS

Case no.	Age/sex	Site	Size (mm)	Mode of presentation
1	66/M	Lower lip	20	Fever blister, ulcerated mass
2*	66/M	Thigh	>25	Sebaceous cyst
3	79/F	Buttock	15	Boil
4	76/F	Buttock	20	Subcutaneous nodule
5†	61/F	Forearm	20 × 12	Pimple
6	23/M	Forearm	20	Nodule

*Epidural metastasis 8 months after excision of primary tumor.
†This patient was tumor free 5 years after operation. Follow-up in all other cases is less than 2 years.
(Courtesy of Warner, T.F.C.S., et al.: Cancer 52:238–245, July 15, 1983.)

abundant in all cases. Ultrastructural study showed electron-dense granules 80–200 nm in size in the tumor cells, as in normal Merkel cells, as well as 10-mm filaments and desmosomes. Four tumors contained filament-rich cytoplasmic spikes resembling the protrusions of normal Merkel cells. Merkel cells of monkey skin exhibited met-enkephalin immunoreactivity on immunocytochemical study. None of the tumors exhibited reactivity to met-enkephalin, β-lipotropin, calcitonin, somatostatin, or neuron-specific enolase.

The paucity of organoid features in Merkel cell tumors helps explain why trabecular carcinoma went so long before being accepted as an entity. The cytologic features permit a diagnosis in most cases, but ultrastructural confirmation should be obtained if possible. The Merkel cell tumor is a distinctive neuroendocrine neoplasm of the skin that probably arises in dermal or follicular Merkel cells. Local recurrence and node metastasis are common, necessitating complete local excision.

▶ [Before the cell line of origin was defined, this undifferentiated carcinoma was termed trabecular carcinoma by Toker (*Arch. Dermatol.* 105:107–110, 1972). Electromicroscopy is required for definitive diagnosis. Other cutaneous neoplasms in the differential diagnosis of Merkel cell tumor include lymphoma, myelogenous leukemia, squamous cell carcinoma, metastatic melanoma, Ewing's sarcoma, neuroblastoma, carcinoid, oat cell carcinoma, medullary carcinoma, and sweat gland carcinoma.—A.J.S.] ◀

4–27 **Immunostaining of Neuron-Specific Enolase as a Diagnostic Tool for Merkel Cell Tumors.** The Merkel cell is a member of the amine-precursor uptake decarboxylation system found mainly in the basal layer of the epidermis. Primary skin tumors thought to arise from the Merkel cell have been described. These cells contain neuron-specific enolase (NSE), an isoenzyme found in a number of neuroen-

(14–27) Cancer 52:1039–1043, Sept. 15, 1983.

docrine cells; thus immunostaining for NSE might be a simple means of identifying this uncommon cell type. Jiang Gu, Julia M. Polak, Susan Van Noorden, Anthony G. E. Pearse, Paul J. Marangos, and John G. Azzopardi (London) performed immunostaining for NSE using the peroxidase-antiperoxidase method in 11 cases of Merkel's cell tumor, including 1 local lymph node metastasis, that had been diagnosed by ultrastructural study. The tumors were removed from the limbs, neck, and face of patients older than age 55 years. Sixteen other skin tumors also were examined.

The tumors were situated in the dermis and extended into the subcutaneous or deeper tissues. The diffuse infiltrate resembled that of malignant lymphoma. Ill-defined anastomosing cords and clusters of cells were observed. The tumor cells had numerous mitoses. Neuron-specific enolase immunoreactivity was found in all tumor cells in each case. Staining was rather weak in 3 cases. Immunoreactivity was uniformly present in the cytoplasm, which formed a rim around the large unstained nucleus. All control sections were negative for NSE immunoreactivity, except for variable, mostly weak activity in some malignant melanomas. Four of the Merkel's cell tumors stained with the Grimelius silver impregnation method, whereas 4 others reacted equivocally and 3 were unreactive.

Merkel's cell tumors can be specifically identified by immunostaining for NSE activity. With adequate fixation, NSE activity can be found in most, if not all, Merkel's cell tumors. The procedure will be diagnostically useful if metastatic oat cell carcinoma of the bronchus and malignant melanoma can be ruled out.

▶ [Very useful tool.—M.C.M.] ◀

14–28 **Primary Neuroendocrine Carcinomas of the Skin (Merkel Cell Tumors): Clinical, Histologic, and Ultrastructural Study of 13 Cases.** Mark R. Wick, John R. Goellner, Bernd W. Scheithauer, J. R. Thomas III, Nestor P. Sanchez, and Arnold L. Schroeter (Mayo Clinic) reviewed the findings in 13 cases of neuroendocrine carcinoma of the skin. All lesions were examined ultrastructurally, and 8 were examined immunohistochemically. All primary tumors were elevated, nodular, red-pink lesions 0.8–4.0 cm in diameter. The neoplastic infiltrate was confined primarily to the dermis and subcutaneous fat. Nests of tumor cells often were seen in dermal lymphatic channels. Rosette formation was noted focally in 2 cases. A polymorphous inflammatory infiltrate was admixed with the tumor cells in about half of the cases. Peripheral cytoplasmic dense-core granules and perinuclear filament whorls were regular ultrastructural features. Immunoperoxidase study showed no serotonin, calcitonin, or ACTH within the tumor cells.

The ages of the 8 men and 5 women ranged from 24 to 84 years. Nine had lesions in sun-exposed areas. One had antecedent hypohidrotic ectodermal dysplasia. Eight tumors metastasized, and 6 spread to regional or distant nodes. Three patients died with visceral metas-

---

(14–28) Am. J. Clin. Pathol. 79:6–13, January 1983.

tases. Most of the 86 reported patients with trabecular carcinoma or Merkel cell tumor of the skin have had primary dermal involvement. The metastatic potential of these tumors requires an early, accurate diagnosis. Most patients have had tumors in sun-exposed areas of skin. The Merkel cell tumor appears to be a neuroendocrine neoplasm. All such lesions must be viewed as potentially aggressive. Wide local excision and close follow-up seem appropriate treatment at present, but further studies are needed to establish the best management of Merkel cell tumors.

▶ [The concurrent presence of perinuclear tonofilaments and dense coarse granules, it must be emphasized, speak strongly against a metastatic small cell carcinoma.—M.C.M.] ◀

14–29 **Benign Adnexal Tumors of Late Occurrence on Verrucosebaceous Nevi of Jadassohn.** Other than basal cell epithelioma, syringocystadenoma papilliferum, various adnexal tumors, such as pilar or sweat gland tumors, may also be associated with sebaceous nevi. D. Bonvalet, Y. Barrandon, C. Foix, and J. Civatte (Paris) report 7 cases, all having appeared in adulthood, that clinically suggested the diagnosis of basal cell epithelioma. Histologic examination showed them to be benign tumors, most likely representing pilar or sweat gland tumors that are not easily identified with precision. Histopathologic study differentiated nodular hidradenoma, chondroid syringoma, trichilemmoma, apocrine cystadenoma, and follicular poroma, respectively.

The variety of tumors associated with Jadassohn's sebaceous nevi clearly illustrates the complex nature of this dysembryoplasia. Among these proliferations 2 types must be distinguished. The first type corresponds to equally dysembrioplastic lesions, more of the nature of dystrophies than true tumors, such as the papilliferous syringocystadenoma and basaloid proliferations. The second type corresponds to truly tumoral proliferations appearing much later, at about 30–40 years of age, and shows evolutive character, such as the basal cell epitheliomas, the rare spinocellular epitheliomas, various benign adnexal pilar or sudoral lesions, with only exceptional malignancy.

4–30 **Clinical and Pathologic Cutaneous Manifestations of Malignant Histiocytosis.** Nathaniel E. Morgan, David Fretzin, Daina Variakojis, and William A. Caro (Univ. of Chicago) reviewed the clinical and pathologic findings in 5 patients seen at 3 centers in 1968–1978 with malignant histiocytosis. One case is described below.

Man, 83, had had congestive heart failure for many years. The right foot and leg were warm, swollen, erythematous, and tender, and the findings persisted despite antibiotic therapy. Papules and nodules with vesicular and ulcerated centers developed on the same extremity; some became hemorrhagic (Fig 14–7). Bacterial cultures of the ulcers were persistently negative. A biopsy specimen of an early nodule showed a patchy dermal infiltrate of large atypical, pleomorphic histiocytes intermixed with plasma cells. Bone marrow examinations disclosed no neoplastic cells. Necrotizing skin lesions pro-

---

(14–29) Ann. Dermatol. Venereol. 110:337–342, 1983.
(14–30) Arch. Dermatol. 119:367–372, May 1983.

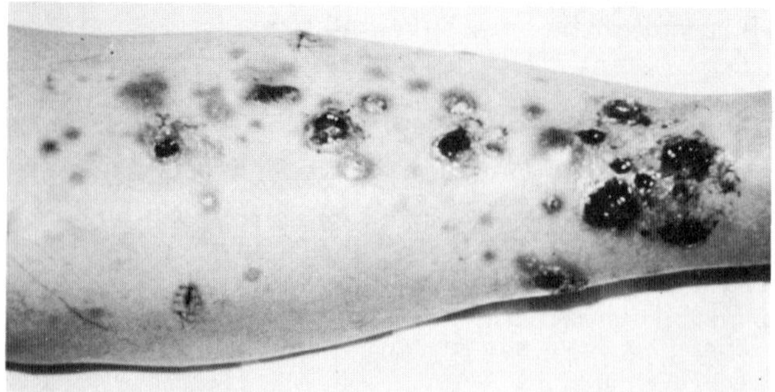

Fig 14–7.—Erythematous papules, nodules, ulcerating nodules, and hemorrhagic ulcers in 83-year-old man with malignant histiocytosis. (Courtesy of Morgan, N.E., et al.: Arch. Dermatol. 119:367–372, May 1983; copyright 1983, American Medical Association.)

gressed in size and number despite prednisone therapy, but remained restricted to the right leg. The patient became weak, lethargic, confused, and jaundiced. Heart failure worsened, and he died in a coma 61 days after admission. At autopsy extensive infiltration of neoplastic histiocytes in the skin of the right lower extremity, lymph nodes, liver, spleen, and lungs was found. Malignant histiocytosis was diagnosed.

The 5 patients studied were aged 12–83 years at the onset of illness. Four patients had papules, nodules, and ulcerated nodules. In 1 patient a herpesvirus infection with secondary infiltration of the lesions by neoplastic histiocytes was discovered at autopsy. Four patients received chemotherapy, but only brief remissions resulted; the longest survival after onset of illness was 7 months. The lesions consisted of epidermal changes, microabscess formation (in 2 cases), sheets and aggregates of tumor cells in the dermis and subcutaneous tissue, and foci of necrosis mixed with inflammatory cell infiltrates.

Cutaneous involvement is present in about 10%–15% of cases of malignant histiocytosis. In rare instances, skin lesions may be the only obvious manifestation of the disease.

▶ [Erythrophagocytosis, a characteristic finding in visceral lesions was only noted in cutaneous lesions in 2 of 5 patients in this study. However, this finding is variable in cutaneous lesions, whereas it is much more consistently observed in the visceral lesions. Therefore, diagnosis is optimally made when skin and other involved organs are available for histopathologic study—M.C.M.] ◀

14–31 **Malignant Eccrine Poroma: Study of 27 Cases.** Eccrine poroma is a generally benign tumor of the intraepidermal component of the eccrine sweat duct. Marcia Shaw, P. H. McKee, D. Lowe, and M. M. Black (St. Thomas's Hosp. Med. School, London) reviewed the findings in 27 cases of malignant eccrine poroma encountered in 1950 to 1981. The clinical features are given in the table. The mean patient age was 62 years. The duration of lesions varied widely. Acral sites were favored. The tumors were observed as verrucous plaques or polypoid growths that often were ulcerated and sometimes bled on

(14–31) Br. J. Dermatol. 107:675–680, December 1982.

CLINICAL FEATURES OF ECCRINE POROMA

Patient	Age	Sex	Site	Duration (years)	Recurrence or metastases
1	82	F	Chin	1	Unknown
2	90	F	Axilla	Unknown	None after 1 year
3	73	F	Calf	2½	Unknown
4	51	M	Sole	⅙	Local recurrence 4 months after 1st excision
5	85	M	Forearm	½	Unknown
6	79	M	Calf	5	No recurrence after 5 years
7	77	F	Unknown	Unknown	Unknown
8	38	F	Back	Unknown	Unknown
9	69	M	Thigh	20	No recurrence after 2 years
10	30	F	Lip	Unknown	Unknown
11	61	F	Foot	40	Metastatic nodes in groin
12	44	M	Heel	1	Recurred and re-excised on four occasions
13	65	M	Shin	Many years	Unknown
14	41	M	Scalp	Several years	Unknown
15	60	M	Leg	Unknown	Unknown
16	75	F	Thigh	20	Unknown
17	65	M	Sole	Unknown	Unknown
18	19	F	Sole	Unknown	Unknown
19	61	M	Palm	20	Recurred and re-excised on three occasions
20	84	M	Hand	8	Unknown
21	45	M	Hand	Unknown	Unknown
22	58	M	Sole	6	Recurred and re-excised 12 years later
23	56	M	Buttock	Unknown	Recurrence after 1 year
24	85	F	Loin	Unknown	Recurrence and metastases in lymph nodes
25	48	M	Foot	Unknown	Unknown
26	72	M	Foot	Unknown	Unknown
27	71	F	Unknown	Unknown	Unknown

(Courtesy of Shaw, M., et al.: Br. J. Dermatol. 107:675–680, December 1982.)

trauma. Six of the 11 patients followed up had recurrences, and 2 had distant metastases. All the tumors contained areas in which the poromatous derivation was apparent. Careful search usually disclosed ductal lumens lined by a periodic acid–Schiff diastase-positive, eosinophilic membrane. In other areas there were more obvious malignant features including distinct nuclear pleomorphism and frequent, often abnormal mitotic figures. Areas of necrosis were frequent. Frankly Bowenoid features were present in 8 cases.

Malignant eccrine porocarcinoma is a rare tumor that is usually found in elderly persons. A long history is typical. Four of the patients in this study had had a tumor present for 20 years or longer, suggesting the possibility of malignant change in a preexisting benign lesion. The clinical features are not especially distinctive. Bowenoid features may be found in an otherwise apparently benign lesion, or the tumor may be frankly malignant with extensive infiltration and sometimes lymphatic spread or infiltration of the perineural space. The preferred treatment is surgical excision. The present limited follow-up experience would indicate that malignant eccrine poroma is a potentially fatal tumor.

▶ [An important review of findings in a series of patients with a rare tumor.—M.C.M.] ◀

15. Photobiology and Phototherapy

15–1 **Alteration of T Cell Subsets and Induction of Suppressor T-Cell Activity in Normal Subjects After Exposure to Sunlight.** Normal subjects who have been exposed to a standard course of treatment to induce tanning in commercial solariums have been found to have depressed delayed hypersensitivity skin test (DTH) responses to dinitrochlorobenzene, reduced lymphocyte counts, and a change in the proportion of T-cell subpopulations in blood as defined by the OKT series of monoclonal antibodies. An increase in suppressor T-cell activity against IgG production in T- and B-cell cultures has also been observed. Peter Hersey, Gregory Haran, Enisa Hasic, and Anne Edwards (Sydney) investigated the effects of exposure to natural sunlight on the immune system in 15 normal subjects. The subjects were asked to sunbathe for 1 hour each day for 12 days over a 2-week period. Tests were conducted before sunbathing and 1 day and 2 weeks after completion of the exposure period. Thirteen age- and sex-matched controls were asked to avoid sun exposure during the same period.

No significant changes were observed in hemoglobin concentrations or total leukocyte, lymphocyte, or neutrophil count in the blood of the test of control subjects. Compared with controls, subjects exposed to sunlight showed significant increases in circulating T cells recognized by OKT8 monoclonal antibodies and a decrease in OKT4-positive T cells. There were no significant changes in the percentage of circulating B lymphocytes in either group. Suppressor T-cell activity against IgG and IgM production as measured in pokeweed mitogen–stimulated cultures of T and B cells was significantly increased. These changes were still observed in many of the test subjects 2 weeks after completion of the exposure period. No significant changes were observed in IgA, IgG, or IgM concentrations in either group throughout the study. Compared with controls, the test subjects showed a trend toward reduction in natural killer cell activity against a melanoma target cell (MM200) 2 weeks after completion of the exposure period. However, this reduction did not appear to be as great as that previously seen in subjects exposed to radiation in solariums.

The differences between the effect of radiation from a solarium and natural sunlight on the immune system may be attributable to the higher dose of ultraviolet A radiation from solariums. In this study, the findings suggest that exposure to sunlight may tend toward the induction of suppressor pathways in response to antigenic stimuli,

(15–1) J. Immunol. 31:171–179, July 1983.

thereby limiting immune responses against tumor cells such as melanoma. Systemic changes in the immune system may be important in the development of malignancy associated with ultraviolet radiation.

15–2 **Immunologic Effects of Solarium Exposure.** Although several studies have shown that the incidence of melanoma is related to exposure to sunlight, this association may be indirect in that tumors often develop at sites not exposed to excessive sunlight. This suggests a "solar factor" that may act systemically to increase the incidence of melanoma. Peter Hersey, Enisa Hasic, Anne Edwards, Margot Bradley, Gregory Haran, and W. H. McCarthy (Sydney, Australia) studied the effects of controlled exposure to ultraviolet (UV) radiation on the immune system in 18 volunteers and 13 age- and sex-matched controls. The test subjects received 12 30-minute exposures to a commercial solarium over a 16-day period. Blood samples were obtained before the tanning course began, on completion of the course, and 2 weeks after completion.

Compared with controls, the test subjects showed a diminished skin test response to dinitrochlorobenzene challenge, a significant decrease in the total white blood cell count, a small but significant drop in blood lymphocyte counts, and changes in the proportions of lymphocyte subpopulations. The mean lymphocyte count remained low 2 weeks after completion of the exposure period. This was associated with a small, though significant, increase in total T-cell numbers as determined by OKT3 antibody attributable to an increase in the OKT8 (suppressor-cytotoxic) subset of T cells. The OKT4 (helper) subset of T cells tended to be decreased at the end of the exposure period, and there was a significant decrease in the ratio of OKT4 to OKT8 cells. Other changes included a significant increase in suppressor T-cell activity against IgG (but not IgA or IgM) production in vitro and a significant reduction in natural killer cell activity against the MM200 target cell. These changes were still observed in some of the test subjects 2 weeks after the exposure period.

The observed effects of exposure to UV radiation could be expected to impair host defenses against tumors, particularly those occurring in the skin. Further, increased suppressor activity against IgG production could be expected to reduce antibody responses to tumors. This could also apply to T-cell-mediated responses if the suppressor activity found in this study is a reflection of a general increase in suppressor activity.

▶ [These two studies convincingly demonstrate a range of immunologic responses occurring in humans following exposure to "physiological" amounts of ultraviolet radiation. The practical significance of these changes remains to be explored, but the authors propose that alteration of defenses against tumors could occur.

The observed difference between the effects of solaria and of natural sunlight are of great interest. It appears that subjects of similar tanning ability were used for the two studies. Immune alterations were greater after solarium exposure: duration and intensity of ultraviolet B (UVB) exposure were calculated to be similar. The authors

---

(15–2) Lancet 1:545–548, Mar. 12, 1983.

propose that the approximately threefold greater ultraviolet A (UVA) exposure in the solarium study may account for the differences which were observed. Other differences in the spectral power distribution may of course be important. The use of predominantly UVB-blocking sunscreens may alter the effective exposure to natural sunlight to a more solarium-like spectrum by allowing prolonged and large UVA exposures. On the other hand, UVA-induced tanning responses, although mainly the result of basal layer melanin and although poorly protective aganst erythema, could perhaps reduce exposure of the vascular contents in the skin including lymphocytes.—R.W.G.] ◀

15–3 **Analysis of Ultraviolet Radiation Doses Required To Produce Erythemal Responses in Normal Skin.** L. A. MacKenzie (Dundee, Scotland) notes that when the abnormality of a skin response to sunlight is expressed as a decreased minimum erythemal dose (MED) on phototesting, it is essential to know the range of response in normal skin. To assess this response to ultraviolet (UV) radiation, the MED values in a group of normal persons were calculated.

The distribution of MEDs already calculated among normal individuals is unlikely to be gaussian. The use of probits in effect converts the cumulative probability curve derived from a gaussian distribution into a straight line, and is equivalent to plotting the observed cumulative proportions on probability graph paper. In any homogeneous group, the distribution of the MED is skewed and is not gaussian (normal), but a gaussian distribution can be fitted to the logarithm of the MED. Using established methods of probit analysis, such "lognormal" distributions were fitted to the observed proportions of erythemal responses to a series of test exposure doses of UV radiation (250–365 nm), providing estimates of the average log MED for normal skin, standard deviations of the distributions, and associated confidence limits.

Factors that might influence the distributions of erythemal doses from the irradiations described in this study include true variations, variations resulting from subjective assessments of erythemal response, limitations set by finite gradation of the basic series of exposure doses, variations in UV dosimetry, and variations in calibrations. There appears to be less variation between the MEDs of individuals at 295 nm than at higher or lower wavelengths. The results of this study refer only to the tests carried out and assessed in the author's photobiology laboratory and do not necessarily have universal significance or application.

15–4 **Statistical Study of Individual Variations in Sunburn Sensitivity in 303 Volunteers Without Photodermatosis.** P. Amblard, J. Beani, R. Gautron, J. Reymond, and B. Doyon (Grenoble, France) examined variations in personal sunburn sensitivity, using erythema as the photobiologic criterion, in a population of 303 normal white subjects, aged 5–89 years, to define the physiologic limits of sunlight sensitivity as a function of biologic factors. Subjects were irradiated with a 2,500-W xenon arc solar simulator with filters fitted. The minimal erythemal dose (MED), the minimal dose needed to elicit intense

(15–3) Br. J. Dermatol. 108:1–9, January 1983.
(15–4) Arch. Dermatol. Res. 274:195–206, December 1982.

erythema (MED++), and the minimal dose eliciting edematous erythema (MOD) were estimated.

High degrees of correlation were obtained among the MED, MED++, and MOD, confirming the usefulness of MED as a photobiologic criterion. The average MED was 889 mJ/sq cm, and the pathologic threshold for total light spectrum irradiation was 347 mJ/sq cm. Significant variations in MED were related to age, sex, complexion, eye color, hair color, and Fitzpatrick skin type. There were no significant differences in average MED for a given type of complexion when hair color and eye-hair factors were varied.

The best photobiologic criterion for sunburn sensitivity is the MED. The biologic factor that most closely reflects individual sunburn sensitivity is complexion, and this factor must be taken into account in studies of ultraviolet therapy and in artificial photoprotection. White persons can be usefully classified as having a light, intermediate, or dark complexion.

▶ [Probit analysis appears to be a useful alternative method for arriving at MED values in a group of normal individuals.

In a very large study Amblard et al. found that the best way of predicting sun sensitivity in an individual was to assess complexion by examination of the untanned buttocks in a good light. It is interesting to note that the authors found a fairly constant arithmetic difference between the MED and the minimal dose resulting in an edematous response (MOD). The relationship could be expressed as follows: MOD = MED + 1,750 mJ/sq cm. This implies that the proportional increase over the MED needed to induce edema is smaller for high-MED subjects than for low-MED subjects. The authors suggest that this may be the result of saturation of the quenching ability of melanin; once this is exceeded (at around the MED), the dose-damage response is similar.—R.W.G.] ◀

15–5 **Sensitization of Near-Ultraviolet Radiation Killing of Mammalian Cells by Sunscreen Agent Para-Aminobenzoic Acid.** Pauline J. Osgood, Stephen H. Moss, and David J. G. Davies (Univ. of Bath, England) note that the wavelengths of sunlight considered to be responsible for erythema and skin cancer formation are in the range of 290–340 nm. Formulated sunscreens usually contain an agent that absorbs in this wavelength region, and one of the most widely used is para-aminobenzoic acid (PABA). Previous work demonstrated PABA sensitization of lethal and mutagenic effects of near-ultraviolet (UV) radiation in a model bacterial system. Sensitization by PABA to 313 nm, near-UV radiation, was examined in mouse lymphoma cells, which do not approximate normal human skin cells. The actual line used was the murine lymphoma cell line L5178Y.

Over the range examined, 0.01%–0.2%, the survival of cells irradiated in PABA plus 5% dimethylsulfoxide (DMSO) was less than that of cells irradiated in PABA alone. In the absence of PABA, DMSO had no effect on cell viability, and survival curves for L5178Y cells irradiated with 313-nm UV radiation, with or without 5% DMSO, were not significantly different. Holding cells in irradiated or nonirradiated PABA solutions for times comparable to those used in the experiments showed no significant loss of survival. Survival for

---

(15–5) J. Invest. Dermatol. 79:354–357, December 1982.

the highest concentration of PABA studied, 0.2%, both with and without DMSO, together with the respective controls, indicated sensitization by PABA of the lethal effect of near-UV radiation, the extent of which, after correction for absorption of UV radiation by PABA, bears a direct relationship to PABA concentration.

These results clearly demonstrate increased cell inactivation by near-UV radiation when PABA is present. However, although these findings may not be taken as evidence that PABA is photocarcinogenic in human skin in vivo, topical pharmaceutical and cosmetic preparations should be screened for their effect on induction of damage by near-UV radiation.

▶ [It is often assumed that human carcinogenesis and aging are delayed by the use of sunscreens. Animal evidence supports this. The relevance of the findings of this study in human skin is not known. As the authors point out, the end point used was cell inactivation, whereas mutation might be more relevant to carcinogenesis. Furthermore, the behavior of mouse cells in vitro does not necessarily predict the behavior of intact human skin. However, Sutherland (*Photochem. Photobiol.* 36:95–97, 1982) has now shown that PABA will sensitize the formation of pyrimidine dimers in DNA of human skin fibroblasts by sunlamp radiation, and it will also cause transformation of these cells to anchorage-independent growth. Oxybenzone did not cause similar changes.—R.W.G.] ◀

15–6 **Response of Human Skin to Ultraviolet Radiation: Dissociation of Erythema and Metabolic Changes Following Sunscreen Protection.** Ultraviolet irradiation of human skin leads to increased epidermal and stratum corneum thickness, an increase in autoradiographic labeling, and an altered distribution of enzyme activities in the epidermis. A. D. Pearse and Ronald Marks (Welsh Natl. School of Medicine, Cardiff, Wales) examined the effects of two commonly used sunscreens on both erythema production and the epidermal response after ultraviolet irradiation in 10 normal subjects, 6 females and 4 males with a mean age of 22 years. Areas of non-sun-exposed buttock skin were irradiated 10 times over 2 weeks at a peak of 313 nm, and the sunscreens Spectraban and Uvistat were then each used by 5 subjects during treatment with a dose sixfold higher than the minimal erythemal dose (MED) of ultraviolet radiation. Other protected sites received 4 and 2 MEDs of ultraviolet radiation. Biopsy specimens were obtained for autoradiographic analysis.

Some histometric and metabolic sequelae of ultraviolet B exposure were observed despite the successful blocking of erythema by the sunscreens. Spectraban was somewhat more effective than Uvistat in preventing erythema at the 6-MED level. Protection from epidermal thickening after ultraviolet exposure was incomplete. A reduction in epidermal succinic dehydrogenase activity after irradiation was not fully prevented by the sunscreens, and the increase in glucose-6-phosphate dehydrogenase activity was not completely blocked.

The reasons for the dissociation between the erythematous response to ultraviolet B and the metabolic changes are unclear, but the latter may be more sensitive indicators of epidermal damage than

---

(15–6) J. Invest. Dermatol. 80:191–194, March 1983.

is erythema. Protection by conventional sunscreens against injury from ultraviolet exposure may be incomplete, and it is not sufficient to use erythema as a marker for sunscreen effectiveness. The findings are particularly significant for patients with photodermatoses, who may experience both short- and long-term effects of ultraviolet exposure despite the use of conventional sunscreens.

▶ [In this study, sunscreens of modest efficacy by U.S. standards were used. The responses observed are the result of interactions between the spectral power distribution of the source, the absorption spectra of the sunscreens, and the action spectra and sensitivities of the responses. Consequently, it is not surprising that different responses were affected differently. However, other studies have shown reasonable correlation between erythemal sun protection factor and protection against other responses such as edema, stimulation or suppression of epidermal DNA synthesis, or changes in epidermal ornithine decarboxylase activity.

It is not clear from the report whether melanization that is likely to occur as a result of 6-MED doses given on 10 out of 14 days could interfere with a microdensitometric measurement of histochemical reaction products.—R.W.G.] ◀

15–7 **Topical Protection Against Long-Wave Ultraviolet A.** The recognition of ultraviolet A (UVA) as a biologically important component of solar ultraviolet radiation has led to interest in developing topical ultraviolet screening agents that, unlike conventional sunscreens containing para-aminobenzoic acid (PABA), protect against UVA. Michael Jarratt, Marcia Hill, and Kenneth Smiles tested alternative agents in 12 men, aged 19–37 years. Test sites were treated after the ingestion of 0.5 mg of 8-methoxypsoralen per kg, followed in 2 hours by exposure to 2–10 J/sq cm of UVA at 320–390 nm. In a subsequent study, 12 men, aged 22–37 years, ingested the psoralen, were treated, and then swam for 5 minutes in a swimming pool before the test sites were exposed to UVA. The preparations evaluated were 5% PABA in alcohol, 10% sulisobenzone in lotion base, 7% PABA ester, and 3% oxybenzone in an anionic emulsion vehicle, and the anionic emulsion vehicle alone.

Erythema in test sites treated with 5% PABA was comparable to that in vehicle-treated sites. Both the PABA ester-oxybenzone preparation and the sulisobenzone lotion provided substantial protection. The 10% sulisobenzone lotion was most protective at 72 hours, and at 48 hours with UVA doses of 8 and 10 J/sq cm. In the substantivity evaluation, the PABA ester-oxybenzone preparation was most protective. The other three treatments were all associated with more erythema at 48 and 72 hours. No significant toxic effects of methoxypsoralen were observed.

Methoxsalen-induced photosensitivity to UVA can be prevented with either a sulisobenzone or a PABA ester-oxybenzone preparation. Bathing tests for substantivity indicated that, for practical purposes, the PABA ester-oxybenzone preparation is more effective. An effective topical UVA screen may protect against such UVA-induced disorders as solar urticaria, polymorphic light eruption, drug-induced phototoxicity or photoallergy, and possibly the deep degenerative changes of solar elastosis.

(15–7) J. Am. Acad. Dermatol. 9:354–360, September 1983.

▶ [This careful study has established that "broad-spectrum" sunscreens containing both PABA (a UVB filter) and benzophenone (a filter of both UVB and UVA) are effective in blocking the action of UVA (to levels as high as 10 J/sq cm) in patients who have ingested methoxsalen for PUVA photochemotherapy. This protection up to 10 J would permit an exposure at noon in Boston of only 50 minutes (approximately 1 J for each 5 minutes of midday sunlight). It is best to encourage PUVA patients to avoid sun exposure during the clearing phase when they are being exposed 2, 3, or 4 times weekly. The peak phototoxic effect varies in different individuals and may occur as long as 72 hours or even 96 hours after a single dose of methoxsalen. Certainly the type of substantive broad-spectrum sunscreens reported here are now readily available in the United States and Europe (Sundown 15, Eclipse 15, Piz Buin 12, Ti-Screen 15, Coppertone Supershade 15, and a few others). These should be routinely used on the face and exposed areas of the body (e.,g., neck, ears, forearms, and legs) by all PUVA patients or, in fact, all patients receiving UVB phototherapy, inasmuch as they also receive inadvertent UVA in sunlight.—T.B.F.] ◀

15–8 **Psoralen-Containing Sunscreen Is Tumorigenic in Hairless Mice.** Lyle E. Cartwright and Joseph F. Walter (Univ. of California, San Diego) note that sunscreens containing 5-methoxypsoralen (5-MOP) are currently being marketed to promote tanning by inducing psoralen-mediated ultraviolet A (UVA) (320–400 nm) melanogenesis. The rationale is that this may prevent ultraviolet B (UVB) (290–320 nm) radiation-induced skin damage. However, mouse studies have shown 5-MOP has the same cutaneous photocarcinogenic potential as 8-methoxypsoralen. In addition, the 5-MOP–containing sunscreen Sun System III (SS-III), when combined with UVA, induces activity of epidermal ornithine decarboxylase, an enzyme associated with tumor promotion.

The authors have investigated whether SS-III has sufficient psoralen concentration to be tumorigenic in hairless mice exposed to chronic, intermittent UVA radiation. For the study SS-III was applied to hairless mice 5 days per week for 20 weeks. After each application, mice were exposed to 2.5–10 J/sq cm of UVA radiation.

All test groups developed atypical squamous papillomas in direct proportion to the dosage of UVA radiation received. A shorter latency period for tumor development was seen with larger UVA doses. Test animals developed invasive squamous cell tumors within 1 year. Control groups (SS-III without UVA and UVA without SS-III) remained tumor free. Animals that received SS-III plus UVA developed persistent skin thickening and increased formation of dermal cysts similar to the results reported with chronic exposure to UVB, a known carcinogenic wavelength.

Over-the-counter sunscreens containing 5-MOP contain sufficient psoralen concentrations to cause cutaneous phototoxicity and photocarcinogenicity in mice. The authors recommend that the use of these sunscreens in humans be discouraged to prevent further ultraviolet-induced skin damage and skin cancer.

▶ [Whether 5-MOP–containing sunscreens can in fact promote pigmentation is not clear. It will be best if clarification is not the result of more widespread use of such agents in the United States. It has been pointed out in correspondence following this study (Magnus I. A., Young, A. R.: *J. Am. Acad. Dermatol.* 10:293, 1984) that oily

---

(15–8) J. Am. Acad. Dermatol. 8:830–836, June 1983.

vehicles may promote photocarcinogenesis by UVB radiation and that this may be the result of increased penetration of radiation. Magnus and Young suggested that a similar effect could account for part of the phototumorigenic effect of the 5-MOP–containing sunscreen in this study. The authors in reply (*J. Am. Acad. Dermatol.* 10:293, 1984) stated that the UVB exposure from the source employed was small and was in the longer, relatively noncarcinogenic wavelength region.—R.W.G.] ◀

15–9 **Cellular Hypersensitivity to UVA: A Clue to The Etiology of Actinic Reticuloid?** F. Giannelli, P. K. Botcherby, B. Marimo, and I. A. Magnus (London) have studied the clinical and cellular responses to long-wave ultraviolet radiation (UVR) (320–400 nm) in patients with idiopathic photodermatoses. One clinical syndrome was distinctive and was called "actinic reticuloid" (AR) because the clinical and histologic findings resembled those in a skin reticulosis of the mycosis fungoides type. Actinic reticuloid has a late onset but causes much discomfort and often imposes severe restrictions on a patient's lifestyle. The researchers selected 6 patients with typical AR from whom fibroblast strains were examined. They also tested patients with xeroderma pigmentosum and Bloom's syndrome and normal volunteers of both sexes by skin biopsy.

Three methods were used to study sensitivity to UVR: (1) exposure of confluent monolayers from skin biopsy specimens to an unfiltered 40-W, blue-black fluorescent light tube and observation of cytopathic effects under Nomarski differential-interference contrast or after Giemsa staining; (2) measurement of UVR effect on uptake of ^{3}H-hypoxanthine into nucleic acids; and (3) assessment of DNA fragmentation with the alkaline elution technique after UVR exposure.

All AR cell strains demonstrated abnormal responses to near UVR; clear cytopathic effects developed during the 24 hours following 8–10-hour exposures to blue-black light. Control cells remained unchanged, as did cells from patients with xeroderma pigmentosum and Bloom's syndrome. The AR cells showed more DNA fragmentation than did control cells when irradiated at room temperature. Abnormal DNA fragmentation in AR cells was also seen when uvasun emission was filtered through 5 mm of "Perspex" (80% transmission at 365 nm and cut-off at 337 nm). This finding provides additional evidence that long-wavelength UVR causes abnormal DNA damage in AR cells.

The authors' observations provide a compelling link between abnormal photosensitivity of the skin in the AR patients and the abnormal photosensitivity of their cultured fibroblasts. The AR cells show abnormal DNA fragmentation only at temperatures high enough to allow enzyme activity during or immediately after UVR exposure. These results suggest a cellular defect in the prevention or repair of some damage caused by free radicals and other photoproducts.

▶ [These observations suggest new possibilities for exploring the pathogenesis of the group of photosensitivity diseases that comprises actinic reticuloid, photosensitive eczema, and persistent light reaction as well as other photosensitivity disorders. It is not yet known whether cells from sites other than the skin are also abnormally

---

(15–9) Lancet 1:88–91, Jan. 15, 1983.

sensitive to UVR. Determination of oxygen dependence of the abnormal sensitivity would lend further support to the authors' hypothesis that AR patients have defective mechanisms for dealing with oxygen radicals.—R.W.G.] ◀

5–10 **Papular Polymorphic Light Eruption: Immunoperoxidase Study Using Monoclonal Antibodies.** J. E. Muhlbauer, A. K. Bhan, T. J. Harrist, J. D. Bernhard, and M. C. Mihm, Jr. (Boston) obtained biopsy specimens of papules in 8 patients with polymorphic light eruption (PMLE) and examined them by immunoperoxidase techniques using monoclonal antibodies. An attempt was made to characterize the infiltrating mononuclear cells in the lesions. The 5 men and 3 women (aged 25–49) had a nonscarring predominantly papular photoeruption induced 1–48 hours after exposure to sunlight.

Routine light microscopy showed mild spongiosis in the epidermis of all papules. Slight basal vacuolization was present in about 50% of the lesions. In adjacent exposed skin, only a few perivenular mononuclear cells were present within the upper dermis. In immunoperoxidase studies, anti-T-cell antibodies stained most of the infiltrating mononuclear cells in papules of PMLE. Staining was confined to cell borders of round cells. Anti-T_3 antibody stained 65%–85% of infiltrating cells. A combination of anti-T_4B and anti-T_8 antibodies stained most of the mononuclear cells in all specimens and were roughly equal to the total number of T_4-positive and T_8-positive cells counted on corresponding sections stained separately with anti-T_4B and anti-T_8 antibodies. Epidermal dendritic and perivenular mononuclear cells stained with anti-T_6 antibody in all lesions. Ia-positive (I_2-reactive) cells represented 40–70% of the dermal infiltrate in papules, exceeding the number of T_6-positive cells in all cases. IgM was detected on rare dermal mononuclear cells in 3 skin lesions.

A dense perivascular mononuclear cell infiltrate is a constant feature of PMLE, and the present findings indicate that most of these infiltrating cells are T cells. The data from this study also provide evidence for a large number of perivascular T lymphocytes in PMLE. Possibly, T cells accumulate in response to antigen formed in a vascular or perivascular location after ultraviolet radiation. Because both T-cell subsets were present in the infiltrate, it is possible that cytotoxic lymphocytes could damage endothelial cells directly, producing the observed vascular injury.

▶ [In this study of Muhlbauer et al., T cells consistently predominated in the infiltrates of papular polymorphic light eruption, although the proportions of the major T-cell subsets were variable. Further exploration of T-cell responses in polymorphic light eruption may be worthwhile.—R.W.G.] ◀

-11 **Study on Cell-Mediated Immunity in Polymorphic Light Eruption.** It has been proposed that polymorphic light eruption (PLE) may be a photoallergic disorder. Irene Horkay, J. Krajczár, E. Bodolay, M. Debreczeni, and A. Bégány (Univ. of Debrecen) assessed immune mechanisms in 55 patients, aged 11 to 67 years, with PLE who had had a sunlight-provoked eruptive disorder for 3 to 31 years. All morpholog-

---

(15–10) Br. J. Dermatol. 108:153–162, February 1983.
(15–11) Dermatologica 166:75–80, February 1983.

ical types of PLE were represented. The eruption could be reproduced in 43 patients. Fifty-eight patients with typical clinical and biochemical features of porphyria cutanea tarda (PCT) were also studied.

Delayed skin tests with PPD were positive in all but 1 of 20 patients with PLE and in 16 of 20 with PCT. Minorities of both groups had positive tests with trichophytin, *Candida* vaccine, and bacterial antigen. All patients with PLE reacted to at least one antigen. Numbers of active and total E rosette-forming peripheral lymphocytes were significantly lower in the active stage of PLE, whereas values were normal during remissions. In active PCT, only total E rosette-forming cells were reduced in number. The proportion of lymphocytes with a dotlike α-naphthyl acetate esterase (ANAE) reaction was significantly reduced in active PLE and normal during remissions.

The findings suggest the involvement of T lymphocytes in some phases of the hypersensitive skin reaction induced by exposure to sunlight. In PCT, humoral immune factors may contribute, mostly secondarily, to maintaining and worsening porphyric hepatopathy. Pathogenetic differences exist between PLE of presumably photoallergic origin and phototoxic PCT.

15–12 **PUVA Therapy in Persistent Light Reaction.** Attila Galosi, Erhard Hölzle, Gerd Plewig, and Otto Braun-Falco (Univ. of Munich) describe the diagnostic procedure in 2 patients with persistent light reaction, and present a modification of the standard schedule of therapy with 8-methoxypsoralen (8-MOP) and ultraviolet A (UVA) (PUVA), which was necessary because of the extreme sensitivity to ultraviolet electromagnetic wavelengths in patients with this photodermatosis.

Man, 76, with skin type III, had, for the past 8 years, severe eczematous changes with tormenting itch on the areas exposed to light. Erythema, strong lichenification, scaling, and scratch effects were found on the face, neck, and back of the hands. The face showed a facies leontina–like aspect. The condition was diagnosed as persistent light reaction with photocontact allergy toward tetrachlorosalicylanilide (TCSA) and tribromosalicylanilide (TBS) and contact allergy toward potassium dichromate, paraphenylenediamine, and benzocaine. Induction of PUVA therapy using 40 mg of 8-MOP was begun and, 2 hours after the patient consumed the tablets, UVA radiation (PUVA 6,000) was introduced. The initial dose of UVA was 0.25 J/sq cm. The patient received 40 PUVA treatments and one cumulative UVA dose of 78 J/sq cm. After 5 months a second PUVA treatment with a cumulative UVA dose of 77 J/sq cm was needed. The patient has been symptom free for 16 months.

In the past year, indications for systemic photochemotherapy have been extended to the treatment of photodermatosis. The principle of this treatment rests most likely on the light protection effect through induction of epidermal hyperplasia with acanthosis and hyperkeratosis, as well as intensive pigmentation, on the immunologic mechanism. It has been shown that dermal lymphocytic infiltrates were destroyed with PUVA therapy. Therefore, this treatment is not only useful for psoriasis but also for lymphomas of the skin and for lichen ruber moniliformis.

(15–12) Hautarzt 33:657–661, December 1982.

An important histologic sign of persistent light reaction is a dense lymphocytic perivascular infiltrate. When using PUVA therapy for persistent light reaction, the high sensitivity to light of these patients in comparison with psoriatic patients must be considered. Therefore, a small initial dose should be used. At the same time, the dose of 8-MOP should be about 10 mg higher. To test the tolerance, radiation of parts of the body is recommended during the initial phase. The radiation dose for the subsequent total body radiation should only be increased when the preceding treatment is tolerated.

Both patients in this study were able, for the first time in 8 years, to resume normal outdoor activities.

▶ [The treatment of "persistent light reaction" is frustrating and unrewarding. These unfortunate people become "light recluses," going out only at night. The use of PUVA therapy has been very rewarding in the treatment of these patients in several centers, and as these authors state, some patients can now live a virtually normal life, outdoors.—T.B.F.] ◀

5–13 **Hydroa Vacciniforme: Induction of Lesions With Ultraviolet A.** Charles L. G. Halasz, Emily E. Leach, Robert R. Walther, and Maureen B. Poh-Fitzpatrick (Columbia Univ.) describe hydroa vacciniforme as a rare photosensitivity disorder with onset in childhood. The distinctive lesion is a vesicle that heals with scarring. Hydroa vacciniforme occurred in a patient in whom an abnormal minimal erythemal dose (MED) to wavelengths of 322–370 nm within the ultraviolet A (UVA) range was demonstrated. Vesicles could be induced only with multiple exposures to UVA.

Woman, aged 22, had a photosensitive skin disorder, which began at age 15 with blistering of the face, scalp, anterior portion of the chest, and dorsa of the hands after exposure to summer sunlight. For the last 3 years the lesions developed during any season when she was exposed to sunlight. The amount of exposure to sunlight necessary to induce lesions varied from a few seconds to a few minutes, depending on light intensity. Within several hours, erythematous macules appeared, developing a small central vesicle usually within 1–2 days. The vesicle ruptured spontaneously, leaving a crust; healing occurred within several weeks, often leaving a pitted scar. Attempts at therapy included application of various topical sunscreens without relief as well as a course of ultraviolet B (UVB) radiation, also without effect. Treatment with oral 8-methoxypsoralen and UVA induced generalized vesiculation after the second exposure.

The patient had an abnormal response to UVA consisting of blanching erythema at the irradiated site within several hours after exposure. The MED was 2.0 J/sq cm. She had a reproducible response over the range of wavelengths of 322–370 nm. The tanning response was poor, but she tolerated UVB treatment without adverse reactions. After about 3 weeks of UVB treatment, the UVA MED increased to 10 J/sq cm. After 4 weeks of UVB treatment, the UVA MED was 20 J/sq cm. At this point, the patient was allowed exposure to sunlight and experienced no response after as much as 20 minutes of exposure, although erythema without vesiculation developed after 30–50 minutes of exposure.

Tolerance to UVA erythema was increased by treating this patient

---

(15–13) J. Am. Acad. Dermatol. 8:171–176, February 1983.

with multiple exposures of UVB. The association of multiple halo nevi, loss of ability to tan, and hydroa vacciniforme has not been reported previously. Whether these are chance associations or linked disorders remains unknown.

▶ [This report of a rare disorder provides a further example of a condition requiring multiple exposures to the provoking wavelengths in order to elicit a clinical lesion on phototesting. It appears that this syndrome is indeed a distinct disorder which cannot be readily grouped with common photosensitivity syndromes.—R.W.G.] ◀

15–14 **Günther's Congenital Erythropoietic Porphyria and Carotenoids: Four-Year Therapeutic Trial.** In this rare disease of autosomal recessive transmission, the hyperproduction of porphyrin is linked to a deficit in uroporphyrinogen III cosynthetase. Clinical manifestations are related to a photosensitivity which result in hypertrichosis and mutilating bullous eruptions associated with hemolytic crises and splenomegaly. Based on reports of the supposed beneficial effects of β-carotene, J. Maleville, J. P. Babin, S. Mollard, C. Martin, Y. Nordmann, and G. Guillet (Bordeaux, France) attempted treatment in a male infant, born at full-term to nonconsanguineous parents.

The child weighed 3,400 gm and was hospitalized at age 24 hours for a hemorrhagic syndrome with melena and red urine, and hepatosplenomegaly. Congenital porphyria was diagnosed. Secondary hemolytic anemia accompanied by severe splenomegaly necessitated repeated transfusions. Results of biologic and enzymatic tests were normal, as were prothrombin rate and electrophoresis. The infant was treated with 50 mg of adenosine monophosphoric acid, which resulted in transient clinical improvement with disappearance of urinary elimination of porphyrins. The child had 1 healthy brother, but a history disclosed the neonatal death of a sibling who had red urine and splenomegaly.

The characteristic cutaneous signs of Günther's disease appear during the first year, progressing in severity with generalized hypertrichosis, distinct erythrodontia and bullous eruptions on exposed areas, and atrophic and mutilating scarring particularly on hands and face. Slight mental retardation is also observed.

For this child, treatment with a carotenoid was instituted when the patient was 6 years of age. The initial dose was 75 mg, followed by 100 mg daily of β-carotene, 25 mg per capsule, or β-carotene, 10 mg, and canthaxanthine, 15 mg (i.e., 25 mg of active carotenoid per capsule). An antisolar cream was added to treatment for external protection. This treatment was followed up regularly during a period of 4 years. Bullous and scabby lesions persisted, with progressive tegmental atrophy.

Although the carotenoid did to some extent diminish the number of blisters, it did not prevent the appearance or evolution of atrophy. This substance merits consideration as an adjuvant in photoprotection, although avoidance of solar exposure is still the essential precaution.

▶ [Carotenoids have not been impressive in the prevention of the devastating effects

---

(15–14) Ann. Dermatol. Venereol. 109:883–887, 1982.

of solar radiation on the skin in Günther's disease, because the action spectrum for the effects is in the visible, not in the ultraviolet range. Nevertheless, because of the lack of toxicity of carotenoids, they should be given to every patient with Günther's disease. Although they are rarely completely effective in erythropoietic protoporphyria, they ameliorate the photosensitivity of most, but not all, patients.—T.B.F.] ◀

15–15 **Hydroxychloroquine Versus Phlebotomy in Treatment of Porphyria Cutanea Tarda.** Both repeated phlebotomies and hydroxychloroquine have been useful in the management of porphyria cutanea tarda (PCT). T. Cainelli, C. Di Padova, L. Marchesi, G. Gori, P. Rovagnati, S. A. Podenzani, E. Bessone, and L. Cantoni compared these treatments over a 1-year period in 62 men with PCT diagnosed from typical cutaneous features and an anomalous porphyrin pattern. None had a family history of porphyria, and none had previously been treated for PCT. All patients acknowledged consuming alcohol in excess of 80 gm daily. Thirty-one patients with a mean age of 50 years received 200 mg of hydroxychloroquine twice weekly for 1 year, and 31 with a mean age of 48 years had phlebotomies of 400 ml twice a month. Both groups were advised to stop drinking.

All 61 patients who completed the study reported reducing their alcohol intake to below 25 gm daily. Both treatments were well tolerated. Mild anemia resulted from the repeated phlebotomies. Cutaneous symptoms improved comparably in the two treatment groups, with regression of phototoxic vesicles, skin fragility, and hyperpigmentation. The serum glutamic oxaloacetic transaminase activities and iron concentrations declined more in the phlebotomy patients. Total urinary porphyrin excretion decreased significantly more in the hydroxychloroquine group at 4 and 8 months, and the uroporphyrin-coproporphyrin ratio was lower in this group at all intervals. The urinary porphyrin pattern had improved more in the hydroxychloroquine group after a year of treatment. Fatty change in the liver and siderosis improved in both groups. Necrosis, inflammation, and fibrosis became worse during treatment in 12 hydroxychloroquine-treated and 8 phlebotomized patients. Cirrhosis developed in 4 and 2 patients, respectively.

Hydroxychloroquine appears to be more effective than repeated phlebotomy in removing porphyrins from patients with PCT. Liver disease improved less in hydroxychloroquine-treated patients in the present study, but this cannot be ascribed to hepatotoxicity from the drug, since factors such as the degree of abstinence from alcohol or hepatitis B virus infection may be important. Further work is needed to determine the safety of long-term low-dose hydroxychloroquine therapy in patients with PCT and concomitant chronic liver diseases.

–16 **Effects of Phlebotomy on Urinary Porphyrin Pattern and Liver Histology in Patients With Porphyria Cutanea Tarda.** C. Di Padova, L. Marchesi, T. Cainelli, G. Gori, S. A. Podenzani, P. Rovagnati, M. Rizzardini, and L. Cantoni investigated urinary porphyrin profiles and liver histology in 35 male alcoholic outpatients with por-

(15–15) Br. J. Dermatol. 108:593–600, May 1983.
(15–16) Am. J. Med. Sci. 285:2–12, January/February 1983.

phyria cutanea tarda (PCT) before and after 1-year phlebotomy. The patients drank 80 gm or more of ethanol daily. They were randomly allocated to phlebotomy or control groups in a ratio of 2:1 (23 men underwent 1-year phlebotomy).

At the end of the 1-year follow-up, all patients had a mean alcohol consumption of less than 25 gm/day. In treated patients, phlebotomy was well tolerated and caused no side effects, except for mild anemia. The skin of the treated patients improved, with regression of phototoxic vesicles, fragility, and hyperpigmentation. The cutaneous symptoms of PCT did not improve in controls, although use of topical protective substances limited the appearance of phototoxic reactions. In treated patients, glutamic oxaloacetic transaminase and γ-glutamyltranspeptidase levels dropped significantly. Other blood parameters did not change after phlebotomy. Screening for urinary porphobilinogen gave negative results in both groups. Phlebotomy produced a significant decline in the urinary total porphyrin excretion rate. No change was recorded in controls. After therapy, the porphyrin pattern improved in 17 of 23 patients, with 5 recovering a normal profile. At the second biopsy, performed after 12 months, 9 (25.7%) men had cirrhosis and 16 (45.7%) of 35 had chronic active hepatitis. Group-by-group analysis indicated that disease in 1 untreated and 3 treated patients was more severe. The degree of fatty liver degeneration and hepatic siderosis decreased significantly in treated patients.

These data confirm that phlebotomy results in marked improvement in the cutaneous and biochemical symptoms of PCT. It appears that regular phlebotomy is well tolerated when it is performed until the attainment of mild anemia. The severity of liver damage does not seem to preclude the favorable response of PCT to repeated phlebotomy. Determination of the porphyrin pattern adds useful information to understanding the course of PCT.

▶ [Most physicians favor repeated phlebotomies for the treatment of PCT, and remissions average about 2½ years. There have been reports of good results, however, in the induction of remission of PCT with the use of hydroxychloroquine (Malkinson, F.D., Levitt, L.: Hydroxychloroquine treatment of porphyria cutanea tarda. *Arch. Dermatol.* 116:1147, 1980). In the comparative study abstracted above, phlebotomy and hydroxychloroquine produced almost equal degrees of improvement, but the liver changes (necrosis, inflammation and fibrosis) became worse in the patients receiving hydroxychloroquine. There remains, however, the question of whether these patients do, in fact, completely give up alcohol. A larger series with more follow-up is needed. It is quite clear from the Milan group's series of PCT patients treated with phlebotomy alone that there was improvement in PCT (clinically and biochemically) even in those patients with rather severe liver damage.—T.B.F.] ◀

15–17 **Immunoreactive Uroporphyrinogen Decarboxylase in Porphyria Cutanea Tarda.** A specific reduction in hepatic uroporphyrinogen decarboxylase activity characterizes porphyria cutanea tarda (PCT), and, in familial PCT, the decrease is due to inheritance of a mutant gene that reduces enzyme activity in all tissues, including the red blood cells. G. H. Elder, Diane M. Sheppard, J. A. Tovey, and A. J. Urquhart (Cardiff, Wales) measured immunoreactive

(15–17) Lancet 1:1301–1304, June 11, 1983.

IMMUNOREACTIVE UROPORPHYRINOGEN DECARBOXYLASE IN HEMOLYSATES*†

	Number of subjects	Immuno-reactive enzyme (arbitrary units/mg haemoglobin)	Ratio of immunoreactive enzyme concentration to enzyme activity	Enzyme activity adsorbed by solid-phase antibody (pmol/min/50 μl)
Familial PCT	7	99 (66–129)‡	8·3 (5·5–11·8) (NS)	4·7 (4·0–6·0) (NS)
Sporadic PCT	6	194 (138–243) (NS)	9·0 (7·5–10·4) (NS)	. .
Controls	7	194 (145–260)	9·0 (8·2–10·38)	4·0 (3·3–5·2)§

*All values represent means and ranges.
†NS denotes not significant as compared with control values.
‡$P < .01$.
§Hemolysates diluted to same activity as hemolysates from patients with familial PCT.
(Courtesy of Elder, G.H., et al.: Lancet 1:1301–1304, June 11, 1983.)

uroporphyrinogen decarboxylase activity by rocket immunoelectrophoresis in hemolysates from 7 unrelated patients having familial PCT, 6 patients with sporadic PCT, and 7 normal subjects. The patients with sporadic PCT had normal red blood cell uroporphyrinogen decarboxylase activity, whereas those with familial PCT had a mean activity of 12.2 picomoles of coproporphyrinogen/minute/mg of hemoglobin, as compared with 21.6 picomoles for controls.

The findings are given in the table. The mean concentration of immunoreactive uroporphyrinogen decarboxylase in hemolysates from patients with familial PCT was about half the normal mean, whereas patients with sporadic PCT had normal concentrations. The concentration of immunoreactive enzyme correlated closely with enzyme activity. The ratio of immunoreactivity to catalytic activity was similar in patients with both types of PCT and in controls. Titration of hemolysates with solid-phase antibody gave further evidence that the specific activity of uroporphyrinogen decarboxylase is unchanged in familial PCT.

Familial PCT is commonly caused by a mutation that does not lead to the production of noncatalytic cross-reactive immunologic material. Familial PCT can be identified by a simple immunoelectrophoretic method that does not involve the measurement of uroporphyrinogen decarboxylase activity. The method is likely to be suitable for routine clinical diagnostic use. Immunochemical studies of the hepatic enzyme defect in sporadic PCT should help to elucidate the pathogenesis of this most common form of human porphyria.

▶ [This new technique will become routine and will be helpful in sorting out familial PCT. PCT is the commonest form of porphyria in the United States, with an estimated incidence of 4:100,000. At the present time at least three types of PCT can be delineated: *(1)* autosomal dominant familial PCT with a decrease in the concentration of both immunoreactive and catalytically active uroporphyrinogen decarboxylase (UD) in red blood cells and presumably in liver; *(2)* sporadic PCT in which the red blood cell enzyme level is normal and reduced activity of UD is *restricted to the liver; (3)*

toxic PCT caused by exposure to polyhalogenated aromatic hydrocarbons, such as hexachlorobenzene and dioxins, for which enzyme measurements have not been reported.—T.B.F.] ◀

15–18 **Bronze Baby Syndrome: New Porphyrin-Related Disorder.** Bronze baby syndrome (BBS) is a rare disorder related to phototherapy for neonatal jaundice; it is characterized by gray-brown discoloration of the skin, serum, and urine. The condition resolves when phototherapy is discontinued. Firmino F. Rubaltelli, Giulio Jori, and Elena Reddi (Univ. of Padua, Italy) examined the mechanism of BBS in 2 newborn infants who were affected after receiving phototherapy for unconjugated hyperbilirubinemia. Spectroscopic studies were done on serum specimens from the infants, and the serum porphyrins were extracted and analyzed chromatographically. The specimens were irradiated in vitro, and the role of porphyrins in inducing discoloration was verified by irradiating normal cord blood serum in the presence of bilirubin and porphyrins.

The absorption spectra of serums from the infants with BBS had features typical of bilirubin as well as an intense band peaking at about 400 nm and broad absorbance in the near-ultraviolet (UV) and the 600–700 nm regions. The latter features were not observed in control serums. The BBS serums had multiband emission spectra with maxima at 585, 619, and 670 nm, indicating that the 400-nm absorption band did not reflect residual hemoglobin in the serum. Porphyrin analyses yielded Cu^{++}-protoporphyrin, Cu^{++}-corproporphyrin, and Cu^{++}-uroporphyrin. Irradiation of diluted serums from the affected infants with visible light led to an increase in the brown color of the solution, disappearance of porphyrin fluorescence, and an increase in absorbance in the near-UV and red spectral regions. Near-total destruction of the porphyrins was confirmed. When normal serum was irradiated in the presence of the porphyrins, the Cu^{++} porphyrins were slowly destroyed, and the spectral changes resembled those seen in the BBS serums. Addition of bilirubin to the solution enhanced the photodestruction of porphyrins.

Serums from infants with BBS contain an abnormally large amount of porphyrins, the chief component being Cu^{++}-protoporphyrin IX. The porphyrins identified appear to lack appreciable photosensitizing efficacy. The simultaneous presence of a high serum concentration of porphyrins and a high level of copper from cholestasis may lead to the formation of Cu^{++} porphyrins, which are converted to brown photoproducts during phototherapy via photosensitization by bilirubin. That the onset of BBS requires hyperporphyrinemia, hyperbilirubinemia, cholestasis, and light treatment explains why the syndrome is so rare.

▶ [Other conditions with high levels of porphyrins may not have photosensitivity or pigmentation (acute intermittent porphyrin and lead intoxications). This curious pigmentation appears to be analogous to jaundice where there is a deposition of bilirubin in the dermis; in this syndrome there is a high dermal level of copper-containing nonphotosensitizing photoporphyrins.—T.B.F.] ◀

(15–18) Pediatr. Res. 17:327–330, May 1983.

15–19 **Phototherapy of Pityriasis Lichenoides.** Mark J. LeVine (Case Western Reserve Univ.) treated 11 patients with chronic pityriasis lichenoides chronica using topically applied bland emollient cream and minimally erythemogenic doses of ultraviolet (UV) radiation from fluorescent sunlamps. The lack of knowledge about the cause of this condition has hampered the development of reliably efficacious therapy. The 3 males and 8 females treated were aged 4–59 years. Duration of asymptomatic lesions of pityriasis lichenoides chronica was 10 months to 15 years. Nine patients received UV exposure 5 times weekly, and 2 received it 3 times weekly. All patients were examined every 2 weeks. After clearance, each patient continued UV exposure as maintenance therapy.

Doses of ultraviolet B (UVB) calculated to produce a faint minimal erythema cleared all exposed lesions in all 11 patients. Complete clearance of all lesions (disappearance of erythema and scale) required an average of 29 treatments at an average UVB dose of 388 mJ/sq cm. The average number of treatments and the average dose at clearance were 45% and 27% higher for females than for males, although these results may be owing to the small sample size. In all patients, the axilla and genitals were not exposed to UV radiation until after a maintenance regimen was started. The lesions in these untreated areas did not resolve until exposed to UV radiation. Symptomatic erythema developed in all patients during maintenance therapy, necessitating a decrease in the UV radiation dose of 30%–50% at clearance.

Despite the present inability to explain the cause of pityriasis lichenoides or the mechanism of action of UV radiation, these results demonstrate the efficacy of artificial UV radiation in the clearance and maintenance therapy of this condition. It is not possible to predict the total number of treatments needed or the length of remission, nor can a direct comparison of efficacy with other available forms of therapy be made.

▶ [Several reports now attest to the efficacy of ultraviolet light therapy for pityriasis lichenoides chronica. Not only UVB but also psoralen and ultraviolet A (PUVA) (*Dermatologica* 159:451, 1979) have been reported to be effective for this condition. Longer longitudinal follow-ups are required to determine the incidence of recurrences. We have seen at least 3 patients who developed recurrence of their disease about 2 years after therapy with PUVA was discontinued. Since the disease is asymptomatic and inconsequential, long-term therapy with ultraviolet light is not warranted if recurrences are frequent.—E.G.] ◀

15–20 **Treatment of Pityriasis Rosea With UV Radiation.** Pityriasis rosea is a common self-limited scaling eruption of unknown etiology. It is generally believed that sunlight or artificial ultraviolet (UV) radiation alleviates the symptoms or alters the course of the disease, or both. Kenneth A. Arndt, Barry S. Paul, Robert S. Stern, and John A. Parrish (Harvard Med. School) conducted a bilateral comparison study to learn more about the efficacy of UVB phototherapy in the

---

(15–19) Arch. Dermatol. 119:378–380, May 1983.
(15–20) Ibid., pp. 381–382.

treatment of this disorder. The 12 women and 8 men reported a generalized eruption for an average of 9.1 days.

Prior to therapy, the minimal erythemal dose (MED) to UVB (290–320 nm) was determined for each patient. Treatments were given to the right side of the body only, with the left side draped and shielded. Treatment started at 80% MED with a 17% increase in UVB exposure daily. After the fifth treatment patients were given the option of having the shielded side treated. Only emollients such as a water-in-oil emulsion or hydrated petrolatum were permitted. (The study was conducted in winter and early spring when inadvertent sun exposure was unlikely to interfere with results of the treatment.)

After 5 days of treatment, 15 of 19 patients noted an improvement of their symptoms. In 9 there was significantly greater improvement in pruritus on the treated side; in the remaining 6 improvement was equal on both sides. Extent of disease in 16 of 20 patients lessened during the study period. In 10 of 20 patients, improvement for extent of disease was significantly greater on the treated side by the end of the therapy period.

Eleven of 20 patients chose to have the previously shielded side treated. After an additional 5 treatments, the two sides were indistinguishable for pruritus and extent of disease. The MEDs had no apparent bearing on subsequent response to therapy.

Five consecutive daily erythemogenic UVB phototherapy exposures resulted in decreased pruritus and extent of disease significantly more often on the treated side than on the untreated side of these patients. The study showed that this therapy seems to be most beneficial to patients receiving treatment within a week after the eruption appears.

► [This may be a useful way of shortening the course of this disease.—R.W.G.] ◄

15–21 **Genetic Toxicity of Psoralen and Ultraviolet Radiation in Human Cells** is discussed by Anders Bredberg (Stockholm). The chief disadvantage of psoralen and ultraviolet A (PUVA) phototherapy for psoriasis appears to be its reactivity with DNA, which may lead to such serious side effects as skin cancer and germ cell mutations. In vitro studies have shown short-lived DNA strand breaks in human fibroblasts with doses of ultraviolet A (UVA) used in clinical practice, but no appreciable mutations. Psoralens readily enter the nucleus and form weak complexes with DNA bases. They are covalently linked with DNA on exposure to UVA, forming psoralen monoadducts and cross-links. Studies in human cells have provided some evidence that these molecules can be removed from DNA to some extent. In vivo studies have given no conclusive evidence that 8-methoxypsoralen alone will cause mutations or chromosomal damage even after penetration into internal organs. Although an increase in DNA and cytogenetic alterations has been reported in cells of psoriasis patients after several years of phototherapy, no increase in malformations or hereditary diseases in the offspring of these patients has been re-

(15–21) Acta Derm. Venereol. [Suppl. 104] (Stockh.) 1–40, 1981.

ported. An excess of tumors has been noted in patients treated with ionizing radiation or arsenic in addition to PUVA and in those with a history of skin cancer.

The genotoxic effects of exposure to PUVA are probably due to an interaction between photoactivated psoralen and DNA. Cytogenetic alterations probably should be viewed as a fairly crude measure of genetic toxicity. Although some genotoxic damage may occur with even a single exposure to PUVA, it is not clear whether this damage increases the genetic risk. It seems reasonable to administer PUVA only to a limited group of patients until treated patients have been observed for some years more. More needs to be learned of the antipsoriatic, mutation-inducing, and tumor-inducing effects of PUVA, and of the repair of various types of lesions.

▶ [It is likely that at least some of the adverse and therapeutic effects of PUVA are due to its reactivity with DNA. Following exposure to UVA radiation, 8-methoxypsoralen forms both monofunctional and bifunctional adducts with DNA. Since bifunctional adducts frequently kill cells, monofunctional adducts may be more mutagenic. PUVA also appears to effect RNA. Long-term exposure to PUVA appears to influence the immune system. The ultimate toxicity associated with PUVA and its relation to dose in humans can be best established by careful prospective study of well-defined cohorts of patients who have been exposed to PUVA, such as the 16-center study of 1,380 patients in the United States.

In spite of a lack of reported malformations or hereditary diseases in PUVA-treated patients, I still advise both male and female patients who are attempting to conceive to discontinue treatment. I do not treat pregnant women with PUVA.—R.S.S.] ◀

16. Pigmentary Disorders

16–1 **Estimate of the Melanocyte Mass in Humans.** Findings suggesting that metabolic products of melanocytes may have biologic effects outside the immediate vicinity of the cells make it of interest to obtain some idea of the overall size of the active melanocyte system. Inger Rosdahl (Univ. of Göteborg) and Hans Rorsman (Univ. of Lund, Sweden) estimated the size of the human melanocyte system as if all active melanocytes in the body were assembled in a single compact organ. The focus was on the epidermal melanocyte population, since the epidermal and follicular melanocytes appear to constitute by far the largest proportion of the pigment-forming melanocytes in the body. The estimates indicated that the epidermal melanocytes constitute the dominant part of the hypothetical "melanocyte organ." In an adult human subject not recently exposed to sunlight, the functional active epidermal melanocytes form an estimated tissue mass of 1.0–1.5 cc. Other melanocytes, such as those in the mucosae, follicles, and eyes, form only a small part of the total melanocyte mass.

It may be possible to diagnose early melanoma metastases by estimating biochemical markers. The most useful metabolite to date is 5-S-cysteinyldopa. Spread of melanoma can be suspected when urinary excretion of this metabolite is 1.5–2-fold greater than the normal mean. Present calculations of the size of the "melanocyte organ" suggest that the excretion level may double with a melanoma metastasis of about 1 cc. Metabolically more active melanoma metastases may be detected even earlier.

▶ [With the Nordic penchant for mathematics, Dr. Inger Rosdahl and Professor Hans Rorsman have produced the remarkable estimate that the total mass of functionally active melanocytes forms a tissue 1.0–1.5 cc. Someone has said that the greatest problems in the world center around three tiny objects: the atom, the ovum, and the melanosome. This relatively small mass of epidermal melanocytes performs a very important task of providing an epidermal melanin density filter constituting in essence, a "photon-proof" vestment, and in the eye, melanocytes guard the inside of the eye by means of pigment in the uveal tract and retinal pigment epithelium. But what possible use are the melanocytes regularly and consistently present in the stria vascularis of the inner ear? There must be another function for melanin in the auditory response in humans; Siamese albino cats, for example, are always deaf. The commonest cause of congenital deafness in humans is Waardenburg's syndrome, but we have not seen a report of the status of melanocytes in the stria vascularis in this disorder.—T.B.F.] ◀

16–2 **Patients Presenting With Addison's Disease Need Not Be Pigmented.** Anthony H. Barnett, Eric A. Espiner, and Richard A. Donald (Christchurch, New Zealand) report findings in 3 consecu-

---

(16–1) J. Invest. Dermatol. 81:278–281, September 1983.
(16–2) Postgrad. Med. J. 58:690–692, November 1982.

tive patients with Addison's disease without increased pigmentation.

CASE 1.—Woman, 59, sustained a fractured sternum. After hospital discharge she experienced nausea, vomiting, and weakness. Upon readmission, her history disclosed a loss of energy over an 8-year period and 1 year of postural dizziness, intermittent nausea and vomiting, and poor memory and concentration. She was drowsy and mildly dehydrated; her supine blood pressure was 80/60 mm Hg; there was no excess pigmentation of the body or buccal mucosa. She had normochromic anemia. With rehydration and administration of steroids, renal function improved and electrolyte values returned to normal. She was given maintenance therapy and discharged; memory function returned to normal.

CASE 2.—Man, 63, had a 6-week history of malaise and a 24-hour history of pleuritic chest pain, weakness, and drowsiness. He had tuberculosis of the spine at age 20 and a "collapse" at age 40. On examination, his blood pressure was 60/0 mm Hg. No increased pigmentation was observed except possibly around the genitalia. His condition was diagnosed as cardiogenic shock secondary to myocardial infarction and suspected adrenal insufficiency. He improved with dobutamine and hydrocortisone treatment, and appropriate replacement therapy led to recovery.

CASE 3.—Man, 63, a smoker with morning cough and sputum, had an x-ray examination that showed a right upper zone opacity. Lobectomy disclosed anaplastic cells and tuberculosis. Five days after treatment with rifampin, isoniazid, and ethambutol was started, he experienced diarrhea and a drop in blood pressure. He had a strong family history of thyroid disorders but not of Addison's disease. He was treated with hydrocortisone, which was quickly reduced to maintenance levels, as well as antituberculosis drugs.

Findings in these patients indicate that, despite the usual textbook descriptions, excess pigmentation is not necessarily a feature of Addison's disease. The symptoms of this disease may date back many years and may be responsible for long periods of mental and physical debility. Care must be taken when using enzyme-inducing drugs, such as antituberculosis therapy, in these patients.

▶ [This report may seem of no interest to a dermatologist who depends on the presentation of increased pigmentation as a guide to searching for decreased cortisol production both in the basal layer and following ACTH stimulation to make the definitive diagnosis of Addison's disease. It is well known that hyperpigmentation is not always present in patients with Addison's disease; the triad of weakness, hypotension, and weight loss with or without hyperpigmentation should prompt the dermatologist to obtain an endocrinologic consultation and biochemical screening for Addison's disease. All of the patients in this report were "of fair complexion," and it is known that skin types I and II will not develop the degree of hyperpigmentation that is so striking in skin types IV and V. In the Japanese (skin types IV and V), for example, the patients develop deep brown generalized hyperpigmentation and often blue-black lesions in the buccal mucosa and the tongue. These New Zealand physicians lament that the "usual textbook descriptions" fail to mention the lack of pigmentation in Addison's disease, but Harrison's *Principles of Internal Medicine* lists hyperpigmentation as a plus or minus among the criteria for Addison's disease!—T.B.F.] ◀

16–3 **The PUVA-Induced Pigmented Macule: A Lentiginous Proliferation of Large, Sometimes Cytologically Atypical, Melanocytes.** Prominent brown macules may develop on light-exposed skin in patients given photochemotherapy for psoriasis. Arthur R. Rhodes,

(16–3) J. Am. Acad. Dermatol. 9:47–58, July 1983.

Terence J. Harrist, and Khosrow Momtaz-T (Boston) have found that at least some types of pigmented macules therapy with psoralen and ultraviolet A (PUVA) are characterized by a lentiginous proliferation of large melanocytes that may be cytologically atypical. Study was made of 11 PUVA-induced pigmented macules (PM) from 7 white men with psoriasis who had received standard PUVA therapy for 4–6 years. The PM were excised from psoriasis-free skin on the groin or buttock. The findings were compared with those in 8 sun-induced pigmented macules (SM) and 5 samples of light-protected skin (LPS) from subjects who did not have psoriasis.

In contrast to the SM, many PM were darkly or irregularly pigmented. A blind histologic study of both routine and L-dopa–incubated tissue sections showed both types of lesion to be "lentigines." Three of 11 PM had slight melanocytic atypism, but none of 8 SM showed this change. The PM had a significantly increased proportion of hypertrophic melanocytes compared with both SM and LPS. Disorganization of the microscopic pigment pattern was marked in some PM (Fig 16–1).

Chronic phototherapy can induce pigmented macules with a lentiginous proliferation of large melanocytes, which in some cases may be slightly atypical. Patients given prolonged PUVA therapy should be continuously monitored for atypical melanocytic lesions. The use of PUVA therapy enhances the incorporation of tritiated thymidine in benign melanocytic nevi in vitro and is associated with intra-

Fig 16–1.—High magnification of mineral oil–covered surface. In PUVA-induced pigmented macule, there are islands of normal epidermal rete pigment pattern *(arrows),* but normal pattern is obscured in many areas by excessive pigment *(arrowheads).* (Courtesy of Rhodes, A.R., et al.: J. Am. Acad. Dermatol. 9:47–58, July 1983.)

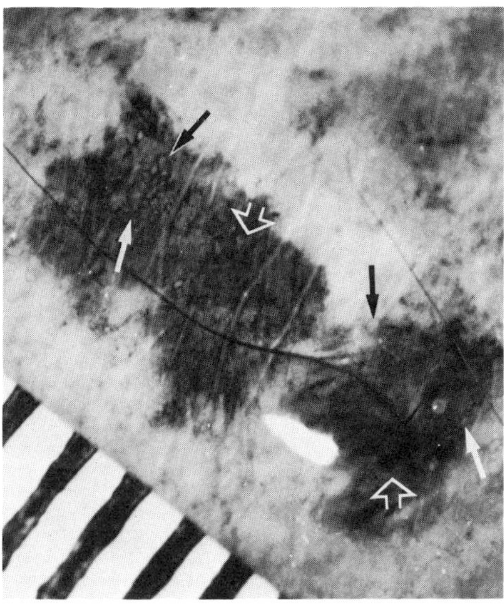

epidermal dysplastic melanocytic changes in nevocellular nevi in vivo.

▶ [The phenomenon of "PUVA lentigo" has been studied in a population of 1,380 psoriatic patients who have received PUVA (Rhodes, A.R., et al.: The PUVA lentigo: an analysis of predisposing factors. *J. Invest. Dermatol.* 81:459–463, 1983). These pigmented macules were observed on the unexposed areas of the buttocks, as this site was an area that had not been previously exposed to sunlight. The presence of PUVA lentigo was noted in 53% of the patients and was associated with a greater number of PUVA treatments and an older age at starting PUVA. It occurred more frequently in males and was less frequently observed in skin types V and VI. The lesions persisted for 1–2 years following cessation of PUVA treatments. Just what is the significance of these pigmented macules? In the report abstracted above, Rhodes et al. compared the PUVA macules (PM) to solar lentigo (SL) and to normal skin. The PM showed an increase in the size of melanocytes and some disorganization of the arrangement and occasional "atypicality" of the melanocytes. During the 10 years since PUVA was introduced, it has not been known to be associated with an increased incidence of primary melanoma, although thousands of patients have been treated. Treatment with PUVA is for difficult disabling psoriasis that is refractory to ultraviolet B (UVB) therapy, and these benign pigmented macules are not a significant risk thus far compared to the benefit. Recently we have seen at the Massachusetts General Hospital the same pigmented macules in a psoriatic patient who had received *only* UVB therapy.—T.B.F.] ◀

16–4 **Lentiginous Eruptions After Photochemotherapy.** Although it is a source of relief to many psoriatic patients, long-term therapy with 8-methoxypsoralen and ultraviolet A (PUVA) may produce less desirable side effects, such as disturbances of the pigmentary system. H. Kietzmann, M. Goos, and E. Christophers (Kiel, Federal Republic of Germany) reported data on 638 psoriatic patients treated with PUVA, of whom 50 required repeated treatment for multiple recurrences. Of these latter, 20 had pigmented skin lesions in regions not

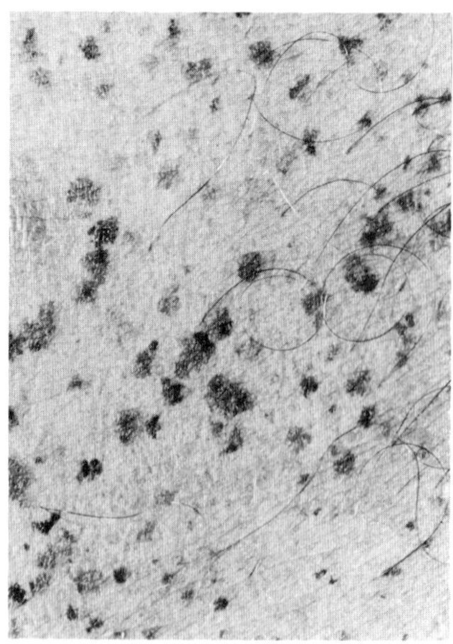

Fig 16–2.—PUVA lentigines showing multiple inhomogeneously pigmented macules with irregular outlines. (Courtesy of Kietzmann, H., et al.: Ann. Dermatol. Venereol. 110:63–67, 1983.)

(16–4) Ann. Dermatol. Venereol. 110:63–67, 1983.

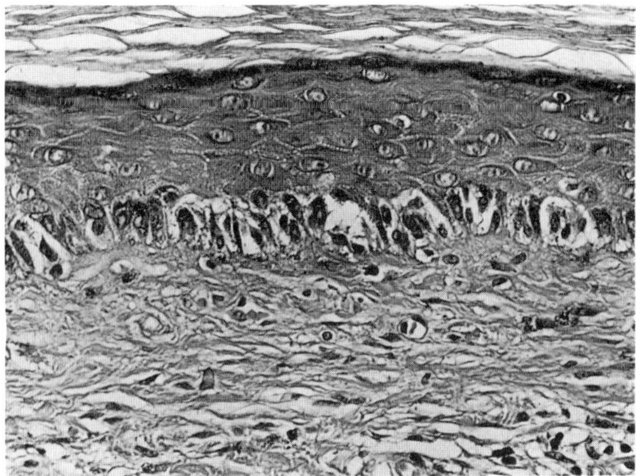

Fig 16–3.—Atypical melanocytic hyperplasia showing linear arrangement of atypical melanocytes in basal cell layer, singly and with a tendency to nesting. Hematoxylin-eosin; original magnification, ×200. (Courtesy of Kietzmann, H., et al.: Ann. Dermatol. Venereol. 110:63–67, 1983.)

normally exposed to the sun (the internal surface of the thighs or inguinal area, but never on the face). These macules varied in color from light brown to almost black; they sometimes showed regular or irregular contour, but were never confluent (Fig. 16–2). No topographic relationship was observed between these pigmented macules and former psoriatic plaques; and it was impossible to establish a precise link between total dose of PUVA, duration of treatment, and appearance of these lesions, which show no tendency toward spontaneous remission after conclusion of treatment.

On histologic examination the epidermis was found to be orthokeratotic and richly pigmented; this hyperpigmentation was not limited to the basal epidermic layer but pervaded the suprabasal layers as well. Notable augmentation of melanocytes was observed in all layers of the affected skin, with morphologically atypical melanocytic hyperplasia in the superior segment of the epidermis. Occasionally a lymphohistiocytic inflammatory infiltration was observed around dermal capillaries. Large numbers of melanophages were observed in the clinically most pigmented lesions (Fig 16–3).

After comparing the histopathologic characteristics of these lesions with other pigmentary disturbances, the authors propose the term "PUVA lentigines," emphasizing the characteristic quantitative modification of the melanocyte population.

The long-term course of PUVA lentigines is unknown. Careful surveillance of such patients is necessary to clarify the significance of these cutaneous alterations and define the risk-benefit ratio of oral photochemotherapy.

▶ [Darkly pigmented macules appear in sun-protected sites of up to half of psoriatic patients treated chronically with PUVA, their frequency being positively associated with a greater number of treatments received and negatively associated with skin types V and VI (*J. Invest. Dermatol.* 81:459–463, 1983). These PUVA-induced macules are characterized histologically by a lentiginous proliferation of relatively hypertrophic, sometimes cytologically atypical, melanocytes (*J. Am. Acad. Dermatol.* 9:47–58, 1983). The long-term course of these relatively "fixed" melanocytic proliferations is being watched closely.—A.R.R.] ◀

16–5 **Spreading Pigmented Actinic Keratosis.** Paul Subrt, Joseph L. Jorizzo, Prapand Apisarnthanarax, Elizabeth S. Head, and Edgar B. Smith (Univ. of Texas, Galveston) describe findings in 4 patients with spreading pigmented actinic keratoses, an only recently described pigmented lesion of sun-exposed areas, in which the histologic appearance is that of actinic keratosis with the additional feature of excessive melanin deposition in the lower epidermis and in the upper dermis. Clinically, the lesion is a brown patch or plaque with a smooth surface, usually larger than 1 cm, that tends to spread centrifugally. Clinical differential diagnoses include seborrheic keratosis and lentigo maligna melanoma.

Case 1.—Woman, 47, had a pigmented facial lesion of 4 years' duration. The lesion measured 3 cm × 4 cm; it was oval and light brown, and appeared as a smooth patch with regular borders on the right malar border. The remainder of the sun-exposed skin showed considerable actinic damage. Cryosurgery was used in treatment.

Case 2.—Man, 66, had a lesion on his nose that was flat and brown; it slowly spread outward over 1 year's time. The lesion, an oval patch 1.5 cm in size, was treated with cryosurgery.

Case 3.—Man, 50, had a brown pigmented facial lesion of 2 years' duration. It was a slightly raised plaque 1.0 cm × 1.2 cm in size. Other sun-exposed areas showed considerable actinic damage. After biopsy, the lesion was treated by cryosurgery.

Case 4.—Woman, 87, had an ulcerated papule on the forehead of 6 months' duration; she had a history of numerous skin malignancies. The lesion on the forehead measured 1 cm, and another brown patch on the nose was 2 cm × 1 cm in size. The forehead lesion was diagnosed as basal cell epithelioma or squamous cell carcinoma. The nasal lesion was diagnosed as spreading pigmented actinic keratosis and was treated with cryosurgery.

Spreading pigmented actinic keratosis appears to be a distinct clinicopathologic entity. Because 4 such patients were seen in only a 3-month period, this lesion may be much more common than the existing literature would indicate; it is probably commonly misdiagnosed as seborrheic keratosis or senile lentigo. The follow-up has been too short to evaluate the efficacy of cryosurgery fully in the 4 patients described.

▶ [This interesting acquired brown facial lesion was first reported in 1978 by James et al. (Spreading pigmented actinic keratoses. *Br. J. Dermatol.* 98:373–379, 1978). There are 4 seemingly "flat" acquired brown lesions of the exposed skin of the face, which on cursory examination appear to be similar and have distinctive features. They were described as follows.

"*(1.)* **Lentigo senilis,** the most frequently observed lesion, has a uniform brown color, is completely flat and without evidence of epidermal change, even when carefully examined with a hand lens and oblique lighting. The lesions may gradually enlarge to 3 to 4 cm or more and completely disappear for one to three years after very short exposures (10 sec) to liquid nitrogen applied with a cotton tip.

"*(2.)* **Seborrheic keratosis** may be indistinguishable in its early stages from lentigo

(16–5) J. Am. Acad. Dermatol. 8:63–67, January 1983.

senilis; usually epidermal change is barely perceptible in seborrheic keratoses when examined with a hand lens and oblique lighting. These lesions almost always recur after short exposures to liquid nitrogen. Treatment is difficult except by excision, which produces a disfiguring scar, or by long exposures (20 to 30 sec) to liquid nitrogen, which results in an unsightly, permanent white macule.

"*(3.)* **Lentigo maligna** is completely flat, without any epidermal alteration, and simulates lentigo senilis except for a distinct variegation of color: brown, dark brown, flecks of black. These lesions should always be biopsied and, if proved histologically, excised with a narrow margin; usually a split-thickness graft is necessary.

"*(4.)* **Spreading pigmented actinic keratosis (SPAK)** is a newly reported lesion described here by the authors; it is not uncommon. It is important to recognize because of its malignant potential and because (as discussed above) treatment with topical 5% 5-fluorouracil cream often results in complete disappearance of the lesion. SPAK is easily distinguished from lentigo senilis and lentigo maligna because of a single feature: the epidermal change. This epidermal change may appear as a slightly verrucous surface perceptible only with a hand lens and oblique lighting; the surface is not shiny, as in lentigo senilis, but the incident light is scattered. Both lentigo maligna and SPAK have a variegated brown to black color, but the border of lentigo maligna tends to be much more irregular and with small pseudopods. In essence, these two variegated pigmented lesions (lentigo maligna and SPAK) should be biopsied; the histologic diagnosis is easily established." (*Br. J. Dermatol.* 98:379, 1978)—T.B.F.] ◀

16–6 **Peutz-Jeghers Syndrome in Children: Report of Two Cases and Review of the Literature.** The Peutz-Jeghers syndrome (PJS) is an association of mucocutaneous pigmentation with gastrointestinal (GI) polyposis that usually appears in childhood. J. A. Tovar, I. Eizaguirre, A. Albert, and J. Jimenez (San Sebastián, Spain) report two new cases of PJS in children and review 68 cases reported during the past two decades. One of the authors' cases, a girl, aged 6 years, was initially seen with repeated GI bleeding and signs of anemia (Fig 16–4). A massive group of hamartomatous polyps was present within the duodenum in this patient.

The sex distribution of the 70 reviewed cases was fairly even. Symptoms tended to occur at ages 5–10 years in male patients and at ages 10–15 years in female patients. Mucocutaneous pigmentation was rarely present in the first 2 years of life. Most patients had a pattern of recurrent episodes of intussusception with pain, vomiting, and obstruction of varying intensity. Many also had GI bleeding or anemia. The polyps often were multiple, and most were jejunoileal in location. Nearly two thirds of patients, however, had gastric or duodenal polyps or both, and one third had colorectal lesions. Fatal malignancies developed in two patients. Three others had gonadal tumors that were successfully treated. Only 16 of the 70 children had not been operated on when last seen.

The clinical picture of PJS in children generally resembles that seen in adults, although the anatomic distribution of polyps differs to some degree. Cancers have occurred in the GI tract, but are not very frequent. The risk of other types of tumor also is increased in patients with PJS. Ovarian, breast, and testicular tumors have been described. Nearly half of the 21 patients with proved malignancy were younger than age 30 years, and 2 were younger than age 16 years.

(16–6) J. Pediatr. Surg. 18:1–6, February 1983.

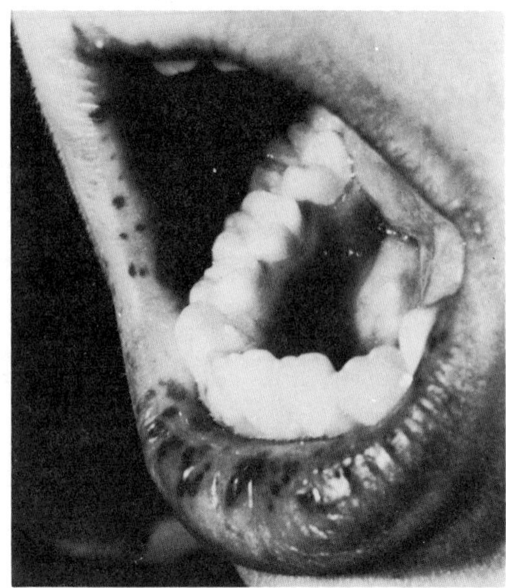

Fig 16–4.—Multiple pigmented spots visible on the lips and inner oral mucosa. (Courtesy of Tovar, J.A., et al.: J. Pediatr. Surg. 18:1–6, February 1983.)

Most episodes of intussusception resolve spontaneously or with nonoperative treatment. Many polyps can be removed endoscopically. When intussusception does not resolve or bleeding or weight loss make surgery necessary, the polyps can be excised by enterotomy and suture ligation, coagulation, or, when necessary, limited intestinal resection. Addition of a Noble-type enteroplication at initial laparotomy should be considered, since most surgical complications are due to repeated intussusception.

▶ [This is an excellent, concise review of the syndrome with 70 references. Probably, its most useful function is an extraordinarily lucid discussion of the risk of malignancy associated with the syndrome. The article is a must for everyone's reference file.—J.C.A.] ◀

16–7 **Persistent Ashen Gray Maculae and Freckles Induced by Long-Term PUVA Treatment.** Prolonged therapy with psoralen and ultraviolet A (PUVA) may be complicated by the development of freckles. L. Kanerva, J. Lauharanta, K.-M. Niemi, T. Juvakoski, and A. Lassus (Univ. of Helsinki) report data on a patient who had PUVA-induced freckles and also developed ashen gray macules.

Man, 42, with recalcitrant psoriasis since age 22 years had received PUVA therapy for about 2 years. Ashen gray macules as large as 1 cm in diameter appeared on the trunk after *130* exposures, with a total ultraviolet A (UVA) dose of 930 J/sq cm. A biopsy specimen showed pigment-containing macrophages in the upper dermis. After 225 exposures, with a total UVA dose of 1,609 J/sq cm, freckles had developed on the thighs (Fig 16–5), upper arms,

(16–7) Dermatologica 166:281–286, 1983.

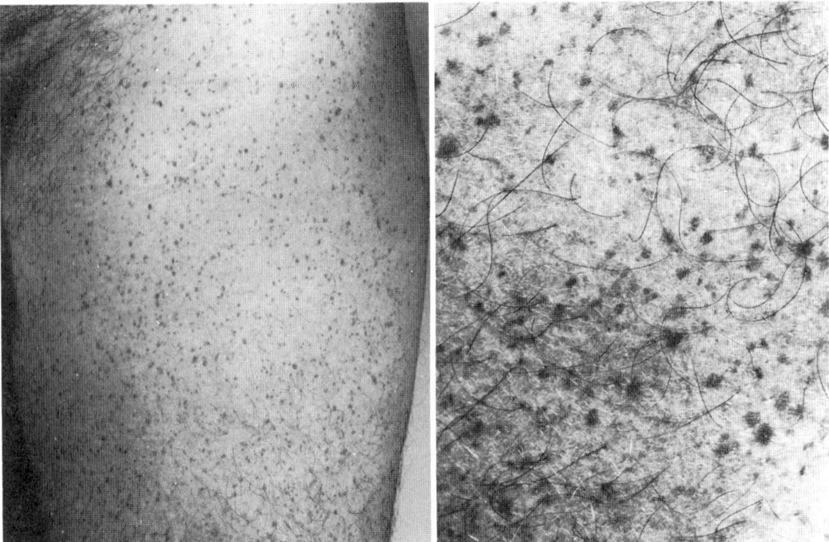

Fig 16–5.—Typical PUVA-induced freckles on left thigh of 42-year-old man. (Courtesy of Kanerva, L., et al.: Dermatologica 166:281–286, 1983; by permission of S. Karger, AG, Basel.)

waist, and buttocks. Several ashen gray macules were present on the upper back, lower stomach, shoulders, and thighs. Patient was healthy apart from psoriasis and was not receiving regular medication. The macules and freckles persisted for 2 years without PUVA therapy, but no further macules developed.

The macules exhibited vacuolar degeneration of some basal keratinocytes and a massive bandlike infiltrate of melanophages in the upper dermis. A moderate perivascular round-cell infiltrate also was noted. No hemosiderin was identified. In the freckles the pigment was markedly increased in the lower epidermis. Electron microscopy showed strong stimulation of melanocytes in both types of lesions. Autophagic vacuoles containing melanosomes were frequently seen in the melanocytes.

The ashen gray macules in this patient presumably represent pigment within dermal macrophages in circumscribed areas. The inflammatory perivascular cells may contribute to the gray hue. The mechanism of formation of PUVA-induced freckles is not clear, but dysplastic changes in both melanocytes and keratinocytes suggest that patients receiving PUVA therapy be closely monitored clinically and histologically.

▶ [Dermal melanin is not excreted or eliminated readily or quickly. Guido Mieschar injected melanin in the dermis of animals and after several months it was still present. The gray-blue macules seen rarely in patients receiving prolonged PUVA therapy (such as the patient presented above, who had had 225 exposures) are usually the result of phototoxic events. The phototoxicity produces damage of the epidermal-dermal junction that leads to "epidermal melanin incontinence," a reaction pattern common to a number of diseases of diverse etiologies including lichen planus, discoid lupus erythematosus, erythema dyschromicum perstans, fixed drug eruption, macular amyloidosis, and incontinentia pigmenti.—T.B.F.] ◀

16–8 **Pigmentary Incontinence in Fixed Drug Eruptions: Histologic and Electron Microscopic Findings.** Shin'ichi Masu and Makoto Seiji (Tohoku Univ., Sendai, Japan) note that pigmentary incontinence is a phenomenon observed in certain inflammatory skin disorders. Clinically, it appears as slate-colored pigmentation; histologically, an accumulation of melanin is observed in the upper dermis. The development of pigmentary incontinence in fixed drug eruption was investigated using biopsy specimens taken at different stages of development from 8 patients. In 5, the drugs concerned were ascertained, and biopsy specimens were obtained at various times after provocative administration of these drugs.

Keratinocytes in various degrees of degeneration were observed in a biopsy specimen obtained 12 hours after drug administration. Melanosomes were intermingled with aggregated tonofilaments in these keratinocytes. In biopsy specimens obtained 24 or more hours after drug administration, the dyskeratotic cells appeared to become more electron-lucent filamentous masses as the condensed nuclei disappeared and the aggregation of tonofilaments loosened. Many macrophages were seen in the epidermis that had phagocytized, in the dyskeratotic cells, and in the Civatte bodies. Some of the filamentous masses appeared to have been digested within the cytoplasm of macrophages in both the epidermis and dermis. Although some of the Civatte bodies contained melanosomes, these melanosomes seemed to disappear. Few free melanosomes were found in the epidermis or dermis. No degenerative changes were observed in the epidermis at 3 hours and within 2–3 months after drug administration or recurrence of erythema.

These findings suggest that, in fixed drug eruption, pigmentary incontinence develops by lymphocytes migrating into the epidermis, with keratinocyte degeneration; macrophages migrating into the epidermis from the dermis, phagocytizing the dyskeratotic cells and Civatte bodies containing melanosomes; macrophages containing phagocytized melanosomes and other materials returning to the dermis. The phagocytized materials are digested in macrophages, but the melanosomes seem to be more resistant to digestion and become phagosomes, or melanosome complexes.

▶ [The phenomenon of epidermal melanin incontinence was fully discussed by Seiji's group in this and in previous articles. These careful studies (some of the final experiments by the illustrious experimental dermatologist, Professor Makoto Seiji) provided the basis for the pathophysiology which is clearly illustrated and described. This important sequence of events is common to a number of diseases of diverse etiologies associated with the clinical term "ceruloderma" and which are dermal melanoses. For a comprehensive discussion of these and other disorders of *dermal* pigmentation consult Fitzpatrick, T.B., et al.: *Biology and Diseases of Dermal Pigmentation.* Tokyo, Univ. of Tokyo Press, 1981, p. 379.—T.B.F.] ◀

16–9 **Malignant Melanoma and Vitiligo-Like Leukoderma: Electron Microscopic Study.** Leukoderma is a somewhat rare, poorly understood phenomenon in patients with malignant melanoma. How-

(16–8) J. Am. Acad. Dermatol. 8:525–532, April 1983.
(16–9) Ibid., 9:696–708, November.

ard K. Koh, Arthur J. Sober, Hidemi Nakagawa, Daniel M. Albert, Martin C. Mihm, and Thomas B. Fitzpatrick treated 8 patients at Massachusetts General Hosp. All had malignant melanoma, and wide-spread areas of hypopigmentation had developed in the preceding 14 years.

Man, 61, had a level II superficial spreading melanoma removed from his back. Two years later, positive findings developed in axillary nodes, followed shortly by hypopigmentation on the face, chest, and middle area of the back (Fig 16–6). Biopsy of a depigmented area several years later showed an absence of melanocytes, whereas normal skin exhibited conspicuous degeneration of keratinocytes and autophagocytosis of melanosomes. Vision was impaired in the left eye 7 years after onset of cutaneous hypopigmentation; examination showed a pigmentary disturbance in the macular region, premacular fibrosis, and a macular hole. The patient was well 10½ years after diagnosis.

Four of the 7 patients in whom biopsies were performed had complete absence of melanocytes, compatible with vitiligo. Ultrastructural studies showed little or no epidermal pigment in hypopigmented areas lacking melanocytes. Some pigment was present in basal keratinocytes in hypopigmented areas with macromelanocytes. Vacuolar degeneration of keratinocytes was observed in normal-appearing skin. All 7 patients studied had ocular abnormalities possibly related to melanoma and leukoderma.

Leukoderma in patients with melanoma is not strictly identical with vitiligo. The distribution of leukoderma is varied and is not clearly related to the primary site of melanoma. All of the present patients had disease in lymph nodes or at distant sites when hypopigmentation was first noted. Their course suggests that progression of disease may be slowed; the patients seem to survive longer than do those with stages II and III disease without leukoderma. Two of the 8 patients survived for 10 years. Larger studies are needed to confirm

Fig 16–6.—A, normal examination of patient with vitiligo-like leukoderma on chest; **B,** examination of same patient under Wood's light. (Courtesy of Koh, H.K., et al.: J. Am. Acad. Dermatol. 9:696–708, November 1983.)

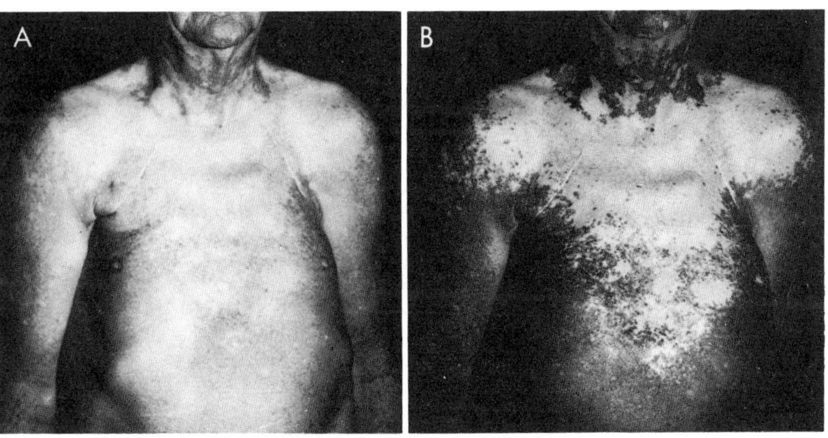

a beneficial prognostic implication of leukoderma in patients with malignant melanoma.

▶ [The term *vitiligo-like leukoderma,* not the term *vitiligo,* is used in the title of these case reports. This is not a semantic debate between the Yale and Harvard schools of thought but an important issue: just what is vitiligo? I recently defined *vitiligo* (Fitzpatrick, T.B., Polono, M.K., Surmond, D.: *Color Atlas and Synopsis of Clinical Dermatology.* New York, McGraw-Hill, 1983) as "an idiopathic, acquired, patterned, circumscribed hypomelanosis of the skin and hair in which other causes of hypomelanosis (postinflammation, chemical, etc.) have been excluded; there is an absence of melanocytes in fully developed hypomelanosis vitiligo macules." Perhaps an additional part of the definition should have included a statement that "the hypomelanotic areas only rarely undergo a partial repigmentation and in 1 or 2 hypomelanotic macules." If we apply this definition (plus the addendum regarding spontaneous repigmentation), the hypomelanosis appearing in patients with coexisting malignant melanoma reported here in the same month by the Yale group is not vitiligo for the following reasons: *(1)* Of the 6 cases with this syndrome, case 6 actually had true vitiligo, as defined above, and not this syndrome. *(2)* There has been spontaneous repigmentation, which was almost complete in case 1. *(3)* The hypomelanotic areas are not truly patterned in these patients, since mirror-image bilateral symmetry is not present, and almost all patients with vitiligo have striking bilateral symmetry. *(4)* When examined by light microscopy and transmission electron microscopy, specimens from 50% of the patients showed the presence of large hypertrophic melanocytes. These melanocytes contained a reduced number of melanosomes, and there were alterations in the shape of melanosomes (i.e., they were spherical rather than ellipsoid).

We have recently completed a prospective study of 52 patients with vitiligo as defined above. Using light and electron microscopy and carefully scanning the hypomelanotic areas, we could not detect the presence of any melanocytes except at the border of the normally pigmented skin and the vitiligo.—T.B.F.] ◀

16–10 **New Observations on Vitiligo and Ocular Disease.** Vitiligo is associated with both Vogt-Koyanagi-Harada syndrome and sympathetic ophthalmia. Michael D. Wagoner, Daniel M. Albert, Aaron B. Lerner, John Kirkwood, Bernadette M. Forget, and James J. Nordlund (Massachusetts Eye and Ear Infirmary, Boston) assessed the occurrence of ocular disease in 226 consecutive patients with vitiligo, 143 females and 83 males aged 2–82 years. The mean duration of vitiligo was 13 years. Many patients were receiving psoralen therapy, and 148 psoriatic patients receiving psoralen plus ultraviolet A therapy also were assessed. In addition, vitiligo was sought in 86 females and 68 males aged 13–80 years who had uveitis. Also evaluated were 57 patients with uveitis secondary to trauma.

Five (3.8%) of 129 patients with idiopathic uveitis had vitiligo. Two others had poliosis or extensive graying of hair at an early age. Five of these 7 patients had anterior uveitis alone. No patient with a known cause of uveitis or posttraumatic or postoperative disease had vitiligo. Eleven (4.8%) of the index patients with vitiligo (4.8%) had active uveitis or were treated for uveitis in the past 2 years. Five of 27 patients with vitiligo associated with cutaneous melanoma had evidence of uveitis. In 3 patients, ocular symptoms began at or shortly after the time that vitiligo appeared; this was also the case in 2 patients with vitiligo not associated with melanoma. Discrete areas

---

(16–10) Am. J. Ophthalmol. 96:16–26, July 1983.

of depigmentation of the choroid and retinal pigment epithelium were seen in 31% of the patients with vitiligo and in 2 psoriatic control patients. About 27% of the patients with vitiligo had hypopigmentation or degeneration of the retinal pigment epithelium, as did 6 psoriatic controls. Acuity of 20/40 or worse was present in 6.5% of eyes in patients with vitiligo. Nine of these 29 eyes were in 5 patients with uveitis.

There is more than a random association between vitiligo and uveitis, and it seems likely that vitiligo is associated with disorders of the retinal pigment epithelium. It is unlikely that simultaneous pigment destruction in the skin and eye is responsible for more than a small proportion of ocular pigmentary disturbances, but all patients with vitiligo should have ocular evaluation. The relationship between vitiligo and retinitis pigmentosa remains unclear.

▶ [A very interesting and important study that positively settles the question of whether abnormal ocular findings occur in patients with vitiligo. All the important controls are here—an especially important control group includes 148 patients with psoriasis who were being treated with PUVA, an "ideal control population" because of similarities in age, racial distribution, and medication regimens" (i.e., PUVA for vitiligo or psoriasis). Chorioretinal scars were present in 30% of the patients with vitiligo and in only 1% of the control group. All patients with vitiligo need an ophthalmologic examination even though only "a small percentage of ocular pigmentary disorders occur." Eye abnormalities rarely result in a decrease in visual acuity; nevertheless, any patient with vitiligo who was started on PUVA or any other treatment without a pretreatment eye examination would be a problem in a court of law.—T.B.F.] ◀

16–11 **Keratinocyte Damage in Vitiligo.** J. Bhawan and L. K. Bhutani performed light and electron microscopic studies on the amelanotic and adjacent normal-appearing skin in 7 females and 2 males with vitiligo. Most were in their second or third decade, but 1 was aged 8 years.

Data from light and electron microscopy were essentially similar in all 9 patients. Light microscopy of normal-appearing skin adjacent to vitiliginous areas showed focal areas of intracellular vacuolation in the lower layers of epidermis, especially in the basal layer. Electron microscopy revealed varying degrees of destructive changes. Many fibrillar masses, similar to amyloid-colloid or colloid bodies, were found both in the epidermis and dermis. Light microscopic examination of the amelanotic skin revealed complete loss of pigment. The stratum corneum was thicker than in normal adjacent skin. The upper dermis of both vitiliginous and normal adjacent skin showed many nerves and nerve endings. Some contained banded structures similar to those seen in nerves in the stroma of cellular blue nevus.

The keratinocyte damage and degeneration observed in these patients was actual and not an artifact of fixation, because keratinocyte damage was found only in clinically normal-appearing skin and not in vitiliginous skin.

▶ [This report confirms the original observations of Moellmann et al. (*J. Invest. Dermatol.* 76:321, 1981) who demonstrated degenerative changes in keratinocytes in the

---

(16–11) J. Cutan. Pathol. 10:207–212, June 1983.

clinically normal-appearing epidermis of patients with vitiligo. If this is, in fact, a specific change limited to patients with vitiligo, it points to pathology outside the melanocyte system. Some, however, believe these changes in the keratinocytes are nonspecific and are not infrequently seen in other disorders of the skin. More controls are needed—especially valuable would be patients with chemical leukoderma. This could clinch the observations of Moellmann and of Bhawan and Bhutani because these changes in keratinocytes should not be found in patients with chemical leukoderma.–T.B.F.] ◀

16–12 **Association of HLA-DR4 With Vitiligo.** Many HLA-associated disorders are now exhibiting stronger associations with antigens of the DR locus. Lynn M. Foley, Nicholas J. Lowe, Ellen Misheloff, and Jawahar L. Tiwari (Univ. of California, Los Angeles) examined the association between vitiligo and DR4 in 48 white patients who were typed for 6 HLA-DR antigens by cytotoxicity testing with B lymphocytes. The control group included 979 normal American white subjects. The only antigen that was significantly more prevalent in the patient group was DR4. Its incidences were 48% in vitiligo patients and 28% in controls. The difference remained significant when the data were corrected for multiple comparisons.

Vitiligo is an acquired idiopathic hypomelanosis that is often familial. It has been reported in as many as 15% of patients with autoimmune disease and has been associated with increases in gastric parietal cell, thyroid, and smooth muscle antibodies. The present finding suggests an increased incidence of vitiligo in persons with HLA-DR4.

16–13 **Cyclophosphamide in Vitiligo.** Vitiligo has special significance in India because of the cosmetic disfigurement it produces in dark-skinned persons. It is of particular concern to unmarried female patients. Immunosuppressive agents have been used in treating this condition because of the presumed role of autoimmunity. B. B. Gokhale and A. P. Parakh (Poona, India) used cyclophosphamide because of its wide margin of safety and reversible side effects and because it can be safely combined with surgery or radiation therapy or both. Patients aged 14–70 years who had not been treated for 6 months (fresh cases) or who had failed to respond to other drugs were given cyclophosphamide. Initial dose was 50 mg twice daily, orally, for adults and 25 mg for younger patients.

Nine of the 16 fresh cases had a good response to cyclophosphamide therapy at 3 months and 4 had a partial response. Eleven of the 17 refractory cases had a good response to cyclophosphamide, and 5 had a partial response. A good response consisted of total repigmentation. Several female patients reported hair loss. Leukopenia was noted in some cases. Menstrual irregularity also was observed. All untoward effects were reversed when treatment was temporarily withdrawn. The response of 1 patient is shown in Figure 16–7.

The results suggest that cyclophosphamide may be useful in patients with vitiligo that has failed to respond to conventional mea-

---

(16–12) J. Am. Acad. Dermatol. 8:39–40, January 1983.
(16–13) Indian J. Dermatol. 28:7–10, January 1983.

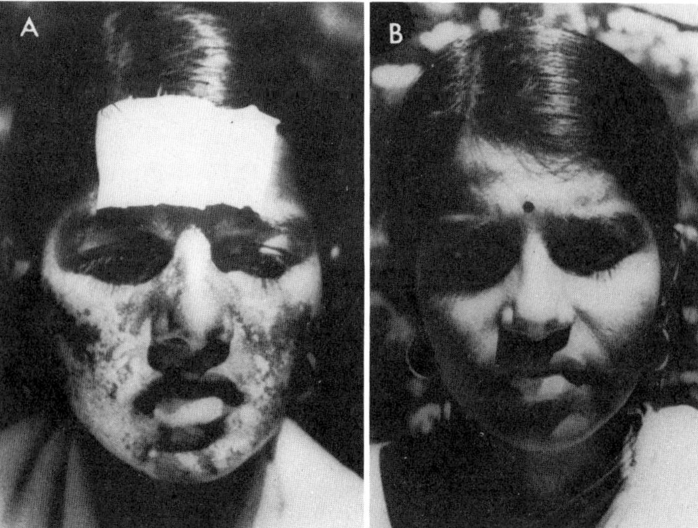

Fig 16–7.—Patient with vitiligo before **(A)** and after **(B)** treatment with cyclophosphamide. (Courtesy of Gokhale, B.B., and Parakh, A.P.: Indian J. Dermatol. 28:7–10, January 1983.)

sures. Treatment must be closely monitored because of the hazards involved in using immunosuppressive drugs.

▶ [Other "immunosuppressive" agents (e.g., corticosteroids and nitrogen mustards) have been partially effective in repigmentation of vitiligo when applied topically. Topical corticosteroids (hydrocortisone acetate 2½%) is a good first treatment for localized macules, especially in children younger than 12 years of age who cannot be treated with PUVA. It is frightening to contemplate the use of cyclophosphamide in a disease such as vitiligo, no matter how desperate the patient is about the social problems; cyclophosphamide can induce cancer, even in young people, and should not be used except for very serious or life-threatening situations.—T.B.F.] ◀

6–14 **Topically Administered Fluorouracil in Vitiligo.** The treatment of some cases of vitiligo remains unsatisfactory. Takuo Tsuji and Toshio Hamada (Osaka Univ., Japan) evaluated topical fluorouracil application, previously used chiefly for premalignant and malignant skin tumors, in 28 patients (7 males) with vitiligo, aged 6–80 years. All had had vitiligo for longer than 2 months. One to five vitiliginous lesions 3–10 cm in diameter, or an area about 5 × 10 cm, were abraded and then treated daily with 5% fluorouracil cream and covered with a polyethylene occlusive dressing. Treatment was continued for 7–10 days, and 5% sulfadiazine sodium in polyethylene glycol was then applied daily until epithelialization was complete.

The treated lesions were completely eroded after 7–9 days of treatment, and epithelialization required 10 days or less. Repigmentation began 1–2 weeks after epithelialization, and occurred within 2

(16–14) Arch. Dermatol. 119:722–727, September 1983.

months in all treated lesions. Two thirds of patients had complete or nearly complete repigmentation in all treated areas, and 5 others had partial repigmentation. Two of the 5 unresponsive patients had segmental vitiligo. Neither epidermal abrasion alone nor topical fluorouracil application alone led to repigmentation in control sites. Three of the 23 responsive patients had a recurrence of vitiligo within 1 year. There was no evidence of toxicity. Only slight burning or pain resulted from the treatment.

Topical fluorouracil therapy can induce repigmentation in lesions of vitiligo in a high proportion of patients, possibly excluding those with segmental-type vitiligo. The treatment effect occurs much more rapidly than with psoralen and ultraviolet A (PUVA) therapy or topical corticosteroid treatment. The mechanism of action of fluorouracil is unclear, but stimulation of epidermal melanocyte division after migration of cells into the affected area and melanocytes derived from hair follicles are both possibilities.

▶ [Paradoxically, almost any trauma can repigment areas of vitiligo. Many treatments have been advocated in the past, including application of caustic phenol. The results in this report look impressive, but the authors did not comment on the amount of scarring that occurred and whether this disappeared with time. The failure of segmental vitiligo to respond is intriguing, but as the authors stated, this disorder may not be the same as vitiligo. Probably many patients with "segmental vitiligo" have, in fact, nevus depigmentosus; a biopsy will differentiate the two: in vitiligo the melanocytes are absent, whereas in nevus depigmentosus melanocytes are present.—T.B.F.] ◀

16–15 **Generalized Vitiligo After Erythroderma.** Robert Allen Schwartz and Marvin G. Trotter describe a patient who developed generalized vitiligo after an exfoliative dermatitis.

Man, 65, a black, had developed pruritic eruptions of the back and groin when he began taking hydrochlorothiazide for essential hypertension. Generalized pruritus with hyperkeratosis of the palms and soles subsequently developed. Chlorthalidone was substituted, and injections of triamcinolone acetate were given, with variable results. A generalized exfoliative dermatitis ensued, and the patient was treated with high doses of prednisone and topical applications of fluorinated corticosteroids. Prostatic adenocarcinoma was discovered. Almost totally depigmented skin and total body alopecia were evident, after several weeks of exfoliative dermatitis, immediately after the patient took a shower (Fig 16–8). Small patches of perifollicular repigmentation were later seen, but the patient remained about 85% vitiliginous. Flares of erythroderma occurred when corticosteroids were tapered over the next 20 months. The cancer was irradiated. Skin biopsy showed no melanocytes. The patient is presently receiving tapering oral prednisone therapy and whole body applications of 0.1% triamcinolone ointment and has multiple long-term corticosteroid effects including cataracts and severe proximal myopathy. Skin biopsies of areas of erythema showed an essentially normal epidermis and a perivascular lymphohistiocytic infiltrate without activated T cells.

Vitiligo is rarely seen as a cutaneous marker of internal malignancy. This is the first known association of generalized vitiligo with prostatic adenocarcinoma. Although postinflammatory hypopigmen-

---

(16–15) Dermatologica 167:42–46, July 1983.

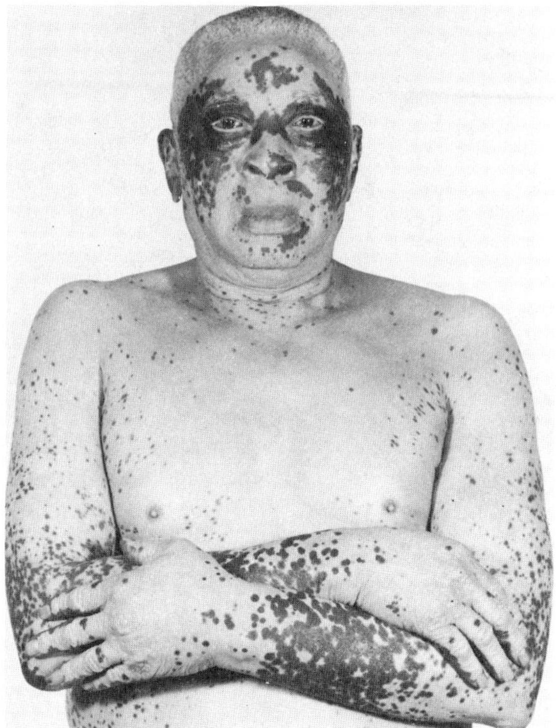

Fig 16–8.—Generalized vitiligo. (Courtesy of Schwartz, R.A., and Trotter, M.G.: Dermatologica 167:42–46, July 1983.)

tation may follow any type of dermatitis, the occurrence of true vitiligo with a dermatitis is unique.

▶ [This patient probably had an exfoliative dermatitis that developed following an allergic reaction to thiazide. The leukoderma that subsequently occurred could be interpreted as a Koebner or isomorphic reaction, a well-recognized phenomenon in persons with vitiligo or in persons with a disposition for the development of vitiligo. Depigmentation in these patients may occur following a severe sunburn or contact dermatitis (irritant or allergic). There was a legal suit in 1970 in which a 33-year-old black patient in a Cleveland VA hospital turned totally white (except for the eyes) following an exfoliative dermatitis that was caused by oral ingestion of a hypnotic (Doriden). This case was never reported in the medical literature, but the medical legal trial was summarized in *Newsweek* (June 22, 1970), which recounted the battle of the dermatologic experts engaged by both the plantiff's and the defendant's counsel.

The association of vitiligo and prostatic cancer is not proved here. The authors rightly state that "its (vitiligo) occurrence with malignancies, beyond a chance association, is unclear." Prostatic carcinoma is very common indeed and is the third most common cause of death in men older than age 55, and the incidence in autopsy studies is 12%–46% with only 1 in 3 being manifest clinically; it would be difficult, if not impossible, to relate the vitiligo in this patient to the prostatic cancer.—T.B.F.] ◀

-16 **"Confettiform" Depigmentation After Treatment of Chloasma With Leucodinine B Ointment.** D. Colomb (Lyon, France) reports

(16–16) Ann. Dermatol. Venerol. 109:899–900, 1982.

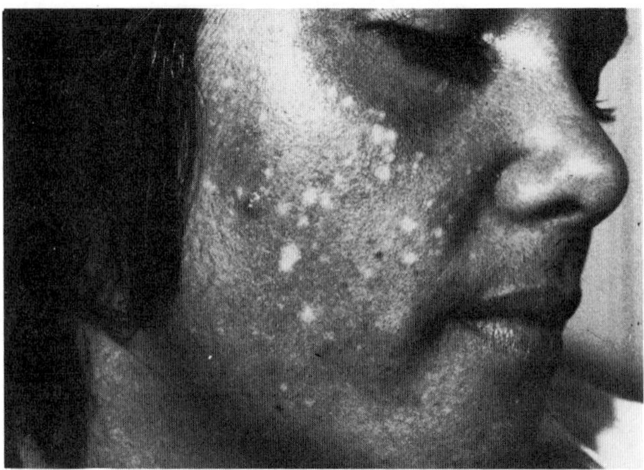

Fig 16–9.—Confettiform leukodermal lesions on right cheek. (Courtesy of Colomb, D.: Ann. Dermatol. Venereol. 109:899–900, 1982.)

on a recent observation of particular interest because it involved a pharmaceutical product. Monobenzyl ether of hydroquinone has been responsible for numerous cases of depigmentation seen in industrial medicine; it is sometimes a component of rubber used in the manufacture of protective gloves. This same substance incorporated into cosmetic preparations has occasionally caused undesirable if not disastrous disturbances of pigmentation. Monomethyl ether of hydroquinone was subsequently heralded as having a slower depigmentative action and as causing no undue side effects or intolerant reactions.

A woman, 33, was seen for a "confettiform" facial depigmentation which had appeared 8 months earlier after application of the ointment Leucodinine B for treatment of a chloasma (Fig 16–9) over a 2-month period. Since there was no sign of spontaneous repigmentation, treatment with 8-methoxypsoralen and ultraviolet A (PUVA) was instituted. After 30 sessions, a 50% repigmentation of the achromatic lesions had occurred. An additional 20 sessions resulted in complete repigmentation.

Investigation disclosed that Leucodinine B contains paramethyloxyphenol in 10% concentration—in fact, monomethyl ether of hydroquinone. It is hoped that publication of this case will lead other dermatologists to report similar observations.

▶ [Study this picture carefully. This same type of disfiguring depigmentation virtually always occurs after some weeks following the treatment of melasma with a preparation available in the United States, namely, Benoquin® or monobenzyl ether of hydroquinone. Despite repeated warnings, dermatologists are still recommending Benoquin for the treatment of melasma, with disastrous consequences—not the least of which are large malpractice claims by these patients. Thus far, we have not seen a published report of confettiform hypomelanoses of this type following prolonged topical applications of unsubstituted hydroquinone, which is available in over-the-counter preparations (e.g., Esoterica, Artra, and Eldoquin).—T.B.F.] ◀

16–17 **Incontinentia Pigmenti Achromians (Ito)** is reported in 3 chil-

(16–17) Arch. Dermatol. 119:391–395, May 1983.

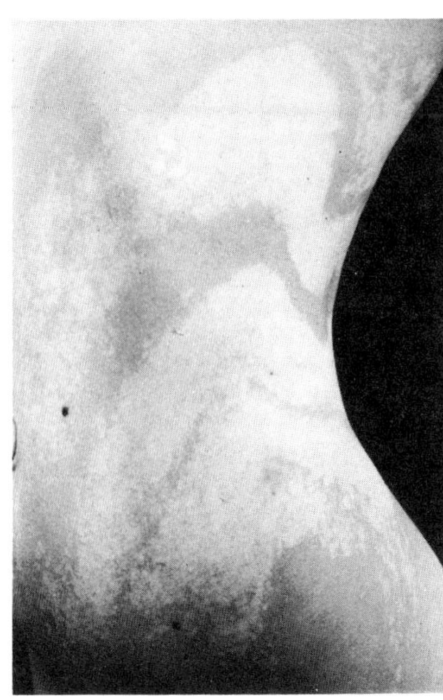

Fig 16–10.—Large, linear or bandlike, irregularly shaped, whorled, hypopigmented macules on left side of trunk. (Courtesy of Takematsu, H., et al.: Arch. Dermatol. 119:391–395, May 1983; copyright 1983, American Medical Association.)

dren by Hideaki Takematsu, Sachico Sato, Minoru Igarashi, and Makoto Seiji (Tohoku Univ., Japan), who also reviewed previously reported cases of which 32 occurred in Japan and 41 in the United States, Europe, Carribean countries, Mexico, and India. One case is reported below.

Girl, 12, showed bizarre pigment changes that had begun as hypopigmented areas on the trunk and extremities during the first months of life. Psychomotor development, growth rate, and body weight were below normal. At 10 months and again beginning at 7 years the patient had seizures that continued despite oral phenobarbital sodium and phenytoin sodium therapy. The pigment changes (Fig 16–10) were also present on the left buttock, inner and flexor aspects of the left thigh, and left leg. Funduscopic examination showed no abnormality. The hair, teeth, and nails were normal. X-ray examination showed scoliosis, lordosis, and spina bifida occulta. The IQ was 77. There were irregular EEG waves in the frontal area. Biopsy of the junction of normal and hypopigmented skin disclosed slight hyperkeratosis and acanthosis.

The ratio of female to male patients has been reported as 2.5:1. Table 1 gives the age at onset and sex of patients with hypopigmented spots for whom sufficient information was available. Table 2 shows the distribution of hypopigmentation and incidence of congenital abnormalities. Fifty-four of the 73 patients had one or more anomalies of the CNS, eyes, musculoskeletal system, hair, skin, teeth, nails, or internal organs.

A clinical relation between incontinentia pigmenti achromians and incontinentia pigmenti is suggested by a distinctive linear or whorled

TABLE 1.—AGE AT ONSET AND INCIDENCE OF SEX OF PATIENTS WITH HYPOPIGMENTED SPOTS

	Hypopigmented Spots	Hypopigmented Spots and Congenital Anomalies	Total
Age of onset			
Birth	8	21	**29**
1 mo	4	9	**13**
2-12 mo	1	8	**9**
1-5 yr	1	5	**6**
5-10 yr	2	4	**6**
10-20 yr	2	1	**3**
Sex			
M	6	13	**19**
F	13	34	**47**

(Courtesy of Takematsu, H., et al.: Arch. Dermatol. 119:391–395, May 1983; copyright 1983, American Medical Association.)

TABLE 2.—DISTRIBUTION OF HYPOPIGMENTATION AND INCIDENCE OF CONGENITAL ANOMALIES

Hypopigmentation	No. of Patients With Congenital Anomalies	No. of Patients Without Anomalies
Torso and extremities	34	9
Torso	11	6
Extremities	3	1
Unknown	6	3
Total	**54**	**19**

(Courtesy of Takematsu, H., et al.: Arch. Dermatol. 119:391–395, May 1983; copyright 1983, American Medical Association.)

pattern of pigment changes and the congenital abnormalities that occur in both disorders. Incontinentia pigmenti achromians is closely related to pigmented nevus and should be categorized as one of the congenital neurocutaneous diseases.

▶ [This is the best review to date on the confusing subject of incontinentia pigmenti achromians (Ito). The subject is confusing because nevus depigmentosus can be congenital or can develop during adolescence and is not, as the authors state, "congenital, constant, and permanent." Furthermore patients with nevus depigmentosus can have associated neurologic and other abnormalities. We prefer to use the eponym *hypomelanosis of Ito* for this syndrome, as suggested by Jelineck. The important message is that a patient presenting with this type of bizarre hypomelanosis should be carefully screened for neurologic and ocular anomalies.—T.B.F.] ◀

16–18 **Prenatal Diagnosis of Oculocutaneous Albinism by Electron Microscopy of Fetal Skin.** Oculocutaneous albinism is an inherited disorder characterized by a congenital decrease or absence of melanin synthesis in the skin, hair, and eyes. At least 6 variants inherited as

(16–18) J. Invest. Dermatol. 80:210–212, March 1983.

autosomal recessive traits have been described. Robin A. J. Eady, David B. Gunner, Alec Garner, and Charles H. Rodeck (London) report the successful prenatal diagnosis of oculocutaneous albinism by ultrastructural study of fetal skin obtained in utero. The parents, who may be distantly related, had a first child who is an albino, and the husband had 2 albino nephews; his great-grandfather was said to have been an albino. Fetal skin was obtained by fetoscopy at 20 weeks' gestation. Melanosome development in hair bulb melanocytes was seen to have progressed no further than stage II; numerous stage IV melanosomes were identified in 4 age-matched control fetuses. The diagnosis was confirmed when the pregnancy was terminated at 22 weeks. Pigment was absent from the retinal epithelium and uvea. The scalp and eyebrow hair was scanty and white. Results of tests for tyrosinase activity were negative.

Oculocutaneous albinism can be detected in the second trimester by ultrastructural study of fetal skin obtained by fetoscopy. Preferably, scalp hair removed at 20 weeks' gestation is evaluated. Pigment was lacking from the ocular structures in this case at a stage of development when ocular melanogenesis is normally active. The apparent lack of tyrosinase activity is not a definitive finding, since the amount of enzyme normally present at this stage may be too low to convert exogenous dopa to melanin. Prenatal diagnosis of oculocutaneous albinism is probably not indicated in temperate regions, where the outlook for albinos is relatively good.

▶ [The problem of albinism is twofold: ocular defects (decrease in visual acuity and nystagmus) and sun intolerance (development of squamous cell carcinoma in subjects exposed to intense sunlight, as in Nigeria). It is probable that the sun damage can be ameliorated or avoided with use of the effective sunscreens now available. The visual problems can be more severe, but there have been some famous albinos. Noah (of the Ark) was alleged to have been an albino and it is certain that W. A. Spooner was an albino. Spooner was head of one of the colleges at Oxford University and is known as the originator of the spoonerism (one example of which is "well-boiled icicle" for "well-oiled bicycle").

The problem with this study is the comparison of the albino fetal skin with the normal fetal skin. The normal fetal skin was obviously obtained from either the scrotum or prepuce or from a fetus with a dark skin type (skin type IV, i.e., tans easily) because of the large number of stage IV melanosomes. A fetus with skin type I or II (not an albino) could very easily have no more than stage I and II melanosomes. In the circumstance *in which the parents are black,* fetal skin with only stage I and II melanosomes would, however, be highly suggestive of a diagnosis of albinism.—T.B.F.] ◀

17. Psoriasis and Related Disorders

17–1 **Decreased Urinary Polyamines in Patients With Psoriasis Treated With Etretinate.** The mechanism of action of retinoids such as etretinate in psoriasis is unclear, but polyamine concentrations are increased in the skin and urine of psoriatics, and reductions have been observed with effective treatment. There is some evidence that polyamines may be important in the regulation of proliferation. Roy C. Grekin, Charles N. Ellis, Nancy G. Goldstein, Neil A. Swanson, Thomas F. Anderson, Elizabeth A. Duell, and John J. Voorhees (Univ. of Michigan) examined urinary values of putrescine, spermidine, and spermine before, during, and after etretinate therapy in 19 patients with more than 20% of the body surface involved with psoriasis or with disabling disease. The 16 men and 3 women were aged 21–70 years. Plaque-type psoriasis was most frequent. Etretinate or placebo was used for 8 weeks in a double-blind design, followed by a crossover phase for placebo patients. Dosages were 1 mg/kg daily for 1 week and 0.5 mg/kg daily in the second week and were then adjusted to maintain a maximum clinical response with tolerable side effects.

All patients but 1 had good to excellent clearing of psoriasis. No patient withdrew because of side effects. There was no significant placebo response. Urinary concentrations of all polyamines declined during etretinate therapy. Decreases preceded significant clinical responses to etretinate. Baseline polyamine concentrations had returned 8 weeks after the end of treatment. Polyamine concentrations in urine tended to increase during placebo administration. The patient who failed to improve clinically had a pattern of polyamine concentrations similar to that of the responsive patients.

The findings accord with the view that etretinate administration inhibits polyamine biosynthesis in patients with psoriasis. Other compounds that can inhibit polyamine synthesis will probably be effective in treatment of psoriasis, and a continued search for such agents is warranted.

▶ [Polyamine levels are increased in the skin and urine of psoriatics. It is a widespread belief that polyamines play a role in the regulation of epidermal proliferation. Grekin et al. clearly demonstrate that etretinate reduces urinary polyamine levels prior to the clinical response. It is thus correctly hypothesized that etretinate works on psoriasis by first inhibiting polyamine synthesis.—R.R.] ◀

–2 **Correlation of Epidermal Plasminogen Activator Activity With Disease Activity in Psoriasis.** J. E. Fraki, G. S. Lazarus,

(17–1) J. Invest. Dermatol. 80:181–184, March 1983.
(17–2) Br. J. Dermatol. 108:39–44, January 1983.

R. S. Gilgor, Patricia Marchase, and Kay H. Singer (Duke Univ.) note that proteinase and exopeptidase activity is increased in rapidly proliferating psoriatic epidermis. Etretinate (Ro-10–9359), an aromatic retinoid, is beneficial in the treatment of psoriasis. Therefore, a double-blind, controlled study of this agent was carried out, and results were correlated with plasminogen activator and disease activity in psoriatic patients. The 8 patients, aged at least 20 years, had more than 20% of their skin involved with psoriasis. All topical and systemic therapy was discontinued 1 week before entering the study. Punch biopsy specimens were taken from involved and uninvolved skin before and during drug therapy with etretinate.

The specific activity of plasminogen activator was 19-fold higher in involved psoriatic epidermis than in uninvolved skin. This activity after 8 weeks of treatment was correlated with the extent of surface involvement with psoriasis at 16 weeks. Six of the 8 patients had a decrease in extent of cutaneous involvement at 16 weeks, and 5 of these had decreases in plasminogen activator activity in the epidermis when compared with pretherapy levels. One patient had a modest diminution in the extent of skin involvement, but the plasminogen activator activity was increased slightly. Two patients had an increase in extent of skin involvement after 16 weeks of therapy, and both had increases in plasminogen activator activity. The plasminogen activator levels in uninvolved skin specimens having low specific activities of enzyme before the start of therapy increased at 8 weeks in 5 patients. But 2 patients with initially high plasminogen activator levels had normal values at 8 weeks and a decrease of skin disease at 16 weeks.

A dramatic increase occurs in the specific activity of plasminogen activator in psoriatic skin when compared with clinically uninvolved skin. The data suggest that the finding of increased plasminogen activator activity in psoriatic plaques is a good indicator of cellular activation in this disease. The correlation of plasminogen activator activity with extent of disease over time in patients given etretinate suggests that plasminogen activator activity may be a useful marker in the study of psoriasis.

17–3 **Calmodulin Levels Are Grossly Elevated in the Psoriatic Lesion.** P. C. M. van de Kerkhof and Piet E. J. van Erp (Univ. of Nijmegen, The Netherlands) note that calcium is a major regulator of intracellular metabolism, with its effects mediated by a specific receptor protein, calmodulin. They measured calmodulin levels in psoriatic lesions, in psoriatic "uninvolved" skin, and in the skin of controls. The patients had chronic, stable, plaque psoriasis that was untreated for 1 month. Biopsy specimens were cut freehand using a razor blade.

The mean calmodulin levels in the psoriatic lesions were about 30 times higher than normal. The calmodulin levels in the "uninvolved" psoriatic skin were not significantly different from those in controls. The grossly increased calmodulin content of the lesions, although not

---

(17–3) Br. J. Dermatol. 108:217–218, February 1983.

the primary genetic expression of psoriasis, may be important in development and maintenance of the overt lesion. Because calmodulin interacts with cellular metabolism at numerous points, it is unwise to speculate in detail regarding pathogenetic pathways. More basic data are clearly needed.

17–4 **Dermatan Sulfate in Urine Reflects the Extent of Skin Affection in Psoriasis.** J. H. Poulsen and M. K. Cramers (Univ. of Aarhus, Denmark) investigated whether urinary glycosaminoglycan excretion, as a measure of connective tissue degradation, can help distinguish between lesions in the dermis and those in other types of connective tissue. A method based on susceptibility to chondroitinases was used to measure the urinary excretion of dermatan sulfate, chondroitin 4/6-sulfate, and heparan sulfate in 15 psoriatic patients and 14 healthy controls aged 21–65 years. None of the patients had been treated. All the glycosaminoglycans were excreted in larger amounts by the psoriatic patients, but hydroxyproline excretion was insignificant in both the patient and the control groups. The absolute increase in excretion of dermatan sulfate was exceeded by the excretion of chondroitin 4/6-sulfate and heparan sulfate. Only the excretion of dermatan sulfate correlated with the extent of skin involvement by psoriasis.

A major part of urinary dermatan sulfate in psoriatic patients may be derived from the skin, and turnover of this fraction may be increased in psoriasis. The increased excretion of dermatan sulfate and chondroitin 4/6-sulfate with normal hydroxyproline excretion distinguishes the pattern of psoriasis from that seen in puberty. Excretion of dermatan sulfate appears to correlate with the extent of skin involvement by psoriasis.

7–5 **Cyclic AMP and Cyclic GMP Production in Normal and Psoriatic Epidermis.** E. Royer, J. Chaintreul, J. Meynadier, B. Michel, J. J. Guilhou, and A. Crastes de Paulet (Montpellier, France) determined cyclic adenosine monophosphate (cAMP) and cyclic guanine monophosphate (cGMP) production in normal and psoriatic (involved and uninvolved) epidermis. After homogenization, epidermal strips were incubated with saturating concentrations of adenosine triphosphate or guanine triphosphate, respectively, from cAMP and cGMP production. Cyclic nucleotides were measured by radioimmunoassay before and after 5, 10, and 20 minutes of incubation. Epidermal biopsy specimens were studied from 7 normal persons and from 13 psoriatic patients.

The production kinetics for both cAMP and cGMP were linear for all tissues studied. A higher level of cAMP was observed in normal skin than in psoriatic skin, as well as in uninvolved compared with involved psoriatic skin. The level of cGMP before incubation was not significantly different in normal epidermis and the psoriatic involved or uninvolved epidermis. Significantly greater cGMP production was

---

(17–4) Clin. Chim. Acta 126:119–126, December 1982.
(17–5) Dermatologica 165:533–543, 1982.

observed after 20 minutes of incubation in psoriatic involved epidermis than in normal skin. The cAMP-cGMP ratio was significantly higher in normal than in psoriatic involved or uninvolved epidermis. No significant difference was observed between involved and uninvolved psoriatic skin in biopsy specimens.

These results indicate that the metabolic balance between cAMP and cGMP is disturbed in psoriatic tissues. The reduction of the cAMP-cGMP ratio observed in psoriatic epidermis could result from decreased adenylate cyclase activity. The abnormalities found for these 2 cyclic nucleotides are consistent with the modifications of cell division and differentiation observed in psoriasis.

17–6 **A Virus-Like Particle Associated With Psoriasis.** Psoriasis is characterized by an increased number of epidermal mitoses and increased DNA synthesis. A relation to certain HLA haplotypes is established, which may act through reducing the threshold for clinical psoriasis in subjects predisposed by other factors, possibly viral infection. A. B. Dalen, L. Hellgren, O.-J. Iversen, and J. Vincent (Univ. of

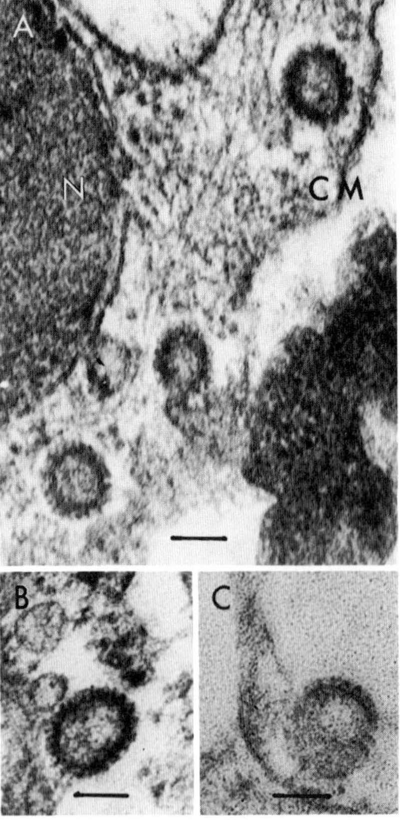

Fig 17–1.—Ultrathin sections from biopsy specimens of psoriatic plaques. **A,** intracytoplasmic spherical bodies; **B** and **C,** extracellular particles coated with surface knobs. Bars indicate 100 nm; original magnification, ×100,000. (Courtesy of Dalen, A.B., et al.: Acta Pathol. Microbiol. Immunol. Scand. [B] 91:221–229, August 1983.)

(17–6) Acta Pathol. Microbiol. Immunol. Scand. [B] 91:221–229, August 1983.

Trondheim, Norway) have now demonstrated virus-like particles by electron microscopy in specimens of psoriatic plaques.

Ultrastructural study of ultrathin sections of biopsy specimens of psoriatic plaques from 10 patients showed intracytoplasmic spherical bodies 110–150 nm in diameter, all with an irregular outer surface. Extracellular particles of similar size containing a regular array of surface projections were also seen in all specimens (Fig 17–1). Cell cultures established from the plaques released particles resembling retrovirus for a prolonged period. They contained a surface protein that bound to concanavalin A and is probably a glycoprotein. A major internal protein and 2 minor proteins were also detected, resembling the pattern of murine type C retrovirus. Virus-like particles were found in the urine of psoriatic patients that had a morphologic appearance different from that of the particles in cell cultures, and a similar difference was found when the latter particles were treated with normal urine. Patients with psoriatic arthritis had serum immune complexes containing distorted particles that could not be morphologically confirmed as being virions. A radioimmunoassay demonstrated common antigens in virus-like particles isolated from cell cultures, urine specimens from psoriatic patients, and immune complexes.

Virus-like particles can be found in cells from psoriatic plaques. It is possible that they are subcellular fragments without genomic viral RNA. If they do represent virus, it must be determined whether they have an etiologic role or are produced as a result of psoriasis.

17–7 **Langerhans Cells in Skin From Patients With Psoriasis: Quantitative and Qualitative Study of T6 and HLA-DR Antigen-Expressing Cells and Changes With Aromatic Retinoid Administration.** Marek Haftek, Michel Faure, Daniel Schmitt, and Jean Thivolet investigated the distribution of Langerhans cells in normal human skin and involved and uninvolved skin of patients with psoriasis before, during, and after systemic aromatic retinoid therapy. Indirect immunofluorescence techniques were used with a monoclonal antibody against human HLA-DR antigens and OKT6. In parallel, enumeration of cells positive for HLA-DR and OKT6 was also performed. Fifteen men with chronic psoriatic plaques of moderate activity were treated with 1 mg of etretinate per kg per day. Control groups consisted of 15 healthy males who received no retinoid and 5 males with other dermatoses treated with same dose retinoid.

Of the 15 psoriasis patients, 12 had good results from retinoid therapy, showing rapid clearing of skin lesions within 6 weeks of treatment. The other 3 had dropped out of the study. In involved psoriatic epidermis, results of monoclonal antibody and indirect immunofluorescence testing showed the distribution of positive cells was disturbed: OKT6-positive cells were reduced in number, as were HLA-DR–positive cells, which were seen in clusters. In control skin sections, a regular pattern of fluorescent dendritic epidermal cells was

---

(17–7) J. Invest. Dermatol. 81:10–14, July 1983.

seen. In normal-appearing human skin, in nonlesional psoriatic skin, but not in diseased psoriatic skin, the number of OKT6-positive cells per epidermal section surface unit was higher than that of HLA-DR–expressing cells. Changes in the number and distribution of cells positive for OKT6 and HLA-DR in involved psoriatic epidermis were corrected by oral retinoid treatment.

The distribution and number of epidermal cells positive for OKT6 and HLA-DR are altered in involved psoriatic skin, and these changes are corrected in healed psoriatic skin after successful oral retinoid treatment. These results suggest the possibility that defects in Langerhans cells themselves may play a role in the pathogenesis of the disease, but the return to a normal Langerhans cell distribution in parallel with lesion improvement with retinoid treatment does not necessarily signify that retinoids exert their action through an effect on the Langerhans cells.

▶ [Although a substantial reduction of OKT6-positive and HLA-DR–positive cells was observed in pretreatment lesional psoriatic skin, significant reduction was also seen in the noninvolved extensor forearm skin of 2 control subjects with palmar keratoses, in 3 control subjects with lichen planus, and in nonlesional psoriatic skin. In each group, values became normal following retinoid therapy.—R.W.G.] ◀

17–8 **Isotretinoin-PUVA for Psoriasis.** Herbert Hönigsmann and Klaus Wolff (Univ. of Vienna) tested isotretinoin, a retinoid, in combination with 8-methoxypsoralen–ultraviolet A (PUVA) photochemotherapy and compared the results with those of etretinate-PUVA therapy in treatment of psoriasis. One of the more serious problems of retinoid treatment is the potential for teratogenic effects. Isotretinoin is cleared from the body as early as 4 weeks after treatment, and contraception is needed for only a month, according to the manufacturers. Sixty patients with severe, widespread psoriasis were randomly assigned to treatment with isotretinoin-PUVA or etretinate-PUVA. Both retinoids were given orally at a daily dose of 1.0 mg/kg 5 days before PUVA therapy was begun, and retinoid administration was continued until the psoriasis cleared completely.

Results showed no significant difference between the two regimens with respect to duration of clearing phase, number of exposures, and cumulative UVA dose. When results in the two patient groups were compared with those in an earlier series of patients treated with PUVA alone, both combinations were superior in effect.

Because isotretinoin can replace etretinate in retinoid-PUVA combination therapy for psoriasis, this treatment can be considered for women of childbearing age provided they have severe psoriasis and take contraceptive precautions for a month after stopping isotretinoin. Etretinate is eliminated more slowly from the body, thus contraception is advised for 1 year after the end of treatment.

▶ [The mechanism of PUVA-retinoid interactions in the treatment of psoriasis is not known. The finding that isotretinoin plus PUVA is as effective as etretinate plus PUVA, although isotretinoin alone is less effective than etretinate, may indicate that there is an interaction that is beneficial rather than an additive effect of two treatments, reti-

---

(17–8) Lancet 1:236, Jan. 29, 1983.

noid and PUVA, working independently. However, a beneficial effect of the isotretinoin-PUVA combination has not been universally agreed upon, and the value of combination treatments requires further substantiation.—R.W.G.] ◀

17–9 **Antipsoriatic Activity of a New Synthetic Retinoid: The Arotinoid Ro 13–6298.** Oral etretinate therapy has been effective in a broad range of severe keratinizing disorders. The oral arotinoid Ro 13–6298 has effects on adult guinea pig skin similar to those induced by etretinate. Dionysios Tsambaos and Constantin E. Orfanos (Free Univ. of Berlin) report the successful use of minute oral doses of Ro 13–6298 in 2 patients with severe, treatment-resistant psoriasis. One patient was a woman, 55, with a 10-year history of generalized psoriasis and joint symptoms that were unresponsive to topical treatment and photochemotherapy. The other patient was a man, 34, with a 10-year history of severe generalized psoriasis and arthropathy that had required frequent hospitalizations. Etretinate therapy had failed in both. The arotinoid was given orally in a dose of 0.002 mg/kg daily for 2 weeks, followed by 0.05 mg daily for 7–8 weeks.

Both patients had progressive improvement in psoriasis starting after about a week of treatment. No new crops of pustules developed, and the existing pustules resolved gradually. Joint function also improved considerably. The psoriasis cleared completely after 7–8 weeks of continuous treatment. The patients remained free of skin lesions after 3 and 6 months, respectively, with no treatment. Joint symptoms, however, recurred shortly after the end of treatment. No intolerable side effects occurred. One patient had a rise in the erythrocyte sedimentation rate during treatment. Histologic studies confirmed the return of a nearly normal epidermis after several weeks of treatment with Ro 13–6298.

It appears that treatment with the oral arotinoid Ro 13–6298 can be effective in patients with severe, treatment-resistant psoriasis and associated joint symptoms. The histologic effects of the agent are similar to those of other oral retinoids. Further studies are needed to define the indications for using this drug and the risks of treatment.

▶ [Ro 13–6298 was an effective antipsoriatic drug in the 2 patients studied, but in a larger study recently published (see abstract below), the medication was less effective and more toxic than Tigason. Obviously more trials are needed before giving the final word on this new retinoid.—R.R.] ◀

–10 **Therapeutic Effect of Arotinoid Ro 13–6298 in Psoriasis.** The arotinoid Ro 13–6298 has exhibited a marked therapeutic effect on chemically induced skin papillomas in mice. F. Ott and J. M. Gieger compared the effect of this agent with that of Tigason (etretinate) in 17 patients (13 men), aged 27–76 years, with severe psoriasis. Fifteen patients had generalized psoriasis vulgaris, 3 with psoriatic arthropathy, and 2 had palmoplantar pustular psoriasis. The patients had previously received Tigason in daily doses of 10–50 mg. Ro 13–6298 was given orally in daily doses of 0.06–0.1 mg for 1–13 months (mean, 5 months).

(17–9) Arch. Dermatol. 119:746–751, September 1983.
(17–10) Arch. Dermatol. Res. 275:257–258, August 1983.

The effect of 0.1 mg of Ro 13–6298 daily on skin lesions in the first 2 months of treatment was equivalent to or, in some cases, better than that achieved previously with 50 mg of Tigason daily. Psoriatic arthropathy did not improve. The treatment was superior overall to Tigason therapy in 4 patients and inferior in 9. In 4 patients the two treatments had comparable effects. All the hypervitaminosis A side effects seen with Tigason also occurred with Ro 13–6298, and some were more frequent and severe after 3–6 months of treatment. Treatment had to be stopped in 2 patients, and in 8 others the daily dose was reduced. No laboratory abnormalities were found.

It appears that Ro 13–6298 is active in psoriatic patients in doses about 500-fold lower than those of Tigason. The margin between clinical efficacy and side effects, however, is small, making Ro 13–6298 potentially less useful than Tigason in the management of patients with psoriasis.

▶ [The goal is to develop a retinoid that will effectively treat psoriasis, yet spare patients the side effects of hypervitaminosis A. Although this new compound, Ro 13–6298, has been shown to be effective in treating chemically induced skin papillomas in mice, the final outcome of this psoriatic study revealed Tigason to be superior in clinical efficacy and degree of side effects. Tsambaos and Orfanos have found this drug to be helpful in 2 psoriatic patients that were previously unresponsive to etretinate (see abstract above).—R.R.] ◀

17–11 **Etretinate Therapy for Psoriasis: Clinical Responses, Remission Times, Epidermal DNA, and Polyamine Responses.** Synthetic derivatives of vitamin A are being increasingly used for treatment of skin disorders characterized by abnormal epithelial cell proliferation. Richard P. Kaplan, Diane H. Russell, and Nicholas J. Lowe conducted a prospective trial of the aromatic retinoid ethylester etretinate in 20 patients with various types of psoriasis vulgaris. All had recalcitrant disease. Ten had erythrodermic psoriasis, 8 plaque-type, and 2 the inverse type of psoriasis vulgaris. The 16 men and 4 women were aged 22–76 years. The initial dose of etretinate was 0.75 mg/kg, and maintenance doses ranged from 0.4 to 1.25 mg/kg. The only other treatment was topical hydrophilic petrolatum or 1% hydrocortisone cream or ointment. Shave biopsy specimens of involved and uninvolved skin were taken before and after 4 weeks of treatment. Polyamines were measured, and epidermal DNA synthesis was assessed with tritiated thymidine.

All types of psoriasis responded clinically within 2 months of the start of etretinate therapy. An average improvement of 62% occurred in patients with erythrodermic psoriasis, and improvement of 44% occurred in those with plaque-type disease. One patient in the latter group became worse. Remissions lasted about 8 weeks in all groups. Arthritis was greatly improved during retinoid therapy in 4 of 7 patients. Side effects were dose dependent. About half the patients exhibited hyperlipidemia, but none of the serum lipid concentrations was more than twice the upper limit of normal. Biopsy specimens taken during treatment showed a decrease in psoriasiform epidermal

---

(17–11) J. Am. Acad. Dermatol. 8:95–102, January 1983.

changes and in lymphohistiocytic infiltration. Concentrations of polyamines decreased during treatment before significant changes in epidermal DNA synthesis. Synthesis of DNA decreased in both involved and uninvolved skin sites.

Etretinate is an effective treatment for various clinical types of psoriasis. Arthritis may also respond to this treatment. Nearly all patients require maintenance therapy. Abnormal liver function and hyperlipidemia are among the possible side effects of this treatment. Polyamine synthesis is normalized early in the course of etretinate therapy before there is any significant change in epidermal DNA synthesis.

▶ [Although etretinate is not uniformly successful in all patients with psoriasis, there is a role for this drug in recalcitrant psoriasis with and without arthritis in selected patients. It is to be hoped that in the near future a new synthetic derivative will achieve a higher ratio of therapeutic to toxic effects than etretinate.—R.R.] ◀

7–12 **Keratin Polypeptide Profile in Psoriatic Epidermis Normalized by Treatment With Etretinate (Aromatic Retinoid Ro 10-9359).** Marie J. Staquet, Michel R. Faure, Alain Reano, Jacqueline Viac, and Jean Thivolet (Lyon, France) studied the variations in expression of epidermal keratins occurring in patients with psoriasis before and during oral administration of etretinate (aromatic retinoid Ro 10-9359), and they compared these findings with those in normal epidermis. Results in 10 men aged 18–45 with clinical psoriasis vulgaris were compared with those in 10 healthy controls of similar age. Etretinate alone was orally administered to patients and volunteers, who ingested 1 mg of retinoid/kg/day. Clinical improvement of psoriatic lesions was observed after 2 weeks of treatment in every patient. Sodium dodecyl sulfate–polyacrylamide gel electrophoresis (SDS–PAGE) densitometric readings were performed on keratins extracted from epidermal cells obtained through trypsinization of skin specimens. Epidermal cells were also tested by immunofluorescence for basement membrane zone antigens and for presence of total keratin and keratin polypeptide (KP).

In psoriasis-involved epidermis, SDS–PAGE analysis showed lower amounts of 67K and increased amounts of 63K and 55K, as compared with findings in normal epidermis. Low proportions of cells expressing 67K and 63K were also noted, with defective expression of these two KPs by suprabasal keratinocytes in psoriasis-involved epidermis. During etretinate administration, a return toward the normal electrophoretic pattern and correction of the defective cellular expression of these two KPs paralleled clinical improvement.

The findings indicate that etretinate, when administered to patients with psoriasis in a dose that corrects clinical and histologic abnormalities, leads to normalization of the abnormal expression of keratins by epidermal cells. The mechanism of action of this modulation of keratin expression is unknown.

▶ [Retinoids tend to normalize keratinization diseases. It is of interest (but not surprising) that the electrophoretic patterns of psoriasis were normalized with etretinate

(17–12) Arch. Dermatol. Res. 275:124–129, April 1983.

therapy. In considering a mechanism of action in psoriasis, one must also take into account the effect of etretinate on neutrophil inhibition (see abstract below).—R.R.] ◀

17–13 **Inhibition of Neutrophil Migration by Etretinate and Its Main Metabolite.** Oral administration of the aromatic retinoid etretinate has helped control psoriasis. The mechanism of the effect is unclear, but a loss of neutrophil migration from dermal capillaries toward the epidermis has been observed. Retinoids are most effective in inflammatory and pustular cases, in which neutrophil migration into the skin is maximal. L. Dubertret, C. Lebreton, and R. Touraine (Creteil, France) used a skin chamber technique to examine the effect of retinoids on neutrophil function in 22 healthy subjects aged 20–25 years. Skin chambers containing autologous serum were placed after removal of the roof of a suction blister and changed at 6, 8, and 24 hours. Etretinate and its metabolite Ro 10-1670 (Met) were administered locally in concentrations of 0.001–0.1 mg/ml, and 6 subjects took Tigason orally in a dose of 1 mg/kg daily for 8 days.

The migration of neutrophils out of the skin was significantly reduced by both etretinate and Met in concentrations of 0.1 mg/ml; the metabolite was significantly more effective. Lower concentrations were ineffective. Systemic etretinate therapy significantly inhibited neutrophil migration out of the skin after 8 days of administration. No changes in phagocytosis or neutrophil bactericidal activity were observed with concentrations of etretinate and Met much greater than those used therapeutically.

The effect of retinoids in inhibiting neutrophil migration from the blood to the skin could be closely related to the antipsoriatic effects of the drugs. The skin chamber method could be helpful in screening new drugs for antipsoriatic activity.

▶ [The antipsoriatic effect of etretinate may in part be attributed to its inhibitory effect on neutrophil migration from vessels to epidermis. This anti-inflammatory hypothesis would explain both the skin and joint responses to the retinoid.—R.R.] ◀

17–14 **Influence of Retinoid Ro 10-9359 on Cell-Mediated Immunity In Vivo.** R. A. Fulton, P. Souteyrand, and J. Thivolet (Lyon, France) used the oral retinoid, Ro 10-9359, to treat 26 patients with psoriasis and 23 patients with other dermatoses (lichen planus, keratosis follicularis, basal cell carcinoma) for 28 days. Intradermal tests to 7 recall antigens were carried out before and after therapy. Dinitrochlorobenzene (DNCB) sensitization was begun at the initiation of retinoid therapy, and challenge tests were made after 28 days.

In the 28 patients who had both psoriasis and other dermatoses and for whom complete data were available, the recall antigen score increased significantly over the 28 days of Ro 10-9359 treatment. The increase in score was also significant when the entire group was subdivided into those with psoriasis (15) and those with other dermatoses (13). Mean scores of spontaneous reactions to DNCB after 14 days of

---

(17–13) Br. J. Dermatol. 107:681–685, December 1982.
(17–14) Dermatologica 165:568–572, 1982.

retinoid therapy in the two treated groups did not differ significantly from scores in the untreated controls. But the mean score of the DNCB challenge after 28 days of retinoid therapy was significantly higher in the untreated, nonpsoriatic group than in untreated controls. Levels of immunoglobulins G, M, A, and E did not alter significantly in the 28 days of retinoid therapy in either group.

These findings demonstrate that the oral retinoid Ro 10-9359 enhances cell-mediated immunity in vivo in various skin diseases. This immune booster effect may explain part of the retinoid's beneficial action in these disorders, and it also suggests how retinoids act to prevent cancer.

17–15 **Goeckerman Regimen in Two Psoriasis Day-Care Centers.** Alan Menter (Baylor Med. Plaza Psoriasis Center, Dallas) and David L. Cram (Univ. of California, San Francisco) used the Goeckerman regimen to treat 300 patients with severe psoriasis. Each patient was evaluated initially and then followed for 1 year or longer to determine skin clearing, side effects, and length of remission. Patients were treated 6 days a week for 6–7 hours daily; all complied completely with the regimen, which was as follows: an initial ultraviolet B (UVB) treatment followed by a tar shampoo, application of 10% liquor carbonis detergens (LCD) in a commercially available oil base to the scalp, and crude coal tar to the general body avoiding the scalp, face, groin, and axillae. The preparation contained 2%–5% crude coal tar with polysorbate 80 (Tween 80), 2.5%, added. Also, 2% or 5% salicyclic acid was added to the tar during therapy to treat thick plaques. Minimal erythemal doses were not determined for each patient, but the initial UVB dose was based on skin type and prior history of ultraviolet light (UVL) exposure and tolerance. After final discharge from each of the 2 centers, patients were encouraged to apply the LCD (in a moisturizing base) or tar gel twice daily and to obtain natural UVL or artificial UVB on a regular basis for 1 month.

Of 300 patients treated, maximum clearing (more than 90%) was achieved in all. Combined average days of treatment to clearing at the 2 centers was 18 days (range, 8–38), resulting in an average stay of 3 weeks. The average total UVB dose per patient per course of treatment was 1.96 J/sq cm. Overall, 90% of the patients remained clear of psoriasis for a minimum of 8 months, and 73% remained clear for 1 year or longer. Arthritis symptoms prior to Goeckerman treatment were noted by 25% of the patients; in follow-up, these symptoms improved or cleared in 85%. A mild degree of folliculitis occurred, particularly in heavyset, hirsute males. This side effect responded to application of antiseptic soaps, topical antibiotics, or Castellani's paint or resolved spontaneously. Some patients occasionally experienced sun burn, and herpes simplex of a transient nature was sometimes observed during therapy.

It would appear that the Goeckerman regimen can clear severe psoriasis in a reasonably short period of time and that it induces excep-

---

(17–15) J. Am. Acad. Dermatol. 9:59–65, July 1983.

tional periods of remission. This treatment can be cost-effective in a psoriasis day-care center and should remain a major choice of therapy for patients with severe or recalcitrant psoriasis.

▶ [The development of the psoriasis day-care centers has added a new dimension to delivery of care on an outpatient basis, and it not only reduces cost of treatment to the patients who otherwise will require hospitalization but also provides a home-like environment and peer support. In the future these benefits should be offered to patients with other chronic diseases requiring intensive therapy on an outpatient basis, such as atopic dermatitis and mycosis fungoides. I am surprised at the long-term remission of 18 months induced by intensive Goeckerman therapy in the day-treatment center and maintenance treatment at home. We certainly have not seen that even in our hospitalized patients receiving similar regimens.—E.G.] ◀

17–16 **Measurement of the Response of Psoriasis to Short-Term Application of Anthralin.** Recent reports indicate that psoriasis may respond to the application of anthralin for short periods, and this would preclude the need for its virtually continuous application as in the Ingram regimen. J. R. Marsden, P. R. Coburn, Janet Marks, and Sam Shuster (Univ. of Newcastle upon Tyne, England) sought to confirm this observation in a series of 36 psoriatic patients, aged 16–67 years, who required inpatient treatment. Thirty had plaque-type psoriasis and 6 had guttate disease. Anthralin was prepared with 0.5% salicyclic acid in an emulsifying ointment. After short-term application of a 2% anthralin preparation for 1 hour, conventional treatment with 0.05%–1.0% anthralin in Lassar's paste was applied to plaques that remained for 21–23 hours. A confirmatory study in 13 patients was followed by optimizing studies to determine the shortest practical time of application and the highest concentration tolerated. Concentrations as high as 8% were applied to half the body for 30-minute periods.

In the confirmatory study, short-term treatment was as effective as conventional therapy in reducing plaque thickness, but burning was worse on the short-term treatment side. Most patients preferred short-term therapy. Times to clinical clearance were comparable with short-term and conventional treatments. The time to clinical clearance correlated closely with the time to reach half plaque thickness. Concentrations of anthralin exceeding 2% did not seem to improve the clinical outcome.

This study confirmed the efficacy of short-term anthralin applications in the treatment of significant psoriasis. The clinical results are comparable with those obtained from continuous treatment. The chief problem has been burning, which is dose related. Although systemic absorption of drug from the high concentrations used in short-term therapy can lead to systemic toxicity such as albuminuria, the practical advantages of short-term therapy are considerable, and it is likely to become the treatment of choice.

▶ [This careful and convincing study confirms anthralin as a highly effective treatment, something Europeans and others have known for years. It also provides convincing evidence of its potential as an outpatient of day-care center treatment. Unfor-

---

(17–16) Br. J. Dermatol. 109:209–218, August 1983.

tunately, anthralin concentrations appropriate for this type of therapy are not marketed in the United States.—R.W.G.] ◀

17–17 **Irritant Reactions to Dithranol in Normal Subjects and Psoriatic Patients.** T. Kingston and R. Marks (Cardiff, Wales) investigated the irritant reaction to dithranol on the normal forearm skin of 40 psoriatic patients and 40 controls using skin contact thermometry to assess the concentration required to irritate 50% of the population tested (ID_{50}). These parameters were calculated for each of 4 skin types.

The threshold concentration that produces a reaction is known as the minimal irritant dose (MID). The ID_{50} value showed that there was no difference between the threshold for irritancy between the patients and the controls considered as a group, but psoriatic patients and controls with skin type I had the lowest threshold for irritancy; this was significantly different from that in all other groups at the 95% confidence limit level for controls only. Blocking the irritant reaction with indomethacin was attempted in 5 dithranol-sensitive subjects, who received 25 mg of indomethacin every 8 hours, 24 hours before repeat patch testing. Five controls were also included. Indomethacin treatment blocked the irritant reaction in 4 patients and raised the irritant threshold in the other; no change occurred in controls.

Skin contact thermometry is an accurate, practical method for assessment of skin irritation caused by dithranol. Further, irritation and inflammation caused by dithranol can be blocked by indomethacin treatment. These findings suggest that dithranol irritation is, at least in part, mediated by prostaglandins and can be blocked by inhibitors of the cyclo-oxygenase pathway.

▶ [These findings support other observations which indicate that type I skin is distinctive in respects other than responses to ultraviolet light. Skin contact thermometry appeared to be a reproducible technique for the evaluation of reactions to dithranol. It would be of interest to know whether different skin types also differ in their ability to acquire tolerance to dithranol with repeated exposure.—R.W.G.] ◀

17–18 **Coal Tar Phototherapy for Psoriasis Reevaluated: Erythemogenic Versus Suberythemogenic Ultraviolet With a Tar Extract in Oil and Crude Coal Tar.** Recent studies have questioned the therapeutic value of coal tar vs. ultraviolet radiation and their relative necessity in phototherapy for psoriasis. Nicholas J. Lowe, Mitchell S. Wortzman, James Breeding, Hala Koudsi, and Linda Taylor (Los Angeles) analyzed the different aspects of tar phototherapy in single-blind paired comparison trials in the University of California, Los Angeles–Wadsworth Dermatology Program.

The effects of 1% crude coal tar (5 subjects) were compared with those of petrolatum (5 subjects) in conjunction with erythemogenic and suberythemogenic doses of ultraviolet B (UVB). A cabinet containing 16 FS72 sunlamp tubes was used. Crude coal tar was clinically superior to petrolatum with suberythemogenic ultraviolet. With erythemogenic UVB, petrolatum was equal in efficacy to crude coal

(17–17) Br. J. Dermatol. 108:307–313, March 1983.
(17–18) J. Am. Acad. Dermatol. 8:781–789, June 1983.

tar. Suberythemogenic UVB was also used adjunctively to compare the effects of a 5% concentration of tar extract in an oil base (4 subjects) to 5% crude coal tar in petrolatum or the oil base without tar (4 subjects). The tar extract in oil plus suberythemogenic UVB produced significantly more rapid improvement than the oil base plus UVB.

Direct bilateral comparison of equal concentrations of tar extract in oil base (5 subjects) vs. crude coal tar in petrolatum in a suberythemogenic UVB photo regimen revealed no statistical differences between treatments. In a study comparing tar extract in oil and the oil base without UVB radiation (5 subjects), the tar extract in oil side responded more rapidly.

The effects of erythemogenic and suberythemogenic UVB, with and without tar extract in oil, on the suppression assay of epidermal DNA synthesis of the hairless mouse were also studied. In this model, erythemogenic doses of UVB produced near maximal inhibition of DNA synthesis with or without coal tars. Suberythemogenic dosages of UVB produced submaximal suppression of DNA synthesis that was enhanced by adjunctive coal tar but not by vehicle. These findings are consistent with the clinical results.

These studies suggest that coal tars combined with suberythemogenic UVB therapy are a practical alternative to the more aggressive UVB therapy without coal tar. This alternative reduces the UVB exposure and thus possible side effects. The question of safety is still unanswered, especially with regard to long-term side effects such as cutaneous carcinogenesis. Presently no data are available on length of remission after treatment with coal tars combined with suberythemogenic UVB.

▶ [A bilateral comparison study may be the most sensitive and practical way of comparing treatment regimes for psoriasis and other generalized disorders, although substantial numbers of patients are still required. The choice of an end point for comparison of results is a major problem, and the credibility of results depends upon an appropriate choice. In our experience, "percent of initial severity" has been a difficult figure to arrive at even by close examination of patients at frequent intervals. It is also not clear how important this figure is. For example, the greatest differences observed by Lowe et al. were seen between treatment with tar oil and oil base and between crude coal tar and petrolatum, both combined with suberythemogenic UVB radiation. Tar oil ("19.6% improvement per week") left one side of 5 patients with a mean of 42% of initial severity at 3 weeks, whereas the oil base ("11.4% improvement per week") left the other side with 60% of initial severity. Although one agent may approximately half-treat patients better than the other agent—indeed it did so at a level of $P < .0005$—it would have been more valuable to know how long each regimen required to cause reasonable (>95%) clearance in exposed skin.

It is interesting that the largest difference in clearing rate, although not the most significant, was seen between oil base and tar oil, with no radiation (12.8% vs. 24.5% per week; $P < .005$ in 5 subjects). Tar may indeed be an adjunctive therapy working independently from UVB radiation, as its phototoxic action spectrum (in the ultraviolet A region) would suggest.—R.W.G.] ◀

17–19 **Topical 8-Methoxypsoralen Photochemotherapy of Psoriasis: Clinical Study.** An interval of 1–2 hours is often allowed between

(17–19) Br. J. Dermatol. 108:519–524, May 1983.

topical application of a psoralen and exposure to ultraviolet A (UVA) in the treatment of psoriasis. K. Danno, T. Horio, M. Ozaki, and S. Imamura (Kyoto Univ.) evaluated a noninterval regimen in a controlled trial in 15 patients with chronic, stable, extensive psoriasis. Thirteen had plaque-type disease and 2 had erythrodermic psoriasis. Mean age was 54 years. Treatment was with a 1% solution of 8-methoxypsoralen in lotion form. Symmetric areas on the trunk were irradiated with UVA either 2 hours after application of the psoralen or within 5 minutes of drug application. Exposures usually were made three times weekly, and the dose of UVA was individualized. Three patients also received topical corticosteroid therapy.

Each patient received a mean of 16 exposures over 5½ weeks, with a mean cumulative energy dose of 16 J/sq cm. Many patients had complete or nearly complete clearing with both 2-hour interval therapy and noninterval treatment. Two patients had only partial improvement. The two regimens were equally effective in most cases. Some patients reported irritation after noninterval therapy, but burning was more frequent with 2-hour interval treatment. Most patients continued to receive treatment once a week with either regimen, and there have been no recurrences during follow-up periods as long as 10 months.

Noninterval treatment with topical psoralen and UVA (PUVA) is an acceptable alternative in the management of psoriasis. It saves time and seems to be as effective as standard treatment with a 1–2-hour delay. Psoralens penetrate rapidly into the epidermis after topical application. It is also possible that some drug remains in the affected skin between treatments. Treatment with PUVA may act in part on psoriasis leukotactic factors in the lesional horny layer, and psoralen would be expected to reach these shortly after being applied.

▶ [Topical psoralen application is remarkably unstandardized. Different groups use concentrations varying from 0.00005% to 1% and vehicles ranging from bath water to ethanol or hydrophilic ointment. All methods appear to cause cutaneous photosensitization and therapeutic benefits. Very dilute aqueous solutions may cause more sensitization than more concentrated solutions in ethanol, presumably because of partition factors and possibly because of surface absorption of radiation by psoralen, which results in a screening effect. It is not surprising that sufficient penetration of psoralen to cause sensitization can occur within 5 minutes of application of a concentrated solution.—R.W.G.] ◀

17–20 **Ophthalmologic Study of Patients Undergoing Long-Term PUVA Therapy.** Results of animal studies have raised concern over ocular damage in patients receiving therapy with psoralen and ultraviolet A (PUVA) for psoriasis. Lena Rönnerfält, Eva Lydahl, Göran Wennersten, Peder Jahnberg, and Monika Thyresson-Hök (Stockholm) performed repeated ophthalmologic studies in 46 patients, 23 of each sex, who had severe, long-standing psoriasis and were followed up for 5–6½ years after the start of photochemotherapy. Thirteen patients had previously received arsenic therapy, and 5, methotrexate. Treatment was with about 0.6 mg of 8-methoxypsoralen per

(17–20) Acta Derm. Venereol. (Stockh.) 62:501–505, 1982.

RESULTS OF LENS EXAMINATION*

Object of examination	Evaluation	Findings† (number of patients, $n = 46$)
Lens capsule		
Pigmentary deposits	Presence noted	11
Pseudo-exfoliation	Presence noted	0
Subcapsular area		
Anterior vacuoles	Presence noted	5
Anterior opacities	Presence noted	2
Posterior vacuoles	Presence noted	15
Posterior opacities	Presence noted	1
Lens cortex		
Punctate opacities	Counted‡	7 (10 opacities or more)
Larger opacities	Presence noted§	14
Zones of discontinuity–zones with a slightly increased light scattering	Counted	25 (1 zone) 19 (2 zones) 2 (3 zones)
Light scattering in the deep anterior cortex–the supranuclear zone	Graded from 1 to 5	16 (grade 3 or more)
Nucleus		
Transparency	Graded from 1 to 5	2 (grade 3 or more)
Colour	Graded from 1 to 5	6 (grade 3 or more)
Punctate opacities	Presence noted	30
Larger opacities	Presence noted§	2

*For each measurement patient is classified according to most affected eye.
†Findings remained unchanged during observation period.
‡In 0.2-mm wide slit beam.
§Marked in schematic drawing of lens.
(Courtesy of Rönnerfält, L., et al.: Acta Derm. Venereol. [Stockh.] 62:501–505, 1982.)

kg and UVA in doses as large as 20 J/sq cm, with a maximal intensity of 365 nm. Most patients received maintenance therapy weekly for about 2 months, and most have received repeated courses of therapy as often as 4 times a year, or continuous treatment once or twice a week.

Three patients had a reduction in visual acuity attributable to senile macular changes; 1 of them also had cortical lens opacities that increased during follow-up. One patient became more myopic during the study. The results of lens examinations are shown in the table.

No ocular side effects were attributed to photochemotherapy in these patients during follow-up for 5–6 years after the institution of treatment. It remains possible that further continuous treatment will carry a risk of such effects. Occlusive ultraviolet opaque spectacles should be used during treatment, and appropriate protective glasses worn for as long as 12 hours after 8-methoxypsoralen ingestion. Patients should be reminded of the importance of wearing the prescribed ocular shielding.

▶ [The size of this cohort (N = 46) is such that only an ocular side effect with a very high incidence would have been likely to be detected. Certainly, given the accelerated cataract formation observed in some animal species treated with PUVA without eye protection and the isolated reports of "PUVA" cataracts in humans who failed to use eye protection, the use of UVA-blocking glasses for at least 12 hours after drug ingestion, whenever patients using psoralen are exposed to UVA, seems prudent.—R.S.S.] ◀

17–21 **Skin Carcinomas and Treatment With Photochemotherapy (PUVA).** Nontherapeutic doses of psoralen with prolonged exposure to ultraviolet A (UVA) have been found to be carcinogenic in animals. Rune Lindskov (Finsen Inst., Copenhagen) reports a 3½-year follow-up of 198 patients given photochemotherapy for more than 3 months, mainly for psoriasis. Treatment was with about 0.6 mg of 8-methoxypsoralen per kg orally, followed after 2 hours by UVA in an initial dose of 0.5–1.0 J/sq cm. The 122 men and 76 women had a median age of 52 years and were examined an average of 43 months after the start of psoralen and UVA (PUVA) therapy. Thirty-eight psoriatic patients treated with methotrexate as well were followed for a mean of 4 years. These patients were matched with 101 control subjects for age, sex, and risk factors.

Seventeen cancers were diagnosed in 10 patients and 9 actinic keratoses in 8. Basal cell carcinomas predominated. More than two thirds of the cancers and 44% of the keratoses were on nonexposed areas of skin. No patient without such risk factors as exposure to ionizing radiation, arsenic treatment, or methotrexate therapy developed carcinoma. The median cumulative doses of UVA were 288 J/sq cm in patients without tumors, 1,058 J/sq cm in patients with keratosis, and 526 J/sq cm in those with cancer. Cancers had occurred in 9% of the control group within 4 years of the most recent examination. All but 1 of the cases of cancer in the control group were basal cell carcinoma.

A relatively large number of skin cancers was found in PUVA-treated patients in this study, but the tumors appeared to be related to the use of potentially carcinogenic treatments other than PUVA, especially ionizing radiation. Carcinogenicity must be considered a possibility until long-term prospective studies have demonstrated the safety of PUVA therapy. A restrictive view seems advisable, particularly toward patients who have been exposed to known carcinogens and those with a history of skin tumors.

▶ [Unfortunately, the small size of the study cohort and the very low exposure to PUVA limit the usefulness of this study. The higher UVA dose received by the keratosis and tumor group suggests a possible dose-related carcinogenic effect for PUVA. Negative results in studies of this size and with this exposure are hardly surprising. There is no good epidemiologic or basic scientific evidence that methotrexate, in doses used to treat psoriasis, is a risk factor for cutaneous cancer.—R.S.S.] ◀

17–22 **Is UVB Treatment of Psoriasis Safe? Study of Extensively UVB-Treated Psoriasis Patients Compared With a Matched Control Group.** Psoriasis was frequently treated with ultraviolet B (UVB) in Scandinavia before the advent of psoralen–ultraviolet A (PUVA) therapy. Olle Larkö and Gunnar Swanbeck (Univ. of Göteborg, Sweden) investigated whether the risk of skin cancer is increased in psoriatic patients extensively treated with UVB. Eighty-five patients who received more than 100 UVB treatments were evaluated and matched with 338 control subjects for sex and age. Prema-

---

(17–21) Acta Derm. Venereol. (Stockh.) 63:223–226, 1983.
(17–22) Ibid., 62:507–512, 1982.

lignant or malignant skin lesions, or both, had occurred in 5.9% of the study group and in 10.1% of the control group, a difference that was not significant. Multiple regression analysis showed a relation between premalignant-malignant skin changes and both advanced age and outdoor work but no correlation with sex, skin type, or travel to southern latitudes.

No increased risk of premalignant or malignant skin changes was apparent in this case-control study of patients treated for psoriasis with extensive use of UVB over many years. Therapeutic doses of UVB are not appreciably greater than those received by subjects who actively sunbathe in the summer in Sweden. A study is underway to compare the erythema-producing UVB doses received in indoor and outdoor work.

▶ [This is not a case-control study. It is a point-prevalence study in a group of patients who had received more than 100 UVB treatments and general population controls. The study is flawed by the small size of the study group and perhaps even more by the relatively low participation rates for both UVB-treated patients and controls (71% and 66%, respectively). Other work suggests that patients exposed to such relatively low numbers of UVB treatments have no detectable increased risk of skin cancer. Fewer than 30 patients in this study had received in excess of 300 UVB treatments, the minimal number of UVB treatments in the multicenter study that was shown to be associated with an increased skin cancer risk. It seems likely that most patients in this group had been treated with doses of UVB that were less erythemogenic than those currently utilized, a fact that further limits the usefulness of this study for assessing the safety of UVB, as it is now used.—R.S.S.] ◀

17–23 **PUVA Therapy Does Not Modify Arsenic Carcinogenesis in Psoriatics.** Ruth Angele, Bernhard Schneider, and Ernst G. Jung (Univ. of Heidelberg) conducted a follow-up examination of 84 psoriatic patients after 4–5 years of psoralen and ultraviolet A (PUVA) therapy to determine the interactions between oral arsenic therapy and PUVA treatment. After skin reaction to ultraviolet radiation and skin type had been determined, each patient was exposed to ultraviolet A (UVA) radiation 2 hours after ingestion of 8-methoxypsoralen.

Seventeen of the 84 patients had a history of exposure to arsenic (oral arsenic therapy was abandoned several years ago). None of the patients had been treated with x-rays, methotrexate, nitrogen mustard, or other cytotoxic agents. Patients were divided into 3 groups: those with psoriasis for more than 17 years who had a history of arsenic exposure, those with psoriasis for more than 17 years who had no history of arsenic exposure, and those with psoriasis for less than 17 years who had no history of arsenic exposure.

Precancerous lesions and malignant tumors were detected in 8 of 84 patients. In 6 patients multiple palmoplantar keratoses were present, which were typical of arsenical keratoses. Five of the 6 were from the first group and 1 was from the second group. This last patient had a possible occupational exposure to arsenic. There was a statistically significant increase in incidence of premalignant and malignant lesions in the first group, compared with the sum of groups 2 and 3.

In this study 35% of patients with psoriasis who were exposed to

---

(17–23) Dermatologica 166:141–145, March 1983.

arsenic experienced palmoplantar keratoses after a latent period of 15–30 years. The authors conclude that PUVA therapy does not modify the late effects of exposure to arsenic and has no mitigating or promoting effect on arsenic carcinogenesis. Arsenic is a complete carcinogen whose carcinogenic potential is not influenced by subsequent PUVA therapy. However, the authors recommend close and painstaking supervision when patients previously exposed to arsenic undergo PUVA therapy.

▶ [This article contains so many methodological flaws that it is perhaps most useful as an illustration of how not to do a study and of the misuse of statistics. The chances of finding a substantial difference between a group of 17 patients with arsenic exposure and the remaining 67 patients without this exposure are, because of sample size, extraordinarily small. The authors fail to provide essential data such as the age and sex of the patients in each group. They fail to provide data on exposure to PUVA in each group. No control group of persons exposed to arsenic but not PUVA is included. A negative finding is not surprising.—R.S.S.] ◀

17–24 **Long-Term Photochemotherapy for Psoriasis: Histopathologic and Clinical Follow-up Study With Special Emphasis on Tumor Incidence and Behavior of Pigmented Lesions.** Photochemotherapy has proved useful in treating psoriasis, but concern continues over the possibility of premalignant or malignant changes being induced. Ann-Marie Ros, Göran Wennersten, and Björn Lagerholm (Stockholm) reviewed data on 250 patients with severe, longstanding psoriasis who received psoralen and ultraviolet A (PUVA) therapy more or less continuously for as long as 7 years, about 50% of them for 5–7 years. Most patients had previously received ultraviolet B (UVB) therapy, and many had traveled south for climate therapy of their disease. The dose of ultraviolet A was increased to a maximum of 20 J/sq cm. Maintenance therapy was given once weekly to most patients. Several patients received repeat courses of PUVA therapy lasting several months, 2 to 4 times per year, or were treated continuously once or twice a week.

The most common acute side effects of PUVA therapy were nausea, pruritus, and paresthesia. The long-term side effects are shown in the table. Slight to moderate lentiginosis was a fairly common finding.

LONG-TERM SIDE EFFECTS CLINICALLY OBSERVED IN PUVA-TREATED PATIENTS

	No. of patients	%
Lentiginosis	82	33
Lentiginosis, profuse	10	4
Hypertrichosis	11	4.5
Actinic elastosis (pronounced)	6	2.5
Actinic keratosis	5	2

(Courtesy of Ros, A.M., et al.: Acta Derm. Venereol. [Stockh.] 63:215–221, 1983.)

(17–24) Acta Derm. Venereol. (Skockh.) 63:215–221, 1983.

No skin carcinomas were observed. The 6 patients with atypical lentigines had received extensive UBV therapy previously, and 3 of them also had received arsenic. Hyperkeratosis, chiefly of the orthokeratotic type, was a frequent skin biopsy finding. Parakeratosis and parahyperkeratosis were rarely observed.

Atypical lentigines appear to be an infrequent complication of long-term PUVA therapy. Whether affected patients are at an increased risk of malignant transformation is unclear, but these patients should be followed up closely. Dark, irregular lentiginous spots that appear during PUVA therapy should be excised. PUVA therapy is effective in the management of severe, long-standing psoriasis. No serious side effects have been observed in patients followed up for as long as 7 years.

▶ [A variety of types of pigmented lesions occur in PUVA-treated patients, usually after at least 1 year of therapy. Lesions range from small lentiginous macules to irregularly formed starlike hyperpigmented lentigines which may be much larger in size and which have recently been studied in some detail (Rhodes et al.: *J. Am. Acad. Dermatol.* 9:47–58, 1983). Rhodes et al. found that pigmented lesions were in every case associated with significant actinic damage (wrinkling, atrophy, scaling, and telangectasia) in neighboring non-sun-exposed skin.—R.W.G.] ◀

17–25 **Skin Vessel Leakage of Plasma Proteins After PUVA Therapy.** Dilatation of dermal blood vessels and damage to vessel walls have been described in both normal and psoriatic skin after psoralen-ultraviolet A (PUVA) therapy. B. Staberg (Finsen Inst., Copenhagen) assessed the local leakiness of the cutaneous microvasculature in healthy subjects after PUVA therapy. Eight male subjects received PUVA therapy with 0.5 mg of 8-methoxypsoralen per kg, followed in 2 hours by 4 to 5 joules per sq cm of UVA, on 2 successive days. An area of abdominal skin was shielded, and changes in skin vessel leakage of ^{125}I-labeled albumin were compared in exposed and unexposed skin areas. Suction blisters were raised in the abdominal skin 30 minutes after injection of the tracer protein.

Most subjects had erythema and edema of the irradiated skin. Suction blisters developed a little more readily in irradiated skin. The relative concentration of injected albumin in suction blister fluid from irradiated skin was only slightly elevated 2 days after PUVA therapy, whereas a significant elevation was found in unirradiated skin. No significant changes were seen in the concentrations of four endogenous plasma proteins (albumin, transferrin, IgG, and α_2-macroglobulin) in serum and blister fluid.

The findings indicate that PUVA therapy can induce an increase in vascular leakage of albumin from the cutaneous vessels. The change is ascribed to an indirect humoral effect. An analogous increase in microvascular permeability has been described in unburned skin areas of dogs with 50% body burns and attributed to the release of chemical mediators of inflammation from the burned skin areas.

▶ [The mechanism and significance of this apparently indirect effect of PUVA therapy is unclear.—R.W.G.] ◀

(17–25) Arch. Dermatol. Res. 275:222–225, August 1983

17–26 **Observations on PUVA Treatment of Psoriasis and on 5-S-Cysteinyldopa After Exposure to UV Light.** Eva Tegner (Univ. of Lund, Sweden) reports data from a follow-up study of 302 patients treated with psoralen and ultraviolet A (PUVA) for widespread psoriasis, mostly of the chronic plaque type, between 1975 and 1981. The mean duration of illness at the time treatment began was 26.5 years. Irradiation at a peak emission of 365 nm was performed 2 hours after administration of 0.6 mg of 8-methoxy-psoralen per kg. The highest initial ultraviolet A (UVA) dose was 4 J/sq cm. Thirty-four patients received maintenance treatment, and 152 received repeated courses of PUVA therapy for relapses of psoriasis. Patients were followed for as long as 5½ years after initial treatment.

All but 4% of the patients had complete clearing or definite improvement after an average of 26 treatment sessions over 7 weeks and a total cumulative UVA dose of 80 J/sq cm. The average remission time without maintenance therapy was 6 months. Treatment was as effective when psoriasis recurred. Complications included severe skin pain lasting as long as 3 months in 5% of patients, and facial seborrheic dermatitis in 6%. Increased serum levels of the melanocytic metabolite 5-S-cysteinyldopa were recorded after 2–3 days of treatment, before an increase in pigmentation was detected. Peak levels occurred after 1–2 weeks when tanning was starting to appear. The change was related to the inflammatory changes induced by PUVA therapy. Skin areas exposed to marked external pressure during UVA radiation showed no delayed erythema or tanning. Squamous cell cancer developed in 1 patient during follow-up.

These findings confirm the effectiveness of PUVA therapy in the management of psoriasis. Patients remained in remission for an average of more than 6 months without maintenance treatment. Comparable benefit was obtained from repeated courses of PUVA therapy. The patient with squamous cell cancer received a total UVA dose of 1,750 J/sq cm, and also had received much UVB radiation for many years. The PUVA therapy can be discontinued after the initial course and resumed for relapse. This approach may improve the long-term safety of the treatment.

▶ [Side effects from PUVA show significant differences in different centers. Severe skin pain and facial seborrheic dermatitis appear to be uncommon in the United States, as are the reproducible visual field defects observed by another European group (Wilkinson, J.D., English, J.: Seminars in Dermatology 2:85–100, 1983). The observation of a pressure effect upon UVA-induced delayed pigmentation and erythema induced by UVA alone is of interest.—R.W.G.] ◀

7–27 **Natural UVB Radiation Received by People With Outdoor, Indoor, and Mixed Occupations and UVB Treatment of Psoriasis.** Although ultraviolet B (UVB) radiation is believed to be effective in the treatment of psoriasis, it also is known to be carcinogenic. O. Larkö (Univ. of Göteborg, Sweden) and B. L. Diffey (Durham, England) assessed the natural UVB exposure of persons with various

(17–26) Acta Derm. Venereol. [Suppl. 107] (Stockh.) 1–68, 1983.
(17–27) Clin. Exp. Dermatol. 8:279–285, May 1983.

occupations in Sweden, and compared the environmental biologically effective UVB (UVB[BE]) doses with the annual radiant exposure to artificial UVB radiation received by psoriatic patients undergoing phototherapy. Personal ultraviolet doses were measured using polysulphone film badges. The UVB(BE) doses were equivalent to the hypothetical dose of monochromatic 297-nm radiation that would produce the same erythemal effect as the solar radiation measured by the film badge.

The average coefficient of variation for the mean dose received by an individual was 20%. Indoor workers received an estimated 6% of the ambient UVB(BE) dose during the summer. For patients who worked outdoors, the therapeutic dose was found to contribute about one third of their total UVB(BE), whereas for those who worked indoors, the therapeutic dose could be 50% to nearly 100% of their total UVB(BE) burden.

A large number of psoriatic patients receive very high UVB(BE) doses and must be carefully followed up. In countries at more southerly latitudes, the fraction of total UVB(BE) received for medical treatment from artificial sources of UV radiation probably is less than that received in Sweden. Hence the relative risk of malignant skin lesions resulting from the added burden of therapeutic UVB compared with solar exposure will be corrrespondingly smaller.

▶ [A large number of factors make it difficult to compare the potential carcinogenicity of exposure to natural and artificial ultraviolet radiation. This study does show that therapeutic ultraviolet radiation can contribute quite significantly to the total UVB exposure experienced by some individuals. The more widespread use of erythemogenic UVB plus emollients in the treatment of psoriasis may substantially increase the cumulative UVB dose received by psoriatic patients. In fact, the median cumulative dose (4 J/sq cm) in this study seems fairly conservative. In our experience, many patients receive 0.5–1 J of UVB per sq cm per treatment, or 20–30 times the original minimal erythemal dose, towards the end of a course of treatment for psoriasis. It is important that the value of maintenance UVB therapy in psoriasis is carefully evaluated in order that cumulative UVB doses are not needlessly increased.—R.W.G.] ◀

17–28 **Comparison of RePUVA and Aromatic Retinoid Ro 10–9359 With Methotrexate in Severe Forms of Psoriasis** is discussed by Asaf L. Mashkilleysson and Nicolas A. Mashkilleysson (Moscow Med. Stomatol. Institute). In the past 10 years psoralen–ultraviolet A (PUVA) therapy has become a widespread method of treatment for psoriasis. However, severe forms of the disease can resist treatment completely or partially. The treatment of 20 PUVA-resistant patients with aromatic retinoid Ro 10–9359 resulted in a considerable improvement of psoriasis and, in some patients, total recovery. It also potentiated a favorable clinical effect of subsequent PUVA-treatment with reduced 8 methoxypsoralen (MOP) dosage.

Aromatic retinoid was especially effective in patients with psoriatic eruptions of palms, soles, face, and scalp. The patients received PUVA treatment with 8-MOP (0.6 mg/kg of body weight)

(17–28) Hautarzt 34:229–230, May 1983.

and, after 2 hours, radiation in an ultraviolet A (UVA) high-intensity cabin. After 14 days PUVA treatment was discontinued and the patients received aromatic retinoid Ro 10–9359 (50 mg daily for 5 days and 75 mg thereafter) for as long as 21 days. Subsequently, PUVA treatment with 50% of the initial dose of 8-MOP was administered. The combination of aromatic retinoid with methotrexate was successfully used in the treatment of 2 patients with particularly severe erythrodermic psoriasis, one also having psoriatic arthritis.

During the first week of treatment with retinoid, 10 patients experienced a definite and 6 patients a moderate improvement, whereas in 4 patients no effect was observed. In the second week, psoriasis in 10 patients had completely healed on palms, soles, face, and scalp. Other areas showed considerable improvement. In 6 patients the treatment was satisfactory and in 4 patients the eruptions had faded and scaling was less. After 3 weeks, 6 patients were symptom free and all other patients showed definite improvement. Ten days after resuming the PUVA treatment, 10 patients in the remission phase together with the symptom-free patients received 3 radiation treatments per week. In 12 patients the maintenance treatment was discontinued and after 8 months no relapse had occurred.

No side effects were observed during retinoid treatment in any of the patients examined.

▶ [Despite the title, this is not a comparison of different forms of treatment, but it does provide further documentation, from Russia, of the beneficial use of a PUVA-etretinate combination in patients with tough psoriasis who were previously resistant to PUVA therapy alone. The combination of methotrexate and etretinate used in 2 patients is potentially hepatotoxic.—R.W.G.] ◀

17–29 **Preliminary Report on the Therapeutic Effect of Khellin in Psoriasis.** Studies of the effects of khellin in vitiligo have been based on the structural isomerism existing between the basic nuclei of khellin and psoralens. Aly Abdel-Fattah, M. Nabil Aboul-Enein, Gamila Wassel, and Bassem El-Menshawi (Cairo) undertook a study of the effects of khellin in a double-blind study of 20 psoriatic patients. The 10 males and 10 females, aged 14–51 years, had had psoriasis of the chronic plaque type for 2–36 years. The disease was unresponsive to conventional measures. Current treatments were withdrawn at least 3 weeks before administration of khellin in a single oral daily dose of 100 mg or placebo in a double-blind design. Treatment was followed in 1 hour by a 15-minute exposure to natural sunlight. Treatment courses of 3 weeks were separated by 9-day intervals over a 4-month period.

Three of the 10 khellin-treated patients showed marked clearing of psoriatic lesions; 4 had moderate remissions; 1 had mild improvement; and 2 failed to respond. None of the 10 controls improved. Responses were characterized by a gradual decrease in scales, flattening of lesions, and reduction in erythema. Six patients remained im-

---

(17–29) Dermatologica 167:109–110, August 1983.

proved during follow-up for three successive winters with no maintenance therapy. Two other patients had recurrences with less severe disease than was present initially.

Khellin has led to improvement in many patients with resistant psoriasis without cutaneous phototoxicity. The findings suggest that the nonpsoralen khellin may be useful in the management of psoriasis.

Khellin has led to improvement in many patients with resistant psoriasis without cutaneous phototoxicity. The findings suggest that the nonpsoralen khellin may be useful in the management of psoriasis.

▶ [It is unfortunate that we in the United States cannot confirm this report on the use of khellin in the photochemotherapy of psoriasis, or a previous report on its use in the successful treatment of vitiligo. Khellin is not a furocoumarin (as are 8-methoxypsoralen and 4.5′,8 trimethyl psoralen), and it is not a photoactive agent—at least it is not phototoxic. Khellin is isolated from the fruit of *Ammi visnaga.* It was introduced into clinical medicine in 1946 because of its direct relaxing action on visceral smooth muscle and coronary arteries. (Anrep, G. V., et al.: *Am. Heart. J.* 37:531–542, 1949). It was removed from the U.S. market by the F.D.A. allegedly because of its toxicity, but we have been unable to ascertain the exact circumstances.—T.B.F.] ◀

17–30 **Benoxaprofen Improves Psoriasis: Double-Blind Study.** The importance of lipoxygenase products in psoriasis could be assessed by treating patients with a lipoxygenase-inhibiting agent such as benoxaprofen, which is also a weak inhibitor of the cyclo-oxygenase pathway. Knud Kragballe and Troels Herlin (Univ. of Aarhus, Denmark) undertook a double-blind, placebo-controlled study of oral benoxaprofen treatment in 40 patients with psoriasis vulgaris. Half the patients received 600 mg of benoxaprofen per day orally. The two groups were comparable demographically and in the extent of involvement. The patients were adults with stable disease. Most had moderate symptoms.

Two study patients failed to complete the trial because of photosensitivity. All but 4 of the other 18 showed considerable improvement on benoxaprofen therapy, whereas only minimal changes occurred in the placebo patients. Improvement in the study group was minimal at 2 weeks but was significant after 8 weeks of treatment. It occurred more rapidly in patients whose lesions were less indurated. About half the patients given benoxaprofen had burning and stinging in exposed skin on sunny days. This effect was not related to improvement in psoriasis. Three placebo patients also reported increased sensitivity to sunlight. Onycholysis developed in a few benoxaprofen-treated patients, but it regressed after treatment was stopped. No significant laboratory abnormalities were found.

Oral administration of benoxaprofen in a dose usually used in treatment of arthritis led to excellent results in three fourths of psoriatic patients in this trial. Photosensitivity was frequent but was well tolerated by most patients and was reversible. The mechanism by which benoxaprofen acts in psoriasis remains to be determined,

---

(17–30) Arch. Dermatol. 119:548–552, July 1983.

but long-term studies on large numbers of patients were warranted. Topical treatment might be attempted to avoid systemic side effects. Lipoxygenase inhibitors may also be effective in the treatment of other inflammatory skin disorders such as cystic acne and nodular prurigo.

▶ [If this study's impressive findings are confirmed by other investigators, lipoxygenase inhibitors could become important therapeutic agents for psoriasis treatment. Unfortunately benoxaprofen is the only effective lipoxygenase inhibitor that has been used in the United States. This agent's toxicity led to its withdrawal from the U.S. market and makes it an unsuitable agent for psoriasis treatment in the general population. If lipoxygenase inhibitors help psoriasis, then dietary manipulation that results in the body's production of lipoxygenase products with less chemotactic effectiveness may also be helpful for this disease.—R.S.S.] ◀

17–31 **Etiology of Psoriasis: Clues Provided by Benoxaprofen.** B. R. Allen and S. M. Littlewood (Queen's Med. Centre, Nottingham, England) studied 24 patients with psoriasis in a double-blind trial of benoxaprofen therapy for cutaneous lesions. Treatment was continued for 8 weeks with additional assessments at 2 and 4 weeks.

Owing to the enforced premature discontinuation of the trial by several participants in both groups, the numbers in each group are small and the figures fail to reach statistical significance. But the data indicate improvement in about 50% of psoriatic patients, irrespective of the extent and severity of the lesions. Benoxaprofen alone is a potent inhibitor of 5-lipoxygenase and is not cytotoxic. Six of 13 patients on benoxaprofen showed very marked improvement.

It is believed that benoxaprofen acts by interfering with the migration of polymorphonuclear leukocytes into the skin through inhibition of leukotriene B_4 synthesis.

▶ [This and several other reports indicate that lipoxygenase inhibitors such as benoxaprofen and meclofenamate may be a step forward in the development of an effective noncytotoxic systemic agent for the treatment of psoriasis.—R.W.G.] ◀

17–32 **Colchicine in Generalized Pustular Psoriasis: Clinical Response and Antibody-Dependent Cytotoxicity by Monocytes and Neutrophils.** Colchicine inhibits polymorphonuclear leukocyte chemotaxis and has suppressed inflammatory responses in animal studies. Hugh Zachariae, Knud Kragballe, and Troels Herlin (Univ. of Aarhus, Denmark) evaluated this drug in 4 patients with generalized pustular psoriasis and erythroderma, a disorder in which neutrophils may be particularly active. The 2 males and 2 females, aged 12–74 years, had acute, generalized pustular psoriasis of the Zumbusch type, confirmed histologically. One patient had had several past episodes and had been treated with methotrexate, systemic corticosteroid administration, and psoralen and ultraviolet A (PUVA). This patient, a boy aged 12 years, received 0.5 mg of colchicine orally twice a day, and the others received 0.5 mg 3 times daily.

(17–31) Br. J. Dermatol. 109(Suppl. 25):126–129, July 1983.
(17–32) Arch. Dermatol. Res. 274:327–333, December 1982.

Three patients were afebrile after a week of colchicine therapy. Two had no pustules at this time, and a third was free of pustules after 2 weeks of treatment. Erythroderma and constitutional symptoms resolved with the pustules. One patient improved only slightly and was withdrawn from treatment. The boy with previous episodes of generalized pustular disease appeared to respond better to colchicine than to earlier measures. One patient reported mild abdominal discomfort during treatment. Leukocyte counts were normal, and no biochemical abnormalities were found. The ability of leukocytes to lyse antibody-coated human red blood cells appeared to decline during treatment, and this was less apparent in the patient who responded least to colchicine therapy.

Three of 4 patients in this study with generalized pustular psoriasis went into complete remission within 2 weeks of the start of oral colchicine therapy, and the antibody-dependent cytotoxicity of leukocytes decreased in the responsive patients. Long-term studies of larger numbers of psoriatic patients with oral low-dose colchicine therapy are needed before the drug can be established as a safe, effective treatment for pustular psoriasis.

▶ [In this short series, the results obtained using colchicine appeared to compare favorably with those of other forms of treatment for this disease, and only minor toxicity was noted.—R.W.G.] ◀

17–33 **Peritoneal Dialysis for Psoriasis: Controlled Study.** Although the clinical impression that peritoneal dialysis is helpful in relieving the signs and symptoms of psoriasis appears to be valid, this has not been demonstrated in a scientifically convincing fashion. Frederick C. Whittier, Dan H. Evans, Philip C. Anderson, and Karl D. Nolph (Univ. of Missouri, Columbia) carried out sham and real trials of peritoneal dialysis in a prospective, double-blind, controlled, crossover study of 5 patients with severe, disabling, plaque-type psoriasis. All 5 had failed to respond to conventional therapy, including methotrexate. The patients were randomly assigned to receive 4 weeks of either sham or real dialysis (48 hours of treatment once a week), followed by 8 weeks of observation. The patients then received 48 hours of the alternative treatment once a week for 4 weeks, followed by another 8 weeks of observation. Topical therapy was not discontinued during the trial.

One of 2 patients who underwent real dialysis in the first treatment period and all 3 who received real dialysis in the second showed a dramatic response. None of the patients had a favorable response to the sham procedure. Two patients who showed 75% body surface clearance had a recurrence 3–6 months later. However, each of these patients has been improved for more than 1 year after repeat uncontrolled dialysis of eight 48-hour treatments over a 4-week period. The other 2 patients who responded showed complete clearing, and 1 remained symptom free for 6 months after therapy. However, the other had a progressive relapse and continued to get worse during sham

(17–33) Ann. Intern. Med. 99:165–168, August 1983.

therapy, but had a transient good response to plasmapheresis with another experimental protocol. One patient continued to have severe, debilitating psoriasis. Three of the 4 improved patients are no longer reclusive and have returned to full-time employment. Two of the patients during a sham procedure and 2 during a real dialysis developed cloudy fluid and abdominal tenderness with presumptive peritonitis that easily cleared with administration of antibiotics and continued dialysis. No other complications were observed.

Peritoneal dialysis may be helpful in patients with severe, debilitating, plaque-type psoriasis that is refractory to conventional and other forms of therapy. Administration of a minimum of eight 48-hour treatments over a 4-week period, with an extension to 12 treatments if the response is poor, is advised. Topical therapy should be continued. Some patients can be expected to have a good response of 75% to complete clearing, though repeat treatments may be necessary to reinduce or maintain remission.

▶ [The costs and risks of peritoneal dialysis are sufficiently great that it is not a promising therapy for psoriasis. Even the patient the authors illustrate as a success would in all likelihood have done as well with ultraviolet B (UVB) and almost certainly would have done better with PUVA or methotrexate, all of which are less costly and in most persons have less associated risk. A controlled trial of hemodialysis, done by investigators who did not develop the therapy, failed to show significant benefit. There is no reason to believe that peritoneal dialysis would work better. This study of 5 patients treated with peritoneal dialysis also fails to show a significant difference between sham and actual dialysis. I believe that the only place for peritoneal or hemodialysis in psoriasis is as a research tool in attempts to identify circulating factors that may be associated with psoriasis. Dialysis is not an appropriate treatment for psoriasis.—R.S.S.] ◀

7–34 **Plasmapheresis in Treatment of Psoriasis: Controlled Clinical Study.** Ole J. Clemmensen, Rud Andresen, and Erik Andersen (Copenhagen) treated 6 patients who had long-standing, moderately active, plaque-nummular psoriasis with either plasmapheresis or sham plasmapheresis once weekly for 7 weeks in a double-blind, controlled trial. Mean age of the patients was 43.5 years, and all 6 had had psoriasis for more than 15 years. Patients were randomly assigned to either genuine or sham plasmapheresis, which was performed with an intermittent-flow blood cell separator.

One of the 3 patients in the plasmapheresis group dropped out after two treatments, but the variation in her disease was still monitored, though at longer intervals. One patient in the sham group was better on each successive evaluation and was almost without symptoms for 6 more months. Another patient in the sham group almost recovered. The other patients either worsened or were unchanged. A decrease in total serum protein concentration and values for other serum fractions was found in patients treated with plasmapheresis. No consistent changes were recorded in hemoglobin concentration, white blood cell count, or thrombocyte count.

This study showed no effect of plasmapheresis in the control of pso-

---

(17–34) J. Am. Acad. Dermatol. 8:190–192, February 1983.

riasis. A larger study might show an effect, but the authors believe the treatment is too expensive to justify a search for marginal benefit.

▶ [The lack of observed effect of plasmapheresis upon relatively mild psoriasis suggests that this treatment may indeed be ineffective. However, it is conceivable that the concomitant free use of topical treatments, including steroids, may have blurred differences that would otherwise have been observed.—R.W.G.] ◀

17–35 **Growth Hormone Levels in Psoriasis.** R. M. MacKie, G. M. Beastall, and J. A. Thomson (Glasgow, Scotland) note the recent report that human growth hormone (HGH) levels are elevated in patients with psoriasis and that therapy with somatostatin, an inhibitor of HGH, is of clinical benefit. Therefore, HGH levels were measured in 9 patients with moderate to severe psoriasis requiring hospitalization. The HGH levels were measured in fasting patients and for 2 hours after administration of 50 gm of glucose.

In 8 of the 9 patients, the basal HGH levels were below the limits of detection and remained suppressed during glucose tolerance testing. In 1 patient with severe palmoplantar pustular psoriasis, the basal HGH level was elevated and was inadequately suppressed after glucose administration.

Previous findings of elevated HGH levels in psoriatic patients could not be confirmed except in 1 patient. The benefits of somatostatin administration may not necessarily be mediated by lowering the HGH level. In addition, in about 70 patients with acromegaly, psoriasis is not a problem, even in those whose HGH levels have been poorly controlled for years.

▶ [Several reports have indicated beneficial results from the use of somatostatin in psoriasis, but the mechanisms are unclear and further confirmation is necessary. This study suggests that somatostatin does not act by decreasing an increased growth hormone level in psoriasis. Somatostatin also suppresses a variety of other hormones, and alteration of epidermal growth factor levels has been proposed as a possible mechanism of action in psoriasis (Ghirlanda et al.: *Lancet* 1:65, 1983).—R.W.G.] ◀

17–36 **Somatostatin Treatment of Psoriasis.** Increased GH concentrations have been reported in psoriatic serums, and remissions of psoriatic skin lesions have been reported to result from treatment with GH inhibitor. J. J. Guilhou, A. Boulanger, G. Barneon, P. Vic. J. Meynadier, J. C. Tardieu, and J. Clot (Montpellier, France) evaluated somatostatin infusion therapy in 18 psoriatic patients (12 men), aged 22–71 years, most of whom had had the disorder for many years. All had active psoriasis at the time of treatment. Five patients had generalized psoriasis or erythroderma, and 10 others had numerous disseminated lesions. No patient had pustular psoriasis. Arthropathy was present in 2 patients. Somatostatin in a 5% glucose solution was infused at the rate of 250 μg/hour for at least 2 days. Twelve patients subsequently received 1-hour infusions twice daily for 10 days. The other 8 patients received a continuous infusion every 2 weeks for a total of three treatments, without brief infusions.

(17–35) Arch. Dermatol. Res. 275:207, June 1983.
(17–36) Ibid., 274:249–257, December 1982.

Six patients had nearly complete clearing 1 month after the start of treatment, and 2 others had partial clearing. Pruritus always responded to treatment within a few days. Five patients were kept free of lesions for 3 months or longer. Two of them received maintenance bromocriptine therapy. Most side effects were well tolerated, but in 2 other patients treatment was stopped because of gastrointestinal difficulty and erythematous papulonodular lesions, respectively. Ultrastructural studies showed enlarged intercellular spaces, deposits of glucidic material, and signs of cell damage after 6 days of treatment. Mitogenic stimulation was significantly depressed, but proportions of T and B cells were unchanged.

Somatostatin infusion therapy may benefit some psoriatic patients, but it appears to be much less important than other established treatments for psoriasis. Because of spontaneous remissions and placebo effects, double-blind studies would be useful in evaluating such drugs as somatostatin and bromocriptine in the treatment of psoriasis.

▶ [The relatively poor response and not insubstantial toxicity produced by somatostatin in this open trial would hardly argue for devoting the resources required for an appropriate double-blind trial that would be needed to test the drug's effectiveness.—R.S.S.] ◀

7–37 **Oral Psoralen Photochemotherapy (PUVA) of Hyperkeratotic Dermatitis of the Palms.** H. Mobacken, K. Rosén, and G. Swanbeck (Univ. of Göteborg, Sweden) examined 5 patients with chronic hyperkeratotic dermatitis of the palms (HDP) without evidence of psoriasis elsewhere. Two patients also had a similar dermatitis on the soles of their feet. Three times a week, each patient ingested 8-methoxypsoralen in a dose of 0.6 mg/kg 1.5 hours before exposure to ultraviolet A (UVA) radiation. The lamp source was either PUVA 180 or UV-A-SUN 2000. The initial UVA dose of 2 J/sq cm was increased to 10 J/sq cm.

All patients responded to treatment. In 3 the lesions cleared completely for the first time in many years (Fig 17–2). In 2, the infiltration and scaling almost disappeared and there were no more fissures. For those patients whose lesions cleared, the mean number of treatments was 20 and mean total UVA dose was 123 J/sq cm. For the improved patients the corresponding figures were 19 treatments and 135 J/sq cm. Recurrences developed in all patients after 1–6 months. Lesions then gradually progressed, and new treatment became necessary in 3 patients. The interval between treatments in these patients was 2, 8, and 9 months, respectively. Results after the second course of treatment were equally good. Two patients had a third course of treatment with similar outcomes. In 3 patients erythema developed on exposed skin during the first course of psoralen and ultraviolet A (PUVA).

This study was not controlled. However, the improvement of chronic lesions irrespective of duration in all patients supports an effect of PUVA treatment. Oral administration of the psoralen was pre-

---

(17–37) Br. J. Dermatol. 109:205–208, August 1983.

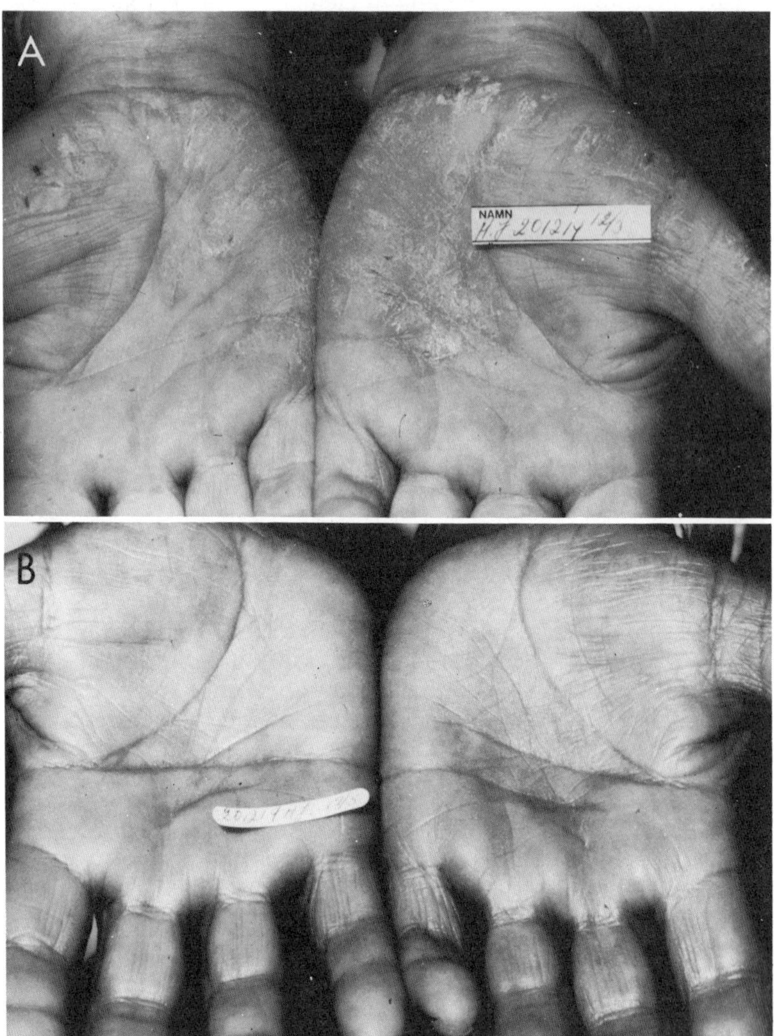

Fig 17–2.—Palms of patient with hyperkeratotic dermatitis of the palms. **A,** before photochemotherapy, and **B,** after photochemotherapy. (Courtesy of Mobacken, H., et al.: Br. J. Dermatol. 109:205–208, August 1983.)

ferred because of the risk of uneven penetration of topically applied photosensitizers.

▶ [Psoralen and ultraviolet A can be an effective alternative in the treatment of hand and foot dermatoses. When pustulation or vesiculation is present, results are not always as impressive as they were in this study.—R.W.G.] ◀

17–38 **Randomized Trial of Etretinate (Tigason) in Palmoplantar Pustulosis.** Erik Foged, Per Holm, Poul Ølholm Larsen, Grete Laur-

(17–38) Dermatologica 166:220–223, April 1983.

berg, Flemming Reymann, Kresten Roesdahle, and Susanne Ullman randomly assigned 50 patients with palmoplantar pustulosis (PPP) to receive 8 weeks of daily treatment with either oral etretinate, 1 mg/kg of body weight, or placebo in a double-blind trial. Median age of the 8 men and 42 women was 55 years. Mean duration of PPP was 3 years. Groups were comparable at allocation. Nine patients withdrew from the trial, and their data were used in analyses of side effects only. The 5 instances of dose reduction (1 on placebo) were retained in all analyses.

Etretinate was superior to placebo with regard to symptoms, difficulty in walking, and overall assessment of efficacy by the physician. This was statistically significant both as a direct treatment effect and as an interaction between treatment and time. With regard to fissures, only the interaction effect was significant. There was some improvement over time in the placebo group as well. Tolerance was less for etretinate than for placebo, chiefly because of side effects to the skin or nasobuccal mucous membranes or both.

The present study confirms previous observations that etretinate is effective in alleviating the symptoms of PPP. Good effect was obtained within 2 weeks, and only pustulation and fissuration improved further between weeks 2 and 8, indicating that it may be possible to reduce doses of etretinate after 2–4 weeks to a lower maintenance level. There were no unexpected side effects, but all patients on etretinate experienced some reactions in the mucous membranes. Changes of liver enzymes were small and equally frequent, but the authors recommend that patients with known liver disease should not be treated with etretinate.

▶ [Etretinate seems to be a viable alternative for treatment of recalcitrant palmoplantar pustulosis. It is to be hoped that the drug will soon be available in the United States for selected disabled patients.—R.R.] ◀

17–39 **Efficacy of Etretinate (Tigason) in Clearing and Prevention of Relapse of Palmoplantar Pustulosis.** A. Lassus, J. Lauharanta, T. Juvakoski, and L. Kanerva (Helsinki) used orally administered etretinate (Tigason®) to treat 40 patients with palmoplantar pustulosis (PPP) in an open trial with a maximum treatment period of 16 weeks. Those who achieved remission were then randomized to receive either a low dose of Tigason or placebo. The original 40 patients included 26 women and 14 men with a mean age of 53.2 years. Initial dose of etretinate was 0.9–1.0 mg/kg/day. In the second phase, which lasted 6 months, a low maintenance dose of 20–30 mg/day (0.14–0.38 mg/kg/day) was used.

During the first phase of treatment 26 (65%) of the 40 patients experienced complete clearing or almost complete clearing of PPP in 10.5 ± 3.6 weeks. Some improvement was seen in 4 of the remaining 14 patients. During 2–4 weeks of treatment, a rapid alleviation of desquamation, infiltration, and pustulation was seen, but erythema disappeared more slowly. After 6 months of maintenance treatment with etretinate, 7 (64%) of 11 patients remained free of lesions, but the difference from results for the placebo group did not attain statis-

(17–39) Dermatologica 166:215–219, April 1983.

tical significance. Relapses occurred after 7.5 ± 1.7 weeks in the etretinate group and after 6.3 ± 2.0 weeks in the placebo group.

Dryness of the lips and nose was the most frequent side effect. Marked hair loss occurred in 4 (10%) of the 40 patients during the first treatment period. During the second treatment period 4 patients suffered hair loss, and all 4 discontinued treatment. All 4 patients were in the placebo group, but 2 of them had shown alopecia during the last weeks of the first treatment period. Desquamation of healthy skin was seen in 10%–13% of patients during the initial 4 weeks of treatment and led to discontinuation in 2 cases. Serum triglyceride levels that were higher than normal were found in 4 patients.

Tigason showed a beneficial effect in most patients with PPP and was better than placebo in preventing relapse of the disease, but intolerable side effects restrict its use in many patients.

▶ [Etretinate is an effective agent in palmoplantar pustulosis. The side effects are usually better tolerated than the symptoms of the disease when the drug is used in severely disabling, recalcitrant disease.—R.R.] ◀

17–40 **Erythroderma: Follow-Up of 50 Cases.** Erythroderma (exfoliative dermatitis) represents a maximal stage of skin irritation due to various underlying conditions. Because the relative importance of different etiologic factors can be affected by changes in environment, Taina Hasan and Christer T. Jansén (Univ. of Turku) reviewed the findings in 50 consecutive patients hospitalized with the diagnosis of erythroderma between January 1973 and December 1980.

The 33 males and 17 females had a mean age at onset of 61.2 years (range, birth to 81 years). Dissemination of the erythroderma to the maximal degree usually took several days or weeks. All patients had itching, which was often disturbing. Balding caused by the erythroderma occurred in 5 patients, and 3 patients had a major nail deformity. About one third of the patients had frequent chills and one fourth were febrile. Lymphadenopathy was frequent, and some patients had hepatomegaly, but splenomegaly was not encountered. The most common laboratory abnormality was a pathologic serum protein

TABLE 1.—CLASSIFICATION OF ERYTHRODERMA CASES BY CAUSE IN PREVIOUS PUBLICATIONS AND IN PRESENT PATIENT SERIES

	Relative incidence (%)			
Etiology	**Wilson**	**Abrahams et al**	**Nicolis and Helwig**	**Present series**
Preexisting dermatosis	48	32	25	42
Drug reaction				
Internal medication	8	11	40	10
External medication	8	3	2	12
Malignancy	10	8	21	4
Undetermined	26	47	12	32

(Courtesy of Hasan, T., and Jansén, C.T.: J. Am. Acad. Dermatol. 8:836–840, June 1983.)

(17–40) J. Am. Acad. Dermatol. 8:836–840, June 1983.

TABLE 2.—DIAGNOSTIC SPLIT-UP IN 21 PATIENTS WITH PREEXISTENT DERMATOSIS AS CAUSATIVE FACTOR OF ERYTHRODERMA

Dermatosis	No. of cases
Atopic dermatitis	7
Psoriasis	5
Seborrheic dermatitis	5
Photosensitive eczema	2
Nummular dermatitis	1
Congenital ichthyosiform erythroderma	1

(Courtesy of Hasan, T., and Jansén, C.T.: J. Am. Acad. Dermatol. 8:836–840, June 1983.)

electrophoresis pattern, which was polyclonal in all cases and almost invariably consisted of an elevated γ-globulin fraction. An abnormally high erythrocyte sedimentation rate was often found. Almost half of the patients had eosinophilia and elevated serum IgE titers. The most frequent causal factor was a preexistent dermatosis (21 patients; 42%) (Table 1), with atopic dermatitis, psoriasis, and seborrheic dermatitis accounting for most of these cases (Table 2). Among the 5 patients whose erythroderma was related to internal medication, the dermatosis was caused by a different drug in each. In 6 patients, it was believed to result from sensitization to topically applied medications. In 2 patients, mycosis fungoides was suspected and histologically verified by repeated biopsies. No etiologic factor could be identified in 16 patients. A follow-up survey at a mean of 6 years (range, 7 months to 20 years) indicated that 17 patients had complete clearance, 12 had a reduction in severity of the disease, and 6 had no change. Ten patients died of causes unrelated to erythroderma. Overall, the best prognosis regarding clearing of the erythroderma was in patients who had an internal drug reaction, though a considerable number of patients with an undetermined cause also had resolution.

The underlying causes of erythroderma do not appear to have changed over the past several decades. Although erythroderma is extremely distressing to patients, most have a favorable prognosis.

18. Urticaria and Mast Cell Disorders

18–1 **Role of Trauma in Spreading Wheals of Hereditary Angioedema.** R. P. Warin (Bristol, England) studied 20 patients with hereditary angioedema (HAO), a disease in which swellings may spread to surrounding tissues. Sixteen of these patients were members of 5 separate families. In 12 patients the C1 esterase inhibitor (C1-INH) was diagnostically low (type A), and in 6 patients (all in 1 family) there was a functional deficiency (type B).

A prodromal rash occurred in 4 patients, all but 1 of whom had other affected relatives. In all 4 patients the prodromal rash was present for 1–4 days before severe attacks of abdominal colic and angioedema occurred, but minor attacks were not always associated with the prodromal rash. The rash was usually widespread (mainly covering the trunk) and consisted of wheals spreading out in an annular fashion. The wheal was just palpable when spreading, but not during the fading stage. Itching was not a feature. The edge of the wheal advanced at a rate of 2–3 mm/hour. Its spread was uneven, and in some sites it was more apparent in one direction. In 2 patients the center of the expanding ring may have corresponded to a site of trauma. Once formed, an angioedematous swelling often spread at a rate of 3–4 mm/hour. A blow on the temple in 1 patient caused swelling of the adjacent eyelid; within 24 hours the swelling had spread across the forehead, and after another 24 hours, to the upper lip. Although many angioedematous swellings develop without any history of preceding trauma, 13 of the 20 patients reported that localized trauma had at some time started a swelling. Abnormal pressure may also initiate the wheals.

The mechanism of the wheal spread is not known, but in HAO a rational explanation may be that, at the central point, complement changes are initiated leading to release of vasoactive substances. These or their tissue effects lead to further complement changes and more vasoactive substances at the periphery. The initiation of the expanding wheal in the HAO prodromal rash can occur not only from localized trauma but also from an acneiform folliculitis.

▶ [The cutaneous alterations preceding the episodes of angioedema in some patients with hereditary angioedema appear as a reticulate and polycyclic erythema that at times may manifest linear urticaria at the periphery (Starr, J. C., Brasher, G. W.: *J. Allergy Clin. Immunol.* 53:352, 1974; Gelfand, J. A., et al.: *N. Engl. J. Med.* 295:1444, 1976; Williamson, D. M.: *Br. J. Dermatol.* 101:549, 1979; Tappeiner, G., et al.: *Br. J. Dermatol.* 102:621, 1980). In this clinical study, the author describes wheals at sites of trauma; the wheals spread rapidly, and urticaria appears at the periphery of the expanding ring. These cutaneous lesions do not itch, an important clinical feature. It

(18–1) Br. J. Dermatol. 108:189–194, February 1983.

is important to point out that spontaneous episodes of classic urticaria are not a feature of hereditary angioedema.—N.A.S.] ◀

18–2 **Lack of Effect of Cimetidine in Chronic Idiopathic Urticaria.** L. J. Cook and Sam Shuster (Royal Victoria Infirm., Newcastle-upon-Tyne, England) carried out a controlled double-blind clinical study of an H_2-receptor blocker, alone and in combination with an H_1-receptor blocker, to treat chronic idiopathic urticaria. Twenty patients with this condition, who were aged 18–62 years, participated in the study. Each patient received all three therapy blocks: cimetidine with placebo, chlorpheniramine with placebo, or cimetidine plus chlorpheniramine. Treatments were administered in a double-blind manner and in a predetermined random order.

Cimetidine alone did not reduce whealing significantly; cimetidine with chlorpheniramine did, but not so much as chlorpheniramine alone. Both patient assessment and clinician assessment agreed on this parameter. For itching, there was a significant change with only chlorpheniramine alone for degree and duration and with both chlorpheniramine alone and in combination with cimetidine for itch severity. For side effects, 4 subjects receiving chlorpheniramine alone and 1 receiving the combination noted drowsiness.

Results of this study show that chlorpheniramine is effective in producing therapeutically useful change in whealing and itch associated with chronic idiopathic urticaria. The results do not agree with those of previous studies that suggested the combination of chlorpheniramine with cimetidine was slightly more effective than either alone in reducing the response to intradermal histamine.

▶ [Inasmuch as chronic idiopathic urticaria-angioedema is a manifestation of a variety of underlying pathobiologic mechanisms and diverse causes, it is not surprising that the therapeutic results vary from study to study. A failing of most therapeutic studies in urticaria-angioedema is the small number of patients evaluated and the short duration of the therapeutic trial.—N.A.S.] ◀

18–3 **Symptomatic Dermographism: Natural History, Clinical Features, Laboratory Investigations, and Response to Therapy.** It has been proposed that symptomatic dermographism may involve an allergic mechanism. S. M. Breathnach, R. Allen, A. Milford Ward, and M. W. Greaves investigated symptomatic dermographism in 31 females and 19 males, mean age 31 years, and 60 age-matched controls. Standard pressures were applied to the upper back at least 48 hours after discontinuance of antihistamine therapy. Thirty patients had intradermal tests with various food and antigen extracts. Twelve patients participated in a double-blind trial of 8 antihistamine regimens including chlorpheniramine, mepyramine, promethazine, ketotifen, trimeprazine, cyproheptadine, hydroxyzine alone, and hydroxyzine plus cimetidine.

The peak age at onset of symptomatic dermographism was in the second and third decades. The mean follow-up was about 5 years. Only 4 mildly affected patients improved spontaneously, and 2 re-

---

(18–2) Acta Derm. Venereol. (Stockh.) 63:265–267, 1983.
(18–3) Clin. Exp. Dermatol. 8:463–476, September 1983.

lapsed. Overall, 20% had a personal history of atopy and 16% reported migraine. Only 1 patient related the onset to scabies infection. Pruritus and whealing usually were most frequent in the evening and tended to occur episodically with relatively symptom-free intervals. The scalp and genitals were less often affected than were other body regions. Hot baths and emotion were frequently cited exacerbating factors; only 10% of patients implicated stress. Dermographometry readily distinguished the patients and the controls. Intradermal tests resulted in immediate positive reactions in 12 of 30 patients, 2 of whom were atopic. No significant laboratory abnormalities were observed on extensive testing of 41 patients. Levels of α-$_1$-antitrypsin were significantly reduced in the patients. All treatments reduced experimental whealing. Clinically, treatment with both hydroxyzine and cimetidine was most effective, followed by hydroxyzine alone and then cyproheptadine. The combination produced the fewest side effects.

The cause of symptomatic dermographism remains unclear, but the reduction in α-$_1$-antitrypsin levels suggests that anabolic steroids may be useful. The most effective treatment in the present trial was with a combination of 40 mg of hydroxyzine and 1,600 mg of cimetidine daily.

▶ [The authors have demonstrated low mean levels of α_1 antitrypsin in some subjects with symptomatic dermographism. This observation is in contrast to the previously reported findings (Doeglas H. M. G., Bleumink, E.: *Arch. Dermatol.* 11:979, 1975) of normal protease inhibitor levels in dermographism. This divergence of results may reflect differences in the patient populations studied or in the severity of the disease. An analysis of the Pi phenotypes of α_1 antitrypsin would be of interest to search for a genetic basis of this inhibitor deficiency in a subset of individuals.

The function of the regulatory protein of the complement system, the inhibitor of the first complement component (C1-INH), is absent in patients with hereditary angioedema and acquired C1-INH deficiency with angioedema (Gelfand, J. A., et al.: *N. Engl. J. Med.* 295:1444, 1976; Hauptmann, G., et al.: *Ann. Intern. Med.* 87:577, 1981), and blood levels of C1-INH return to normal after the administration of impeded androgens. On the basis of these observations, the authors suggest treatment with this class of therapeutic agent. This form of therapy remains unreported in individuals with dermographism and should be used with caution, if at all, owing to side effects.—N.A.S.] ◀

18–4 **Greater Inhibition of Dermographia With a Combination of H_1 and H_2 Antagonists.** Lyndon E. Mansfield, Joseph A. Smith, and Harold S. Nelson (Army Medical Center, El Paso, Texas) measured the dermographic response in 11 subjects with dermographia and chronic urticaria at baseline and after treatment with an H_1 antihistamine, an H_2 antihistamine, and the combination. Subjects were randomly assigned to receive in each 1-week period a 3-day course of chlorpheniramine (8 mg 4 times per day), cimetidine (300 mg 4 times per day), or the combination of the two.

There was no difference between the responses during the single-agent periods. Both agents caused some suppression when compared with the unmedicated period. Seven of 11 subjects had a decrease in

(18–4) Ann. Allergy 50:264–265, April 1983.

histamine cutaneous responses compared with baseline after chlorpheniramine, 4 of 11 during cimetidine therapy, and 10 of 11 with the combination of agents. Seven of 11 patients felt that their urticarial symptoms were less severe during the combination therapy.

The results replicate those of 2 similar studies that reported a beneficial effect of an H_1 and H_2 combination in treatment of dermographia.

18–5 **Nonfamilial, Vibration-Induced Angioedema.** Vibratory angioedema is a rare form of physical angioedema first described in familial form. Stanislaus Ting, Bernhard E. F. Reimann, David O. Rauls, and Lyndon E. Mansfield (William Beaumont Army Med. Center) report a nonfamilial case of vibration-induced angioedema in a Mexican-American boy with an elevated plasma histamine concentration.

Youth, 16, was seen for recurring attacks of prolonged swelling of the hands that followed riding a motorcycle or mowing grass. Symptoms had occurred for 3 months. Physical examination yielded normal findings, and there was no family history of allergy or angioedema. Skin tests with routine aeroallergens and foods were negative. The whealing response to intradermal codeine was normal, as was the skin test response to histamine. A methacholine test was negative. Dermatographism was not demonstrated, and a test for pressure urticaria was negative. No active serum factor was found on Prausnitz-Küstner passive transfer study.

Prolonged angioedema occurred at various body sites when an electric vibrator was used, contrasting with the transient erythema and whealing seen in family members and normal control subjects. The plasma histamine concentration increased during stimulation in the stimulated arm only. In stimulated skin, most mast cells had released their granules. Gradually increasing vibration exposures were carried out, and the patient became increasingly able to tolerate the stimulus. He was finally able to ride a motorcycle and mow the lawn without swelling of the fingers. Symptoms remained absent after 6 months. The patient continued to desensitize himself for 5 minutes every 5–7 days.

The pathogenesis of vibratory angioedema is unknown, but its clinical and histologic features, the histamine release, and the ability to develop tolerance suggest that it is a nonimmunologic immediate-type hypersensitivity reaction. The clinical problem in the present case was eliminated through development of tolerance to vibration.

▶ [A single patient with idiopathic vibration-induced angioedema was successfully treated with increasing exposures to vibration and subsequent intermittent maintenance exposures to remain asymptomatic. This type of therapy offers an alternative to the administration of antihistamines. It should be noted that vibration-induced angioedema may occur after several years of occupational exposure to vibration (Wener, M. H., et al.: *Ann. Intern. Med.* 98:44, 1983).—N.A.S.] ◀

18–6 **Exercise-Induced Anaphylaxis.** Physical stimuli can provoke anaphylaxis in sensitive persons, and Sheffer and Austen recently described anaphylaxis following exercise. Vanee Songsiridej and W. W. Busse (Univ. of Wisconsin, Madison) encountered 9 subjects with ex-

---

(18–5) J. Allergy Clin. Immunol. 71:546–551, June 1983.
(18–6) Clin. Allergy 13:317–321, July 1983.

ercise-induced anaphylaxis during the past year. The importance of exercise as a stimulator of symptoms was not always initially apparent. Symptoms developed after 20–30 minutes of exercise. All patients had prodromal features, usually including palmar pruritus, and cessation of exercise was followed by gradual recovery. All patients had urticaria, and 6 had some respiratory difficulty. Two had severe reactions including hypotension and loss of consciousness. The reactions were infrequent and unpredictable. Symptoms did not seem to be related to the intensity of exercise, or to the time of day or ambient temperature. Specific foods were not implicated. All patients were young and healthy. Five had allergic rhinitis, 2 had asthma, and 4 had a family history of atopy.

The mechanism of this type of reaction is unclear, but histamine and other mast cell–related vasoactive substances may be involved. Further study of the events triggering mast cell–mediator release is needed. Exercise-induced anaphylaxis is not a rare disorder, and it can be life-threatening. No effective prophylactic measures are known. Patients should be instructed in the self-administration of epinephrine and should be advised to stop exercising if prodromal symptoms develop. In addition, they would be wise to exercise with a partner who is able to administer epinephrine.

▶ [This report adds additional individuals with exercise-induced anaphylaxis to the literature. Of importance to the dermatologist is the fact that all of the afflicted individuals experience pruritus and urticaria-angioedema. This condition has been noted to be a form of physical allergy distinct from cholinergic urticaria. Histamine was released into the circulation after experimental challenge (Sheffer, A. L., et al.: *J. Allergy Clin. Immunol.* 71:311, 1983).—N.A.S.] ◀

18–7 **Testing for Hepatitis B Virus in Patients With Chronic Urticaria and Angioedema.** Chronic urticaria and angioedema (CUA) may affect as many as 20% of persons during their lifetimes, yet the cause of these disorders is established in no more than 20% of cases. As a relation between acute urticaria and hepatitis B virus (HBV) has been recognized, George A. Vaida, Maury A. Goldman, and Kurt J. Bloch (Harvard Med. School) sought serologic markers of HBV infection in serum from 85 (75%) of 114 consecutive patients with CUA seen from February 1980 through December 1981.

Fifteen (17.6%) of the patients had serologic evidence of exposure to HBV. Of these, 13 were found to have antibody to hepatitis B surface antigen (anti-HBs) and 2 had hepatitis B surface antigen (HBsAg). No patient had both HBsAg and anti-HBs in the same sample of blood. Of the 13 patients with anti-HBs, 6 had urticaria alone, 3 had CUA, and 4 had angioedema alone. The serum samples containing HBsAg were obtained from 1 patient with urticaria alone and 1 with CUA. In 2 patients who had HBsAg in their serum, chronic persistent hepatitis was diagnosed, suggesting a causal relation between CUA and HBV infection. None of the 15 patients had a history of previous blood transfusions or of hepatitis. Four were involved in occupations that might be associated with an increased prevalence of

---

(18–7) J. Allergy Clin. Immunol. 72:193–198, August 1983.

exposure to blood and blood products. The median duration of CUA in these 15 patients was 35 months, which is fairly long.

In this series the incidence of current and previous HBV infection was several times higher than that reported for the general population. Further investigation of the relation between CUA and HBV infection is warranted.

▶ [To the list of diseases associated with recurrent (chronic) urticaria-angioedema can be added chronic active hepatitis. In one instance, biopsy examination of an urticarial skin lesion showed changes suggestive of cutaneous necrotizing vasculitis. It is of interest that 15.3% of patients with chronic episodes of urticaria-angioedema had antibody to hepatitis B surface antigen, suggesting a possible relation.—N.A.S.] ◀

18–8 **Cold Urticaria Associated With Infectious Mononucleosis.** L. Y. Frank Wu, Wesley Mesko, and Bruce H. Peterson (St. Vincent Hosp., Indianapolis) evaluated 2 patients with cold urticaria associated with infectious mononucleosis and reviewed 3 case reports of patients with this syndrome.

Case 1—Man, 26, presented with a 1-week history of pruritus, erythema, urticaria, and lip swelling that first appeared after ingesting cold foods and later occurred after exposure to cold air or contact with cold surfaces. Presence of cold urticaria was confirmed by a positive response to an ice cube test. A Mono Spot test was positive. Results of cryoglobulin determination, antinuclear antibody, and rapid plasma reagin tests were negative 2 days after disappearance of cold urticaria. Fluorescent antibody titers for Epstein-Barr virus (EBV) were 1:40 in the acute phase and 1:80 in the convalescent phase. The patient chose not to use medication, and cold urticaria disappeared 3 days after initial visit.

Case 2—Male, 17, had a 4-day history of generalized pruritus, urticaria, and numbness of his tongue upon cold exposure. His younger brother had infectious mononucleosis 3 weeks earlier. The patient later developed sore throat and increased malaise. Presence of cold urticaria was confirmed by a positive response to an ice cube test. A Mono Spot test was positive. Fluorescent antibody titer for EBV was 1:640, and tests for cryoglobulin were positive.

Reports of 3 similar patients (1 female and 2 males) involved patients who were in the age group that develops infectious mononucleosis. One patient had atopy; one had urticaria and angioedema as well as systemic anaphylaxis and other cold-related symptoms. One patient had cryoglobulins in his serum but no cold agglutinins, whereas another patient had a reverse pattern of absence of cryoglobulins and presence of cold agglutinins. The third patient had cryoglobulins and cryofibrinogens.

The accumulated information indicates that the urticarias induced by cold are a result of degranulation of mast cells and the release of chemical mediators. Mechanisms by which cold stimulates mast cell degranulation vary with different types of cold urticarias. Urticaria and other skin eruptions occur in about 5% of patients with infectious mononucleosis. Cold sensitivity in this patient group may be more common than was previously thought.

(18–8) Ann. Allergy 50:271–274, April 1983.

▶ [Infectious mononucleosis was associated with transient acquired cold-induced urticaria-angioedema in a small number of individuals. Importantly, one or more types of cryoproteins, including cryoglobulins, cryofibrinogens, or cold agglutinins, were present in each patient. The cold sensitivity may antedate the symptoms and signs of infectious mononucleosis.—N.A.S.] ◀

18–9 **Association of Chronic Urticaria and Angioedema With Thyroid Autoimmunity.** Chronic urticaria has been associated with hyperthyroidism, though none of the patients in whom this association was observed were studied for thyroid autoimmunity. Arthur Leznoff, Robert G. Josse, Judah Denburg, and Jerry Dolovich describe the clinical and laboratory findings in 17 patients with idiopathic chronic urticaria and angioedema (CUA) and elevated serum titers of thyroid microsomal antibodies (TMAs), identified among 140 consecutive patients with chronic urticaria, with or without angioedema, seen over a 4-year period.

All 17 patients had persistently elevated serum TMA titers of 1:1600 or greater. The patients were aged 12–71 years, and all but 2 were female. The CUA had been present for 3 months to 12 years. Follow-up ranged from 3 to 46 months. All 17 patients had daily flare-ups of urticaria, and all experienced recurrent episodes of angioedema. Antihistamines failed to control urticaria and angioedema in 9 patients, and prednisone was prescribed to reduce the severity of disease, but not to suppress it completely. One patient had life-threatening occurrences of angioedema involving the airway. No patient had a history suggestive of cold urticaria or cholinergic urticaria, and in none did food, drugs, or other identifiable causes precipitate the disease. In 2 patients, however, aspirin potentiated the disease; avoidance of salicylate, benzoate, and food dyes did not produce remission. Coexistent diseases were not temporally related to CUA. One patient had already-proved allergic disease. In 4 patients, skin biopsies showed dermal edema and a sparse, perivascular, mononuclear cell infiltrate with no vasculitis and no IgG, IgA, IgM, or C3 deposits. Few immunologic abnormalities were observed in the 17 patients. Low titers of antinuclear antibodies (ANA) were seen in 3 serum samples, slightly depressed C4 concentrations were found in 2, and weakly elevated concentrations of circulating immune complexes were present in 5. Intracutaneous injection of 3 patients' serums into volunteers did not elicit local whealing. Three patients had evidence of hyperthyroidism when first seen. One of these required thiourea therapy, and his CUA disappeared after 2 months of treatment. The second patient had a spontaneous return of euthyroid function, but her CUA subsided only after treatment with 0.2 mg of levothyroxine sodium per day for 3 months. The third patient remained mildly hyperthyroid without treatment and with persistent CUA. Fourteen patients were euthyroid when first seen. Five of 7 showed improvement or disappearance of CUA, usually within 2 months, when treated with 0.2 mg of levothyroxine sodium per day. Three of the euthyroid patients became hypothyroid during the observation period. The CUA subsided

(18–9) Arch. Dermatol. 119:636–640, August 1983.

in 2 of these after 2 months of treatment with 0.2 mg of levothyroxine per day. Once begun, levothyroxine was continued in all patients whose urticaria improved, as it is an appropriate treatment for autoimmune thyroiditis as well as hypothyroidism.

Since the cause of CUA is infrequently diagnosed, the presence of thyroid autoimmunity in 12.1% of the subjects in this study—and in 17.3% of the female subjects—is of clinical importance. Patients, especially females, with persistent urticaria and recurrent angioedema should be examined for thyroid autoimmunity.

▶ [The recognition of an association between recurrent (chronic) urticaria-angioedema and autoimmune thyroid disorders with elevated levels of thyroid microsomal antibodies adds another group of medical disorders to the list of diseases to be sought in patients with recurrent urticaria-angioedema. Of note is the observation that other thyroid function studies, such as triiodothyronine uptake and thyroxine levels are usually normal and thyroglobulin antibodies are absent. It was disappointing to note that the treatment of the underlying thyroid disease was not associated with consistent remission of the urticaria-angioedema.—N.A.S.] ◀

18–10 **Chronic Urticaria in Childhood: Natural Course and Etiology.** A number of immunologic and other factors have been implicated in the pathogenesis of chronic urticaria, but most affected persons have no identifiable cause. Alan Harris, Frank J. Twarog, and Raif S. Geha (Harvard Med. School) reviewed the findings in 94 children younger than age 16 years with urticaria that had been present for 6 weeks or longer. All were followed for at least 2 months. The sex distribution was equal, as was the age distribution within the pediatric range. Median age at onset of urticarial symptoms was 6.8 years. Seventy-nine patients had urticaria alone, 9 had angioedema alone, and 6 had both. Six patients also had arthralgia. Atopic disease was not significantly more frequent than in control subjects.

Precipitating factors were suspected by patients or parents in nearly two thirds of cases. Six patients were lymphopenic, and 17 had a sedimentation rate of more than 20 mm in the first hour. Possible underlying disorders are listed in the table. A presumptive cause of

POSSIBLE UNDERLYING DIAGNOSIS IN 94 CHILDREN WITH CHRONIC URTICARIA

Etiology	Number of Patients
Physical	
Cold	8
Infectious	
Sinusitis	1
Hepatitis	1
Immunologic	
Juvenile rheumatoid arthritis	1
Arthralgia with positive ANA	1
Complement defect (low CH_{50})	1
Allergic	
Food	2
Unknown	79

(Courtesy of Harris A., et al.: Ann. Allergy 51:161–165, August 1983.)

(18–10) Ann. Allergy 51:161–165, August 1983.

urticaria was identified or suspected in 15 patients. Eight patients had cold urticaria. The median duration of urticarial symptoms in 52 patients followed for a year or longer (mean, 2 years) was 16 months. Urticaria resolved more frequently in girls than in boys and in children younger than age 8 years, but the differences were not significant. The outcome could not be related to the presence of angioedema, a history of atopy, or associations of urticarial symptoms with food, medication, physical agents, or other factors.

Chronic urticaria in children appears to be a benign disorder, usually of unknown cause. Only systemic symptoms such as those suggesting infection or collagen vascular disease warrant an extensive work-up. If a specific cause is not identified, primary management includes an H_1 antihistamine. Continuous administration is most effective, and tachyphylaxis to the soporific effect of the drug usually develops. Addition of an H_2 antagonist is sometimes helpful. Systemic corticosteroid therapy is reserved for severe or acute exacerbations.

▶ [In this study of recurrent chronic urticaria in 94 children, causes were suspected or found in only 15 individuals, of whom 8 had cold urticaria. As has been recognized previously in adults, extensive laboratory evaluation is unnecessary in most children. A careful history and physical examination provide better clues to suspected causes.—N.A.S.] ◀

18–11 **Histologic Studies of Chronic Idiopathic Urticaria.** Sheila Farkas Natbony, Mildred E. Phillips, Jules M. Elias, H. P. Godfrey, and Allen P. Kaplan (SUNY Stony Brook) obtained skin biopsy specimens from 43 consecutive patients with chronic idiopathic urticaria and from 7 normal controls to quantitate the various cells present in this condition and to determine which ones predominate. Minimal duration of urticaria was 8 weeks; maximal duration was 4 years. Two 4-mm punch skin biopsies in two adjacent sites that were part of the same urticarial lesion were performed in each subject.

Histologic results indicated that normal skin from controls contained a small number of cells infiltrating the dermis, with minimal accumulation around small venules. By comparison, patients with chronic urticaria had an infiltrate evident throughout the dermis, which was more prominent in the superficial region beneath the epidermis. There were also obvious areas of infiltration surrounding small venules. Cellular infiltrates of chronic urticaria consisted of mononuclear cells, mast cells, eosinophils, and neutrophils. Basophils were not seen in chronic urticaria. No difference in the mean number of neutrophils, eosinophils, or basophils was seen when the urticarial and control populations were compared. The major differences noted were that patients with chronic urticaria had a four-fold increase in the number of mononuclear cells surrounding small blood vessels, and the number of mast cells was increased 10-fold.

Chronic urticaria is characterized by a nonnecrotizing perivascular lymphocytic infiltrate with an accumulation of mast cells. The origin is unknown. Patients with vasculitis and urticaria are considered to

---

(18–11) J. Allergy Clin. Immunol. 71:177–183, February 1983.

be a separate subpopulation in which the cause and pathogenesis of hive formation is probably different.

▶ [The data on numbers of infiltrating cells in chronic idiopathic urticaria are reported as mean numbers of cells. It is conceivable that this form of analysis obscures different patterns of cell infiltration, which might be expected in an entity with more than one possible molecular pathobiologic mechanism. Of interest, however, is the observation of increased numbers of mast cells. In this consecutive study, it should be noted that 1 of 43 patients had urticaria as a manifestation of necrotizing vasculitis. At the present time the prevalence of necrotizing vasculitis in patients with chronic idiopathic urticaria remains unknown.—N.A.S.] ◀

18–12 **Treatment of Bullous Mastocytosis With Disodium Cromoglycate.** Bullous mastocytosis is a rare variant of mastocytosis in which bullae predominate. It occurs early in childhood and can be complicated by ulceration and infection. Previously, treatment has been symptomatic. Elizabeth A. Welch, Joseph C. Alper, Hendrick Bogaars, and David S. Farrell (Brown Univ.) report the successful use of oral disodium cromoglycate therapy, as described by Soter, in two children with bullous mast cell disease, both of whom had failed to respond to conventional treatment.

Girl, aged 9 months, had developed recurrent crops of erythematous, pruritic, urticarial papules and vesicles on the abdomen and groin at age 5 months. She had otherwise been well. There was a strong family history of asthma and seasonal rhinitis. The entire trunk and groin were involved by age 6 months, when biopsy showed dermal mast cell infiltration and a subepidermal bulla. Cyproheptadine therapy produced no change in the eruption. Episodes at age 8 months were associated with vomiting and diarrhea and with extensive bulla formation and widespread erosions. Areas of pink pap-

Fig 18–1 (left).—Healing and active lesion.
Fig 18–2 (right).—Close-up showing scotch-grained surface.
(Courtesy of Welch, E.A., et al.: J. Am. Acad. Dermatol. 9:349–353, September 1983.)

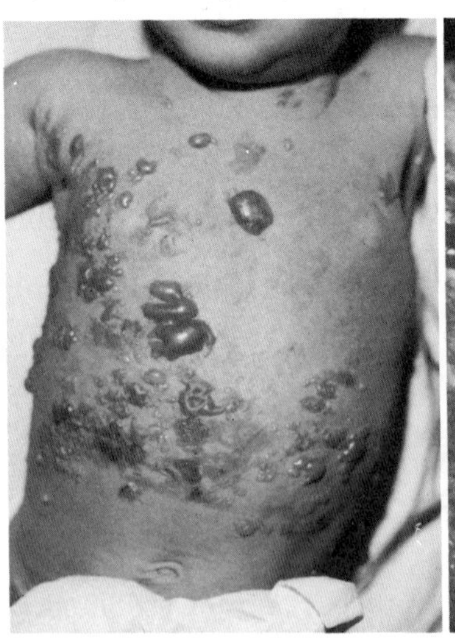

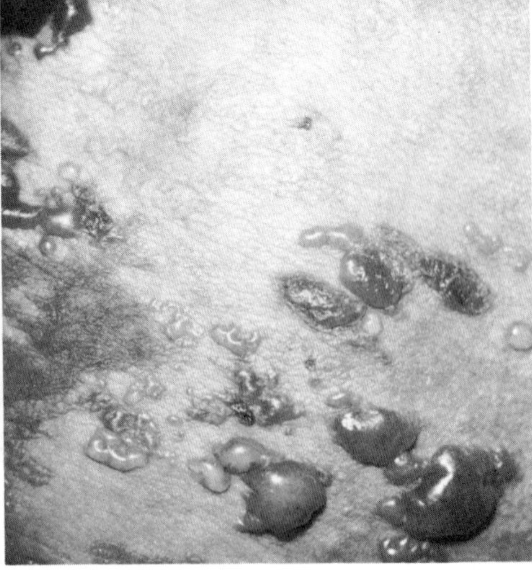

(18–12) J. Am. Acad. Dermatol. 9:349–353, September 1983.

ules and leather-grained skin were surmounted by numerous 0.2–1-cm clear bullae and erosions (Figs 18–1 and 18–2). Dermatographism was observed. On topical treatment with Burow's solution and oral administration of cyproheptadine and disodium cromoglycate, the latter in a dose of 5 mg every 12 hours, new bullae stopped forming and the erosions began to re-epithelialize. A further episode associated with persistent fever was complicated by gram-positive coccal infection, which responded to dicloxacillin therapy. Only an occasional bulla occurred in the next year. The infant has received disodium cromoglycate orally in daily doses of 160–200 mg.

A number of clinical features distinguish bullous mastocytosis from other forms of mastocytosis and from primary blistering disorders. Systemic involvement may or may not be present in bullous mastocytosis. Many patients improve spontaneously after a few years, but serious medical complications can occur in the active phase of disease, and it can significantly impair psychosocial development of the child. Adverse effects from oral disodium cromoglycate therapy for mastocytosis have not been described. The risk-benefit ratio would seem to be highly favorable, but use of the drug should be closely monitored.

▶ [This clinical report documents the efficacy of the oral administration of disodium cromoglycate in the control of bullous skin lesions in two children with mastocytosis. It is important to note that side effects have not yet been reported after the oral administration of this drug, which makes it an attractive therapeutic consideration in patients of all ages with mastocytosis.—N.A.S.] ◀

19. Vascular Lesions

19–1 **Moist Wound Healing Under Vapor Permeable Membrane.** Joseph C. Alper, Elizabeth A. Welch, Michael Ginsberg, Hendrick Bogaars, and Patricia Maguire (Providence, R.I.) studied 10 ambulatory patients with unilateral and 8 with bilateral ulcers of various etiologies to determine the effects of keeping a wound bed moist under a water vapor and oxygen permeable membrane (VPM). In the bilateral group, VPM healing was compared with that achieved with use of a debriding enzyme ointment and 10% benzoyl peroxide in the same patient.

The healing rate achieved with VPM was significantly faster than that achieved with the control substances ($P < .05$). In the unilateral group, 2 patients with ulcers to the bone or into the joint capsule, and 1 in whom grafting failed had ulcer healing without surgery with the VPM treatment. Healing with VPM failed in 2 patients. All healing occurred despite gross bacterial contamination. Cellulitis developed in 3 patients treated with VPM, but all 3 responded to standard therapy with either semisynthetic penicillin or cephalexin.

These results indicate that VPM-treated ulcers heal significantly faster than control ulcers treated with standard measures. On the average, VPM-treated ulcers healed 2.6 times faster than controls did, even though the larger and/or deeper ulcer was selected for VPM therapy. Also, these good results were achieved in most patients managed on an outpatient basis.

▶ [Striking improvements in ulcer healing have been reported with the use of vapor permeable membranes of which several types are presently in use (e.g., Duoderm, Tegoderm, Opsite). Upon initial encounter, the technique of wound occlusion, which would promote increased bacterial growth, appears to be the opposite of that needed to encourage healing. Nonetheless, moist wounds seem to heal faster than dry wounds in part because epithelia appear to have an easier time migrating over moist surfaces than over dry surfaces.—A.J.S.] ◀

19–2 **Sympathectomy in Treatment of Chronic Venous Leg Ulcers.** R. Don Patman (Baylor Medical Center, Dallas) observes that it has been estimated that 10 times as many persons have chronic venous disease of the lower extremities as have arterial disease with leg symptoms. Twenty-three patients with refractory, chronic, recurrent postphlebitic ulcers who underwent lumbar sympathectomy were studied. They were aged 23–74 years; 60% were women. The patients had undergone 47 prior operations directed at controlling ulcers, including skin grafts, wide local excision with grafting, and various localized or extensive vein ligations, strippings, or both.

(19–1) J. Am. Acad. Dermatol. 8:347–353, March 1983.
(19–2) Arch. Surg. 117:1561–1565, December 1982.

At the time performance of sympathectomy was entertained, no further operation directed at control of venous hypertension seemed to be indicated, and all patients had optimal conservative management for 4–32 months. After sympathectomy and without change of any other therapy, all ulcers healed within 2–6.5 months after operation. During follow-up of 2.5–11 years, 18 patients remained free from ulcers. One patient died after 3 years without ulcer recurrence. Four patients had recurrence; in 3, recurrent ulceration promptly healed after resumption of their previous regimens. In only 1 patient did the ulcers remain refractory, except under sedentary conditions.

Sympathectomy should not be used indiscriminately in this condition. Perfect-flawless compression therapy is the single most important principle in management of ulcerations of the legs associated with postphlebitis syndrome. Sympathectomy is a simple and effective adjunctive method of surgical management for the occasional patient with long-standing, recurrent, intractable postphlebitic ulceration. It does not preclude or replace classic therapy that assists in control of the altered fluid dynamics responsible for the ulcerations.

▶ [This article is interesting, and it is possible that sympathectomy may be beneficial in helping to heal refractory venous stasis ulcers. However, this study does not prove the point because of one major flaw: an inappropriate control group. Each patient was used as his or her own control, the control period being a varying amount of time spent with aggressive, *outpatient* therapy. The treatment period consisted of the sympathectomy and the postoperative, *inpatient* treatment (length of time not specified) followed by discharge. The appropriate control group would have been an equal number of patients admitted to the hospital for the same length of time with the same topical therapy as the patients who underwent sympathectomy. The real cause of healing may have been only the enforced bed rest during inpatient and outpatient convalescence.—J.C.A.] ◀

19–3 **Frostbite Injuries: Rational Approach Based on Pathophysiology.** Robert L. McCauley, David N. Hing, Martin C. Robson, and John P. Heggers observe that the breakdown products of arachidonic acid have been implicated as mediators of progressive dermal ischemia in both cold and thermal injuries. Increased tissue survival can be demonstrated experimentally with preservation of the dermal microcirculation by use of antiprostaglandin agents and thromboxane inhibitors. A protocol designed to decrease production of thromboxane locally and prostaglandins systemically was used to treat frostbite in 38 consecutive patients (28 males), aged 2 months to 46 years, at the University of Chicago's Burn Center in January 1982.

All patients treated by this protocol healed without major tissue loss of the affected areas. Two patients with acute second-degree frostbite showed progression of their injury to third-degree frostbite, with development of hemorrhagic blisters. Both patients healed without further tissue damage and no tissue loss. One other patient with deep second-degree frostbite of the ears showed some tissue necrosis, but reconstruction was unnecessary. Average hospital stay for acute frostbite patients was 5.6 days, and that for patients with subacute frostbite (seen more than 24 hours after exposure) was 6.9 days.

(19–3) J. Trauma 23:143–147, February 1983.

Although success was uniform in this study, the patients were not prospectively randomized. However, previous experimental and clinical data implicating prostaglandins and thromboxane in progressive dermal ischemia are quite strong. Further, nontreatment of these patients in such a study is unjustifiable.

▶ [This article presents interesting but unsubstantiated data which could have implications for other vaso-occlusive disorders. One problem in this report is that a control group was not used. Also, the patients were treated with, in addition to aspirin, the prostaglandin inhibitor, debridement of clear blisters, topical application of *Aloe vera,* elevation and splinting of the affected part, intravenous penicillin, and daily hydrotherapy. The study needs to be repeated using a control group being treated the same *except* for the use of the antiprostaglandin agent.—J.C.A.] ◀

19–4 **Direct Immunofluorescence in Pyoderma Gangrenosum.** F. C. Powell, A. L. Schroeter, H. O. Perry, W. P. D. Su (Mayo Clinic and Found.) performed direct immunofluorescence studies in 51 patients with pyoderma gangrenosum. Biopsy specimens were taken from the peripheral erythematous zone of the lesion. The cause of this disorder remains unknown, but several studies report disordered immune responses in patients with pyoderma gangrenosum.

In 31 (61%) patients, a positive result was obtained on direct immunofluorescence, and those with multiple biopsy specimens had a higher positive yield (13 [18%] of 16) than did those with a single biopsy specimen (20 [57%] of 35). Perivascular or intravascular deposition of immune reactants was the most frequent pattern, present in 27 of 31 patients with positive results on immunofluorescence; IgM and C3 were the reactants seen most frequently. Both superficial and deep vessels were involved in equal numbers. Arteriolar fluorescent involvement was found frequently. In 41 patients another disease was associated with the pyoderma gangrenosum; however, the presence or type of associated disease did not influence the immunofluorescent findings. In only 1 of 30 controls was there vascular fluorescence (C3).

When biopsies are performed on perilesional erythematous skin, most specimens of pyoderma gangrenosum yield positive results on direct immunofluorescence, although previous studies have generally reported negative results. In these patients, the intense vascular fluorescence involving both superficial and deep vessels suggests immune-mediated damage of these vessels. When considered with the lymphocytic vasculitis in these patients, the presence of immune reactants in and around the vessels suggests that vascular damage may be significant in the pathogenesis of pyoderma gangrenosum.

▶ [These authors imply that the presence of immunoreactants in superficial and deep vessels in the erythematous areas adjacent to the ulcers of pyoderma gangrenosum "support[s] a vasculitis pathogenesis." In our opinion this statement is too strong. To use healthy volunteers' normal skin for comparison with a zone of erythema about an ulcer is not a real control. Zones of erythema surrounding other non-pyoderma-gangrenosum ulcers would be more useful. Inflamed vessels, it seems, are sites of deposition of immunoreactants. Although these findings are interesting, we believe they are still very circumstantial evidence.—M.C.A.] ◀

(19–4) Br. J. Dermatol. 108:287–293, March 1983.

19–5 **Pyoderma Gangrenosum and Crohn's Disease: Eight Cases and a Review of the Literature.** Pyoderma gangrenosum is an uncommon, progressive, ulcerative cutaneous disorder of obscure cause and is associated with a number of chronic debilitating diseases such as ulcerative colitis. It has been considered to be rare in association with Crohn's disease. David J. Schoetz, Jr., John A. Coller, and Malcolm C. Veidenheimer (Lahey Clinic Med. Center, Burlington, Mass.) reviewed 961 cases of Crohn's disease seen between 1957 and 1980 and found 8 cases associated with pyoderma gangrenosum, for an incidence of 0.8%. Average age at which Crohn's disease was diagnosed was 30 years. Two patients were first seen with both Crohn's disease and pyoderma. In the other 6 patients, pyoderma developed an average of 7.3 years after the onset of Crohn's disease. Crohn's disease was diagnosed histologically in 5 patients. Five patients had ileocolitis, 2 colitis, and 1 ileitis. In 6 patients only the legs were involved by pyoderma. Only 1 patient had a definite history of trauma preceding pyoderma. The activity of pyoderma paralleled that of the bowel disease in 5 patients. Three patients had extraintestinal manifestations of Crohn's disease, and 2 patients had involvement of the anus. Four patients had intralesional as well as systemic corticosteroid therapy. Local measures were used to prevent secondary infection. The most important factor in the outcome was control of the underlying bowel disease.

Pyoderma gangrenosum is a clinical diagnosis. It may be seen in otherwise healthy persons, but most often a debilitating condition is present, most prominently inflammatory bowel disease. The pathophysiologic nature of pyoderma is unclear. Close correlation between the activity of Crohn's disease and the course of pyoderma was apparent in most patients in this study. Treatment is directed to the bowel disease. Both medical control of the disease and bowel resection lead to improvement of the pyoderma in many patients. Local measures such as debridement and topical antibiotic therapy are used where indicated to prevent secondary local septic complications.

19–6 **Pyoderma Gangrenosum and Monoclonal Gammopathy.** Frank C. Powell, Arnold L. Schroeter, W. P. Daniel Su, and Harold O. Perry (Mayo Clinic and Found.) reviewed the records of 8 patients with pyoderma gangrenosum and monoclonal gammopathy seen during a 12-year period to clarify the relationship between the 2 conditions.

In 7 of the 8 patients, pyoderma gangrenosum preceded the detection of monoclonal gammopathy; in 1, onset of both conditions was noted simultaneously. Seven patients had an IgA gammopathy and 1 had an elevated IgM level. Four had λ light chains and 4 had κ light chains. The bone marrow in 5 of 8 patients showed an increased number of plasma cells. Light chains were found in the urine in 3 pa-

---

(19–5) Dis. Colon Rectum 26:155–158, March 1983.
(19–6) Arch. Dermatol. 119:468–472, June 1983.

tients. Follow-up examinations ranged from 6 months to 11 years. One patient died of multiple myeloma after 6 months, but all of the others retained characteristics of benign monoclonal gammopathy. All cutaneous lesions were typical of pyoderma gangrenosum, and their duration varied from 3 months to 13 years. All lesions had raised, tender, bluish borders with undermined edges and were located mainly on the buttocks, thighs, and lower legs, except for 2 patients, in whom they were widely disseminated. Direct immunofluorescent microscopy, done in 5 patients, yielded positive results in 3, showing granular deposition of C3 at the basement membrane. Some patients responded well to sulfapyridine treatment, whereas others responded to dapsone and prednisone. Clofazimine, thalidomide, and cromolyn sodium were without benefit. Melphalan administration and plasmapheresis in 1 patient resulted in improvement. Three patients had thyroid gland abnormalities, and 3 had arthritis; none had ulcerative colitis.

Reports of the incidence of monoclonal gammopathy with pyoderma gangrenosum vary. In the present study, pyoderma gangrenosum preceded the detection of monoclonal gammopathy, except in the 1 patient. The most effective treatment for the skin lesions in these patients was that commonly used in pyoderma gangrenosum: administration of sulfapyridine, dapsone, and prednisone or a combination of these drugs. In patients with resistant skin lesions, it may be worthwhile to treat the paraproteinemia in an effort to control the lesions.

▶ [The two abstracts above describe two different associations of pyoderma gangrenosum (PG). One group of 8 cases was associated with Crohn's disease, the most common finding being ileocolitis. The PG responded best to treatment of the Crohn's disease and tended to recur with exacerbations of the intestinal problem. The overall incidence of PG is about 1% in patients with Crohn's disease. One fourth of the patients (2) presented simultaneously with PG and Crohn's disease, whereas in the remaining 6, PG appeared an average of 7 years later.

In the second group there was no bowel disease but an associated monoclonal gammopathy. The PG presented before the gammopathy in 7 cases and simultaneously in 1 case. The gammopathy was of the IgA class in 7 patients and IgM in 1. Most monoclonal gammopathies are IgG, with 10% IgA and 10% IgM. One patient developed multiple myeloma, the other 7 remained as benign gammopathies. The authors found about 12% of patients with PG had a gammopathy.

In PG the sex ratio is usually one, whereas 7 of 8 patients in this second series were males. Both articles list some of the many associated diseases. Both indicate that the histology of PG is generally nonspecific, and both indicate that the pathogenesis of PG is unknown. An immunoelectrophoresis as well as a bowel evaluation should be part of the PG workup.—R.M.] ◀

19–7 **Kasabach-Merritt Syndrome in Infants.** Kasabach-Merritt syndrome consists of thrombocytopenia, microangiopathic hemolytic anemia, and acute or chronic consumption coagulopathy associated with a rapidly enlarging hemangioma. Nancy Burton Esterly (Children's Meml. Hosp., Chicago) describes 4 infants with large hemangiomas and hematologic abnormalities.

Boy, aged 7 weeks, had a cavernous hemangioma at birth that gradually

---

(19–7) J. Am. Acad. Dermatol. 8:504–513, April 1983.

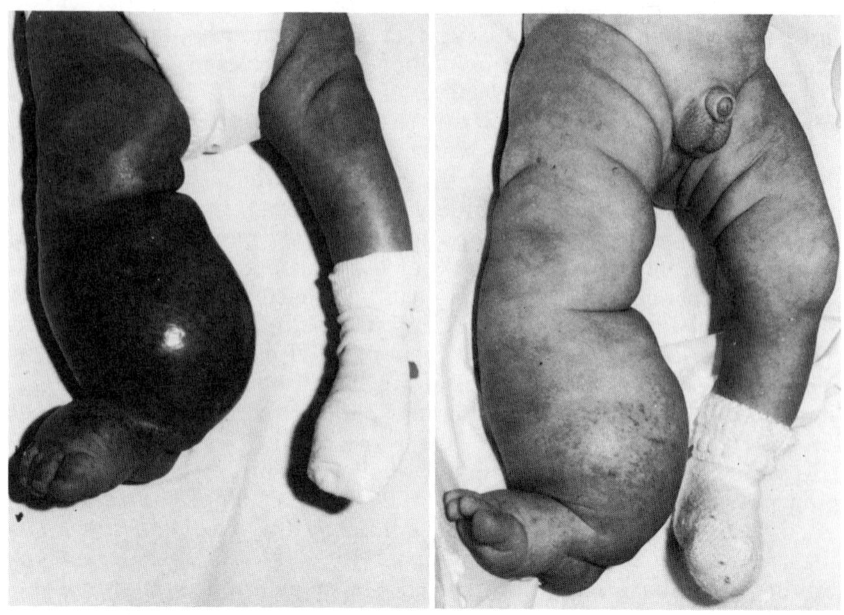

Fig 19–1 (left).—Hemangioma of right leg at age 10 weeks.
Fig 19–2 (right).—Same hemangioma at age 8 months.
(Courtesy of Esterly, N.B.: J. Am. Acad. Dermatol. 8:504–513, April 1983.)

enlarged. The compressible mass extended from the right ankle to below the knee. The hemoglobin concentration was 10.8 gm/dl, and platelet count was 87,000/cu mm. Prednisone, 2 mg/kg/day, was prescribed. By age 10 weeks, the leg had enlarged several centimeters (Fig 19–1), and was firm to palpation, and ecchymoses and petechiae were visible in the taut skin over the hemangioma. A compressible, 3-cm inguinal mass was felt on the right side. The hemoglobin concentration was 8.9 gm/dl; platelet count, 9,000/cu mm; fibrinogen, 85%; factor V, 64%; prothrombin time (PT), 15.8 seconds; and partial thromboplastin time (PTT), 52.8 seconds. The prednisone dosage was increased to 3 mg/kg/day. At age 3 months, leg edema was significantly decreased, petechiae had disappeared, and the groin mass was smaller and softer. The platelet count was 35,000/cu mm; fibrinogen, 51 mg/dl; fibrin split products, greater than 10; PT, 16.5/11.3 seconds; and PTT, 46.5 seconds. At age 7 months, all laboratory results were normal, and prednisone was discontinued at age 8 months. The right leg, although larger and firmer than the left, was less discolored and the circumferential measurement was decreasing (Fig 19–2). At age 1 year, the boy was standing and walking despite the hemangioma, which was regressing.

Kasabach-Merritt syndrome occurs primarily during the first few weeks; the median age in one report was 5 weeks, but older children and adults can also be affected. In some patients, the coagulopathy has been aggravated or precipitated by operations or angiography, and in gravid women, by delivery or therapeutic abortion. Mortalities have ranged from 20% to 30%. Findings that are suspect include pallor, spontaneous petechiae and ecchymoses, rapid change in size and appearance of the hemangiomatous mass, prolonged bleeding from abrasions, hematuria, hematochezia, epistaxis, and oozing from the umbilicus or circumcision site in infants. Hemangiomas may take on the appearance of cellulitis. Petechiae and ecchymoses, initially concentrated in the skin overlying and adjacent to the hemangioma, may spread to other areas. The following screening tests are suggested: hemoglobin and hematocrit determinations, blood smear, PT, PTT, or both, platelet count, fibrinogen concentration, and fibrin split products.

Most hemangiomas involute spontaneously and hematologic abnormalities resolve without therapy. If the hemangioma enlarges rapidly and the platelet count drops precipitously, prednisone (2–4 mg/kg/day) may prevent further growth of the lesion and effectively palliate the condition, for prednisone increases platelet survival time. Systemic corticosteroid therapy should be tried for 2–4 weeks. In the presence of thrombosis and bleeding, heparin in a dosage of 100 units/kg every 4 hours should be given until bleeding ceases, the platelet count is stable, and the coagulation defect is controlled.

► [A very large hemangioma may be associated with consumption coagulopathy (Kasabach-Merritt syndrome). Esterly describes the very difficult course of 4 infants with this problem and emphasizes treatment aspects. The management of this problem is a challenge for the combined efforts of dermatologist, pediatrician, hematologist, and surgeon. Often the course of the consumption coagulopathy is self-limited, and the hemangioma undergoes spontaneous resolution. Various approaches to therapy are reviewed.—A.R.R.] ◄

19–8 **Unilateral Dermatomal Superficial Telangiectasia: Nine New Cases and Review of Unilateral Dermatomal Superficial Telangiectasia.** Jonathan K. Wilkin, J. Graham Smith, Jr., David A. Cullison, Gerald E. Peters, Louis J. Rodriquez-Rigau, and Christopher L. Feucht note that unilateral dermatomal superficial telangiectasia (UDST) may be congenital or acquired. Acquired UDST may occur coincident with physiologic states of estrogen increase, including puberty and pregnancy in women and adrenarche in men. Acquired UDST may also occur in estrogenized pathologic states such as chronic hepatic disease in alcoholism. The occurrence of UDST during estrogenized states, the dermatomes of distribution, and the presence of anemic halos suggest kinship with arterial spiders. Findings were reviewed in 9 newly reported UDST patients.

The patients ranged in age from 21 to 83, and 7 were women. One woman, aged 31, had a rash on her left leg since age 12. She had numerous fine, threadlike telangiectasias on the posterior left leg. The redness of the lesion intensified during her 2 pregnancies, returning to the usual state after delivery. Another woman, aged 21, had skin lesions on her upper right arm, which became intensely red during her first pregnancy at 17 years. Skin biopsy showed only superficial dermal telangiectasia. In another woman, also aged 21, an eruption developed on the right arm and neck during her first and second pregnancies. Threadlike telangiectasias were found.

A fourth woman, aged 28, had a rash during her 3 pregnancies that

---

(19–8) J. Am. Acad. Dermatol. 8:468–477, April 1983.

resolved after delivery. The telangiectasias usually faded to a marked degree. In a woman aged 31, a red dermatosis developed at age 12. The rash was aggravated during 2 periods of birth control use. The oldest patient, a man aged 83, had an extensive red rash of unknown duration. Two granddaughters and 1 greatgranddaughter had similar lesions. The patient's entire left side had numerous erythematous macules and threadlike telangiectasias.

A woman, aged 26, reported that the skin of her left shoulder, upper left chest, and left arm had been redder in color than skin elsewhere since birth. The redness appeared to intensify over the years. The patient had irregular menses. Her telangiectasia persisted until the third month of pregnancy, only to return 2 weeks after delivery. The seventh woman, aged 25, had a red eruption of the skin 2 weeks before examination, at which time she was 3 months pregnant. Six weeks after delivery, the telangiectasia was barely visible. The ninth patient, a man aged 49, had an asymptomatic red rash on the left arm present from birth. Physical examination showed erythematous macules and telangiectasias.

From these findings in 9 patients and those previously reported in 37 patients, it would appear that UDST and some instances of benign, generalized telangiectasia may be local and universal forms of the same pathologic process in the cutaneous microvasculature.

▶ [Unilateral nevoid telangiectasia syndrome (UNTS) is most often seen associated with states in which estrogen levels are elevated, e.g., puberty, pregnancy, liver disease, and estrogen hormone therapy. Estrogen has long been implicated in the appearance of spider angiomata and palmar erythema in both physiologic (pregnancy) and pathologic (liver disease) conditions. Accordingly, most studies have postulated that UNTS lesions represent a congenital, localized abnormality which somehow renders the vasculature more susceptible to estrogen.

Uhlin and McCarty (*Arch. Dermatol.* 119:226–228, 1983) recently studied a 20-year-old woman who first developed UNTS when she began to use oral contraceptives and whose lesion became more prominent during a subsequent pregnancy. Biopsy specimens from lesional and nonlesional skin were assayed for the presence of estrogen and progesterone receptors. Neither receptor was demonstrable in nonlesional skin, whereas significant levels of both receptors were found in lesional skin. A previous study had confirmed the very low or absent level of estrogen receptors in normal skin (*J. Clin. Endocrinol. Metab.* 50:76–82, 1980), but progesterone receptors have not been studied in normal skin. If confirmed, Uhlin and McCarty's findings would explain the putative local estrogen sensitivity. Stimulation of receptors by high maternal estrogen levels or even the normal, low levels present prepubertally would provide a unifying hypothesis to explain those rare presentations as well.

More than a mere curiosity, UNTS offers promise as a model for the study of hormone receptors in other vascular anomalies. (Comment prepared by Dr. Mark S. Bernhardt.)] ◀

19–9 ***Ulex europaeus* I Lectin as a Marker for Tumors Derived From Endothelial Cells.** *Ulex europaeus* agglutinin I (UEA-I), a lectin with specific affinity for some 1-fucose moieties, specifically detects human endothelial cells in various normal tissues. Markku Miettinen, Harry Holthofer, Veli-Pekka Lehto, Aaro Miettinen, and Ismo Virtanen (Univ. of Helsinki) compared the usefulness of fluorochrome-labeled UEA-I with that of factor VIII–related antigen in

---

(19–9) Am. J. Clin. Pathol. 79:32–36, January 1983.

demonstrating endothelial cells in tumors of vascular origin. The immunofluorescence microscopy technique was employed.

The endothelial cells of large vessels of cavernous hemangiomas were uniformly stained with both the antibody to factor VIII–related antigen and with UEA-I; the latter marker demonstrated more clearly the small vessels of capillary hemangiomas. This marker also showed much stronger fluorescence in pyogenic granulomas and was preferable for demonstrating angiosarcomas. Both markers permitted visualization of Kaposi's sarcomas and hemangiopericytomas. The tumor cells of malignant melanomas, anaplastic carcinomas, and fibrosarcomas did not stain positively, but the blood vessels were clearly visualized.

Ulex europaeus agglutinin I appears to hold promise as a marker for endothelial cells in both benign and malignant endothelial proliferations. It may have applications both in routine surgical pathologic practice and in studies of the possible endothelial origin of certain neoplasms.

▶ [Products from various beans and grain substances termed lectins have been found to bind specifically to unique membrane carbohydrates such as mannose, fucose, or *N*-acetylglucosamine. By using panels of these lectins, it is possible to determine the composition and sequence of surface carbohydrates. The implications of this article is that tumors of endothelial cell origin share the sugar molecule fucose in a terminal position on one of the surface membrane components and that this relationship is not present in tumors of nonendothelial origin.—A.J.S.] ◀

20. Viral Infections

20–1 **Human Papillomavirus: Frequency and Distribution in Plantar and Common Warts.** The human papillomaviruses (HPV) cause a variety of cutaneous warts and mucosal papillomas, and evidence is accumulating that the type of HPV influences the clinical and pathologic findings and the course of these lesions (table). A. Bennett Jenson, Simone Sommer, Charles Payling-Wright, Franklin Pass, Clifton C. Link, Jr., and Wayne D. Lancaster examined cutaneous warts for HPV by electron microscopy and with type- and genus-specific antiserums prepared from both HPV and bovine papillomavirus. Twenty-four plantar warts and 35 common warts excised from 44 patients, aged 18–32 years, were studied. The indirect fluorescent antibody and peroxidase-antiperoxidase tests were used.

Papillomavirus particles were seen in both the granular and the keratinized layers of the warts. Half the plantar warts and just over half the common warts showed HPV on electron microscopic examination. Immunologic tests were positive in 58% of the plantar warts and 68% of the common warts. Half of the plantar warts and 11% of the common warts were definitely due to HPV type 1 (HPV-1). These warts were more clinically aggressive than those caused by other types of HPV, and they contained more virus. In several cases the presence of HPV-1 was confirmed by molecular hybridization studies. The interval between clinical discovery of a wart and its removal did

HUMAN PAPILLOMAVIRUS TYPES*

Virus	Type of lesion
HPV-1	Plantar warts
HPV-2	Common warts
HPV-3	Flat warts
HPV-4	Common and plantar warts
HPV-5	Pityriasis-like lesions in epidermodysplasia verruciformis
HPV-6	Anogenital warts
HPV-7	Meat handler warts
HPV-8	Pityriasis-like lesions in epidermodysplasia verruciformis

*Adapted from Howley, P.M.: Papovaviruses: search for evidence for possible association with human cancer, in Phillips, L. (ed.): *Viruses Associated With Human Cancer*. New York, Marcel Dekker, 1982.

(Courtesy of Jenson, A.B., et al.: Lab. Invest. 47:491–497, November 1982.)

(20–1) Lab. Invest. 47:491–497, November 1982.

not correlate with the presence or absence of detectable virus. All the HPV-1-positive lesions, however, were removed within 10 months, suggesting a more rapid or more symptomatic clinical course.

It appears that HPV-1 produces aggressive lesions containing large amounts of virus, regardless of anatomical site. The natural course of warts seems to be more closely related to HPV type than to location of the lesions.

▶ [This study suggests that in the future the classification of warts will be based on the type of human papillomavirus (HPV) rather than on anatomic location; HPV-1 was found to be present in plantar and common warts and determined their natural course. It appears that HPV-5 and HPV-8 are carcinogenic, and they are associated with epidermodysplasia verruciformis; HPV-16 is also carcinogenic and is associated with flat warts of the cervix which are precursors of invasive cancer of the cervix.—E.G.] ◀

20–2 **Humoral and Cell-Mediated Immunity to Human Papillomavirus Type 1 (HPV-1) in Human Warts.** At least 8 types of human papillomavirus (HPV) have been described, and available data suggest a relationship between the morphologic characteristics of papillomas and the type of virus involved. J. L. Kienzler, M. Th. Lemoine, G. Orth, N. Jibard, D. Blanc, R. Laurent, and P. Agache (France) examined the immune response of papilloma carriers to HPV type 1 (HPV-1). The study group included 85 male and 77 female patients, aged 6–72 years. From one to 40 warts were present in each patient. Some lesions were removed surgically and examined histologically and by immunofluorescence, using guinea pig antiserums to the various HPV types. Humoral immunity studies were carried out with a highly purified preparation of HPV-1 as antigen. Cell-mediated immune studies were performed with the capsid polypeptides of HPV-1 as antigen.

Subjects with myrmecia had antibodies to HPV-1 in 39% of instances. Significantly fewer subjects with common warts, flat warts, and anogenital warts had antibodies. Antibody was found in about 10% of control subjects. Average titers did not differ significantly in the various clinical groups. Delayed hypersensitivity testing showed no differences between carriers of the various papilloma types. New or increased production of antibody to HPV-1 was observed chiefly in myrmecia carriers. New delayed hypersensitivity reactions to HPV-1 were observed in 33%–56% of all groups of papilloma carriers. There was some evidence of an association of HPV-1 with myrmecia, of HPV-2 with common warts, and of HPV-3 with flat warts.

These findings confirm the presence of common antigenic determinants in the various human papillomavirus types. Cell-mediated immunity to an HPV-1 capsid antigen has been found in myrmecia carriers, and at least in France, myrmecia appears to be preferentially associated with HPV-1. Valid studies of the immune response in HPV infections require well-defined antigens and clinically well-characterized lesions.

▶ [Another step is taken to associate the clinicoanatomic presentation of warts with the specific papillomavirus, and although common antigens are found among the

---

(20–2) Br. J. Dermatol. 108:665–672, June 1983.

different strains, purified antigens may make it possible to distinguish among them in the future. This is important, since some of these strains have been ascribed carcinogenic potential. Although HPV-1 (associated with plantar warts) and HPV-2 (associated with common warts) seem to carry no carcinogenic potential, other types, such as HPV-5, -8, and -16, do.

A recently published retrospective study that evaluated the incidence of carcinoma in situ (CIS) in patients with condyloma acuminata demonstrates a higher incidence than expected for CIS, suggesting that condyloma acuminata also carries a carcinogenic potential (*Arch. Dermatol.* 120:476, 1984). Unfortunately, no identification of HPV strains was performed. It is possible, however, that future studies can identify the patients with condyloma acuminata carrying the potential of malignant degeneration by using these modern techniques of purifying antigens for papillomavirus.—E.G.] ◀

20–3 **Abnormalities of the Uterine Cervix in Women With Vulval Warts: Preliminary Communication.** Genital warts are common in women attending clinics for sexually transmitted diseases. P. G. Walker, N. V. Colley, C. Grubb, A. Tejerina, and J. D. Oriel (Univ. College Hosp., London) studied 50 women, seen at a clinic for sexually transmitted diseases, who had vulval condyloma acuminata. Cytologic and colposcopic examinations were carried out to detect cervical infection by human papillomavirus (HPV), epithelial abnormalities indicative of cervical intraepithelial neoplasia (CIN), or both. Cytologic evidence of wart virus infection was obtained in 23.5% of 34 evaluable patients. Four had cell changes consistent with CIN, and 2 had both types of change. Colposcopy showed changes of wart virus infection alone in 11 patients, changes of CIN in 8, and evidence of both conditions in 9. Fourteen of the 20 women with cervical changes indicative of wart virus infection had no exophytic condylomas. The results of cervical cytologic and colposcopic examination with regard to wart virus infection were not in close agreement.

Both HPV infection of the cervix and changes of CIN were prevalent in this group of women with vulval condyloma acuminata. Half the subjects had evidence of cervical infection by HPV, and more than one third had epithelial abnormalities consistent with CIN types 1 or 2. Cervical intraepithelial neoplasia is known to be related to early age at first intercourse and to multiple sex partners, and patients with vulval warts may share these features. The relation between wart virus infection and CIN is uncertain. Some lesions of CIN may regress spontaneously, but some, if untreated, develop into carcinoma in situ or even invasive cancer. Adequate cervical smears should be obtained from women with vulval warts and possibly from the female sex partners of men with penile condylomas. Persistently abnormal cytologic findings warrant referral for colposcopy.

▶ [As the authors comment in this article, evidence is accumulating that suggests that human papillomavirus (HPV) may have a causal role in the development of cervical cancer, acting either alone or in concert with other agents. More recently, for example, evidence was presented that the presence of a strain of HPV (type 16) correlates with the presence of abnormal mitotic figures in flat warts of the cervix and that this type of flat wart is a precursor of invasive cancer of the cervix (*N. Engl. J. Med.* 310:880, 1984).—E.G.] ◀

(20–3) Br. J. Vener. Dis. 59:120–123, April 1983.

20–4 **Treatment of Extensive Virus Warts With Etretinate (Tigason) in a Patient With Sarcoidosis.** J. Boyle, D. C. Dick, and Rona M. Mackie (Glasgow, Scotland) report a case of sarcoidosis complicated by extensive warts that responded dramatically to oral treatment with etretinate.

Man, 22, was seen in 1965 with erythema nodosum and 2 years later de-

Fig 20–1 (top).—Gross hyperkeratosis of hand before treatment.
Fig 20–2 (bottom).—Marked response after etretinate therapy.
(Courtesy of Boyle, J., et al.: Clin. Exp. Dermatol. 8:33–36, January 1983.)

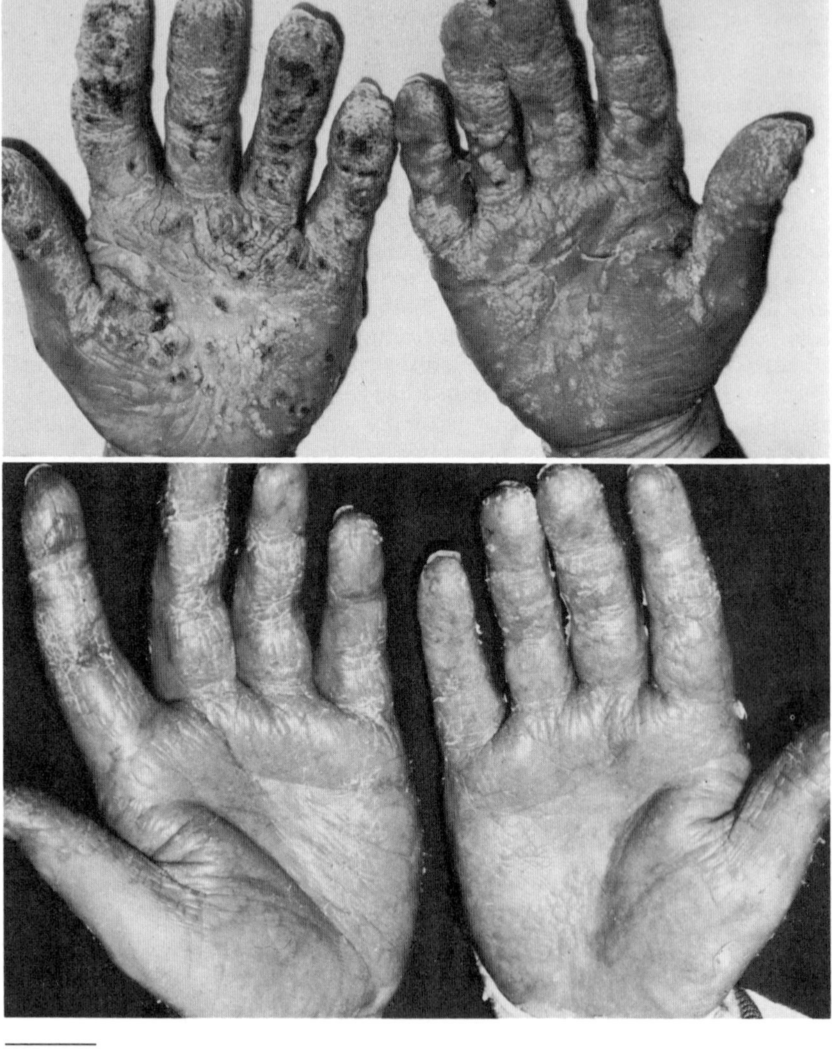

(20–4) Clin. Exp. Dermatol. 8:33–36, January 1983.

veloped bilateral hilar lymphadenopathy with pulmonary infiltration. Raised, reddish purple lesions were observed on the arms, thighs, and trunk, and biopsy revealed a few well-defined, noncaseating tubercles consistent with a diagnosis of sarcoidosis. Treatment of the pulmonary lesions with prednisolone (10 mg/day) was begun in 1970, with a gradual reduction in dosage over the next 6 years. Between the onset of sarcoidosis and the start of corticosteroid therapy, troublesome common warts had developed on the patient's hands. Two years after this therapy, there was such rapid and extensive spread of multiple large warts that repeated diathermy with general anesthesia was required. However, no improvement was observed. The patient had numerous filiform warts on the neck and beard area and massive and disabling confluent hyperkeratoses covering both hands, including the dorsal and palmar surfaces, and both wrists (Fig 20–1). Painful fissures caused such discomfort that he became unemployed. After withdrawal of corticosteroid therapy, there was no roentgenographic evidence of progressive pulmonary sarcoidosis. Routine hematologic and biochemical tests gave normal results, and chemotaxis and serum immunoglobulin concentrations were normal. However, cutaneous anergy to purified protein derivative, *Candida albicans, Trichophyton rubrum,* and mumps antigen could be demonstrated. Neither transfer factor nor a short course of levamisole restored immune function to normal. However, within 2 weeks of the start of etretinate treatment (100 mg/day) there was a dramatic reduction in the degree of hyperkeratosis on the hands (Fig 20–2). Maximum improvement was attained after 1 month of treatment, at which time the epidermis was relatively smooth. The facial warts disappeared; only depigmented areas remained. The improvement has been maintained, although the dosage of etretinate has been reduced to about 30 mg/day. The patient experienced the usual side effects associated with etretinate, i.e., cheilitis, skin thinning, and hair loss, but only to a mild degree.

Although etretinate has no role in the management of simple warts, it may be of value in the treatment of multiple warts associated with immunosuppression.

▶ [These are impressive results which are presumably due to etretinate, although it is conceivable that spontaneous regression of the warts could have played a role, since the patient was not receiving systemic steroids (and was therefore conceivably not as strongly immunosuppressed) at the commencement of therapy with etretinate. Even though there was evidence of anergy at the start of therapy, these tests were not repeated to determine whether the patient had become immunocompetent during treatment and after sarcoidosis had gone into remission. In view of the similar reports regarding the effectiveness of etretinate in epidermodysplasia verruciformis (*N. Engl. J. Med.* 302:1091, 1980), the observations made on this patient with sarcoidosis sound convincing. Since recurrences followed discontinuation or reduction of etretinate, the risks of long-term therapy with this drug have to be carefully considered.—E.G.] ◀

20–5 **Using the Laser to Treat Vulvar Condylomata Acuminata and Intraepidermal Neoplasia.** The incidence of genital condylomata appears to be increasing, especially in sexually mature persons. Several complications can occur, and many types of treatment have been recommended for vulvar lesions. Alex Ferenczy (McGill Univ., Montreal) evaluated use of the CO_2 laser in 55 women seen during a 2-year period with condyloma acuminata of the vulva, urethral mea-

(20–5) Can. Med. Assoc. J. 128:135–138, Jan. 15, 1983.

tus, and anal region, and in 11 others with multicentric vulvar intraepidermal neoplasia. The respective mean ages for these two groups were 25 and 38 years. Nearly 90% of the women with condylomata had extensive lesions that had failed to respond to conservative treatment measures. Twelve of these patients had vaginal as well as vulvar lesions, 10 had cervical involvement, and 9 had disease in the perianal region or anal canal. Three had urethral meatal lesions. In the second group, vulvar intraepidermal neoplastic lesions had been present for 1–9 years. Lesions were extended by laser to 3–4 mm beyond the visible lesion margins. Power densities of 500–750 W/sq cm were used to destroy epidermal lesions, and mucosal lesions were treated with 380 W/sq cm.

Eighty-seven percent of women with condylomata required only one laser treatment to clear the lesions for a year or longer. Four of the 7 patients with residual condylomata were immunosuppressed. Two patients required a third treatment. Eight of the 11 women with intraepidermal neoplasia of the vulva were free of disease for at least 1 year after a single treatment. Perioperative bleeding in 2 cases was readily controlled by electrocoagulation. Two women had severe pain. Two with extensive disease had vulvar stricture or synechia formation.

Laser surgery was less successful in this series than in others, which had reported success rates as high as 95%, but it was generally superior to other forms of treatment. Laser treatment is recommended in extensive cases, where it is cost-effective. Since extensive condylomata and intraepidermal neoplasia are not common in routine gynecologic practice, it probably is best to refer these patients to a hospital-based unit.

▶ [This open study shows success in treating condyloma acuminata of the vulva with the CO_2 laser. The rates of persistence or recurrence were 13% and 5%, respectively. The author claims that success is dependent on careful examination (with a colposcope) and thorough treatment of all identifiable lesions.

The discrepancy between this report and the one that follows might be explained on the basis of design and location. The study by Billingham and Lewis was a bilateral comparison study of CO_2 laser and electrocautery, and the warts were located in the perianal region. In the study by Ferenczy, on the other hand, all treatments were done with the CO_2 laser, and most of the warts were located in the vulva although three patients also had perianal warts (all of which cleared). Even though the study design by Billingham and Lewis sounds more convincing, their results are difficult to accept. They observed that warts recurred in all patients during the postoperative course, and most of the warts treated with CO_2 laser recurred faster than the ones treated with electrocautery. It is conceivable that the high recurrence rate was induced by intraanal lesions shedding virus to the perianal region (see abstract below).—E.G.] ◀

20–6 **Laser Versus Electric Cautery in the Treatment of Condylomata Acuminata of the Anus.** Condyloma acuminata of the anus is an increasing problem, and the warts frequently persist or recur after treatment. Richard P. Billingham and F. Gary Lewis (Seattle) compared laser treatment with conventional electrical cautery in a series of 38 patients seen between 1979 and 1981 whose warts were consid-

---

(20–6) Surg. Gynecol. Obstet. 155:865–867, December 1982.

ered to be too extensive for office treatment. All patients were treated in an outpatient surgical unit under general anesthesia. Warts on one side of the anus were cauterized electrically, and those on the other side were treated with the laser. Residual warts were detected using an operating microscope and treated. Warts detected during follow-up examination were treated in the office with the electric cautery or, rarely, bichloracetic acid.

Several patients had more severe postoperative pain on the laser-treated side. Nearly all recurrent warts were first noted on the laser-treated side. In 28 patients who were followed up for an average of 25 weeks, the average interval from initial treatment to the absence of warts was 16 weeks. Six patients required reoperation because of the rapid growth of new warts. The average time between operations in this group was 6 weeks.

The laser has not replaced electric cautery as the chief surgical treatment of anal warts. Recurrences were more frequent after laser treatment in the present study, and pain often was more marked than with electric cautery treatment. In addition, laser treatment is more costly. The use of magnification seems to help in identifying the smallest warts at the time of surgery. It is hoped that advances in immunotherapy will eventually replace the surgical treatment of condyloma acuminata.

▶ [These are interesting results that show an advantage of electrocautery over CO_2 laser in the treatment of perianal warts. Unexpectedly, pain was more common and severe in the laser-treated side. We are still hoping that a more effective and less radical approach will be developed to treat these extensive lesions. Injectable interferon might answer our prayers (see abstract below).—E.G.] ◀

20–7 **Intralesional Human Fibroblast Interferon in Common Warts.** Some patients with common warts have severe, protracted problems despite treatment by chemical or surgical destruction of the lesions. Wart regression now is regarded as an immunologic phenomenon, and immunotherapy reportedly is effective. Michihito Niimura (Jikei Univ., Minato-ku Tokyo) examined the response of common warts to intralesional injections of human fibroblast interferon in a double-blind study. Eighty patients with bilateral common warts on their extremities received weekly intralesional injections of either human fibroblast interferon or an albumin-lactose placebo. A dose of 0.1×10^6 IU of interferon was injected into warts on one side and placebo into those on the matching extremity. No more than 10 weekly injections were given.

In the 64 patients who completed the study, more than 81% of interferon-treated extremities were cured or responded effectively, compared with 17% of placebo-treated lesions. In all, 42 actively treated extremities and 7 treated with placebo were cured of warts. The average number of interferon injections required for cure was 5.9. No adverse effects on renal, hepatic, or hematopoietic functions were observed. Pigmentation followed regression of warts in 3 instances.

(20–7) J. Dermatol. 10:217–220, June 1983.

Encouraging clinical responses to intralesional interferon therapy were observed in this series. The treatment may prove especially useful when other measures have failed. New delivery systems or other dose regimens might increase the value of interferon therapy for warts.

▶ [This is the first double-blind study demonstrating the effectiveness of intralesional human fibroblast interferon in common warts. Minimal local inflammatory reaction was observed in the interferon-treated side, but otherwise no side effects were seen. Subcutaneous injections might prove to be as effective in the future where the patient can inject the interferon with minimal supervision.—E.G.] ◀

20–8 **Scissor Excision of Anogenital Warts.** John M. Gollock, Kenneth Slatford, and Jennifer M. Hunter (Edinburgh) evaluated the method of scissor excision of anogenital warts described by Thomson and Grace. Saline containing 1:300,000 epinephrine is infiltrated in the volume (no larger than 150 ml) needed to separate the warts and permit their accurate removal with scissors. The procedure was done in the hospital with general anesthesia. Intra-anal warts were removed by using a Park anal retractor, with injection of saline-epinephrine solution into the submucous plane. If an area of confluent warts was excised, the defect was repaired with 3-0 Dexon sutures. Diathermy has not been necessary for hemostasis.

Thirty-four patients were treated by this method. The 24 men and 10 women had a mean age of 27 years. Warts had been present for a mean of 5 months, and most patients had had various treatments such as podophyllin and freezing with liquid nitrogen. Fourteen had extension of the warts to surrounding areas. The only surgical complication was bleeding in 1 patient, which was readily controlled with a suture. The mean inpatient stay was 3 days; only 6 patients were hospitalized for 5 days or longer. Half the patients did not require a narcotic analgesic postoperatively. Twenty of the 28 patients followed required no further treatment or only a single podophyllin application. There were 3 definite recurrences, and 1 patient required further operation. Mean follow-up was 6 weeks.

Scissor excision appears to be an excellent treatment for anogenital warts. The primary cure rate in this series was 71%, and the recurrence rate was 9%. Females are treated as readily as males by this method. The mean hospital stay of 3 days could easily have been shortened.

▶ [This study confirms the previous report by Thomson and Grace (*J. R. Soc. Med.* 71:180, 1978) on the effectiveness of scissor excision for anogenital warts. Although theirs was not a controlled study, Gollock et al. achieved cure and relapse rates (71.4% and 9.3%) that compare with other modalities of treatment. The lack of tissue destruction to adjacent areas minimizes scarring; however, morbidity is high, as is shown by the following: 50% of the patients required sedation; all of them required general anesthesia; and the average hospitalization was 3 days. This drastic approach is hardly warranted for small anogenital warts and probably should be reserved for intractable ones.—E.G.] ◀

20–9 **Treatment of Anogenital Warts: Comparison of Trichloroacetic Acid and Podophyllin Versus Podophyllin Alone.** G. Gabriel

---

(20–8) Br. J. Vener. Dis. 58:400–401, December 1982.
(20–9) Ibid., 59:124–126, April 1983.

and R. N. T. Thin (London) undertook a double-blind comparison of podophyllin alone and combined with trichloroacetic acid in men with anogenital warts who had not been treated in the preceding 3 months. Treatment was with 25% podophyllin in industrial methylated spirits or podophyllin with 50% trichloroacetic acid. Treatment was given weekly. The solution was left on for 4 hours after the first application, 12 hours after the second, and then 24 hours. Patients with persistent warts after 6 weeks were treated with 100% trichloroacetic acid or by cryocautery.

Twenty-nine of 60 patients in the trial were treated with podophyllin alone, and 31 with both agents. The groups were clinically comparable. Twenty patients treated with podophyllin alone and 21 treated with both drugs were free of warts at 6 weeks. Nine and 10, respectively, remained free of warts at 3 months. Fewer applications were needed by patients treated with both podophyllin and trichloroacetic acid. Five of these patients had superficial ulceration or excessive soreness. No side effects occurred in patients treated with podophyllin alone.

Podophyllin alone was as effective as combined podophyllin–trichloroacetic acid therapy in clearing anogenital warts in men in this study, and side effects occurred only with combined treatment. The routine use of combined treatment is not recommended.

▶ [The only advantage for the combined therapy was that fewer applications were required. Otherwise, cure rates were comparable and side effects were more frequent with the combination of trichloroacetic acid–podophyllin. According to the authors, therefore, trichloroacetic acid doesn't add any therapeutic benefit and should not be used in combination with podophyllin.—E.G.] ◀

20–10 **Bleomycin in the Treatment of Recalcitrant Warts.** Bleomycin is gaining popularity in treatment of warts, but its efficacy has not been examined in well-controlled studies. Steven M. Shumer and Edward J. O'Keefe (Univ. of North Carolina) evaluated bleomycin in a double-blind, placebo-controlled crossover study of recalcitrant warts treated unsuccessfully by conventional methods. Patients were assigned alternately to placebo or bleomycin groups and were treated by intralesional injections of bleomycin, 1 unit/ml, or saline at 2-week intervals. If warts persisted after two injections, patients were changed to the alternate group and retreated with 1 or 2 further injections. Forty patients entered the study.

None of the 55 warts treated with placebo were resolved. Of the 151 warts treated with bleomycin, 123 showed complete resolution after 1 or 2 injections. Sixty percent of plantar warts, 94% of periungual warts, and 95% of warts at other sites were cured, a total cure rate of 81% by 1 or 2 injections. Eighty-two warts resolved after 1 injection and 41 warts resolved after 2 injections. No warts have recurred; 8 patients have been followed up for 6–12 months without evidence of recurrence. Most patients experienced moderate pain on injection. It was of short duration and was similar in both groups.

(20–10) J. Am. Acad. Dermatol. 9:91–96, July 1983.

Local pain, erythema, and swelling for 24–72 hours often occurred. During the first week after bleomycin injection, blackening, thromboses, and eschar developed. In the area of wart resolution, there was no sign of pigmentary change or scar after treatment with bleomycin. Some patients with periungual warts experienced significant local tenderness and swelling that took 5–7 days to resolve. In general, patient acceptance was favorable compared with acceptance of past treatments.

Bleomycin is unequivocally effective in treatment of warts, but the propriety of its use remains uncertain. Bleomycin has antitumor, antibacterial, and antiviral activity which may be related to its ability to bind to DNA, causing strand scission and elimination of pyrimidine and purine bases. The authors have restricted the use of bleomycin to recalcitrant warts in adults and believe that long-term safety requires further follow-up.

▶ [This is a controlled study that shows the efficacy of intralesional bleomycin for warts, especially for perianal warts, which are usually recalcitrant to other modalities. Although I agree with most of the authors' observations, the pain experienced by most of my patients has been intense, not only during the injection but for 2–4 days after, especially on plantar warts.

This study, however, has to contend with a negative report by Munkvad et al. (see abstract below) that showed no clinical benefit of intralesional bleomycin in saline or oil suspension compared with placebo in a double-blind study. Cure rates of 18% and 23% were obtained with bleomycin in saline and oil suspension compared with 40% for the placebo group. It is difficult to reconcile these conflicting results. The main difference seems to be in the amount of bleomycin injected; the authors of the study abstracted above injected from 0.2 to 1.0 ml of bleomycin solution (1 unit/ml), depending on the size of the wart; Munkvad et al. injected from 0.1 to 0.4 ml of 1% solution of bleomycin. Further studies are required.—E.G.] ◀

20–11 **Locally Injected Bleomycin in the Treatment of Warts.** Bleomycin has an affinity for squamous epithelium, and it has been widely used to treat skin tumors. M. Munkvad, J. Genner, B. Staberg and H. Kongsholm evaluated the effects of bleomycin in saline and oil suspensions in the treatment of warts resistant to conventional measures. A total of 62 patients with 108 warts were included in the trial. Warts on the hands and feet and mosaic warts were included, but children younger than age 14 years and pregnant women were excluded. Bleomycin in saline or oil or saline alone was administered in a double-blind design. A 0.1-ml volume of 1% bleomycin solution or saline was administered with a jet injector after the wart was pared down. As many as 4 injections were given, and the treatment was repeated 3 times at 2-week intervals.

Cure rates of 18% and 23%, respectively, were obtained with bleomycin in saline and oil suspension. Cure rates exceeding 40% were obtained in the placebo group, and these results were significantly better than those obtained in the bleomycin-treated patients. Adverse effects such as pain, swelling, and bleeding occurred in 19 patients.

Bleomycin had no apparent advantage over placebo in the treatment of resistant warts in this study. In view of the risk of toxic side

---

(20–11) Dermatologica 167:86–89, August 1983.

effects from bleomycin, its use in the treatment of warts is not recommended.

▶ [This negative study has to be reconciled with previous uncontrolled studies showing the efficacy of the treatment as well as with the double-blind, controlled study done by Shumer and O'Keefe (see abstract 20–10) that showed cure rates as high as 95% for recalcitrant warts.—E.G.] ◀

20–12 **Acyclovir Halts Progression of Herpes Zoster in Immunocompromised Patients.** Because acute herpes zoster can produce chronic pain and there is always the danger of visceral dissemination in immunocompromised patients, an effective treatment for such patients is important. Henry H. Balfour, Jr., Bonnie Bean, Oscar L. Laskin, Richard F. Ambinder, Joel D. Meyers, James C. Wade, John A. Zaia, Dorothee Aeppli, L. Edward Kirk, Anthony C. Segreti, Ronald E. Keeney, and the Burroughs Wellcome Collaborative Acyclovir Study Group report the results of a multicenter, randomized, placebo-controlled, double-blind trial of intravenous acyclovir therapy (1,500 mg/sq m of body surface area per day) in 94 immunocompromised patients with acute herpes zoster.

The patients were primarily white, and males outnumbered females. Fifty-two patients had localized cutaneous zoster at entry into the study, and 42 had disseminated cutaneous disease. Although there was a wide range of ages in all categories, median age of patients with localized cutaneous zoster was lower than that of patients with disseminated cutaneous zoster. Zoster progression events occurred significantly less often in patients with localized (P = .006) or disseminated cutaneous zoster (P = .03) treated with acyclovir than in those who received placebo. Such progression events included an increase in area of the primary dermatome rash, new dermatome involvement, development or progress of cutaneous dissemination, and development of visceral zoster. Only 1 of the 52 patients with localized or disseminated cutaneous zoster treated with acyclovir showed severe progression, compared with 11 of the 42 patients receiving placebo (P = .0005). None of the 52 acyclovir recipients, but 8 of the 42 placebo recipients, were regarded as representing treatment failures (P = .0005). Among patients with localized zoster, those with a longer duration of disease at entry into the study had a significantly shorter time to scabbing and resolution of pain. Among the patients whose rash was present for 3 days or less at entry, visceral or progressive cutaneous zoster developed in 1 of 23 acyclovir recipients, compared with 8 of the 25 placebo recipients (P = .02). Of those whose rash had been present for more than 3 days at entry, none of 29 acyclovir recipients and 3 of 17 placebo recipients developed visceral or cutaneous dissemination (P = .05). Time to total scabbing was significantly shorter in patients who had cutaneous disseminated zoster at entry and were treated with acyclovir than in those who received placebo. Resolution of pain was faster in patients receiving acyclovir, but not significantly. Patients with disseminated cutaneous

(20–12) N. Engl. J. Med. 308:1448–1453, June 16, 1983.

zoster treated with acyclovir had significantly faster clearance of virus from vesicles than did placebo recipients. Acyclovir was well tolerated, and there were no significant blood chemistry or clinical abnormalities.

The results demonstrate that acyclovir is effective in preventing the progression of localized or disseminated cutaneous herpes zoster in immunocompromised patients.

▶ [This well-controlled study demonstrates very clearly the efficacy of intravenous acyclovir in preventing progression of herpes zoster in immunocompromised patients when compared with placebo, even if the treatment is started 3 days after the onset of the clinical manifestations. These results compared favorably with previous reports of the use of vidarabine and interferon for immunocompromised hosts with similar complications of herpes zoster.

The effect of this therapeutic intervention in prevention of postherpetic neuralgia is still not clear, since the differences between intravenous acyclovir and placebo were not significant. It might require longer intravenous infusions or combination with other therapeutic agents to prevent this sequela.

Intravenous acyclovir has been shown to be very effective in controlling dissemination and reducing morbidity of Kaposi's varicelliform eruption induced by herpes simplex virus in patients with eczema and in other susceptible hosts, and it seems to be the drug of choice for this complication of herpes simplex virus infection. More recently, two patients with eczema herpeticum were treated with oral acyclovir and showed good clinical response, suggesting that this route of administration of acyclovir may also be effective (*Br. Med. J.* 288:531, 1984).—E.G.] ◀

20–13 **Treatment of First Episodes of Genital Herpes Simplex Virus Infection With Oral Acyclovir: Randomized Double-Blind Controlled Trial in Normal Subjects.** Most patients with first episodes of genital herpes do not require hospitalization, and an effective outpatient treatment would be of value. Yvonne J. Bryson, Maryanne Dillon, Michael Lovett, Guillermo Acuna, Stephen Taylor, James D. Cherry, B. Lamar Johnson, Edward Wiesmeier, William Growdon, Terri Creagh-Kirk, and Ronald Keeney undertook a double-blind, placebo-controlled trial of oral acyclovir treatment of first-episode genital herpes infections in 48 young adults. Actively treated patients received acyclovir in a dosage of 200 mg five times per day orally for 10 days. Patients were assessed at least eight times until healed and were then assessed monthly. About half the patients had primary herpes simplex infections, and these were equally distributed in the acyclovir and control groups. Herpes simplex virus type 2 was isolated from the lesions of 43 subjects and type 1 virus from the lesions of the other 5.

The duration of virus shedding from genital lesions was significantly reduced in acyclovir-treated patients. New lesion formation was significantly less in the acyclovir group. Symptoms were less severe and lasted a shorter time in patients given acyclovir. No adverse reactions were observed. Recurrence rates in subjects followed for 4–9 months were comparable in the acyclovir and placebo groups and exceeded 50% in both. Only 1 of the 5 patients with herpes simplex type 1 infection had a recurrence.

Oral acyclovir therapy significantly reduced new lesion formation

---

(20–13) N. Engl. J. Med. 308:916–921, Apr. 21, 1983.

and ameliorated symptoms in patients in this study with first episodes of genital herpes. The clinical course was shortened by about a week. Studies of oral treatment in pregnant women near term are planned in the hope of avoiding section delivery by eliminating virus from the maternal genital tract. Studies of prophylaxis in patients with frequent recurrences of infection are under way. Oral acyclovir treatment of first-episode genital herpes does not appear to prevent recurrences.

▶ [This report, as well as the one by Nilsen et al. (*Lancet* 2:571, 1982), attests to the effectiveness of oral acyclovir in the treatment of primary genital herpes. Not only was viral shedding reduced, but clinical improvement was also significant. Nilsen et al. also treated recurrent genital herpes and showed similar results except that the effect on lesion progression was less pronounced in the recurrent process than in the primary infection. It seems therefore that oral acyclovir is effective in primary as well as recurrent genital herpes and has a definite advantage over topical acyclovir. Unfortunately, recurrences are not prevented with oral treatment, and prophylactic therapy is probably required. The safety and efficacy of this approach remains to be determined.—E.G.] ◀

20–14 **Successful Treatment of Herpes Labialis With Topical Acyclovir.** Recurrent herpes simplex infections in the area of the mouth (herpes labialis) occur in as many as 20% of young adults. A. Paul Fiddian, Jane M. Yeo, Ronald Stubbings, and Donald Dean evaluated the effectiveness of topically applied cream containing 5% acyclovir, an antiviral drug with highly specific activity against herpes simplex virus types 1 and 2, in a double-blind, placebo-controlled study of 49 patients with frequent recurrences of herpes labialis. The cream was applied 5 times a day for 5 days. After each treated episode, patients were rerandomized to receive acyclovir or placebo for their next recurrence.

The percentage of lesions in first episodes that failed to progress beyond the papule stage was significantly greater in patients treated with acyclovir than in those receiving placebo, regardless of whether treatment was begun before or after vesicles had developed. The development of new lesions was not affected by acyclovir, though this was infrequent in both groups. First episodes and all episodes treated with acyclovir had significantly shorter times to first formation of ulcer or crust and to complete healing in all patients. Treatment with acyclovir reduced the duration of all symptoms and the proportion of patients who developed itching in first episodes, though the difference between groups was not significant. Two patients treated with placebo and 4 treated with acyclovir developed flaking of the skin in the area where the cream was applied. Treatment did not have to be discontinued in any patient. Acyclovir cream is well tolerated and effective in the treatment of recurrent herpes labialis.

▶ [This study is the first one to show a significant clinical benefit with topically applied acyclovir. According to the authors, there was a significant reduction of total healing time and duration of symptoms compared with placebo; and if treatment was started before the onset of vesicles, these could be aborted, presumably preventing infectivity of active lesions. This is in contrast with previous studies in which topical

(20–14) Br. Med. J. 286:1699–1701, May 28, 1983.

acyclovir did not produce significant improvement of clinical parameters even though reduction of viral shedding had been noticed. Corey et al. (*N. Engl. J. Med.* 306:1313, 1982) and Spruance et al. (*J. Infect. Dis.* 146:85, 1982) used acyclovir ointment for recurrent genital herpes and herpes labialis, respectively, and were unable to show significant response, especially among females. To reconcile these disparate results, the authors claim that their use of an acyclovir cream that contained propylene glycol as the solvent seemed to result in better penetration of the skin and hence in optimization of the antiviral effect of the drug. This study obviously requires confirmation.

Interestingly, no virologic studies were performed in the patients to determine if decreased viral shedding and/or increased clearance accompanied their clinical response. Future studies should include viral cultures, and patients treated with this new antiviral agent should be monitored closely for the development of resistant strains, which has already been reported. In the meantime, judicious use of acyclovir is recommended.—E.G.] ◀

20–15 **Topical Acyclovir in Treatment of Initial Genital Herpes.** Acyclovir has low toxicity and high activity in vitro against herpes simplex virus types 1 and 2, and intravenous therapy has been effective in initial episodes of severe genital herpes. R. N. Thin, Joan M. Nabarro, J. Davidson Parker, and A. Paul Fiddian (London and Beckenham, England) undertook a double-blind placebo-controlled trial of topical acyclovir in outpatients aged 16 and older with initial attacks of typical genital herpetic lesions. Eighteen of 40 patients applied 5% acyclovir in a polyethylene glycol base 5 times daily, whereas 22 used the base alone. The 2 groups were clinically similar except for more patients with ulcers alone in the study group. All 6 patients with

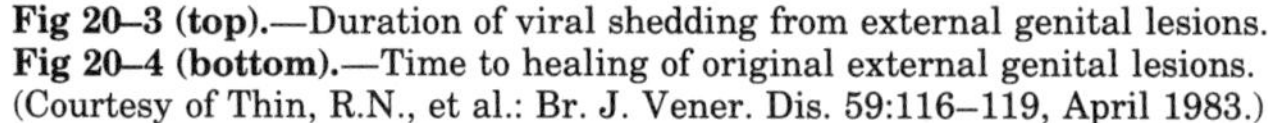

Fig 20–3 (top).—Duration of viral shedding from external genital lesions.
Fig 20–4 (bottom).—Time to healing of original external genital lesions.
(Courtesy of Thin, R.N., et al.: Br. J. Vener. Dis. 59:116–119, April 1983.)

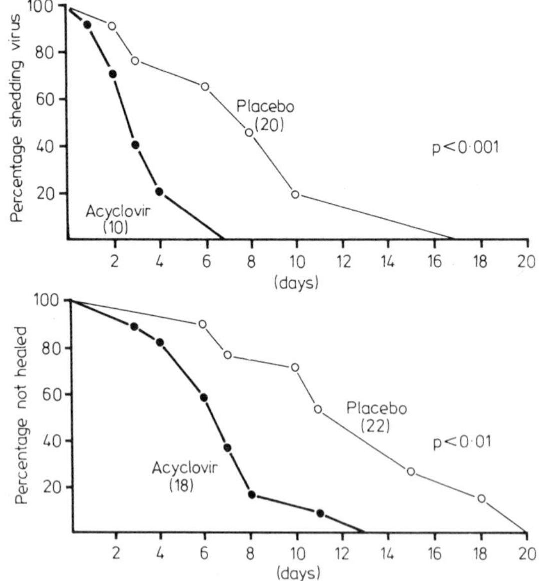

(20–15) Br. J. Vener. Dis. 59:116–119, April 1983.

crusts already present were in the placebo group. Virus was confirmed at entry to the study in 14 acyclovir-treated patients and 20 placebo patients.

The duration of viral shedding was substantially less in the acyclovir group (Fig 20–3). Healing occurred appreciably more rapidly in the study group (Fig 20–4). New lesions developed in 6% of acyclovir-treated patients and in 45% of placebo patients. Symptoms lasted longer in the placebo recipients. No patient reported side effects.

Topical acyclovir appears to be a safe and, at least in the short term, effective treatment for moderately severe initial attacks of genital herpes in outpatients. Shortening of the period of viral shedding by acyclovir therapy is advantageous to patients and probably has epidemiologic importance. A topical acyclovir cream and oral acyclovir administration are currently under study.

▶ [Another controlled study that hails the effectiveness of topical acyclovir in the treatment of primary herpes infection, specifically herpes progenitalis. Although the beneficial effect of topical acyclovir for primary herpes infection requires no further confirmation, its effectiveness in recurrent infections requires corroboration. Although it is true that viral shedding is reduced, the evidence for clinical response is still controversial. The vehicle in which the acyclovir is contained seems to have a significant effect on percutaneous penetration with propylene glycol and dimethyl sulfoxide enhancing both its absorption and its beneficial effect. Further confirmation of this phenomenon is expected in the future. For the practitioner, the best advice is to use topical acyclovir according to the guidelines stipulated by the FDA and the drug insert and to await further developments to insure that we do not create resistant strains that will make ineffective one of the genuine antiviral drugs.—E.G.] ◀

20–16 **Herpetic Whitlow: Epidemiology, Clinical Characteristics, Diagnosis, and Treatment.** Herpetic whitlow is a herpes simplex virus infection of the distal phalanx, seen mainly in medical personnel and in patients with herpetic gingivostomatitis or genital herpes. It is considered uncommon in infants and children, in whom it has been described only in association with gingivostomatitis or severe trauma. Henry M. Feder, Jr., and Sarah S. Long report 7 cases of herpetic whitlow, 5 occurring in pediatric patients and 2 in pediatric residents. In 2 pediatric cases, both involving young infants, herpetic whitlow occurred as the sole manifestation of herpes simplex infection, without preceding injury and without identification of an autogenous or exogenous source of virus. In 2 other infants, a whitlow developed following exposure to oral herpes, and an adolescent patient had a lesion associated with genital herpes. The affected pediatric residents had had contact with herpes simplex infection. One had intubated a neonate who had overwhelming herpes simplex type 2 viremia, and the other had pierced his thumb with a lancet contaminated with this organism.

The whitlow is a painful, pus-producing infection of the distal part of a finger or toe. Patients with herpetic whitlow typically have pain and tingling or burning of a distal phalanx, followed by digital swelling and erythema. There may be fever, adenopathy, lymphangitis, and constitutional symptoms. Then vesicles appear and usually co-

(20–16) Am. J. Dis. Child. 137:861–863, September 1983.

alesce. They last about 10 days and are followed by crusting. About one fifth of patients have recurrences, which usually are less severe than the initial infection. The initial episode usually occurs during a primary herpes simplex infection. The manner of inoculation is variable. The diagnosis can be rapidly confirmed by the Tzanck test or culture. Serologic tests usually are not helpful. The treatment of herpetic whitlow is symptomatic. Pain may be relieved with analgesics or by aspirating tense vesicles, but deep incision or debridement should be avoided. Local application of an idoxuridine solution may be helpful.

▶ [This study provides a good characterization of herpetic whitlow in children and adults, and it should serve as a reminder to all practitioners, since the condition is often misdiagnosed and mistreated. In some cases the source of infection is not apparent, a fact that stresses the importance of high suspicion for any painful, pus-containing, inflammatory lesion of the fingers or toes. Since Tzanck preparation is such an accessible tool to establish a rapid diagnosis, herpes should be rarely missed.

The authors suggest that idoxuridine (40% in dimethyl sulfoxide) can be helpful in shortening the course of the disease. This obviously requires confirmation since a controlled study on the effectiveness of topical idoxuridine in dimethyl sulfoxide for genital herpes didn't show significant effects on the duration of symptoms, new lesion formation, healing time, or rate of recurrence (*JAMA* 248:953, 1982). It is probable that similar ineffectiveness can be shown in herpetic whitlow if controlled studies are performed. Since strains resistant to idoxuridine have been demonstrated, it might be better to avoid such therapy until further conclusions are drawn.—E.G.] ◀

20–17 **Complement Deposition in the Skin of Patients With Herpes-Associated Erythema Multiforme.** An association of erythema multiforme (EM) with herpes simplex is well established. In most cases EM follows a recurrent herpes simplex lesion due to type 1 virus. Ronald Grimwood, J. Clark Huff, and William L. Weston (Univ. of Colorado) studied 10 patients with recurrent herpes-associated EM (HAEM) who had typical skin lesions, with or without mucosal lesions. All had fixed erythematous papules that evolved into iris or target lesions that were distributed symmetrically, usually over extensor surfaces, and resolved within 4 weeks. Biopsy specimens of early lesions were examined by immunofluorescence in an attempt to demonstrate granular C3 at the dermoepidermal junction.

A mononuclear infiltrate was present around superficial vessels and along the dermoepidermal junction. The basal cells exhibited hydropic degeneration. Necrotic keratinocytes were scattered throughout the epidermis. All 10 patients had granular C3 along the basement membrane zone and in papillary vessels. No patient exhibited deposits of C1q or C4. Only 1 patient did not exhibit 1+ staining for properdin.

The findings of granular C3 and properdin staining in the skin of patients with HAEM suggest activation of complement by the alternate pathway. The detection of herpes antigens in early skin lesions and of the herpes viral genome in an incomplete or latent form would clarify the possibility of viral activation of the alternate complement

(20–17) J. Am. Acad. Dermatol. 9:199–203, August 1983.

pathway in HAEM. Immune complexes occur in patients with EM, but they are of doubtful pathogenetic significance.

▶ [On the basis of immunofluorescence studies, the authors propose a different pathogenetic mechanism to explain erythema multiforme secondary to herpes simplex infection. They hypothesize that herpes virus induces C3 receptors in the infected cell, and, upon cleavage of C3 to C3b, the alternative pathway is activated to produce cell lysis. This theory presupposes that viral antigen remains on the skin of these patients developing erythema multiforme in order to initiate the complement cascade; this remains to be proved.—E.G.] ◀

20–18 **HLA Antigen Frequency in Erythema Multiforme and in Recurrent Herpes Simplex.** D. Middleton, T. H. Hutchinson, and J. Lynd (Belfast) determined the human leukocyte antigen (HLA) frequency in a group of patients with erythema multiforme and in a separate group with recurrent herpes simplex to determine whether either disease had any antigens whose frequency deviated from that in a normal population. Twenty-nine patients with erythema multiforme and 29 with herpes simplex were tissue typed for HLA-A and HLA-B antigens.

In both groups, HLA-B15 occurred more frequently than in controls ($P<.05$). After correction for the number of antigens compared, only the P value for the erythema multiforme group remained significant. In the erythema multiforme group, HLA-B15 was present in 4 (28.6%) of 14 patients whose disease was associated with herpes simplex, and in 3 (20%) of 15 patients with no herpes simplex association.

In Northern Ireland there is little immigration, thus the population has remained relatively homogeneous. Since the frequency of HLA-B15 was similar in those patients of the erythema multiforme group with associated herpes simplex and in those without herpes association, it is unlikely that the increase in B15 in patients with erythema multiforme is due to the fact that some of them also have herpes simplex.

▶ [The bottom line is that HLA antigens are not helpful in identifying erythema multiforme secondary to other factors from erythema multiforme induced by herpes virus infection. As with other diseases, HLA antigens should not be considered the only parameter to establish associations, and on many occasions they can't substitute for the chronology of events that a good history can provide.—E.G.] ◀

20–19 **Erythema Multiforme: Microvascular Damage and Infiltration of Lymphocytes and Basophils.** Erythema multiforme is an acute, self-limited, often recurrent inflammatory disorder of the skin and mucous membranes, which has been considered to be a hypersensitivity reaction to a variety of agents such as drugs and infectious organisms. Immune mechanisms have been implicated in its pathogenesis. Marcia G. Tonnesen, Terence J. Harrist, Bruce U. Wintroub, Martin C. Mihm, Jr., and Nicholas A. Soter (Harvard Med. School) examined the sequence of changes in recurrent erythema multiforme by examining 1-μm tissue sections by the immunofluorescence method in 5 patients who had an acute, self-limited eruption with at

---

(20–18) Tissue Antigens 21:264–267, March 1983.
(20–19) J. Invest. Dermatol. 80:282–286, April 1983.

least one target lesion. The 3 males and 2 females were aged 16–44 years. Four patients had had episodes of postherpes erythema multiforme for 2 months to 17 years, and 1 had had recurrent idiopathic erythema multiforme for 3 years. The last patient and 2 of those with postherpes involvement were followed during the development of lesions.

An initial red papule was followed by a vesicle surmounting the papule and then by a target (iris) lesion. Clinically normal skin exhibited focal endothelial cell swelling. The red papule was characterized by endothelial cytoplasmic swelling, vacuolation, and nuclear hypertrophy with luminal obliteration of superficial venules. In vesicular and target lesions the venular changes were more marked, with endothelial cell necrosis, and deeper venules were involved. Lymphocytes were present around venules and in the lower epidermis in the earlier lesions. Venule damage correlated with degree of lymphocyte infiltration. Hypogranulated basophils were seen around venules in the later lesions. Fibrin deposits were present within and beneath the vesicles. Deposits of IgM and C3 were present in papules and vesicles.

Some of the findings in erythema multiforme resemble those in cutaneous delayed-type hypersensitivity, suggesting a role for cell-mediated immunity in the pathogenesis of the former. Antigen-specific, antibody-dependent cytotoxicity may be a mechanism of cell-mediated tissue injury in recurrent erythema multiforme.

21. Miscellaneous Disorders

21–1 **Immunodeficiency in Female Sexual Partners of Men With Acquired Immunodeficiency Syndrome.** Carol Harris, Catherine B. Small, Robert S. Klein, Gerald H. Friedland, Bernice Moll, Eugene E. Emeson, Ilya Spigland, and Neal H. Steigbigel (Bronx, N.Y.) studied 7 female sexual partners of men with acquired immune deficiency syndrome (AIDS) to determine whether the current outbreak may be caused by a transmissible biologic agent and whether development of the syndrome may be preceded by immunologic abnormalities with or without a prodromal illness. All of the men were drug abusers.

One of the 7 women had the full-blown syndrome, another had an illness consistent with the prodrome of AIDS (generalized lymphadenopathy, lymphopenia, and a decreased ratio of helper to suppressor T cells), and 4 others had generalized lymphadenopathy or lymphopenia with or without a decreased ratio of helper to suppressor T cells. Only 1 woman had no abnormalities. Five women were Hispanic (Puerto Rican), 1 was black, and 1 was white. Their ages ranged from 23 to 39 (mean, 31). All of the women stated that they maintained an exclusively heterosexual relationship with their partners. All denied the use of intravenous drugs or inhalants, or contact with drug paraphernalia.

These findings suggest that AIDS may be transmitted sexually between heterosexual men and women.

▶ [The implications of this report are far reaching. Up to now most of the "innocent bystanders" acquiring the disease have been children born to mothers who are at high risk for AIDS because of their promiscuity and drug abuse. Hemophiliacs have also proved to be at risk because of their required blood transfusions. If females that are not promiscuous or drug abusers can be infected by their heterosexual male partners by sexual intercourse, the incidence of this disease among "innocent bystanders" is going to multiply several fold. It will have to be assumed that the offspring of these mothers will be also at a higher risk of developing AIDS.—E.G.] ◀

21–2 **Kawasaki Syndrome in the United States.** During the 4½-year period from July 1976 to December 1980, the Centers for Disease Control (CDC) received reports of 669 suspected cases of Kawasaki syndrome (KS) in persons in 43 states, Puerto Rico, and the Virgin Islands. Of these reports, 593 (89%) satisfied the CDC case definition of KS, and 523 (78%) also indicated that a serologic test or throat culture showed no evidence of infection with group A β-hemolytic streptococci. David M. Bell, David M. Morens, Robert C. Holman, Eugene S. Hurwitz, and Miriam K. Hunter (Centers for Disease Control, Atlanta) reviewed the epidemiologic characteristics, clinical and lab-

---

(21–1) N. Engl. J. Med. 308:1181–1184, May 19, 1983.
(21–2) Am. J. Dis. Child. 137:211–214, March 1983.

oratory features, and associated complications in these 523 patients.

During the period studied, the average annual incidence was 0.59 cases per 100,000 children younger than age 5 years. Males of all childhood ages were affected more often than females, with a male-female ratio of about 1.6:1. There were 4.07 cases per 100,000 Asian or Pacific Islander children, 0.68 case per 100,000 black children, 0.52 case per 100,000 Hispanic children, and 0.41 case per 100,000 white children. Most cases occurred in children younger than age 5 years (median, 2.3 years). Four patients (0.8%) experienced a second episode of KS. In 55% of the patients, onset of KS was during the period from February through May ($P<.001$). A smaller peak was observed during November and December, when 37% of the other cases occurred ($P<.001$). Complications frequently reported included arthritis or arthralgias (27%) and cardiac abnormalities (22%). Six patients (1.2%), all younger than age 5 years, died. Investigation by the CDC of four outbreaks (mean duration, 3.8 months) uncovered no evidence of person-to-person transmission or a point source of exposure.

The findings confirm earlier reports of a significantly higher incidence of KS in children younger than age 5 years, males, and children of Asian ancestry and suggest that some cases may be caused by an exogenous agent or toxin that is most prevalent in the late winter and spring. It is also likely that host, environmental, or other cofactors are important determinants of susceptibility.

▶ [Several points are worth noting from this epidemiologic study of Kawasaki syndrome (KS) in the United States: *(1)* the diagnosis may require time for evolution and the exclusion of other diseases; *(2)* coronary aneurysms were present in 13.4% of cases evaluated for this complication; *(3)* a normal ECG does not exclude significant coronary artery disease, and there may be an occasional false-negative with the use of echocardiography; *(4)* the late winter–early spring peak occurrence has no explanation, nor does a secondary peak in the late fall; and *(5)* secondary episodes occur but are rare. The etiology of KS is still unknown, despite extensive studies in the United States and Japan.—A.R.R.] ◀

21-3 **Infantile Acropustulosis.** First described in 1979, infantile acropustulosis is an uncommon pustular dermatosis in children that does not respond to routine therapies. Robert F. Findlay and Richard B. Odom (Letterman Army Med. Center, San Francisco) report a new case of infantile acropustolosis and compare the findings with those in cases previously reported.

Boy, aged 22 months, was examined for an extremely pruritic rash of about 10 months' duration. It consisted of numerous, discrete, 1–3-mm, vesiculopustular lesions on the hands and feet, with fewer lesions on the wrists, ankles, upper extremities, trunk, and face. Excoriations were also observed, though no distinct burrows were detected. Areas of previous involvement exhibited residual hyperpigmentation with slight scaling. There were no mucosal abnormalities. The rash occurred sporadically at 2–4-week intervals, with the eruption appearing in crops that persisted for 6–12 days before resolving spontaneously. Laboratory tests gave normal results. Biopsy of a pustular lesion revealed a well-circumscribed, subcorneal pustule extending to the lower part of the epidermis. Polymorphonuclear leukocytes admixed with

(21–3) Am. J. Dis. Child. 137:455–457, May 1983.

fibrinoid material predominated within the cavity. The subjacent papillary dermis exhibited a mild, primarily perivascular, lymphoid infiltrate. Tissue stains for fungi and bacteria showed none. The biopsy findings were consistent with those in previously reported cases of infantile acropustulosis. Dapsone therapy (2 mg/kg/day) was begun in two divided doses. The patient responded dramatically, with marked symptomatic relief occurring within 24–36 hours and complete resolution of the pustules and pruritus within 72 hours. Therapy was maintained at this dosage for several months without complications. Withdrawal of the drug resulted in a prompt and severe exacerbation of the eruption. Rapid relief was obtained with reintroduction of dapsone. A later interruption in treatment resulted in a similar, though less intense, recurrence. Dapsone was then administered at a lower dosage (1 mg/kg/day) and provided good control. When the patient was aged 2½ years, dapsone was successfully discontinued without recrudescence of the disease.

The clinical findings in this and in the 13 cases previously reported are remarkably similar. All patients were aged 1 year or younger at onset of disease, 12 were black, and 12 were male. The lesions consist of 1–3-mm, pruritic vesiculopustules erupting in crops and located primarily on the distal parts of the extremities, with scattered lesions on the forearms, proximal portions of the extremities, trunk, face, and scalp. The eruptions occur as intermittent exacerbations and remissions, with progressive improvement and resolution between ages 2 and 3 years. Bacterial, fungal, and viral cultures are universally negative. The differential diagnosis includes scabies, impetigo, candidiasis, erythema toxicum neonatorum, transient neonatal pustular melanosis, subcorneal pustular dermatosis, pustular psoriasis, and dyshidrotic eczema. The severe pruritus, appearance and location of the lesions, normal findings on various laboratory studies, and results of cutaneous biopsy should lead to the correct diagnosis. Dapsone is the only drug with demonstrated efficacy.

▶ [Any dermatosis thought to be compatible with scabies should have a scraping confirmation of the diagnosis. For instance, acral pustulosis may have a presentation almost identical to scabies except that in acral pustulosis, skin lesions appear in crops and heal spontaneously, whereas in scabies the skin lesions are usually additive. Dapsone appears to be effective therapy, but recurrence is common when therapy is temporarily discontinued. Acral pustulosis appears to be a real disease and, unfortunately, is still poorly understood. Although dapsone appears to be effective therapy, the burden of disease must be balanced against the toxicity of the drug. First, do no harm!—A.R.R.] ◀

21–4 **Barrier Properties of Newborn Infant's Skin.** V. A. Harpin and N. Rutter (Nottingham, England) examined the barrier properties of the skin in 223 studies in 70 newborn infants of 25–41 weeks' gestation, aged from 1 hour to 26 days. Percutaneous drug absorption was studied by observing the blanching response to solutions of 1% and 10% phenylephrine applied to a small area of abdominal skin.

Infants of 37 weeks' or more gestation had a minimal or no response to phenylephrine application, indicating low skin permeability to the drug. Skin water losses were low. Infants of 33–36 weeks' gestation had a mild degree of skin permeability to phenylephrine in the

(21–4) J. Pediatr. 102:419–425, March 1983.

first few days of life, but this became less marked by 1 week of age. Skin water loss was slightly higher than in term infants, but fell to normal within a week. Infants of 30–32 weeks' gestation had high skin permeability to phenylephrine initially, but this fell steadily in the early neonatal period. By 2 weeks of age the blanching response had virtually disappeared. Skin water losses mirrored drug permeability. Infants of less than 30 weeks' gestation had very high skin permeability to phenylephrine, and skin water loss was high. Infants who were small for gestational age had skin barrier properties similar to those of appropriately grown infants of the same gestation. To assess skin damage caused by application of 2 different adhesive materials, an adhesive tape or ring was placed on the leg or abdomen of 11 infants. Thirty minutes after removal of the tape or ring, water loss was greater in every infant studied; the final level was between 2 and 6 times that from adjacent undamaged skin.

The blanching response to phenylephrine is a good indicator of percutaneous drug absorption; lack of blanching indicates a lack of absorption rather than failure to respond by vasoconstriction. The skin of mature newborn infants is an effective barrier against water loss and drug absorption. In preterm infants, when adhesive tape, monitoring probes, or electrodes are removed, the outermost layer of epidermis is stripped off, weakening the skin barrier. Therefore, the application of adhesive tape should be confined to as small an area of the newborn's skin as possible; also, monitoring devices using surface probes and electrodes should be in contact with as small an area of skin as is consistent with their function.

► [Previously published work has shown that skin of very premature newborns is an ineffective barrier to water loss, compared with skin of full-term newborns, and that barrier function is usually normal by 2 weeks of age. The classic studies of Nachman and Esterly demonstrated that a blanching response to a topically applied vasoconstricting agent like phenylephrine occurs in preterm newborns, but not in full-term infants. However, abnormal reactivity of the vasculature (vs. enhanced absorption) might account for this finding. The studies by Harpin and Rutter demonstrate an identical blanching response in skin of full-term newborns, but only if the skin is pretreated with tape stripping. These studies emphasize the dangers of adhesives on skin of premature newborns, whose barrier function is already compromised.—A.R.R.] ◄

21–5 **Juvenile Hyaline Fibromatosis** is a rare disease characterized by skin lesions, muscle weakness, and flexion contractures of large joints. Although it occurs sporadically, it has been described in siblings. Both multiple large tumors and small pink or pearly papules are found in the head and neck region and on the trunk of these patients. A. Y. Finlay, S. D. Ferguson, and P. J. A. Holt (Cardiff, Wales) report data on a young boy with this disorder.

Boy, 4, born to unrelated Indian parents in the United Kingdom, had small spots at the sides of the nose at birth and enlargement of the gums at age 18 months. Motor development was delayed; he could not arise unaided until age 2½ years. Small plaques were noted about the nasal alae at age 2 years (Fig 21–1), and small pearly papules were seen on the upper lip, neck, and

---

(21–5) Br. J. Dermatol. 108:609–616, May 1983.

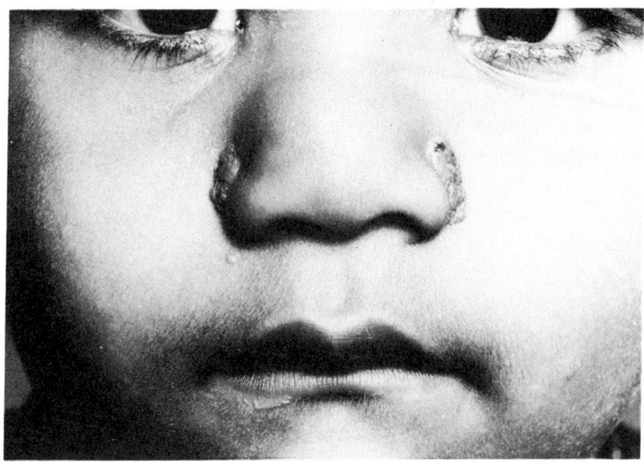

Fig 21–1.—At age 2 years boy had small plaques around alae nasi and papules on upper lip and bridge of nose. (Courtesy of Finlay, A.Y., et al.: Br. J. Dermatol. 108:609–616, May 1983.)

mastoid region (Fig 21–2). Gross gingival enlargement also was noted. Marked shoulder girdle weakness was present. Mental development was normal. Muscle biopsy specimens showed mild fiber atrophy and some hypertrophied fibers. There was osteolytic lesion in the distal left humerus. A biopsy specimen from the retroauricular papular eruption showed hyalinized eosinophilic material in the upper dermis. There was a patchy perivascular mononuclear cell infiltrate in the dermis. The hyaline material also was found in the gingiva. The disease has progressed in the past 18 months. Growths had

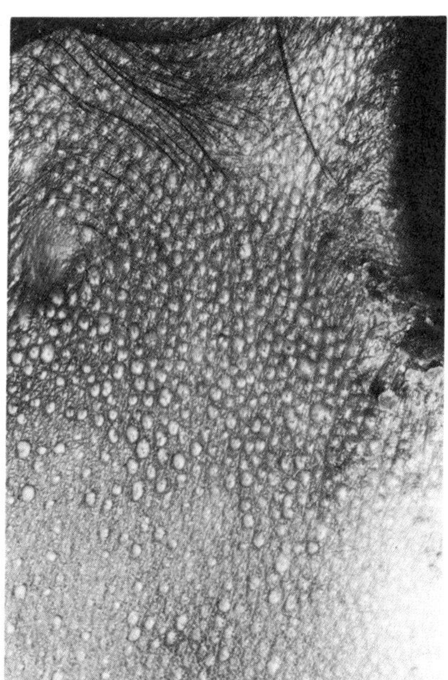

Fig 21–2.—Multiple papules coalescing over mastoid region at age 4 years in boy shown in Fig 21–1. (Courtesy of Finlay, A.Y., et al.: Br. J. Dermatol. 108:609–616, May 1983.)

to be removed from the nostrils, and gingivectomy was necessary on 2 occasions. Some improvement in muscle strength occurred.

Small pearly papules on the face and neck are the most common skin lesions in juvenile hyaline fibromatosis. There also may be translucent nodules on the fingers and nose and in the retroauricular regions as well as large subcutaneous tumors, most commonly in the scalp. Joint contractures are often present. Delayed motor development was a significant feature in the present case, but it has not been well characterized.

Treatment of the condition has not been satisfactory. Significant spontaneous regression seems unlikely. The tumors are characterized by "chondroid" cells within an eosinophilic ground substance. Juvenile hyaline fibromatosis may be a connective tissue disorder with aberrant synthesis of glycosaminoglycans by fibroblasts.

▶ [This is a well-written, concise, clinical review of this unusual syndrome. The authors of this article contacted the authors of other reports, and they present follow-up data concerning these published cases. Thus, new prognostic data are presented. We await more definitive biochemical findings on cultured fibroblasts from these patients.—J.C.A.] ◀

21–6 **Eradication of Scabies With Single Treatment Schedule.** David Taplin, Carmen Arrue, Jane Graham Walker, William I. Roth, and Alicio Rivera evaluated treatment with 1% gamma benzene hexachloride (GBH) lotion in patients living on 2 adjacent islands, part of the districts of San Blas, Republic of Panama. Scabies had been present in epidemic proportions for about 18 months despite careful daily personal hygiene. No treatment had been given. On one island every person had a single overnight application of 1% GBH lotion; on the other island, only clinically active disease was treated. Exposure to the medication lasted for 16–20 hours. Head-to-toe applications were used except in nursing mothers.

On the island on which all of the inhabitants were treated, 74 of 178 examined had clinical scabies. The cure rate was more than 98%; only 1 person was affected on reexamination at 10 and 21 weeks. On the other island, on which only clinically active disease was treated, 140 persons used the lotion; disease prevalence was reduced by only 50% at 10 weeks.

This experience indicates that eradication of scabies from a population requires the treatment of all contacts, even those who are not clinically infected. Treatment of the entire population at risk at one time is best. Coexisting pyoderma should also be treated; a second treatment for scabies may be necessary after the pyoderma resolves. A less aggressive approach may reduce the extent of the problem, but leaves a substantial reservoir for reinfestation. No adverse effects resulted from a single application of 1% GBH lotion. Mass eradication at one time may not be feasible in large or urban populations, but it is important to treat family contacts who may be incubating scabies.

▶ [This study provides a very strong argument for treating nonpregnant, noninfant contacts, as well as clinically infected individuals with scabies, with 1% gamma ben-

(21–6) J. Am. Acad. Dermatol. 9:546–550, October 1983.

zene hexachloride. The effectiveness of a single course of therapy strongly suggests that clothes and furniture are not frequent reservoirs of scabies infestation. Unfortunately, there are few data that adequately compare 1% gamma benzene hexachloride and croamitin with respect to safety or efficacy.—R.S.S.] ◀

21–7 **Experimental Canine Scabies in Humans.** The self-limiting nature of canine scabies in man has suggested that the canine type of *Sarcoptes scabiei* is host specific and cannot burrow or suvive on human skin. Stephen A. Estes, Barbara Kummel, and Larry Arlian investigated whether this is the case by applying adult female *S. scabiei* var. *canis* mites to human skin for 96 hours in an experimental chamber and examining the resultant lesions histologically. The mites were collected from crusted lesions of a dog with scabies.

Of the 28 mites applied, 16 were recovered alive at 96 hours, 8 from each of the hosts. The prototype lesion was an erythematous, variably edematous, papular burrow (Fig 21–3). One host developed vesicles with erythematous bases. The host inflammatory response lagged behind the progress of some burrows. Pruritus developed in both subjects within 24 hours, but declined over time. Mineral oil preparations of epidermal shave biopsy specimens showed continuing deposit of eggs throughout the burrow (Fig 21–4). In each host a single egg was seen to hatch, with successful emergence of a larva within 24

Fig 21–3 (left).—Edematous vesicles produced in 96 hours by canine scabies on human skin. Note pigmented material along course of burrow *(arrow)*.

Fig 21–4 (right).—Mineral oil epidermal shave biopsy preparation demonstrating burrow containing adult female mite, feces, and eggs; original magnification, ×16.

(Courtesy of Estes, S.A., et al.: J. Am. Acad. Dermatol. 9:397–401, September 1983.)

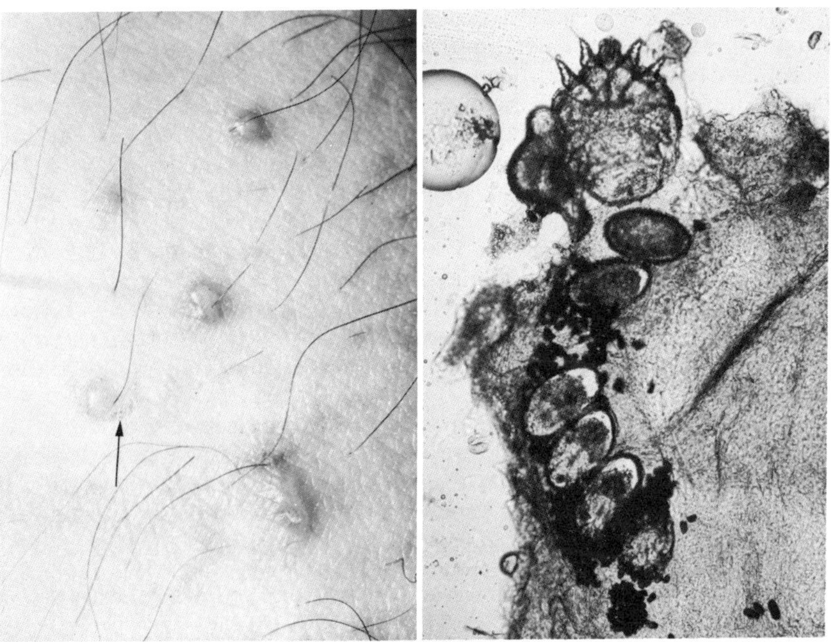

(21–7) J. Am. Acad. Dermatol. 9:397–401, September 1983.

hours. Skin biopsies showed mites and eggs within the stratum corneum, epidermal spongiosis, mononuclear exocytosis, and an intense perivascular mononuclear cell infiltrate within the dermis.

These observations indicate that canine *S. scabiei* can survive in human skin for at least 96 hours and that the nutritional needs of the mites are satisfied in human skin. The mites are capable of burrowing and of depositing eggs that hatch in human skin. It has been suggested that continuous interbreeding between the strains of mites that infest man and domestic animals may occasionally produce a strain that is well adapted to man and is perhaps responsible for intermittent human epidemics.

▶ [Ingenious experimental inoculation of canine scabies in human subjects was performed to determine whether mites could survive and produce an inflammatory reaction. It seems that this parasite is very adaptable and can survive in many different host environments, and occasionally it might be the source of infestation in some of our patients with scabies.—E.G.] ◀

21–8 **Sweating Efficiency in Acclimated Men and Women Exercising in Humid and Dry Heat.** A. J. Frye and E. Kamon (Pennsylvania State Univ.) compared thermoregulatory function and the density of active sweat glands in equally fit men and women exposed to humid and dry heat. Four acclimated men and 4 women exercised at 30% of maximal oxygen uptake in both a hot-humid environment, with a dry-bulb to wet-bulb temperature ratio of 37/30 C, and in a hot-dry environment, with a temperature ratio of 48/25 C. Peak density of sweat gland activity was determined first by stimulation with methacholine. Three-hour heat stress tests were carried out.

No differences in rectal temperature or heart rate were found between the sexes in either environment. Both men and women had significantly lower total-body sweat rates and chest sweat rates in humid heat than in dry heat, and women maintained lower sweat rates in humid heat. Sweating efficiency, determined as the ratio of required to observed sweating, was significantly greater in the women. No such differences were apparent on dry heat testing. In women, sweat gland activity per unit of surface area on the chest relative to maximum activity was higher in dry heat than in humid heat, as was sweating efficiency, but sweat gland flow on the chest was similar in the two settings. In men, sweat gland flow was higher in dry heat, while sweating efficiency was similar in the two settings. In both environments, men recruited fewer available sweat glands than did women.

Women appear to conserve body water through improved sweating efficiency when exposed to humid heat, but men have a larger reserve for increased sweating in more severe dry heat, when evaporation is not restricted. Men who are exposed to humid heat reduce their sweat gland flow without an improvement in sweating efficiency.

▶ [Horses sweat, gentlemen perspire, and women glisten. This article confirms a commonly-held notion among experienced runners that acclimated trained female runners tolerate humid heat better than acclimated trained male runners. In this arti-

---

(21–8) J. Appl. Physiol. 54:972–977, April 1983.

cle, female runners were noted to sweat more efficiently in humid heat than male runners. Vive la difference.—A.R.R.] ◀

21–9 **Surgical Treatment of Primary Hyperhidrosis: A Report of 42 Cases.** Primary or idiopathic hyperhidrosis is best managed surgically, preferably by the supraclavicular approach. Harry Bogokowsky, Sam Slutzki, Leon Bacalu, Raphael Abramsohn, and Michael Negri reviewed the results of upper dorsal sympathectomy by the supraclavicular approach in 42 patients seen between 1977 and 1982 with primary hyperhidrosis. The 27 females and 15 males were aged 16–58 years. All patients reported social embarrassment and interference with everyday tasks, including writing. About a third had become withdrawn, and some exhibited aggressive behavior. Bilateral sympathectomies were done in a single session. The excision was done below the stellate ganglion and included T2 and T3.

All 84 hands were dry immediately after operation, and only 1 patient had a significant recurrence of sweating on follow-up for as long as 5 years after operation. Three others had mild sweating that was much more tolerable than before operation. Transient compensatory hyperhidrosis of the chest and abdomen was noticed by 15 patients. Plantar hyperhidrosis occurred in all patients at various times after operation. Complications were infrequent and minor. Two patients had a small pneumothorax not requiring chest drainage. No patient had Horner's syndrome or neural pains in the chest and upper limbs.

Bilateral upper dorsal sympathectomies by the supraclavicular approach yielded satisfactory results in all but one of these 42 patients with primary hyperhidrosis. The operation greatly improved the quality of the patients' lives.

▶ [Hyperhidrosis is a vexing problem for both the patient and the physician called upon to manage this problem. Oral agents have either been ineffective or had unacceptable side effects. Although the patients in this series seem to have had good immediate results, a report on long-term follow-up would be of value.—A.J.S.] ◀

21–10 **Histopathologic, Ultrastructural, Immunologic, and Virologic Study of Gibert's Pityriasis Rosea** was undertaken by J. L. Bonafé, J. Icart, M. Perpère, F. Oksman, and D. Divoux (Toulouse, France). Direct and indirect immunofluorescence studies were performed (serum antibodies to cutaneous structures), as well as ultrastructural examination of biopsy material, inoculation of homogenized skin specimens for 3 different types of cellular structures, and titration of serum antibodies were related to various viral antigens such as A and B influenza, para-influenza 1, 2, 3, adenovirus, respiratory syncytial virus, *Mycoplasma pneumoniae,* ornithosis-psittacosis, Q fever, herpesvirus, varicella-zoster virus, and Epstein-Barr virus (EBV). None of the histologic investigations of biopsy specimens taken from 15 patients (aged 5–46 years) disclosed any new elements when compared with classic descriptions.

During the course of Gibert's pityriasis rosea (GPR), a focal or total epidermal necrosis is evident; the cellular necrosis leads to exoserosis,

---

(21–9) Arch. Surg. 118:1065–1067, September 1983.
(21–10) Ann. Dermatol. Venereol. 109:855–861, 1982.

occasionally creating intraepidermal cavities. No acantholytic dyskeratosis was observed, although multinucleated keratinocytes were encountered in 1 case. The hyperkeratosis may alternately take the form of orthokeratosis or parakeratosis; the parakeratotic zones correspond to the elimination of necrotic material from epidermal cells. The phenomena of epidermal necrosis and dermal inflammation seem most intense in the phase of initial plaques. Immunologic findings were normal except in cases of recurrent GPR in which direct immunofluorescence studies showed a fixation of IgM and IgG at the level of the basal membrane.

All results of viral investigations were normal; no viral infective agent could be incriminated as the cause of GPR. However, about 50% of the patients were found to have antibodies to the "early antigen" of EBV. Although a direct participation of EBV cannot be suggested on the basis of this study, this viral profile may be interpreted as proof of a particular immunologic disturbance or an endogenous reactivation of EBV infection linked to a triggering factor yet to be determined.

▶ [Viral etiology for pityriasis rosea has been postulated largely on the basis of the increased numbers of cases seen in spring and fall. Evidence against a viral etiology is the failure of household contacts to develop the disease. Without a comparable control group, the finding of antibody to EBV in half the patients is not evaluable.—A.J.S.] ◀

21–11 **Recent Upper Respiratory Tract Infection and Pityriasis Rosea: Case-Control Study of 249 Matched Pairs.** Pityriasis rosea is an inflammatory dermatosis of unknown cause that runs an acute, self-limited course. An earlier study indicated recent or concurrent infection and a history of asthma, hay fever, or atopic dermatitis in many patients. Tsu-Yi Chuang, H. O. Perry, D. M. Ilstrup, and L. T. Kurland (Mayo Clinic and Found.) matched 249 of 939 patients from a previous study with control subjects on the basis of age, sex and year of diagnosis. The clinical features of the study patients were similar to those of the original group of 939. Immunization in the preceding month was reported by 4% of cases and 5% of controls. A history of atopy was obtained from 14% of cases and 12% of controls. Asthma was insignificantly more frequent in the cases. Infection had occurred in the preceding 3 months in 12% of cases and 6% of controls. The difference was due chiefly to upper respiratory tract infection, which occurred in 8% of cases and 2% of controls. A positive throat culture was obtained in nearly half of the infected patients.

The findings do not substantiate an autoimmune cause for pityriasis rosea. Recent upper respiratory tract infection appears to be closely associated with the development of pityriasis rosea in a small proportion of patients. Some studies have suggested an infectious cause for the disease; RNA viruses have been described in lesions of pityriasis rosea, and "epidemics" have been reported. Pityriasis may have multiple causes.

(21–11) Br. J. Dermatol. 108:587–591, May 1983.

▶ [We have always considered pityriasis rosea as one of the viral exanthems, and this exhaustive survey would support an infectious etiology. Perhaps the simplest way to prove this is to attempt the experiment performed by Dr. Udo Wilde in 1927 (Wilde, U.: *Arch. Dermatol. and Syph.* 16:185) in which he was able to produce a generalized eruption resembling pityriasis rosea by dermal injection of serum obtained from blisters of the primary plaque and from the secondary lesions.—T.B.F.] ◀

21–12 **Histopathology of Pityriasis Rosea Gibert: Qualitative and Quantitative Light Microscopic Study of 62 Biopsies of 40 Patients.** Renato Panizzon and Peter H. Bloch (Univ. of Zurich) reviewed the biopsy findings in 40 patients, 24 women and 16 men, with pityriasis rosea Gibert (PRG). The clinical diagnosis was agreed

FREQUENCY AND INTENSITY OF 31 HISTOLOGIC CRITERIA OF PITYRIASIS ROSEA GIBERT IN 62 BIOPSY SPECIMENS

Criteria	Intensity	Frequency	%
Papillomatosis	+	62	100
Spongiosis	+ to ++	62	100
Exocytosis	+	62	100
Homogenization of the papillary collagen	+	62	100
Inflammatory infiltrates of the superficial plexus	+ to ++	62	100
Inflammatory infiltrates in the reticular dermis	+	62	100
Erythrocytes in the papillary dermis	+ to ++	62	100
Decrease/absence of the granular cell layer	++ to +++	61	98
Inflammatory infiltrates in the papillary dermis	+	61	98
Absence of elastic fibers in the papillary dermis	+	60	97
Dilated capillaries	+	60	97
Acanthosis	+	59	95
Edema in the papillary dermis	+	59	95
Swelling of endothelial cells	+	59	95
Nuclear debris	0 to +	59	95
Parakeratosis	+	57	92
Intracellular edema in the epidermis	+	57	92
Disintegration of the basal layer	0 to +	57	92
Melanine in the upper dermis	+	56	90
Alcian-blue-pos. material in the reticular dermis	+	56	90
Erythrocytes in the epidermis	+	54	87
Intraepidermal vesicles	+	53	85
Dilated superficial plexus	0 to +	53	85
Intracorneal exudate	0 to +	50	81
Hyperemia in the papillary dermis	0 to +	44	71
Intracorneal microabscesses	0 to +	34	55
Hyperkeratosis	0 to +	33	53
Eosinophils in dermal infiltrates	0 to +	29	47
Mitoses in the epidermis	0.5/HPF	24	39
Dyskeratosis	0 to +	16	26
Hyaline bodies	0 to +	15	24

HPF = High power field.

Single plus indicates slight intensity; + +, medium; and + + +, strong.
(Courtesy of Panizzon, R., and Bloch, P.H.: Dermatologica 165:551–558, 1982.)

(21–12) Dermatologica 165:551–558, 1982.

on independently by at least two dermatologists. Biopsy specimens were taken an average of 9 days after the onset of PRG. The frequency of the histologic abnormalities is given in the table. A majority of the biopsy specimens showed eczema-like changes, whereas most of the rest exhibited parapsoriasis en plaques–like changes. Older lesions tended toward the latter appearance and also were characterized by more frequent microabscesses and exudates in the corneum and by the appearance of granular cells. In addition, eosinophils were found in the inflammatory infiltrate in the older lesions.

There are no pathognomonic histologic features of PRG, but the diagnosis is suggested by an absence or decrease of the granular cell layer, often without parakeratosis; extravasation of red blood cells into the papillary dermis and epidermis; and the presence of homogenized collagen in the papillary dermis. The differences between recent and older lesions are not striking except for an increase in eosinophils in older lesions. The appearance of PRG may be more like that of parapsoriasis en plaques in older cases.

▶ [This article emphasizes that PRG must be included in the list of disorders that are often associated with intraepidermal Pautrier-like microabscessess.—M.C.A.] ◀

21–13 **Frequency of Desquamative Gingivitis in Skin Diseases.** A. Sklavounou and G. Laskaris (Univ. of Athens) studied the frequency of desquamative gingivitis in patients with chronic bullous dermatoses, e.g., cicatricial pemphigoid, pemphigus vulgaris, bullous pemphigoid, and lichen planus, based on examination of a large series of patients in each disease group. The series included 453 patients seen from 1972 to 1981. The groups included 157 patients with pemphigus vulgaris, 62 patients with bullous pemphigoid, 55 patients with a chronic vesicular disease that usually involved the oral and other mucous membranes, and 179 patients with lichen planus.

The frequency of desquamative gingivitis in all patients is shown in the table. Analysis of the clinical data revealed that, of the 4 skin diseases, cicatricial pemphigoid appeared as desquamative gingivitis in 63.6% of the patients. Desquamative gingival lesions were less frequent in lichen planus (25%) and in pemphigus vulgaris (18.4%) pa-

FREQUENCY OF DESQUAMATIVE GINGIVITIS (DG) IN 453 PATIENTS WITH SKIN DISEASE*

Underlying disease	*No. of cases*	*Females*	*Males*	*Mean age*	*DG*
Pemphigus vulgaris	157	97 (61.8%)	60 (38.2%)	54	29 (18.4%)
Bullous pemphigoid	62	39 (62.9%)	23 (37.1%)	65	2 (3.2%)
Cicatricial pemphigoid	55	33 (60%)	22 (40%)	65	35 (63.6%)
Lichen planus	179	115 (64.2%)	64 (35.7%)		45 (25%)
Total	453	284 (62.6%)	169 (37.3%)		111 (24.5%)

*Patients with pemphigus vulgaris and bullous pemphigoid without oral lesions are also included. (Courtesy of Sklavounou, A., and Laskaris, G.: Oral Surg. 56:141–144, August 1983.)

(21–13) Oral Surg. 56:141–144, August 1983.

tients. Most patients with desquamative gingivitis were females (72.9%). Identification of the underlying causes of desquamative gingivitis is of utmost importance and is dependent on clinical, histologic, and immunologic criteria.

▶ [The authors review the incidence of desquamative gingivitis, which they note is not a true disease state but a primarily clinical manifestation of four dermatological entities—pemphigus vulgaris, bullous pemphigoid, cicatricial pemphigoid, and lichen planus. They recommend clinical observation, gingival biopsy, direct immunofluorescent studies of perilesional and normal gingival specimens, and indirect immunofluorescent examination of serum for epithelial antibiodies associated with pemphigus vulgaris, cicatricial pemphigoid, and bullous pemphigoid. A recent study by Leonard et al. (*Br. J. Dermatol.* 110:307–314, 1984) points out the presence of oral lesions in linear IgA disease (as well as ocular lesions).—R.M.] ◀

21–14 **Lymphocytotoxicity for Oral Mucosa in Lichen Planus.** A subpopulation of T cells with cytotoxic activity has been identified in patients with lichen planus (LP), and OKT-8-positive lymphocytes have been demonstrated in oral and cutaneous lesions of LP. Miklós Simon, Jr., Georg Reimer, Michael Schardt, and Otto Paul Hornstein (Univ. of Erlangen-Nürnberg, Federal Republic of Germany) investigated whether peripheral blood lymphocytes are cytotoxic for syngeneic oral epithelial cells in LP. Twenty-three patients with histologically confirmed LP of the skin, oral mucosa, or both partipated in the study. The 12 men and 11 women had a mean age of 45 years. Mean duration of disease was 5 years. No patient was receiving immunosuppressive therapy when studied. Ten dermatology patients without mucosal involvement and 8 healthy subjects of similar sex and age were studied as controls. Twelve of the study patients had lesions of LP on both the skin and the mucous membranes. Substantial in vitro lymphocytotoxicity was observed with effector lymphocytes for ^{51}Cr-labeled syngeneic oral epithelial tissue culture cells in patients with LP in a modified ^{51}Cr release macroassay. The difference from controls was significant.

A significant lymphocytotoxic effect of peripheral blood lymphocytes from LP patients on autologous epithelial cells has been demonstrated. These lymphocytes are presumably involved in the pathogenesis of LP. The lymphocytotoxicity observed is probably generated by sensitized effector lymphocytes through specific recognition of foreign antigenic structures on syngeneic oral target cells.

▶ [Monoclonal antibodies have been instrumental in identifying the OKT-8-positive lymphocytes in oral and cutaneous lichen planus, suggesting that their cytotoxic activity might play a central role in the pathogenesis of lichen planus. Using an in vitro assay, these authors now demonstrate that similar cytotoxic activity is present in the peripheral blood lymphocytes of these patients. It remains to be determined whether injecting these lymphocytes in vivo will induce lichen planus. For ethical reasons, an animal model will have to be used, and I'm not aware that this disease occurs in animals.—E.G.] ◀

21–15 **Oral Manifestations of Chronic Graft-Versus-Host Reaction.** The graft-versus-host reaction (GVHR) is a multisystem immunologic phenomenon probably related to the antigen-dependent proliferation

---

(21–14) Dermatologica 167:11–15, July 1983.
(21–15) JAMA 249:504–507, Jan. 28, 1983.

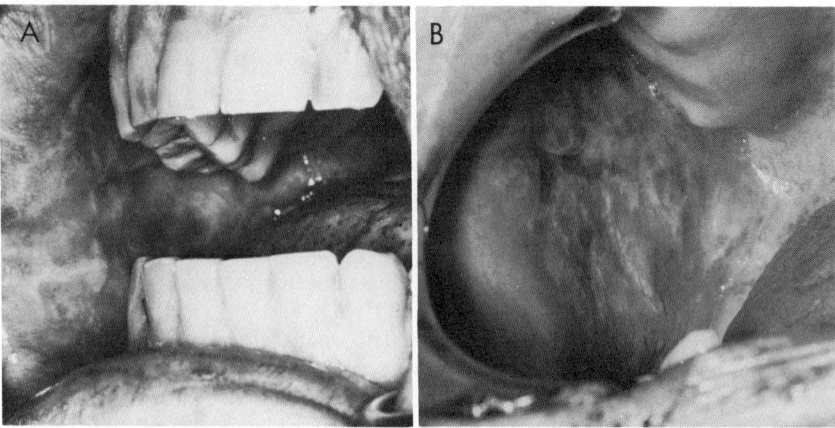

Fig 21–5.—A, lichenoid keratosis involving buccal mucosa and gingiva in 22-year-old man diagnosed as having acute lymphocytic leukemia. **B,** identical lesions in same areas in 33-year-old man who was diagnosed as having anaplastic anemia. (Courtesy of Rodu, B., and Gockerman, J.P.: JAMA 249:504–507, Jan. 28, 1983; copyright 1983, American Medical Association.)

of thymus-dependent donor lymphocytes, which give rise to effector cells reactive with host tissues. Cutaneous manifestations are the most important indicator of GVHR and its extent. Brad Rodu and Jon P. Gockerman (Univ. of Alabama) report data on 2 cases of chronic GVHR in which the oral findings contributed to diagnosis. One case is described below.

Man, 22, had complete remission of acute lymphocytic leukemia after chemotherapy. After conditioning and total body irradiation, he underwent bone marrow transfusion from a sibling donor. An abdominal rash developed 25 days later, and a skin biopsy showed acute GVHR, which responded to prednisone therapy. Subsequently, mild cytomegalovirus and mild herpes zoster infection developed, and there was progressive motor neuropathy of the lower extremities.

A skin biopsy performed on day 194 showed minimal changes of chronic GVHR. A lichenoid keratosis had developed in the buccal mucosa on about day 80 and had extended to the gingiva, tongue, and labial mucosa (Fig 21–5). Biopsy specimens showed lymphocytic infiltration of periductular areas of the minor salivary glands and periductal fibrosis. The mucosa exhibited vacuolar degeneration of the basal cell layer and collections of small lymphocytes in the lamina propria, some infiltrating the epithelium and associated with epithelial cell necrosis. The oral mucosal lesions resolved gradually on treatment with prednisone and azathioprine.

Oral manifestations of chronic GVHR can precede other manifestations by some time. The diminution or exacerbation of oral lesions may closely reflect the successful treatment or progression of GVHR. Cultures can rule out a viral etiology of oral lesions, and toxic reactions to most drugs can be excluded 35–40 days after the start of treatment.

▶ [The finding of a lichen planus–like mucosal change is of interest because of the similar lichen planus–like changes seen in skin (see Touraine, R., et al.: *Br. J. Der-*

matol. 92:589–590, 1975; Saurat, J., et al.: *Br. J. Dermatol.* 92:591–592, 1975). Other patients develop scleroderma-like changes (Spielvogel, R., et al.: *Arch. Dermatol.* 113:1424–1428, 1977). As bone marrow transplantation becomes more widely used (in treatment of leukemia, aplastic anemia, reconstitution of immune deficiencies), these eruptions will undoubtedly become a more troublesome problem.—A.J.S.] ◀

21–16 **Griseofulvin in Treatment of Three Cases of Oral Erosive Lichen Planus.** Of the 6 reported patterns of lichen planus involving the oral mucosa, the atrophic, erosive, and bullous forms are the most troublesome and are generally refractory to currently available therapies. Treatment of cutaneous lichen planus with griseofulvin, a fungistatic agent derived from a species of *Penicillium,* has been described, but there are few reports of its efficacy against oral lesions. Thomas B. Aufdemorte, Richard L. De Villez, and Donald R. Gieseker (Univ. of Texas, San Antonio) describe 3 cases of oral erosive lichen planus that responded dramatically to treatment with griseofulvin.

Woman, 68, had a 2-year history of erosive lichen planus. Examination revealed multiple, diffuse, markedly erosive, erythematous lesions with peripheral lacy striae involving the lips, tongue, buccal mucosa, floor of the mouth, and alveolar ridges. One cutaneous lesion characteristic of lichen planus was also seen on the volar surface of the left wrist. Histologic examination confirmed the diagnosis of erosive lichen planus. The lesions did not respond to Benadryl elixir, topically applied corticosteroids, or antibiotics. The patient's medical history was significant only for diabetes mellitus and essential hypertension, compatible with Grinspan's syndrome. A course of griseofulvin microsize (500 mg twice daily) was begun. After 3 weeks the patient reported improvement of the oral symptoms, though clinical examination revealed no objective change. The areas of erosion were seen to be resolving at 6 weeks, and at 8 weeks clinical remission was complete. The erythematous, erosive, or ulcerative lesions had completely resolved, but areas that were initially white, plaque-like, or reticular persisted. The cutaneous lesion remained, but it was not as pruritic and healed with hyperpigmentation after 2 months. The dose of griseofulvin was reduced by 50% at 3 months, and the drug was discontinued at 12 months. There has been no exacerbation over a 15-month follow-up.

Complete remission without exacerbation occurred in 2 of the patients, and the third has shown continuing improvement. Objective improvement became evident after 6–10 weeks of treatment. There were no significant hematologic, hepatic, or other side effects, and complete blood counts and blood chemistries were normal at 1- and 6-month intervals during therapy. However, all patients reported mild, transient gastrointestinal discomfort during the first 2 days of griseofulvin, and 1 patient had a mild headache. These effects disappeared within 2–4 days. Further trials of griseofulvin in the treatment of severely symptomatic oral lichen planus appear to be warranted.

▶ [These 3 cases do little to prove a therapeutic effect for griseofulvin in the treatment of oral erosive lichen planus. In fact, there are still no well-executed controlled

---

(21–16) Oral Surg. 55:459–462, May 1983.

studies that demonstrate griseofulvin's efficacy for lichen planus. Why griseofulvin would be expected to help lichen planus remains a mystery.—R.S.S.] ◀

21–17 **Colchicine in Treatment of Acute Febrile Neutrophilic Dermatosis (Sweet's Syndrome).** S. Suehisa, H. Tagami, F. Inoue, K. Matsumoto, and K. Yoshikuni (Hamamatsu, Japan) note that Sweet's syndrome is characterized by a massive polymorphonuclear leukocyte (PMN) infiltration in the dermis, with increased chemotactic activity of the peripheral blood PMNs in the acute stage. Colchicine was used to treat 3 patients with Sweet's syndrome.

All 3 patients had typical skin lesions. In addition, oral aphthosis was noted in 2, and an erythema nodosum–like lesion was found on the left lower leg in 1. Histologic examination of the latter lesion disclosed features of thrombophlebitis. Treatment with oral colchicine was started with 1.5 mg daily, and clinical improvement was observed within 2–5 days in all patients. Two patients stopped taking the drug after 7 days. In the third patient, the dosage was gradually reduced to 0.5 mg daily over a 3-week period to prevent recurrence. The increased erythrocyte sedimentation rate and positive findings for C-reactive protein returned to normal after treatment. Improvement in these patients after colchicine treatment may be due to a mechanism similar to that occurring after colchicine therapy in patients with Behçet's disease or necrotizing vasculitis.

▶ [These patients' symptoms, including the presence of aphthosis in 2 of the patients, suggest that the diagnosis is far from secure. In at least 1 case, Behçet's disease seems a more likely diagnosis than Behçet's syndrome. No mention is made of the presence of associated myeloproliferative disease, which is especially frequent in males with Sweet's syndrome. In spite of this study's shortcomings, the fact that neutrophils are prominent in Sweet's syndrome makes colchicine a logically possible alternative to systemic corticosteroids in the treatment of this disease. This report provides some—but not definitive—proof that colchicine is, in fact, effective.—R.S.S.] ◀

21–18 **Marjolin's Ulcer: The LSU Experience.** Marjolin's ulcer is a skin cancer arising in an area of chronic injury or irritation. Its biologic behavior is thought to be more aggressive than that of the more common types of skin cancer. The best initial surgical management remains controversial. Louis H. Barr and John W. Menard (Louisiana State Univ.) reviewed the management of 37 cases of Marjolin's ulcer seen at two treatment centers between 1950 and 1980. The mean age at presentation was 64 years, and the mean interval from injury to the diagnosis of malignant neoplasm was 36 years. Burn injury was reported by half of the patients, and chronic stasis ulcers of the lower extremity by about a third. All lesions but 2 were squamous cell cancers.

Five of the 16 patients whose cancers were managed by wide excision and skin grafting had recurrences. Nine of the 13 patients followed up for 5 years or longer remained free of disease. Only 2 patients have died of metastatic disease. Of 18 patients undergoing amputation for treatment of larger lesions, 3 have had recurrences

---

(21–17) Br. J. Dermatol. 108:99–101, January 1983.
(21–18) Cancer 52:173–175, July 1, 1983.

and died of metastatic disease. Six of the 8 total recurrences involved regional lymph nodes. One of these patients survived, without disease, following lymphadenectomy. Two patients who refused primary treatment died of unrelated causes after a year. One recently seen patient with advanced basal cell cancer involving the regional nodes underwent radiotherapy and subsequent above-the-knee amputation.

Marjolin's ulcer is a virulent form of skin cancer. Metastatic disease and death both are more frequent in patients initially seen with lower extremity lesions, possibly because of more frequent, clinically occult regional metastasis at the time of the first examination. Regional node dissection is not, however, necessary in most cases of Marjolin's ulcer. Recurrences have been more frequent after wide excision than after amputation, but they usually were of a local nature and were easily managed.

▶ [This is a very valuable review to stress, once again, the significance of chronic skin ulcers. Dermatologists must constantly be aware of the development of malignancies with the potential to metastasize in these lesions. Early biopsy of any suspicious lesion is strongly suggested.—J.C.A.] ◀

21–19 **Bacteremia Associated With Decubitus Ulcers.** Several recent studies have indicated the potential of decubitus ulcers for giving rise to bacteremia. Charles S. Bryan, Christopher E. Dew, and Kenneth L. Reynolds (Columbia, S.C.) reviewed findings in 102 patients with decubitus ulcers seen in a 5-year period at 4 hospitals in the Columbia, S.C., area with 104 episodes of bacteremia. The rate of bacteremia was highest at a teaching Veterans Administration hospital. Males predominated among the patients, and the mean age was 64. About two thirds were internal medicine patients. Paraplegia was present in 23%, and another 23% had neurologic deficits from cerebrovascular disease.

Other sites of infection were documented during hospitalization in 86% of the patients. The decubitus ulcers were considered to be the "probable" source of bacteremia in 51 episodes and the possible or unlikely source in 53 episodes. In both groups, bacteremia tended to occur after relatively prolonged hospitalization. The sites of ulcers were similar in the 2 groups, but patients in whom decubitus ulcers were the probable source of bacteremia were more likely to have multiple ulcers and to require surgical debridement. The most common blood isolates were *Proteus mirabilis, Staphylococcus aureus,* and *Escherichia coli.* Only *Bacteroides* species correlated with the probable origin of bacteremia from decubitus ulcers. The overall mortality was 55%, with about half of the deaths attributed to infection. Mortality either related or unrelated to bacteremia was comparable in both groups of patients. Apparently, appropriate antimicrobial therapy was not associated with lower mortality, nor did the use of individual antimicrobials or various combinations influence mortality. Mortality was insignificantly higher in patients having ulcer debridement.

(21–19) Arch. Intern. Med. 143:2093–2095, November 1983.

Patients with decubitus ulcers and bacteremia have a poor outlook. Although many deaths are due to other causes, decubitus ulcers should be prevented when possible and treated early and aggressively should they develop. Broad antimicrobial coverage seems indicated after culture results are obtained. Further debridement should be done when necessary, and coexisting osteomyelitis should be sought.

▶ [This article does not address the incidence of bacteremia in an unselected population of patients with decubitus ulcers. Support for this point is the 60-fold difference in incidence of bacteremic episodes in the 4 hospitals studied. Rather, groups of patients with decubiti who are at high risk for developing bacteremia are defined. Prolonged hospitalization, multiple ulcers, and presence of neurologic disease seemed to be the most important predisposing factors. The common theme among these factors might be general debility. As suggested by the authors, the development of cutaneous ulcers in these high-risk patients should be treated as early and aggressively as possible in an attempt to decrease the significant mortality rate.—J.C.A.] ◀

21–20 **Treatment of Keloids With Excision and Postoperative X-Ray Irradiation.** Anders Enhamre and Hans Hammar (Karolinska Inst., Stockholm) reviewed the results of excision of keloids with postoperative superficial irradiation in 47 patients in whom 62 keloids were treated in 1971–1979. Thirty-nine lesions developed after operations and 13 after trauma. Acne scarring, burn injury, and ear piercing were less frequent factors. Seven patients were aged 15 and younger when treated. All but 2 patients were followed for a year or longer after treatment. Irradiation was usually begun within 3 days after excision, and most patients so treated received a single dose of 1,000–1,200 rad. Patients treated later usually received fractionated doses totaling 1,000–1,500 rad.

Fifty-six lesions in 42 patients showed an excellent response to excision and irradiation. Results were comparable with single-dose and fractionated regimens, and the outcome did not depend on the interval from excision to irradiation. Neither patient age nor age of the lesion influenced the outcome. Pruritus and hyperesthesia were relieved in most cases. Hyperpigmentation in the area of treatment was a complication in 16 patients. Telangiectases were seen in 5 patients, and atrophy was seen in 2.

Satisfactory results were obtained in 88% of keloids treated by excision and postoperative irradiation in this series. Small keloids and lesions in the head-neck region responded best. The results are not strictly dependent on the interval between excision and irradiation, permitting convenient transfer of the patient after operation. In the future, radiotherapy may be optimized for the most appropriate treatment of lesions in different regions of the body.

▶ [The study is interesting but suffers from two problems: *(1)* there are no photographs, and *(2)* only 1 of the 47 patients was black. The data, therefore, might not have as much relevance to the keloid problem in the United States. Also, there is no discussion at all about the possibility of carcinogenesis.—J.C.A.] ◀

21–21 **Chronic Radiation Dermatitis From Radioactive Gold Jewelry.** L. William Luria, H. Berman, and S. Satchidanand (Buffalo

---

(21–20) Dermatologica 167:90–93, August 1983.
(21–21) N.Y. J. Med. 83:741–743, April 1983.

Gen. Hosp.) recently encountered 3 patients with chronic radiation dermatitis of the hands affecting areas that had been in contact with gold jewelry. Radioactive gold had contaminated the local gold supply, and the two pieces of jewelry tested proved to be radioactive. At present the problem appears to be primarily limited to New York State. The jewelry had been worn for periods of 15 months to 18 years. The rings were not worn after the patients noticed skin dryness, cracking, and bleeding. Chronic radiation dermatitis was diagnosed by biopsy in all 3 patients. The disorder begins with atrophic changes and may progress to telangiectasia, a wartlike keratosis, ulceration, and, ultimately, carcinoma. Several workers recommend conservative treatment in early cases, but others suggest excision to prevent carcinoma. All the authors' patients had wide excision of the clinically involved skin, with a 2-mm margin around all lesions, and full-thickness skin graft reconstruction. Healing was uncomplicated.

Chronic radiation dermatitis is the result of repeated "suberythemal" doses of ionizing radiation. Atrophic changes are seen initially, but later there are proliferative epidermal alterations and, in time, malignant changes. Malignancy usually occurs 20–25 years after exposure. Squamous cell cancer is the most common type. Excision of a suspicious lesion is indicated if suspect jewelry cannot be tested and the lesion does not respond to conservative measures. Wide excision with full-thickness skin graft reconstruction and close follow-up are recommended if chronic radiation dermatitis is confirmed.

1–22 **Chondrodermatitis Nodularis Chronica Helicis Treated With Curettage and Electrocauterization: Follow-up of a 15-Year Material.** Debate continues regarding the most appropriate treatment for chondrodermatitis nodularis chronica helicis (CNCH), a distinct, not uncommon, clinical entity characterized by a small tender nodule on the lateral aspect of the outer ear (Fig 21–6) that causes considerable distress. N. Kromann, H. Hoyer, and F. Reymann (Finsen Inst., Copenhagen) report the results of a follow-up study of 142 patients with CNCH who were treated principally by curettage followed by electrocauterization (see Fig 21–6) from 1965 through 1979. Adjunctive therapies in some cases included irradiation, intralesional injection of a triamcinolone crystal suspension, and freezing with carbon dioxide. Mean interval between treatment and follow-up was 7.1 years.

Of the 142 patients, 97 (68%) were male and 45 (32%) were female, a considerably higher proportion of women than previously reported in the literature. Multiple unilateral nodules were present in 3.5% of patients; no patient had bilateral involvement. The lesions were located on the preferred sleeping side in 78% of patients. Recurrence of the tumor more than 3 months after initial treatment occurred in 36 (25%) of the 142 patients. Among the 78 patients who were reexamined, 24 (31%) had a recurrence. In these patients the mean interval between treatment and recurrence was 2.1 years, with 50% of recur-

---

(21–22) Acta Derm. Venereol. (Stockh.) 63:85–88, 1983.

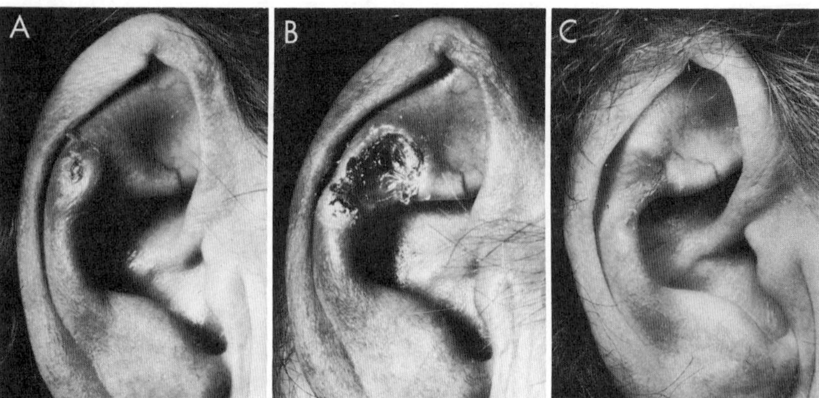

Fig 21–6.—Typical lesion of anthelix. **A,** before curettage-electrocauterization; **B,** 2 weeks after procedure; and **C,** 6 months after procedure. (Courtesy of Kromann, N., et al.: Acta Derm. Venereol. [Stockh.] 63:85–88, 1983.)

rences occurring during the first year after treatment. The recurrence rate for 1 person-year during the follow-up period was 0.04. Histologic examination of the primary tumor in 109 cases suggested basal cell carcinoma in 2 and squamous cell carcinoma in 1. However, there was no clinical suspicion of malignancy and no relapse after initial treatment. One uncharacteristic nodule treated as CNCH that reappeared 6 weeks later was histologically diagnosed as a squamous cell carcinoma.

Usually, CNCH can be diagnosed on the basis of its clinical presentation: appearance of a nodule on a typical location and extreme tenderness to pressure. Histologic examination is performed primarily to exclude malignancy. In this series the recurrence rate after routine curettage and electrocauterization was similar to that for more elaborate surgical procedures, such as excision of an ellipse of skin and subjacent cartilage. Thorough cauterization of all chondritic tissue remaining after curettage is important to the success of the procedure. Cosmetically, this simple technique gives a very satisfactory result (see Fig 21–6).

▶ [Chondrodermatitis nodularis chronica helicis is a pesky nuisance and is not uncommon in cardiologists (stethoscope) and telephone operators (earphones) and nuns (in the old days they wore a hood). This must be one of the largest reported series, and the treatment results are good. However, intralesional steroids are very effective and are less traumatic and scarring. If intralesional steroids fail, this Danish technique is probably a better option than surgery.—T.B.F.] ◀

21–23 **Generalized Pruritus and Systemic Disease.** Generalized pruritus (GP) can be the presenting feature of systemic disease, but the frequency of such disease in patients with GP is uncertain. Gary R. Kantor and Donald P. Lookingbill (Pennsylvania State Univ.) reviewed data on 44 patients with GP who had extensive, symmetric

(21–23) J. Am. Acad. Dermatol. 9:375–382, September 1983.

SYSTEMIC DISEASE IN GP CASES

Systemic disease	Known by patient at time of clinic visit	Diagnosed by workup at time of clinic visit	Subsequently diagnosed	Total
Thyroid	3	1	1	5
Diabetes mellitus	4	0	0	4
Parathyroid	0	0	0	0
Kidney	0	2*	0	2
Liver	0	1*	2	3
Hodgkin's disease	0	0	0	0
Hematologic malignancies	1	0	0	1
Other cancer	2	1*	1†	4
Adrenal‡	0	0	1*	1
Total	10	5	5	20 (14 patients)§

*Diseases possibly related to patient's GP.
†Patient with colon carcinoma and metastatic liver disease.
‡Information volunteered by patient and subsequently confirmed by patient's internist. Routine questionnaire did not include inquiry about adrenal disease.
§Four patients had two systemic diseases and 1 patient had three.
(Courtesy of Kantor, G.R., and Lookingbill, D.P.: J. Am. Acad. Dermatol. 9:375–382, September 1983.)

pruritus in the absence of primary skin lesions. Forty-four age- and sex-matched patients with psoriasis served as controls. The patients were followed for 1–6½ years.

Systemic disorders were found in 30% of the patients with GP and in 23% of the control group. Five patients with GP had multiple systemic disorders. Kidney disease, liver disease, hypothyroidism, and internal malignancy were more frequent in the GP patients, whereas diabetes and hypertension were more frequent in the psoriatic group. A relation of systemic disease of GP was suspected in 6 patients. The time of diagnosis of systemic disease in the GP and control groups is compared in the table. In two thirds of cases, GP persisted to the last follow-up or until death. Patients with persistent itching had a much higher rate of systemic disease than those in whom pruritus subsided. Patients with a history of psychiatric difficulty had a particularly high incidence of persistent itching. The mean duration of pruritus in patients in whom it subsided was 42 months, and the mean duration to last follow-up in those in whom it persisted was 67 months.

Systemic disease has been found in 16%–50% of patients presenting with GP. A probable temporal relation between systemic disease and GP was found in 14% of the authors' patients and in none of the psoriatic controls. In 4 patients, systemic disease was diagnosed after presentation, and in 2 of them, 1 with metastatic colonic cancer in the liver and 1 with adrenal failure, a probable relation to GP was established.

▶ [The authors of this interesting study found 6 out of 44 patients with generalized pruritus to have a temporally associated systemic disease. The youngest of the 6 patients was 69 years old, and the authors caution against attributing persistent itching in the elderly to such factors as "dry skin," or "old age." The recommended workup for persistent generalized pruritus includes a complete blood count with differential, chest x-ray, thyroid and liver profiles, and determinations of levels of blood urea nitrogen and creatinine. I wonder if a stool guaiac wouldn't be a simple inexpensive test to add to the list. Needless to say, a careful physical examination might be helpful.—R.M.] ◀

21–24 **Skin Tags: A Cutaneous Marker for Colonic Polyps.** Earlier identification of patients who are at an increased risk for development of adenomatous colonic polyps may lead to the earlier diagnosis or prevention of colonic cancer. James Leavitt, Irwin Klein, Fred Kendricks, Judith Gavaler, and David H. VanThiel attempted to determine whether skin tags may be a marker for colonic polyps. Skin tags were sought in 100 consecutive male patients who were referred for colonoscopy during a 6-month period, all for suspected colonic disease. The 94 evaluable patients had an average age of 54.5 years. Adenomatous polyps were found in 36 patients. Ten others had colonic cancer, and 5 of these had adenomatous polyps as well. Simple skin tags were observed in 48 patients. The relative risk of colonic polyps in patients with skin tags was 13.8, a significant association. The presence of skin tags was an 80% sensitive and 77% specific for identifying patients at risk for colonic polyps. The association was unaffected by the exclusion of patients with colonic cancer. The association was not attributable to a difference in the age-related presence or absence of either skin tags or colonic polyps.

The finding of skin tags may identify persons potentially at risk for colonic polyps and colonic cancer. Further evaluation may be warranted in persons with skin tags.

▶ [This is potentially a very important paper. However, the study group utilized in this report was comprised of people who already had symptoms that suggested colonic disease. The study needs to be repeated in the general population. Of course, it will be difficult to subject normal people without gastrointestinal symptoms to colonoscopy. A cooperative study will probably have to be done in order to get enough patients for statistical significance. Only then will the true risk of colonic polyps in the general population of individuals with skin tags be known.—J.C.A.] ◀

21–25 **Acute Myelomonocytic Leukemia Presenting as Xanthomatous Skin Eruption.** Skin and mucosal infiltrates are a recognized feature of monocytic leukemias. J. R. O'Donnell, P. Tansey, P. Chung, A. K. Burnett, J. Thomson, and G. A. McDonald (Glasgow, Scotland) report data on a case of acute myelomonocytic leukemia in which skin infiltration by xanthomatous nodules was the presenting feature.

Man, 44, had multiple yellowish nodules on the trunk and limbs (Fig 21–7) for 6 weeks. There was no family history of disordered lipid metabolism. Hemoglobin concentration was 8 gm/dl. A blood smear showed 40% blast cells, and an iliac crest biopsy specimen led to a diagnosis of acute myelomonocytic leukemia. Lipid studies were negative. Bone marrow remission was induced by chemotherapy, but the xanthomatous lesions did not resolve entirely. Hemorrhagic skin infiltration was present after 2 courses of consolidation chemotherapy were completed. The patient died suddenly. Biopsies of skin lesions performed before antileukemic therapy was started showed a high concentration of triglyceride and cells resembling macrophages with prominent mitotic figures. Cells resembling myeloid precursors were scattered throughout the lesions. Electron microscopy showed closely packed cells

(21–24) Ann. Intern. Med. 98:928–930, June 1983.
(21–25) J. Clin. Pathol. 35:1200–1203, November 1982.

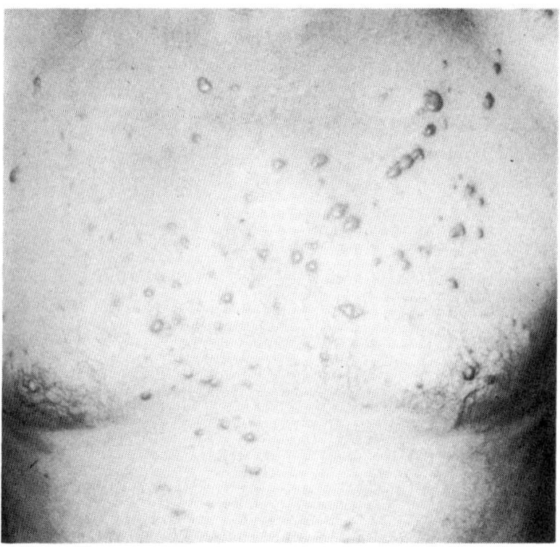

Fig 21–7.—Xanthomatous lesions on upper trunk of 44-year-old man. (Courtesy of O'Donnell, J.R., et al.: J. Clin. Pathol. 35:1200–1203, November 1982.)

with a number of organelles including fat vacuoles, lysosomes, and randomly disposed microfilaments.

The microscopic appearances in this case indicated a degree of cellular pleomorphism and mitotic activity that suggested neoplasia rather than eruptive xanthoma or infective granuloma. Electron microscopy showed no specialized intercellular junctions, indicating a nonepithelial origin of the tumor. The leukemic monoblasts in this case may have been capable of phagocytosing lipid to a degree that resulted in xanthomatous nodule formation in the skin. Autopsy was not done. The skin lesions decreased in size and number during treatment but persisted during bone marrow remission, and they may well have provided a "sanctuary" for leukemic cells during this period.

▶ [An interesting "first case" observation in which the xanthomatous skin lesions were the presenting complaint.—R.M.] ◀

1–26 **Acute Febrile Neutrophilic Dermatosis (Sweet's Syndrome) and Myeloproliferative Disorders.** Philip H. Cooper, Donald J. Innes, Jr., and Kenneth E. Greer (Univ. of Virginia) report 4 cases of patients with both neutrophilic dermatosis (ND or Sweet's syndrome) and a hematologic disorder. Acute febrile ND consists of abrupt onset of red, tender, cutaneous plaques on the face, extremities, and upper part of the trunk, with fever, malaise, and neutrophilic leukocytosis. Histologically, ND has distinctive, dense, dermal infiltrates of neutrophils. Response to systemic corticosteroid therapy is dramatic. The authors also review reports of 12 similar cases and compare their 4 patients, who had leukemia or preleukemia and ND (LND), with otherwise healthy persons who had ND (idiopathic ND; IND).

CASE 1.—Man, 49, had skin lesions, fever, night sweats, weight loss, and

(21–26) Cancer 51:1518–1526, Apr. 15, 1983.

multiple, red, cutaneous plaques over the body. Differential diagnosis included ND. Hematologic findings showed preleukemia. Treatment with prednisone resulted in marked improvement in cutaneous eruptions after 6 weeks. Several months later the skin lesions recurred, and the patient received a diagnosis of leukemia or lymphoma.

CASE 2.—Man, 72, developed tender, red, pustular papules on the face, arms, upper part of the trunk, thighs, and legs. The clinical impression suggested ND. Hematologic findings were consistent with preleukemia or a cellular phase of myelofibrosis. Prednisone therapy was begun, and skin lesions cleared in 2 weeks. Treatment with oxymetholone was begun. The skin lesions returned on the lower part of the legs. Preleukemia was found on bone marrow biopsy. The patient died soon thereafter with severe pancytopenia.

CASE 3.—Woman, 27, was pregnant and had acute myelomonocytic leukemia. Twelve days after starting cytosine arabinoside therapy she had tender, red plaques, fever, and malaise. A diagnosis of LND was considered. Prednisone therapy resulted in rapid disappearance of tenderness and malaise and in skin clearing. The patient delivered a healthy baby, but died 3 months later.

CASE 4.—Man, 29, had a remission of acute myelomonocytic leukemia. One month later, tender, red, vesicular plaques appeared on the forehead and hands. A diagnosis of LND was considered. Prednisone therapy produced improvement of the skin eruptions within hours. One week later LND recurred. Lesions again cleared with prednisone. After yet another LND episode, the patient died in leukemic blast crisis.

The most characteristic finding on skin biopsy for LND was a dense, nodular, patchy, or bandlike dermal infiltrate composed primarily of mature-appearing neutrophils. The epidermis appeared to be normal. Although lesions of LND more frequently had vesiculobullous appearances or location on mucous membranes, no consistent difference between LND and IND for cutaneous signs, symptoms, histologic findings, and response to therapy were found. The most common hematologic condition associated with LND was acute myeloid or myelomonocytic leukemia. Moderate to severe anemia was present in 9 of 10 patients whose first episode of LND preceded the discovery of the hematologic condition by 8 months or less.

The presence of anemia is the most obvious and readily detectable difference between LND and IND. The possibility of an underlying myeloproliferative disorder should be considered in all patients with ND. Leukemia-associated ND should not be confused with infectious complications in patients known to have myeloproliferative disorders.

▶ [The authors report 4 cases of Sweet's syndrome associated with myeloproliferative disorders. The identifying factors suggesting a myeloproliferative disorder were anemia (not usually present in Sweet's syndrome on presentation), a lower than normal white blood count and an atypical smear. The underlying disorders in these cases were either acute myeloid or myelomonocytic leukemia. Sweet's syndrome may now be considered as a possible presenting manifestation of a leukemia.—R.M.] ◀

21–27 **Nonrashes: IV. Audible Signs of Cutaneous Disease** are discussed by Jeffrey D. Bernhard (Harvard Med. School). Dermatologic disorders associated with audible signs are listed in the table. A hoarse patient with a red, swollen ear may have relapsing polychon-

---

(21–27) Cutis 31:189–190, February 1983.

DISEASES WITH CUTANEOUS AND AUDIBLE SIGNS*

Hereditary Disorders
- Lipoid proteinosis†
- Pachyonychia congenita
- Farber's syndrome
- De Lange's syndrome (feeble, low-pitched, growling cry)

Bullous Diseases
- Pemphigus vulgaris†
- Erythema multiforme

Infectious Diseases
- Histoplasmosis
- Laryngeal papillomas
- Candidiasis
- Secondary syphilis
- Epidemic typhus (dysphonia due to cranial nerve paralysis)

Inflammatory and Connective Tissue Diseases
- Relapsing polychondritis†
- Lupus erythematosus
- Dermatomyositis (dysphonia)
- Angioedema (difficulty speaking)

Infiltrative
- Amyloidosis (hoarseness or difficulty speaking due to infiltration of tongue)

Granulomatous
- Sarcoidosis

Endocrine
- Hypothyroidism†

Neoplastic
- Eruptive keratoacanthomas

*Hoarseness unless otherwise indicated.
†Audible change may be of major diagnostic significance.
(Courtesy of Bernhard, J.D.: Cutis 31:189–190, February 1983.)

dritis rather than cellulitis. A dysphonic patient may have dermatomyositis rather than lupus. The association of hoarseness with bullae suggests pemphigus rather than pemphigoid. Dysphagia may be a feature of histoplasmosis and candidiasis. Patients with angioedema or infiltrative processes such as amyloidosis may have difficulty speaking because of a swollen tongue. Uncommon causes of hoarseness include laryngeal involvement in xanthoma disseminatum, progressive nodular histiocytoma, and generalized eruptive keratoacanthoma. Laryngeal cancer may itself be associated with cutaneous signs and must be ruled out in any patient with persistent hoarseness not proved to have another cause. Patients with such painful disorders as herpetic gingivostomatitis, infectious pharyngitis, aphthous stomatitis, and Behçet's syndrome may be reluctant to speak during clinical evaluation.

▶ [This article presents a delightful concept that is well expressed and amazingly extensive. It provides a new way to think about old problems. May I, on Dr. Bernhard's invitation, add the usual ghost in the closet to his very complete list, to wit, psychogenic aphonia, which may accompany other cutaneous complaints (organic or psychogenic).—R.M.] ◀

21–28 **Pruritic Urticarial Papules and Plaques of Pregancy (PUPPP)** is a benign dermatosis that must be distinguished from other dermatoses of pregnancy. It is characterized by a rash of urticariform papules and plaques appearing in the third trimester on the abdomen and proximal thighs. The lesions, which are intensely pruritic, resolve before or a few weeks after delivery. J. Noguera, A. Moreno, and J. M. Moragas (Univ. of Barcelona, Spain) reviewed the findings in 14 cases of PUPPP seen between 1975 and 1981. This disorder appears to be the most common dermatosis developing during pregnancy. The patients' ages ranged from 17 to 32 years.

Lesions developed initially on the abdomen in all cases; in 6 they extended toward the gluteal region and thighs and in 4 toward the thorax (table). Initial erythematous papules changed to small urticariform plaques. The condition was diagnosed in 5 patients at term. The median time required for resolution was 3 weeks. No laboratory abnormalities were noted. All deliveries were normal. Two women have had subsequent pregnancies not complicated by PUPPP. Oral steroid therapy was helpful in patients with pronounced pruritus. Topical fluorated corticoids were very helpful in all cases. Some patients had only a lymphohistiocytic infiltrate around superficial dermal vessels, but most had epidermal lesions as well, including focal spongiosis and acanthosis. Three showed foci of parakeratosis. No immunoglobulin deposits were detected in the 9 cases studied.

No maternal or fetal mortality has been associated with this dermatosis. The histologic findings in PUPPP are nonspecific. Some le-

Clinical Characteristics of Patients With PUPPP

Age	Degree of pruritus	Distribution	Onset of pregnancy (month)	Clearing time after delivery	Therapy*
17	Severe	Trunk, abdomen, buttocks, legs	8	1 week	Topical cs 20 mg/d
22	Intense	Trunk, abdomen	7	4 days	Baby powder
30	Intense	Trunk, abdomen	9	2 days	Topical cs
29	Intense	Abdomen	8	–	Oral cs
20	Severe	Abdomen, buttocks, legs	8	1 week	Oral cs topical cs 20 mg
26	Moderate	Abdomen	8	6 days	None
25	Moderate	Abdomen, trunk	8½	7 days	Oral cs 20 mg, antihistaminic topical cs
25	Severe	Abdomen, trunk buttocks	8½	6 days	Antihistaminic, topical cs
30	Severe	Abdomen, trunk, legs, buttocks	8	10 days	Topical cs
21	Intense	Abdomen trunk, buttocks	9	3 days	Topical cs
20	Moderate	Abdomen	8	3 days	Topical cs, antihistaminic
32	Intense	Abdomen,trunk	9	5 days	Topical cs, antihistaminic
22	Severe	Abdomen, trunk, buttocks legs	9	7 days	Topical cs antihistaminic
23	Moderate	Abdomen, trunk	9	3 days	topical cs antihistaminic

(Courtesy of Noguera, J., et al.: Acta Derm. Venereol. [Stockh.] 63:35–38, 1983.)

(21–28) Acta Derm. Venereol. (Stockh.) 63:35–38, 1983.

sions resemble the toxin erythema found in many dermatologic disorders, whereas others, with epidermal involvement, bear some resemblance to papular dermatitis of pregnancy.

▶ [The phenomenon of PUPPP is well described. Although the etiology remains uncertain, we may all take comfort from the absence of fetal and maternal mortality, the tendency to resolution after delivery, the often good response to topical steroids, and the possibility of future pregnancies without recurrence.—R.M.] ◀

21–29 **IgA Deposits in Skin in Alcoholic Liver Disease.** A selective increase in serum IgA concentration is observed in patients with chronic alcoholic liver disease, and deposit of IgA along the perisinusoid areas has been described in alcoholic liver injury. Martin A. Swerdlow, Kokendra N. Chowdhury, Vinod Mishra, and Hymie Kavin (Michael Reese Hosp.) examined the frequency and consistency of IgA deposit in the skin in alcoholic liver disease. Liver and skin biopsy specimens were obtained simultaneously from 19 patients with established alcoholic liver disease and from 8 with non-alcohol-related liver disorders and examined by standard immunofluorescence and immunoperoxidase methods. All but 5 of the patients with alcoholic liver disease had a "continuous" pattern of IgA deposit in the liver, and 12 of the 14 also had IgA deposits in the superficial cutaneous capillaries. Studies with antibody to human C3 showed granular deposit in 9 of the 12 patients with IgA deposits in the skin. None of the control specimens had deposits of IgA or C3 in the skin or characteristic IgA deposits in the liver.

The findings support a correlation between deposit of IgA in the livers of patients with alcoholic liver disease and IgA deposit in cutaneous capillaries. The mechanism of IgA deposit at either site is unclear. Alcoholic injury of the intestinal mucosa may lead to increased production and release of IgA into portal venous blood. Further, IgA may be transported from hepatocytes into the bile. Excess IgA in the liver could lead to a spillover into the systemic circulation and deposit of IgA in the dermal capillaries and the renal mesangium. The finding of IgA deposits in the superficial cutaneous vessels can aid the diagnosis of acute and advanced alcoholic liver disease.

21–30 **Isolation of an Elastase-Like Enzyme From Skin Lesions With Sweet's Syndrome.** Kazuko Hamanaka, Kenji Ishizu, Sumiyoshi Takasugi, and Naotika Toki (Univ. of Hiroshima) attempted to isolate protease from skin lesions in patients with Sweet's syndrome to clarify the pathogenesis of this syndrome from the viewpoint of protease theory. Casein and Azo-albumin were used as substrates to measure proteolytic activity. A skin sample was received from a woman aged 58 years diagnosed to have Sweet's syndrome. The sample was cleaned thoroughly, homogenized, and dialyzed to obtain the protein sample.

It was found that 1 mg of skin extract from the lesion of the patient with Sweet's syndrome possessed 20 units of caseinolytic, 18.1 units of Azo-albumin hydrolytic, 85 units of elastolytic, and 10 units of AC-

---

(21–29) J. Am. Acad. Dermatol. 9:232–236, August 1983.
(21–30) Dermatologica 166:181–185, April 1983.

Tyr-OEt esterolytic activities. Extracts from healthy skin removed at mastectomy possessed almost the same proteolytic and esterolytic activities as that of the patient with Sweet's syndrome, but only a trace amount of elastolytic activity. A major protein band was found in segments 12 to 15 and a minor band was found at segment 20 on polyacrylamide gel disk electrophoresis. Proteolytic and esteolytic activities were present in both protein bands. Elastolytic activity was present in only the minor protein band. By further dialysis, an elastase-like enzyme with specific activity of 680 elastolytic units/mg of protein was partially purified.

From these results it is assumed that elastase-like enzymes in this study originated in neutrophil granules dispersed in lesions with karyorrhexis. One of the characteristic histologic findings in skin lesions in a patient with Sweet's syndrome is a marked perivascular infiltrate of neutrophils with karyorrhexis.

21–31 **Clinicopathologic Spectrum of Lymphomatoid Papulosis: Study of 31 Cases.** Although lymphomatoid papulosis usually follows a protracted, recurrent, but benign course, several patients with subsequent lymphoid malignancy have been reported. Nestor P. Sanchez, Mark R. Pittelkow, Sigfrid A. Muller, Peter M. Banks, and R. K. Winkelmann reviewed data on 31 cases of lymphomatoid papulosis seen since 1965 at the Mayo Clinic. The patients had a papular-nodular eruption that often underwent vesiculation, pustulation, and necrosis and subsequently healed, often with scarring. There was evidence of a dermal infiltrate of large pleomorphic cells with hyperchromatic nuclei and variable cytoplasm, suggestive of lymphoid malignancy.

Fig 21–8.—Histopathologic features of lymphomatoid papulosis, showing superficial and deep dermal infiltration by atypical, pleomorphic cells. Hematoxylin-eosin; original magnification, ×100. (Courtesy of Sanchez, N.P., et al.: J. Am. Acad. Dermatol. 8:81–94, January 1983.)

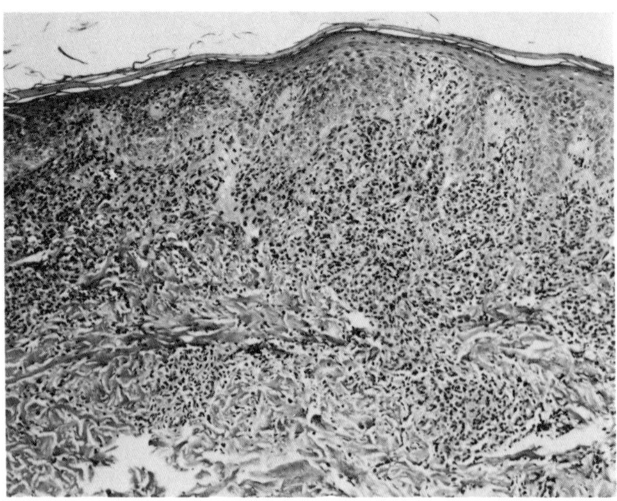

(21–31) J. Am. Acad. Dermatol. 8:81–94, January 1983.

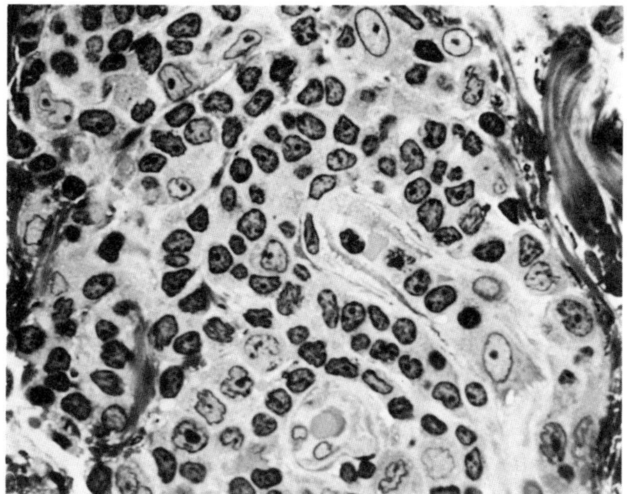

Fig 21–9.—Spurr-embedded section showing pleomorphic character of infiltrate; original magnification, ×1,000. (Courtesy of Sanchez, N.P., et al.: J. Am. Acad. Dermatol. 8:81–94, January 1983.)

The 20 men and 11 women in the study had a median age of 35 at the outset. The median duration of the eruption was 9 years. The trunk and extremities were predominantly affected. Eruptions of papules were not associated with signs of systemic illness in most cases. Six patients had a lymphoid malignancy 1–36 years after the onset of lymphomatoid papulosis. Three had non-Hodgkin's lymphoma, 2, mycosis fungoides, and 1, nodular sclerosing Hodgkin's disease. Three patients had systemic neoplasia, and 5 had endocrinopathies. Delayed hypersensitivity skin testing showed normal results in 8 patients in the study. The histologic appearances are shown in Figures 21–8 and 21–9. Immunofluorescence microscopy showed granular deposits of IgM and C3 about the vessels in 2 of 9 cases. The clinical course was not influenced by chemotherapy of the lymphoid malignancies.

The data indicate that, with adequate follow-up, some patients with lymphomatoid papulosis may be shown to have malignant lymphomas. Lymphomatoid papulosis appears to be a distinctive lymphocytic perivascular reaction which, like all lymphoid reactive processes of the skin, can be associated with or evolve toward a lymphoproliferative state. The condition ranges from the usual chronic reaction with benign destructive lesions to the occasional syndrome related to lymphoma.

1–32 **HLA-B15 Association With Erythema Multiforme.** Madeleine Duvic, Emily G. Reisner, Deborah V. Dawson, and Eleanor Ciftan (Duke Univ.) describe erythema multiforme (EM) as a cutaneous reaction that develops after numerous infections, the administration of

(21–32) J. Am. Acad. Dermatol. 8:493–496, April 1983.

certain drugs, or the occurrence of various neoplastic and inflammatory disorders in some individuals. A prospective study was made of 38 HLA specificities of the A, B, and C series in 16 white patients with EM and in 140 white controls. The provocative factor for EM was also evaluated.

Seven (44%) of the 16 patients had the HLA-B15 antigen, as did only 7% of the 140 controls and 11.6% of the Eighth International Histocompatibility Workshop controls, both comparisons having high statistical significance. In 5 of 9 patients with herpes preceding EM, a positive finding for HLA-B15 was obtained. A subgroup consisted of 9 patients with recurrent EM who had antecedent herpes simplex and 3 who had uncertain flare factors. Six of these 12 patients had the B15 antigen. There was no HLA antigen association found for 10 black patients with EM compared with 23 black blood donors.

The observation that erythema multiforme may develop after a variety of infections, the use of certain drugs, or the occurrence of various inflammatory conditions suggests that it may be a host-specific immune response. Herpesvirus is the most commonly recognized etiologic agent for EM. This study is the first report of an HLA association in EM. Although B15 antigen activity is significantly increased in these patients, the presence of the antigen is not necessary for disease expression and may reflect linkage to immune response genes of the HLA-D locus.

21–33 **Erythema Annulare Centrifugum: Review of 24 Cases With Special Reference to Its Association With Underlying Disease.** John M. Mahood (Sheffield, England) reviewed the findings in 24 new cases of erythema annulare centrifugum seen between 1976 and 1981. The condition is defined as a persistent erythema in the form of annular, circinate, gyrate, or serpiginous lesions, starting as a papule and usually enlarging slowly, with central clearing. Vesiculation can occur, but frank blistering is unusual. Histologically there is a fairly tight-knit, upper dermal, perivascular, mononuclear cell infiltrate and no marked epidermal abnormalities.

The 14 females and 10 males had a mean age at presentation of 53 years. The trunk was involved in three fourths of cases, the lower limbs in 55%, the upper limbs in 32%, and the face and neck in 14%. Five of the 23 living patients continue to have active disease. The mean duration in those in whom the disease resolved was 20 months or, excluding 1 patient, 11 months. Nearly two thirds of patients were not using drugs. Two patients had mild strokes during the study period, 1 had duodenal ulceration, and 1 had active gingival infection. In none of these patients did the eruption respond to treatment of the systemic disorder. Several other patients had long-standing disease antedating the eruption. There was no evidence of malignancy during a mean follow-up of 6 years from onset.

Extensive investigation of cases of erythema annular centrifugum does not seem to be warranted. It is possible that an association with

---

(21–33) Clin. Exp. Dermatol. 8:383–387, July 1983.

underlying disease has been suspected because many cases are not reported unless such an association is present.

▶ [Twenty-four cases of erythema annulare centrifugum were studied over a 5-year period, and no evidence of consistent associated underlying disease was found. The author suggests that extensive workup does not appear to be warranted. Where listed,the workups of these patients were not particularly extensive—only 3 had "extensive radiological investigations," and only 50% had chest x-rays. Sixty-seven percent cleared by 1 year, 83% by 2 years, and 94% by 3 years. A longer follow-up or more extensive investigation, especially of patients with persistent disease, would be more supportive of the assertion that there is no underlying disease or malignancy.—R.M.] ◀

21–34 **Immunofluorescence and Histochemical Studies of Localized Cutaneous Amyloidosis.** P. Norén, P. Westermark, G. G. Cornwell, III, and Wendy Murdoch note that lichen amyloidosus (LA) and macular amyloidosis (MA) are 2 forms of localized cutaneous amyloidosis in which the amyloid occurs as larger and smaller deposits in the papillary dermis. The amyloid in LA and MA was examined by indirect immunofluorescence, using antibodies to previously characterized amyloid fibril proteins. Skin specimens obtained from 8 patients with LA, 3 with MA, and 1 with clinical and histologic findings of both LA and MA were studied. Several punch biopsies of affected skin were performed on each patient under local anesthesia.

In all biopsies, amyloid deposits were limited to the papillary dermis. In LA, large lumps dominated. The amyloid in MA consisted of groups of small, faceted bodies intermingled with pigment-containing cells. Similar small bodies were also found, together with larger deposits, in the patient with both LA and MA and in 1 patient with LA. In all patients with LA and MA, the amyloid reacted with antisera to IgG, IgA, IgM, and C3. Anti-IgM and anti-C3 antisera gave a brighter fluorescence pattern than anti-IgA and anti-IgG antisera did. There was no reaction of the amyloid with antisera to amyloid fibrill proteins of the AA, AL, Ae_t, or ASc_I type. The antikeratin antiserum resulted in a bright fluorescence of all portions of the epidermis except for the stratum corneum, which reacted weakly or strongly in small areas.

These results indicate that the amyloid of LA and MA is different from other known types of amyloid. Protein AP, which was demonstrated in amyloid of MA and LA, is present in all forms of amyloid and is of unknown significance. Antiserum to keratin did not react with the larger homogeneous amyloid bodies, but showed a weak reaction with some small deposits.

▶ [Findings in the article present controversy as to the origin of amyloid in lichen amyloidosus and macular amyloidosis. Previously it has been reported that the material reacts with anti-keratin antiserum.—M.I.M.] ◀

1–35 **Dilated Pore and Pilar Sheath Acanthoma: Clinical and Histologic Diagnosis.** Günther Klövekorn, Winfried Klövekorn, Gerd Plewig, and Hermann Pinkus report clinical and histologic data on

(21–34) Br. J. Dermatol. 108:277–285, March 1983.
(21–35) Hautarzt 34:209–216, May 1983.

dilated pores in 54 biopsy specimens from 45 patients from Munich and 39 biopsy specimens from 36 patients from Detroit. The dilated pore of Winer is a relatively common benign adnexal tumor originating from the outer hair root sheath, mostly next to the sebaceous gland and rarely from the terminal hair follicle. It is found mostly in chronically light-damaged skin of the face. The dilated pores appear as round, oval, basin-shaped, crater-shaped, or tunnel-shaped indentations of the skin. Three-dimensional reconstructions of the tumor show that 4 different types of dilated pores can be identified: (1) the hair follicle type, characterized by funnel-shaped configuration and long vertical expansion with a marrow diameter; (2) the balloon-shaped type, roundish with a comedo frequently with narrow ostium, and with horn cell masses firmly pressed together; (3) the multichamber type, identified by communicating chambers, cystic cavities, and node-shaped excrescences of the infundibulum epithelia; and (4) the basin-shaped type, an open tumor with a broad base and wide ostium; only the lower part is filled with horn cell masses. The dilated pore is a tumor sui generis and not a trichoepithelioma.

A second benign adnexal tumor, the pilar sheath acanthoma of Mehregan and Brownstein, was observed in 11 biopsy specimens from 11 patients from Munich and in 9 biopsy specimens from 9 patients from Detroit. This tumor is noteworthy because it is usually located on the upper lip or the forehead. It originates mostly from the sebaceous gland follicle. The tumor epithelium is acanthotically diffused with plump papillomatosis. Because of the elevated margin in pilar sheath acanthoma, the basaloma is the most important feature in the differential diagnosis. Further considerations apply to dilated pores, scars, dilated comedos, and trichoepitheliomas. The histologically differential diagnosis includes trichoepithelioma, trichoepithelioma-like basaloma, trichofollicularoma, the inverted follicular keratosis, the tumor of the follicular infundibulum, trichilemmona, keratinized trichilemmoma, and scars. Esthetically disturbing lesions can be excised.

21–36 **Granuloma Faciale: Treatment With the Argon Laser.** David B. Apfelberg, David Druker, Morton R. Maser, Harvey Lash, Bart Spence, Jr., and David Deneau (Palo Alto Med. Found., Palo Alto, Calif.) used the argon laser to treat the plaques of granuloma faciale in three patients. The laser used in this study produced intense light in the blue-green spectrum, 480–520 nm. Spot or aperature size varied between 1 and 5 nm. Power range varied from 0.6 to 1.8 W. Pulse duration most frequently used was 20 seconds. Total laser exposure averaged 100–125 J/sq cm of treated area.

CASE 1.—Woman, 63, initially seen in 1975 had undergone injection of triamcinolone acetonide in the granuloma faciale, but it later recurred. The lesion resolved with the use of topical adrenal steroids. Several other plaques then developed. Laser treatment of 3 plaques resistant to intralesional adre-

---

(21–36) Arch. Dermatol. 119:573–576, July 1983.

nal steroid therapy promptly resolved these plaques, which have not recurred in 23 months of follow-up.

CASE 2.—Man, 42, had 1 plaque diagnosed as granuloma faciale, which showed partial resolution with triamcinolone acetonide treatment. Full recurrence of this particular plaque and the development of another led to argon laser treatment. Resolution of both plaques was rapid and persistent, with no recurrence over 21 months of follow-up.

CASE 3.—Woman, 48, had multiple lesions on both cheeks and was diagnosed as having granuloma faciale. Several lesions had been injected with triamcinolone acetonide with no improvement. Minimal improvement was achieved with intralesional steroids. With argon laser therapy prompt disappearance of the lesions occurred without recurrence over 5 months of follow-up.

Granuloma faciale is an uncommon benign skin disorder consisting of asymptomatic single or multiple reddish brown plaques, usually present on the face of adults. Thus far all treatments with the argon laser by these authors have resulted in total and complete resolution of plaques of granuloma faciale hypertrophic scar formation or recurrence, although a whitish collagenous scar remains in the skin. Sequential biopsies have confirmed resolution of the inflammatory process.

▶ [Why argon laser would have a beneficial effect on controlling the inflammatory aspect of granuloma faciale is unclear. Argon laser's usefulness in lightening plaques that include superficial vascular proliferation is not surprising.—R.S.S.] ◀

21–37 **Seborrhea Is Not a Feature of Seborrheic Dermatitis.** J. L. Burton and R. J. Pye (Bristol, England) measured the sebum excretion rate from the forehead skin in 44 patients aged 18–88 years with classic seborrheic dermatitis and in 200 controls. Sebum excretion was measured by the modified gravimetric method.

The mean sebum excretion rate was normal in the 29 male patients and significantly reduced in the 15 women. Because sebum excretion varies with age and sex, the patients were also divided into 3 age groups for each sex: 20–39 years, 40–59 years, and 60–79 years. Values did not differ from normal in men, and in the female groups, sebum production remained decreased significantly. Dividing patients clinically into those with mild, moderate, and severe seborrheic dermatitis found no relationship between sebum production and disease severity.

These findings suggest that the term seborrheic dermatitis is a misnomer, because the disease is not associated with seborrhea, and in women older than age 40, sebum excretion was significantly reduced. Further evidence that seborrhea is not essential to seborrheic dermatitis is that a dose of estrogen sufficient to suppress sebum secretion produces no improvement in patients with seborrheic dermatitis. "Dermatitis of the sebaceous areas" is a more accurate term.

▶ [That sebaceous gland secretion is not increased in seborrheic dermatitis should come as no great surprise. For example, acne, which is usually associated with se-

---

(21–37) Br. Med. J. 286:1169–1170, Apr. 9, 1983.

borrhea, does not occur more frequently in patients with seborrheic dermatitis, or vice versa. The observation of a *decrease* in sebum secretion in women with seborrheic dermatitis compared with control subjects is of interest, but the authors do not discuss the implication of or speculate upon the reason for this difference.—P.E.P.] ◀

21–38 **Porokeratosis (Mibelli): Treatment With Topical 5-Fluorouracil.** The cause of porokeratosis is unknown. All forms are resistant to treatment, and malignancies have arisen in a number of affected patients. Sharon G. McDonald and Edward S. Peterka (Peoria, Ill.) report data on a patient with classic porokeratosis of Mibelli who was treated successfully with topical 5-fluorouracil.

Man, 42, had a gradually enlarging lesion on the dorsum of the right thumb. Radiotherapy had been given for croup in infancy. No family member had a similar lesion, although several males, including the patient, had palmar and plantar hyperkeratosis. The lesion (Fig 21–10) was about 2 cm in diameter and had irregular borders marked by a keratotic ridge. A biopsy specimen of the ridge showed a cornoid lamella of parakeratotic cells within a keratin-filled sulcus. A biopsy specimen from the center of the lesion showed moderate hyperkeratosis and irregular acanthosis. A mononuclear cell infiltrate surrounded dilated vessels in the papillary dermis. Treatment with undiluted 5-fluorouracil solution containing 500 mg in 10 ml under occlusion, given twice daily, produced ulceration and flattening of the lesion within 5 weeks. Treatment was discontinued for 4 weeks and then resumed for 2 weeks. The site was clear after 2 years.

Treatment with concentrated 5-fluorouracil under occlusion deserves a trial in patients with classic porokeratosis of Mibelli, especially if surgical removal would lead to loss of function or unacceptable scarring. Retinoids may offer a potentially superior

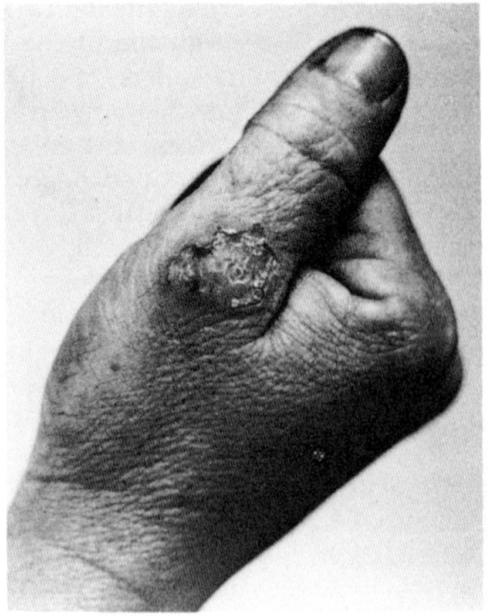

Fig 21–10.—Lesion before treatment showing sulcus within bordering keratotic ridge. (Courtesy of McDonald, S.G., and Peterka, E.S.: J. Am. Acad. Dermatol. 8:107–110, January 1983.)

(21–38) J. Am. Acad. Dermatol. 8:107–110, January 1983.

treatment, particularly in patients with disseminated or disabling lesions.

▶ [This is an especially curious case in that the patient had both palmar-plantar hyperkeratosis and porokeratosis. Could this have been porokeratosis related to sun exposure, rather than porokeratosis of Mibelli? If this is the case, the response to topical 5-fluorouracil is less surprising.—R.S.S.] ◀

21–39 **Dermatitis Artefacta in Mother and Baby as Child Abuse.** An increasing number of abused children who are harmed in unusual ways have been described. The prognosis has been poor. David P. H. Jones (Univ. of Colorado) reports the second known instance of child abuse in the form of factitious skin lesions identical with the lesions seen in the mother.

Girl was born to a mother, aged 19, who was married because of the pregnancy, but who was pleased to be pregnant. She had been physically abused as a child. Two attempts at self-poisoning had been made during the pregnancy. Discrete, dug-out facial lesions 4 mm in diameter, surrounded by scar tissue, were seen on the baby at age 4½ weeks. The lesions were of different ages. The mother attributed them to various causes that seemed unlikely, and her own forearm and lower legs were covered with numerous scars of lesions of the same dimensions. Improvement occurred over 6 months of supportive psychotherapy with the parents. The mother did not deny the origin of the lesions on the infant, but no frank discussion took place. At age 1 year the child's weight fell and the mother was seen to be handling her roughly. New lesions appeared on the baby's face at age 18 months. The infant was quiet and slow to move or respond, and she avoided gaze fixation. Language and social development were delayed. She improved rapidly when removed from the home. Her social behavior and language improved slowly over several months as the child continued in foster care with the same family.

An association between self-injurious behavior and child abuse is evident in this case. The diagnosis of dermatitis artefacta requires recognition of the disorder and a high index of suspicion. Abuse was not confined to the skin in this instance. Unusual forms of child abuse tend to occur where the parents have personality disorders. Such parents may have more disturbed personalities than those who lose control and impulsively harm their children, and such parents may be less accessible to psychiatric treatment.

▶ [Some physicians may not allow themselves to admit that child abuse (physical, sexual, and/or psychological) happens in their own patients. Dermatitis artefacta is a special case in which individuals may not be aware of their own activities. Therefore, confronting parents who are inducing lesions of dermatitis artefacta in their own children may help little. Intensive supportive therapy is required, and if it is not effective, the child needs to be taken out of the home and placed in protective services. The baby in this report did well when removed from the mother's custody.—A.R.R.] ◀

21–40 **Psychosomatic Concepts in Dermatology: A Dermatologist-Psychoanalyst's Viewpoint** is presented by Caroline S. Koblenzer (Univ. of Pennsylvania). Many of the theories of somatization developed since the time of Freud have used the skin as an example. The skin forms a channel for preverbal communication, where unexpressed

---

(21–39) Br. J. Psychiatry 143:199–200, Aug. 1, 1983.
(21–40) Arch. Dermatol. 119:501–512, June 1983.

feelings may be experienced and observed. Whatever the process of symptom development, the onset of disease depends on complex interactions between biologic, social, and psychological factors. There is extensive evidence for the occurrence of stress-related pathophysiologic changes in a variety of organ systems, including the skin. A classification of psychocutaneous disease is presented in the table, which lists a broad range of disorders. Antidepressants are therapeutically useful where indicated. Indications for major tranquilizers are limited, and anxiolytics should generally be restricted to the control of acute anxiety from transient inner or environmental stress or from somatic illness. Chronic anxiety responds best to individual psychotherapy. Psychiatric referral may be considered where the response to treatment is unsatisfactory, no underlying physical cause can be implicated, and the illness is significantly disrupting the patient's life.

Among the conditions of strictly psychological origin, dermatitis artefacta often is seen in psychotic or borderline patients who use their lesions to obtain attention and nurturing and to maintain contact with others. Trichotillomania in young children generally runs a benign course. Patients with neurotic excoriations usually are obsessive. The psychogenic purpura syndrome is clearly a modern version of stigmatization. Psychogenic factors appear to be strongly implicated in chronic urticaria, generalized and anogenital pruritus, and alopecia areata. Many other dermatologic states may be influenced

Classifications of Psychocutaneous Disease

- Conditions strictly psychological in origin:
  - Dermatitis artefacta
  - Delusions related to the skin
  - Compulsive habits (neurotic excoriations, liplicking, trichotillomania)
  - Obsessional thoughts (parasitophobia, syphilophobia, cancerophobia)
  - Glossodynia and glossopyrosis
  - Psychogenic, purpura syndrome
- Conditions in which strong psychogenic factors are imputed
  - Chronic urticaria
  - Generalized pruritus
  - Pruritus of the anogenital region
  - Alopecia areata
  - Hyperhidrosis
- Conditions probably dependent on genetic or environmental factors whose course may be affected by emotional stress:
  - Atopic dermatitis
  - Psoriasis
  - Dyshidrotic eczema[37(pp 165-167),77]
  - Acne vulgaris
  - Seborrheic dermatitis
  - Lichen simplex chronicus
  - Lichen planus
  - Recurrent herpes simplex

(Courtesy of Koblenzer, C.S.: Arch. Dermatol. 119:501–512, June 1983.)

by emotional stress. A significant emotional component can be suspected where the response to conventional therapy is less than expected or the symptoms seem to be disproportionate to the manifest disease.

▶ [An extensive review of the psychosomatic approach to dermatological problems. Organic mechanisms remain to be described.—R.M.] ◀

21–41 **Psychiatric Symptoms in Dermatology Patients.** Relations may exist between psychiatric and cutaneous disorders with respect to psychosomatic mechanisms, hypochondriasis or delusions related to the skin, psychiatric symptoms due to disfigurement, symptoms related to drugs used in treatment of skin disease, or production of both skin lesions and psychiatric disorder by systemic diseases. J. E. Hughes, B. M. Barraclough, L. G. Hamblin, and J. E. White (Southampton, England) used the General Health Questionnaire (GHQ) to screen 196 consecutive new dermatology outpatients and 40 patients admitted consecutively to dermatology beds. Patients with high scores on the 30-item GHQ completed the Wakefield Self-Assessment Depression Scale.

High GHQ scores were found in 30% of the outpatients and 60% of the dermatology inpatients. Fifteen percent of the outpatients and 33% of the inpatients had high Wakefield scores. Several of the outpatients with high GHQ scores reported that their psychiatric symptoms had preceded the skin disease. Five felt that their skin disorder had become worse because of emotional factors. Hypochondriacal preoccupation with trivial lesions accounted for 2 referrals. More than two thirds of patients with lesions on the face or hands had high GHQ scores. High scores were associated with such disorders as acne, eczema, and psoriasis. The highest scores were in 4 alopecic patients. High scorers frequently reported sleeplessness, avoidance of other persons, and cessation of party-going and of participation in hobbies. Two thirds of 21 patients receiving high-potency corticosteroids had high GHQ scores, compared with a little more than one third of those receiving low-potency corticosteroids. There were no cases of systemic disease causing both psychiatric disturbance and skin lesions.

Dermatologic outpatients appear to have psychiatric disorders more often than the general population, and dermatology inpatients have such disorders more often than general medical inpatients. Psychiatric disorder was especially prevalent among patients in this study who had acne, eczema, psoriasis, or alopecia. High GHQ scores were associated with extensive lesions on exposed body surfaces and with the topical use of high-potency corticosteroids. Counseling or psychotropic drug therapy may be helpful to dermatology patients with depression or anxiety, even when these are explicable as a reaction to the stress of severe skin disease.

▶ [The GHQ is "a screening instrument designed to be used in a medical setting to detect neurotic symptoms." The authors state in their discussion that "disfigurement, stigma, and the inconvenience resulting from severe skin disease were the most fre-

---

(21–41) Br. J. Psychiatry 143:51–54, July 1983.

quent causes of psychiatric symptoms reported by these patients." This emphasizes the need for sympathetic understanding, and reassuring management of our patients. The occurrence of "exacerbation of a skin disease by psychological factors was reported by a smaller number of patients, but objective investigation of this phenomenon was beyond the scope of our study."—R.M.] ◀

21–42 **Autoerythrocyte Sensitization.** Autoerythrocyte sensitization has been reported in more than 100 patients, but little attention has been given this disorder in children. To provide a definition of this disorder in the pediatric age group, A. N. Campbell, Melvin H. Freedman, and P.D. McClure (Univ. of Toronto) reviewed their experience with 6 children who had autoerythrocyte sensitization seen between 1978 and 1982. An illustrative case report is presented.

Girl, 12, underwent removal of an accessory navicular bone from her right foot. Two years later she fractured the navicular tubercle. This was followed by a painful, swollen bruise of the left knee, which resolved slowly. She sprained her ankle 1 year later and was treated with a cast. Within 3 months, painful and discolored swelling of the foot had developed, and a diagnosis of "sympathetic dystrophy" was made. The foot remained painful, and the girl was admitted for investigation. A diagnosis of juvenile rheumatoid arthritis was considered, and aspirin therapy for 2 months produced some relief from symptoms. Three months later the patient fell on her left wrist and was treated with a volar plastic cast for a suspected fracture of the scaphoid. Pain and swelling of the hand developed rapidly, with altered sensation in the median nerve distribution. Swelling and ecchymosis of the entire forearm were observed upon removal of the cast, but exploration of the carpal tunnel revealed no abnormality. One month later painful bruises developed on the left upper arm and face. Venography of the arm revealed no vascular malformations. Intradermal injection of 0.1 ml of autologous red blood cells elicited a tender bruise 2.5 cm in diameter in 12 hours. A skin biopsy of one of the lesions revealed a perivascular lymphocytic infiltrate associated with hemosiderotic granules, indicating previous hemorrhage. Because of the emotional problems that became apparent during the patient's many hospital admissions, a psychiatric examination was arranged. It revealed that she had an unhappy home life because of family conflicts and that she was intensely preoccupied by her illness. Psychotherapy over 6 months resulted in complete resolution of symptoms.

It is believed that autoerythrocyte sensitization is more common in children or young teen-agers than was previously reported. Typically the skin lesion is a painful, erythematous bruise that appears after minor trauma or operation and often involves an area not associated with the injury. The skin manifestations can be debilitating and can recur unpredictably over an indefinite period. Somatic symptoms may be associated with the bruising. All too often, multiple detailed investigations are carried out before the diagnosis is made. Intradermal injection of autologous red blood cells may or may not yield a "positive" ecchymotic reaction. Psychotherapy is usually the only effective treatment in pediatric patients.

▶ [This syndrome was reviewed authoritatively and thoroughly by Ratnoff in 1980 (*Semin. Hematol.* 17:192, 1980). No clear-cut organic mechanism has been consistently found, and most cases have had significant emotional concomitants. The pres-

(21–42) J. Pediatr. 103:157–160, July 1983.

ent study found no specific organic mechanism, and the aûthors indicate that psychotherapy may be very helpful. They argue for early diagnosis and psychotherapy and indicate that multiple investigations may prolong the problem.—R.M] ◀

21–43 **Skin Thickness in Patients With Acromegaly and Cushing's Syndrome and Response to Treatment.** J. K. Ferguson, R. A. Donald, T.S. Weston, and E. A. Espiner (Christchurch, New Zealand) assessed skin thickness (ST) radiologically in 22 patients with acromegaly and in 17 with Cushing's syndrome. The age ranges of the patients and the 55 controls were comparable. Skin thickness, used to determine endocrine changes, was measured by the original method of Meema et al.

The mean ST in male controls was 1.6 mm and that in female controls, 1.4 mm. The difference between sexes was significant. The mean ST in acromegalics at diagnosis was 2.3 mm in males and 2.1 mm in females. Acromegalic ST was significantly greater than normal in both males and females. No significant relationship was found between ST and either growth hormone (GH) level at diagnosis or duration of symptoms before diagnosis. The change in ST in patients treated successfully was significant for males and females. Growth hormone levels in these patients were less than 5 μg/L. The mean time between the 2 measurements was 6.1 years. Skin thickness values determined in patients with GH levels of less than 5 μg/L were within the normal range, whereas ST values in patients with post-treatment GH levels greater than 5 μg/L were above normal. A highly significant correlation was observed between log plasma GH concentration and ST values. In patients with Cushing's syndrome, ST in those who were untreated was significantly reduced from normal. The mean ST was 0.95 mm. Mean time between measurements was 4.5 years. The mean ST in patients after bilateral adrenalectomy was 1.14 mm, whereas after other forms of treatment the mean ST was 1.4 mm. This difference was not significant.

The measurement of ST is a useful screening test for both acromegaly and Cushing's syndrome, and it provides an objective assessment of the clinical response to treatment.

▶ [This is a nice demonstration of changes in skin thickness in acromegaly and Cushing's syndrome, with reversion toward normal after satisfactory treatment. The question comes to mind as to whether growth hormone could be successfully used to treat patients with extensive skin atrophy from topical steroid therapy, especially if continued topical therapy is indicated or necessary.—R.M.] ◀

(21–43) Clin. Endocrinol. (Oxf.) 18:347–353, April 1983.

Subject Index

A

Abdominal lipohypertrophy
  after insulin, 136
Abuse
  child, dermatitis artefacta in mother and baby as, 397
Acanthoma
  dilated pore and pilar sheath, 393
Acne, 21 ff.
  chloracne, fume inhalation, 36
  after 13-*cis*-retinoic acid, 22
  conglobata, 13-*cis*-retinoic acid in, 21
  cystic
    androgen excess in, 26
    isotretinoin in, 23
  Propionibacterium acnes resistance to antibiotics in, 30
  pyogenic granuloma-like, after isotretinoin, 24
  sebum secretion in, sustainable rates, 26
  testosterone levels in women with, 27
  vulgaris
    azelaic acid cream in, 33
    benzoyl peroxide in, 32
    erythromycin in, 32
    propionibacteria in, 31
  vulgaris, in women, 28 ff.
    androgens in, plasma, 28
    prednisolone and estrogen in, 29
Acromegaly
  skin thickness in, 401
Acropustulosis
  in infant, 364
Actinic
  keratosis (*see* Keratosis, actinic)
  reticuloid, etiology of, 254
Acyclovir, 355 ff.
  in herpes, genital, as initial treatment, 356, 358
  in herpes labialis, 357
  in herpes zoster, 355
Addison's disease
  pigmentation in, 267
Adrenal
  abnormalities in hirsutism, 166
  cortex function, effects of corticosteroids on, 127
AIDS
  immunodeficiency in female sexual partners of men with, 363
  Kaposi's sarcoma and, 227
Albinism
  oculocutaneous, prenatal diagnosis, 286
Alcohol
  -induced flushing, suppression by histamine antagonists, 126
Alcoholic liver disease
  cutaneous IgA deposits in, 389
Allergens
  garlic, 120
  IgG and IgE antibodies to, in atopic dermatitis, 107
Allergic dermatitis
  garlic causing, 120
Allergy
  contact, 2,4-dinitro-1-chlorobenzene, immune status in, 120
  risk, and infant feeding, 110
Alopecia areata, 168 ff.
  diphencyprone in, 169
  minoxidil in, 171
  photochemotherapy in, 168
Amebiasis
  skin, 51
Amelanotic
  lentigo maligna melanoma, dermatitis-like plaque in, 197
Amniotic fluid
  cells in epidermolytic hyperkeratosis, 163
cAMP
  in psoriasis, 291
Amyloidosis
  of skin, immunofluorescence and histochemistry in, 393
ANA-negative systemic lupus erythematosus, 81
Anaphylaxis
  exercise causing, 326
Androgen
  excess in cystic acne, 26
  plasma, in acne vulgaris in women, 28
Angiitis
  hypersensitivity, due to heat-activated photocopy paper fumes, 119

Angioedema
hepatitis B virus in, 327
hereditary, wheals of, and trauma, 323
thyroid autoimmunity and, 329
vibration-induced, 326
Anogenital (*see* Warts, anogenital)
Anthralin
in psoriasis, 300
Antibiotics
Propionibacterium acnes resistance to, in acne, 30
Antibody(ies)
against reticulin and gluten in dermatitis herpetiformis, 65
anticentromere, and scleroderma variants, 93
antigliadin, in dermatitis herpetiformis, 64
antinuclear antibody-negative systemic lupus erythematosus, 81
anti-Sm, in SLE, 83
anti-*Toxoplasma* IgM, 89
to C3 in SLE, 75
-dependent cytotoxicity, and colchicine, 313
to DNA in SLE, 75
gliadin, in dermatitis herpetiformis and pemphigoid, 62
IgG and IgE, to allergens in atopic dermatitis, 107
monoclonal (*see* Monoclonal antibodies)
to organisms producing fungal infections, 147
Anticentromere antibody
scleroderma variants and, 93
Antigen(s)
histocompatibility, in nevomelanocytes and malignant melanoma, 205
HLA, in erythema multiforme and herpes simplex, 361
HLA-DR, in psoriasis, 293
pemphigoid, heterogeneity of, 57
pemphigus-like, in urine, 56
Antigliadin antibodies
in dermatitis herpetiformis, 64
Antinuclear antibody
-negative systemic lupus erythematosus, 81
Anti-Sm antibodies
in SLE, 83
Anti-*Toxoplasma* IgM antibodies, 89
Anus
condylomata acuminata, laser vs. electric cautery in, 350
Argon laser
in granuloma faciale, 394
Aromatic retinoid (*see* Retinoid, aromatic)
Arotinoid Ro 13-6298
in psoriasis, 295 ff.
Arsenic
carcinogenesis, and PUVA, 306
Arthritis
-dermatosis syndrome, bowel in, 98
rheumatoid, D-penicillamine in, fatal polymyositis after, 140
Athlete's foot
gram-negative, antifungal activity of *Pseudomonas aeruginosa* in, 148
Atopic
dermatitis (*see* Dermatitis, atopic)
eczema, oral evening-primrose-seed oil in, 111
subjects, IgE production by mononuclear cells in, 106
Atrophy
of left side of body and right side of face in scleroderma, 94
Autoerythrocyte sensitization, 400
Autoimmunity
thyroid, in urticaria and angioedema, 329
Azelaic acid cream
in acne vulgaris, 33

B

Bacteremia
decubitus ulcer and, 379
Basophils
in erythema multiforme, 379
BCG
in immunotherapy of leprosy, 178
BCNU
in mycosis fungoides, 237
Benoxaprofen
in psoriasis, 312 ff.
Benzoyl peroxide
in acne vulgaris, 32
Biofeedback training
in Raynaud's phenomenon, 96
Biopsy
skin
fetal, in prenatal exclusion of Herlitz syndrome, 72
of relatives in dermatitis herpetiformis, 70
repeat, in SLE, 81
Blastomycosis
skin, 152
Bleomycin (*see* Warts, bleomycin in)
Blister
fluid
from bullous skin, collagenase and elastase in, 61
in pemphigoid, lymphocytes in, 57
formation, suction-induced, in insulin-dependent diabetes, 73
Bowel-bypass syndrome
without bowel bypass, 98

Brain
  Trichophyton dissemination to, 145
Brominated swimming pools
  dermatosis and, 122
Bronze baby syndrome
  as porphyrin-related disorders, 262
Bullous
  pemphigoid (*see* Pemphigoid, bullous)
  mastocytosis, disodium cromoglycate in, 332
Bypass
  bowel-bypass syndrome without bowel bypass, 98

C

Calmodulin
  elevation in psoriasis, 290
Cancer
  in dermatitis herpetiformis, incidence, 71
  skin, papillomavirus type 5 DNA in, after immunosuppression, 217
Candidal diaper dermatitis
  nystatin in, 156
Candidiasis, 154 ff.
  mucocutaneous, ketoconazole in, 154
  vaginal, clotrimazole and econazole in, 155
Captopril
  drug eruptions, 136
Carcinogenesis
  arsenic, and PUVA, 306
Carcinoma
  basal cell, curettage and electrodesiccation in, 222
  skin, 220 ff.
    basal cell, metastases, 224
    basal cell, recurrence, multivariate risk score, 221
    neuroendocrine (*see* Merkel cell tumors)
    PUVA in, 305
    squamous cell, recurrent, 220
Carmustine
  topical, in mycosis fungoides, 237
Carotenoids
  Günther's erythropoietic porphyria and, 258
Cell(s)
  amniotic fluid, in epidermolytic hyperkeratosis, 163
  endothelial, tumors from *Ulex europaeus* I lectin marking, 342
  hypersensitivity to UVA, 254
  Langerhans, in psoriasis, 293
  -mediated
    immunity (*see* Immunity, cell-mediated)
    lympholysis defect in atopic dermatitis, 103
  Merkel (*see* Merkel cell)
  mononuclear (*see* Mononuclear cells)
  T cell (*see* T cell)
Cervix
  abnormalities, and vulval warts, 347
Chancroid
  trimethoprim-sulfametrole in, 48
Chemotaxis
  neutrophil, in cystic acne, isotretinoin in, 23
Chemotherapy
  flag sign of, 171
  photochemotherapy (*see* Photochemotherapy)
Child abuse
  dermatitis artefacta in mother and baby as, 397
Children, 90 ff.
  hyaline fibromatosis, 366
  incontinentia pigmenti achromians, 284
  infant
    acropustulosis, 364
    dermatitis in, seborrheic and atopic, 108 ff.
    feeding, and allergy risk, 110
    Kasabach-Merritt syndrome, 339
    leprosy (*see* Leprosy, in infant)
  nevi on scalp, dysplastic, in melanoma-prone families, 184
  newborn
    barrier properties of skin of, 365
    hyperkeratosis, epidermolytic, 163
    lupus erythematosus (*see* Lupus erythematosus, in newborn)
  pemphigus, juvenile, 54
  Peutz-Jeghers syndrome, 273
  rheumatic disease, nailfold abnormalities in, 90
  scleroderma, systemic, 91
  Staphylococcus aureus infection, office treatment, 42
  urticaria, natural course and etiology, 330
Chloracne
  fume inhalation, 36
Cholestasis
  vitamin K-dependent coagulation factors and, 133
Chondrodermatitis
  nodularis chronica helicis, curettage and electrocauterization in, 381
Churg-Strauss granuloma
  systemic disease and, 99
Cimetidine
  in urticaria, idiopathic, 324
Cirrhosis
  liver, after vitamin A intoxication, 132

13-*cis*-retinoic acid, 21 ff.
  in acne, 22
    conglobata, 21
  sebum secretion after, 22
  in T cell lymphoma, 239
  toxicity in ichthyosis, 131
Cloasma
  leucodinine B in, "confettiform" depigmentation after, 283
Clotrimazole
  in candidiasis, vaginal, 155
Coagulation factors
  vitamin K-dependent, and cholestasis, 133
Coal tar phototherapy
  in psoriasis, 301
Colchicine
  in psoriasis, 313
  in Sweet's syndrome, 378
Cold urticaria
  infectious mononucleosis and, 328
Collagen
  implants, injectable, 142
Collagenase
  activity in blister fluid from bullous skin, 61
Colonic polyps
  skin tags for, 384
Comedones
  open, pigmentation of, ultrastructure, 35
Complement
  C3
    antibodies to, in SLE, 75
    dermatitis herpetiformis and, 67
  deposition in herpes-associated erythema multiforme, 360
Condylomata acuminata, 349 ff.
  of anus, laser vs. electric cautery in, 350
  vulva, laser in, 349
Connective tissue disease
  immunosuppression vs. prednisolone in, 87
Contact
  allergy, 2,4-dinitro-1-chlorobenzene, immune status in, 120
  dermatitis (*see* Dermatitis, contact)
Corticosteroids
  effects on adrenocortical function, 127
Coumadin
  skin necrosis after, 132 ff.
Crohn's disease
  pyoderma gangrenosum and, 338
Curettage, 222 ff.
  in carcinoma, basal cell, 222
  in chondrodermatitis nodularis chronica helicis, 381
  in epithelioma, basal cell, 222 ff.
    midfacial, 222
Cushing's syndrome
  skin thickness in, 401
Cutaneous (*see* Skin)
Cyclophosphamide
  in vitiligo, 280
Cyclosporine
  in T cell lymphoma, and Sézary syndrome, 235
Cyproterone acetate
  action on skin due to metabolite, 34
5-S-Cysteinyldopa
  after ultraviolet, 309
Cystic (*see* Acne, cystic)
Cytology
  lung, in mycosis fungoides, 232
Cytotoxicity
  antibody-dependent, and colchicine, 313

D

Dandruff
  miconazole nitrate and selenium disulfide for, 125
Dapsone
  in brown recluse spider bite, 128
  in dermatitis herpetiformis, 67
Death in melanoma
  stage I, predictors of, 206
  thin, with metastases, 202
Decubitus ulcer
  bacteremia and, 379
2'-Deoxycoformycin
  in T cell lymphoma of skin, 236
Depigmentation
  "confettiform," after leucodinine B in cloasma, 283
Dermatan sulfate
  psoriasis and, 291
Dermatitis
  artefacta in mother and baby as child abuse, 397
  atopic, 103, 107
    cell-mediated lympholysis defect in, 103
    diagnosis, in infant, 108 ff.
    disodium cromoglycate in, 113
    food hypersensitivity in, 110
    of hand, 112
    IgG and IgE antibodies to allergens in, 107
    mononuclear cell infiltrate in, 104
    thymopoietin pentapeptide in, 114
  chondrodermatitis nodularis chronica helicis, 381
  contact
    allergic, garlic causing, 120
    diphenhydramine hydrochloride causing, 118
  diaper, candidal, nystatin in, 156

herpetiformis, 61 ff.
antibodies against reticulin in, 65
antigliadin antibodies in, 64
cancer incidence in, 71
case review, 70
collagenase and elastase in blister fluid in, 61
C3 in, 67
dapsone in, 67
gliadin antibodies in, 62
gluten in, 65 ff.
gluten in, circulating antibodies against gluten, 65
gluten in, dietary gluten withdrawal, 66
gluten in, gluten challenge, 65
gluten in, gluten-restricted and gluten-free diet, 67
immune complexes in, 63
immunoglobulin A and, 67
intestinal mucosa in, 65
with lupus erythematosus, 68
renal involvement in, 63
skin biopsies in relatives, 70
irritant, in psoriasis, and glycosaminoglycans, 123
-like plaque in lentigo meligna melanoma, 197
of palms, hyperkeratotic, PUVA in, 317
radiation, from radioactive gold jewelry, 380
seborrheic, 108 ff.
diagnosis, in infant, 108 ff.
in neuroleptic-induced parkinsonism, 142
seborrhea contrasted with, 395
whirlpool-associated, *Pseudomonas aeruginosa* in, 43
Dermatologist
-psychoanalyst's viewpoint, 397
Dermatology
patients, psychiatric symptoms in, 399
psychosomatic concepts in, 397
Dermatomal
telangiectasia, 341
Dermatomyositis, 88 ff.
methylprednisolone pulse therapy in, 88
toxoplasmosis in, 89
Dermatophytosis
ketoconazole vs. griseofulvin in, 149
Dermatosis
-arthritis syndrome, bowel in, 98
brominated swimming pools and, 122
febrile neutrophilic (*see* Sweet's syndrome)
IgA linear, 85
Dermis
glycosaminoglycans, in psoriasis, 123
Dermographism, 324 ff.
H_1 and H_2 antagonists inhibiting, 325
symptomatic, study of, 324
Diabetes mellitus
insulin-dependent, suction-induced blister formation in, 73
scleredema adultorum and, 101
Dialysis
peritoneal, in psoriasis, 314
Diaper dermatitis
candidal, nystatin in, 156
Digital ischemia
heated gloves for, 97
2,4-Dinitro-1-chlorobenzene contact allergy
immune status in, 120
Diphencyprone
in alopecia areata, 169
Diphenhydramine hydrochloride
contact dermatitis due to, 118
Disodium cromoglycate
in atopic dermatitis, 113
in mastocytosis, bullous, 332
Dithranol
irritant reactions to, and psoriasis, 301
DNA, 217 ff.
antibodies in SLE, 75
epidermal, after etretinate in psoriasis, 296
papillomavirus type 5, in skin cancer after immunosuppression, 217
repair in actinic keratosis, 217
D-penicillamine
in rheumatoid arthritis, fatal polymyositis after, 140
Drug eruption
captopril causing, 136
fixed, pigmentary incontinence in, 276
Dysplastic nevi
melanocytic, with melanoma, 181
on scalp of prepubertal children from melanoma-prone families, 184

E

Eccrine poroma
malignant, case review, 344
Econazole
in candidiasis, vaginal, 155
Eczema
atopic, oral evening-primrose-seed oil in, 111
Ehlers-Danlos syndrome, type IV, 157 ff.
biochemical characterization of variants, 158
pregnancy complicated by, 157
Elastase
in blister fluid from bullous skin, 61
-like enzyme in Sweet's syndrome, 389

Electric cautery
  in chrondrodermatitis nodularis chronica helicis, 381
  in condylomata acuminata of anus, 350
Electrodesiccation, 222 ff.
  in carcinoma, basal cell, 222
  of epithelioma, midfacial basal cell, 222
Electron microscopy, 276 ff.
  of leukoderma, vitiligo-like, 276
  of melanoma, malignant, 276
  of pigmentary incontinence in fixed drug eruptions, 276
  in prenatal diagnosis of albinism, 286
  in prenatal exclusion of Herlitz syndrome, 72
Electrophoresis
  lipoprotein, in ichthyosis vulgaris, 161
Endothelium
  cells, tumors from, *Ulex europaeus* I lectin marking, 342
Enolase
  neuron-specific, and Merkel cell tumors, 241
Enzyme
  elastase-like, in Sweet's syndrome, 389
  -linked immunosorbent assay of antigliadin antibodies, 64
Eosinophilic fasciitis
  eosinophilotactic activity in, 94
Eosinophilotactic activity
  in eosinophilic fasciitis, 94
Epidermis
  DNA after etretinate in psoriasis, 296
  intraepidermal tumors, laser in, 349
  plasminogen activator, and psoriasis, 289
Epidermolytic
  hyperkeratosis, 163
Epithelioma, basal cell, 222 ff.
  curettage in, 224
  midfacial, curettage and electrodesiccation in, 222
Epithelium
  lesions, keratin polypeptide to discriminate benign and malignant, 219
Erythema, 391 ff.
  annulare centrifugum, and underlying disease, 392
  migrans, relationship to Lyme disease, 47
  multiforme, 360 ff.
    herpes-associated, complement deposition in, 360
    HLA antigen in, 361
    HLA-B15 and, 391
    lymphocytes and basophils in, 361
  nodosum leprosum, 179
  response, ultraviolet dose required to produce in normal skin, 249
  sunscreen protection and, 251
Erythemogenic ultraviolet
  coal tar and, 301
Erythrocyte
  autoerythrocyte sensitization, 400
Erythroderma
  follow-up of cases, 320
  vitiligo after, generalized, 282
Erythromycin
  in acne vulgaris, 32
Erythropoietic porphyria
  Günther's, and carotenoids, 258
Estrogen
  for acne vulgaris in women, 29
Etretinate
  in ichthyosis of Sjögren-Larsson syndrome, 162
  in lymphoma of skin, 238
  neutrophil migration inhibition by, 298
  in pemphigus, benign familial, 59
  in psoriasis (*see* Psoriasis, etretinate in)
  in pustulosis, palmoplantar, 318 ff.
  in warts, viral, and sarcoidosis, 348
Evening-primrose-seed oil
  oral, in atopic eczema, 111
Exercise
  anaphylaxis due to, 326
  sweating efficiency during, 370
Eye disease
  vitiligo and, 278

F

Face
  midfacial epithelioma, curettage and electrodesiccation in, 222
  right side, atrophy in scleroderma, 94
Fasciitis
  eosinophilic, eosinophilotactic activity in, 94
Favre-Racouchot syndrome
  radiotherapy and, 35
Febrile neutrophilic dermatosis (*see* Sweet's syndrome)
Feeding of infant
  allergy risk and, 110
Fetoscopy
  in prenatal exclusion of Herlitz syndrome, 72
Fibroblast
  interferon in warts, 351
  synthesizing glycosaminoglycan in systemic scleroderma, 92
  -type intermediate filaments in pigmented nevi and malignant melanoma, 206

Fibromatosis
hyaline, juvenile, 366
Flag sign
of chemotherapy, 171
Fluorescent monoclonal antibody
in lymphogranuloma venereum, 49
5-Fluorouracil
in porokeratosis of Mibelli, 396
in vitiligo, 281
Flushing
alcohol-induced, histamine antagonists suppressing, 126
Food
hypersensitivity in atopic dermatitis, 110
Freckles
after PUVA, 274
Frostbite injuries
pathophysiology of, 336
Fume inhalation chloracne, 36
Fungal infection
antibodies to organisms producing, 147

G

Gammopathy
monoclonal, and pyoderma gangrenosum, 338
Garlic
allergic contact dermatitis due to, 120
Genetic
toxicity of psoralen and ultraviolet radiation, 264
Genital
anogenital (*see* Warts, anogenital)
herpes, acyclovir in, as initial treatment, 356, 358
Gibert's pityriasis rosea (*see* Pityriasis rosea, Gibert)
Gingivitis
desquamative, in skin disease, 374
Gliadin
antibodies in dermatitis herpetiformis and pemphigoid, 62
Gloves
heated, for digital ischemia, 97
Gluten
in dermatitis herpetiformis (*see* Dermatitis, herpetiformis, gluten in)
Glycosaminoglycan
fibroblasts synthesizing in systemic scleroderma, 92
in psoriasis, 123
Gm immunogenetic markers
in Kaposi's sarcoma, 230
cGMP
in psoriasis, 291
Goeckerman regimen
in psoriasis, 299
Gold jewelry
radioactive, radiation dermatitis from, 380
Graft
-vs.-host reaction, oral manifestations of, 375
Granuloma
faciale, argon laser in, 394
necrotizing, cutaneous extravascular, and systemic disease, 99
pyogenic granuloma-like acne after isotretinoin, 24
Trichophyton mentagrophytes, 145
Gray maculae
after PUVA, 274
Griseofulvin
in dermatophytosis, 149
in lichen planus, oral erosive, 377
Growth hormone
in psoriasis, 316
Günther's erythropoietic porphyria
carotenoids and, 258

H

H_1 and H_2 antagonists
inhibiting dermographism, 325
Hand
atopic dermatitis of, 112
Head
melanoma, incidence, 189
Healing
moist wound, under vapor permeable membrane, 335
Heat
humid and dry, sweating efficiency during exercise in, 370
Hemorrhagic
proctitis due to lymphogranuloma venereum, 49
Heparin
skin necrosis due to, 134
Hepatic (*see* Liver)
Hepatitis B virus
in urticaria and angioedema, 327
Herlitz syndrome
prenatal exclusion, 72
Herpes, 355 ff., 360 ff.
-associated erythema multiforme, complement deposition in, 360
genital, acyclovir in, as initial treatment, 356, 358
gestationis, 60 ff.
etiology and pathogenesis, 60
features, clinical and histologic, 60
labialis, acyclovir in, 357
neuralgia after, pimozide in, 129

simplex, HLA antigen in, 361
zoster, acyclovir in, 355
Herpetic whitlow
study of, 359
Hidradenitis suppurativa
surgery of, 38
Hirsutism, 165 ff.
idiopathic, adrenal abnormalities in, 166
in polycystic ovary syndrome, peripheral tissue events in, 165
Histamine antagonists
H_1 and H_2, suppressing alcohol-induced flushing, 126
Histiocytosis
malignant, skin manifestations of, 243
sea-blue, familial, ultrastructure in, 160
Histocompatibility antigens
in nevomelanocytes and malignant melanoma, 205
HLA
antigen in erythema multiforme and herpes simplex, 361
-B15 and erythema multiforme, 391
-DR antigen in psoriasis, 293
-DR4, and vitiligo, 280
in Kaposi's sarcoma, 230
typing in neonatal lupus erythematosus, 78
Hodgkin's disease
pruritus in, 234
Homosexual men (*see* Kaposi's sarcoma, in homosexual men)
Hormone(s)
growth, in psoriasis, 316
Humoral immunity
to papillomavirus type 1, 346
Hyaline fibromatosis
juvenile, 366
Hydroa vacciniforme
ultraviolet A and, 257
Hydroxychloroquine
in porphyria cutanea tarda, 259
Hyperhidrosis
surgery of, 371
Hyperkeratosis
epidermolytic, 163
Hyperkeratotic
dermatitis of palms, PUVA in, 317
Hyperostosis
retinoid, 131
Hypersensitivity
angiitis due to heat-activated photocopy paper fumes, 119
cellular, to UVA, 254
delayed, repeated skin tests in, 121
food, in atopic dermatitis, 110
Hypertension
portal, after vitamin A intoxication, 132
Hypertrichosis lanuginosa
acquired, 167

I

Ichthyosis, 161 ff.
refractory, 13-*cis*-retinoic acid toxicity in, 131
of Sjögren-Larsson syndrome, etretinate in, 162
vulgaris, X-linked recessive, 161
Ig (*see* Immunoglobulin)
Imaging
of melanoma with ^{131}I-monoclonal antibodies, 211
Immune
complexes in dermatitis herpetiformis, 63
status in 2,4-dinitro-1-chlorobenzene contact allergy, 120
Immunity
cell-mediated
to papillomavirus type 1, 346
in polymorphic light eruption, 255
Ro 10-9359 and, 298
humoral, to papillomavirus type 1, 346
thyroid autoimmunity in urticaria and angioedema, 329
Immunocompromised patients
acyclovir for zoster in, 355
Immunocytochemistry
of Merkel cell tumors, 239
Immunodeficiency syndrome, acquired (*see* AIDS)
Immunofluorescence
of amyloidosis, cutaneous, 393
direct, in pyoderma gangrenosum, 337
Immunogenetic markers
Gm, in Kaposi's sarcoma, 230
Immunogenetic study
in SLE, familial, 80
Immunoglobulin
A
antigliadin antibodies in dermatitis herpetiformis, 64
deposits in skin in alcoholic liver disease, 389
dermatitis herpetiformis and, 67
dermatosis, linear, 85
E, 104 ff.
antibodies to allergens in atopic dermatitis, 107
assays, isotopic and enzymatic, in nonallergic subjects, 104
in dermatitis, in infant, 108

    production by mononuclear cells, 106
  G
    antibodies to allergens in atopic dermatitis, 107
    antigliadin antibodies in dermatitis herpetiformis, 64
  M antibodies, anti-*Toxoplasma,* 89
Immunohistochemistry
  of lymphoma of skin, 234
Immunologic effects
  of solarium exposure, 248
Immunologic study
  of Gibert's pityriasis rosea, 371
Immunoperoxidase study
  of light eruption, polymorphic, 255
Immunosorbent assay
  enzyme-linked, of antigliadin antibodies, 64
Immunosuppression
  in connective tissue disease, 87
  papillomavirus type 5 DNA in skin cancer after, 75
Immunotherapy
  in leprosy, 178
Implants
  collagen, injectable, 142
Incontinentia pigmenti achromians, 284
Infant (*see* Children, infant)
Infectious mononucleosis
  urticaria and, cold, 328
Inoculation blastomycosis, 152
Insulin
  abdominal lipohypertrophy after, 136
  -dependent diabetes, suction-induced blister formation in, 73
Interferon
  fibroblast, in warts, 351
  leukocyte A, in Kaposi's sarcoma in homosexual men, 228
  lymphoblastoid, in malignant melanoma, 214
Intestine
  small, mucosa in dermatitis herpetiformis, 65
Intoxication
  vitamin A, portal hypertension and cirrhosis after, 132
Intraepidermal tumors
  laser in, 349
Iodine-131
  -monoclonal antibodies for melanoma imaging, 211
Irradiation (*see* Radiation)
Ischemia
  digital, heated gloves for, 97
Isotretinoin, 23 ff.
  neutrophil chemotaxis in cystic acne after, 23
  in psoriasis, 294
  pyogenic granuloma-like acne after, 24
Ixodes dammini spirochete
  natural distribution, 46

J

Jadassohn nevi
  verrucosebaceous, tumors on, 243
Jewelry
  radioactive gold, radiation dermatitis from, 380
Juvenile (*see* Children)

K

Kaposi's sarcoma, 226 ff.
  AIDS and, 227
  Gm immunogenetic markers in, 230
  HLA in, 230
  in homosexual men
    early lesions, 226
    leukocyte A interferon in, 228
  staging classification, 229
Kasabach-Merritt syndrome
  in infant, 274
Kawasaki syndrome
  case review, 363
Keloid
  excision and radiotherapy in, 380
Keratin
  polypeptide
    to discriminate benign and malignant epithelial lesions, 219
    profile after etretinate, 297
Keratinocyte
  damage in vitiligo, 279
Keratosis
  actinic
    DNA repair in, 217
    spreading pigmented, 272
  solar, lichenoid, prevalence and immunology, 218
Ketoconazole
  in candidiasis, mucocutaneous, 154
  in dermatophytosis, 149
  liver reactions during, 138
  in mycosis, systemic, 153
Khellin
  in psoriasis, 311
Kidney
  involvement in dermatitis herpetiformis, 63
  transplant, immunosuppression for, papillomavirus type 5 DNA in skin cancer after, 217

L

Langerhans cells
 in psoriasis, 293
Laser, 349 ff.
 argon, in granuloma faciale, 394
 in condylomata acuminata
  of anus, 350
  of vulva, 349
 in intraepidermal neoplasia, 349
Lectin
 Ulex europaeus I, marking tumors from endothelial cells, 342
Leg ulcer
 venous, sympathectomy in, 335
Leishmanial infections
 in travelers, 50
Lentiginous, 268
 eruption after photochemotherapy, 270
 melanocyte after PUVA, 268
Leprosy, 175 ff.
 immunotherapy with *Mycobacterium leprae* and BCG, 178
 in infant, 175 ff.
  in Ethiopia, 176
  after maternal lepromatous leprosy, 175
 lepromatous
  erythema nodosum leprosum in, 179
  T-cell unresponsiveness reversal in, 176
 skin infiltrates of, 177
 T-cell phenotypes in, 177
Leucodinine B
 in cloasma, "confettiform" depigmentation after, 283
Leukemia
 myelomonocytic, presenting as xanthomatous skin eruption, 384
 T cell, virus identification in patient, 232
Leukocyte
 A interferon in Kaposi's sarcoma in homosexual men, 228
Leukoderma
 vitiligo-like, electron microscopy of, 276
Lichen planus
 differentiation from lupus erythematosus, 84
 lymphocytotoxicity of oral mucosa in, 375
 oral erosive, griseofulvin in, 377
Lichenoid
 solar keratosis, prevalence and immunology, 218
Light
 eruption, polymorphic, 255 ff.
  cell-mediated immunity in, 255
  papular, immunoperoxidase study, 255
 microscopy in Gibert's pityriasis rosea, 373
 reaction, persistent, PUVA in, 256
Lipohypertrophy
 abdominal, after insulin, 136
Lipoprotein
 electrophoresis in ichthyosis vulgaris, 161
Lithium
 skin conditions after, 139
Liver
 cirrhosis after vitamin A intoxication, 132
 disease, alcoholic cutaneous IgA deposits in, 389
 histology after phlebotomy, 259
 reactions during ketoconazole, 138
Lung
 cytology in mycosis fungoides, 232
 metastases, solitary, in high-risk melanoma patients, 215
Lupus erythematosus, 75 ff.
 with dermatitis herpetiformis, 68
 discoid, variant of, 83
 lichen planus differentiation from, 84
 in newborn, 77 ff.
  HLA typing in, 78
  in successive pregnancies, 77
 systemic, 75 ff.
  ANA-negative, 81
  antibodies to DNA and C3 in, 75
  anti-Sm antibodies in, 83
  classification, revised criteria, 75
  familial, 79 ff.
  familial, immunogenetic study, 80
  familial, in males, 79
  mild, plasma exchange in, 85
  pregnancy during, 76
  skin biopsies in, repeat, 81
 verrucous, ultrastructure of, 83
Lyme disease, 44 ff.
 early manifestations, treatment, 45
 relationship to erythema migrans, 47
 spirochetal etiology of, 44
Lymph nodes
 Trichophyton dissemination to, 145
Lymphoblastoid
 interferon in malignant melanoma, 214
Lymphocytes
 in blister fluid in bullous pemphigoid, 57
 in erythema multiforme, 361
 subpopulations in atopic dermatitis, and TP-5, 114
Lymphocytotoxicity
 for oral mucosa in lichen planus, 375

Lymphogranuloma
  venereum, causing hemorrhagic proctitis, 49
Lymphokine
  pemphigoid and, bullous, 57
Lympholysis
  cell-mediated, defect in atopic dermatitis, 103
Lymphoma
  skin
    correlation of features in, 234
    etretinate in, 238
  T cell, 235 ff.
    (*See also* Mycosis fungoides)
    13-*cis*-retinoic acid in, 239
    cyclosporine in, and Sézary syndrome, 235
    retrovirus-associated, 230
    skin, 2'-deoxycoformycin in, 236
Lymphomatoid papulosis
  clinicopathology, 390
  PUVA in, 128
Lymphomatous vasculitis
  of skin, and leukemia virus, 232
Lymphotoxicity
  of oral mucosa in lichen planus, 375
Lysogeny
  in *Staphylococcus aureus,* 41

M

Macula
  gray, ashen, after PUVA, 274
Macule
  pigmented, due to PUVA, 268
Malignancy (*see* Cancer)
Marjolin's ulcer
  experience with, 378
Mastocytosis
  bullous, disodium cromoglycate in, 332
Melanocyte
  lentiginous, after PUVA, 268
  mass, estimation of, 267
  nevomelanocytes, HLA and mononuclear inflammatory infiltrate in, 205
Melanocytic (*see* Nevi, melanocytic)
Melanoma, 181 ff.
  familial atypical multiple mole-melanoma syndrome, 181 ff.
    phenotypic variation, 182
    segregation analysis, 181
  head, incidence, 189
  high-risk patients, solitary lung metastases in, 215
  ^{131}I-monoclonal antibody imaging of, 211
  lentiginous, acral, clinicopathology, 196
  lentigo maligna, amelanotic, dermatitis-like plaque in, 197
  malignant, 187 ff.
    electron microscopy of, 276
    epidemiology in Germany, 193
    fibroblast type intermediate filaments in, and neurofilaments absence in, 206
    HLA and mononuclear inflammatory infiltrates in, 205
    interferon in, lymphoblastoid, 214
    with melanocytic nevi, acquired, favorable prognosis, 203
    preinvasive and invasive, survival, 187
    recurrent, prognostic parameters, 209
    risk, skin factors in, 188
    skin, excision, metastases after, 208
    skin markings in, 198
    skin, resection margin for, 212
    skin, update in Hawaii, 191
    stage II, postsurgical management, 213
    staging, proposal for, 198
    thin, biologic behavior, 202
    thin, metastases of, 201 ff.
    thin, metastases and death in, 202
  multiple, and atypical melanocytic nevi, 183
  neck, incidence, 189
  nodular, radiotherapy in, 0–7–21, 216
  -prone families, dysplastic nevi on scalp in children of, 184
  skin
    geographic distribution in Queensland, 190
    incidence and reporting of, 188
    with melanocytic nevi, dysplastic, 181
    recurrence, late, 207
    uvea in, 195
  stage I
    death in, predictors of, 206
    prognosis and anatomical location, 200
    prognosis and surgical results in, 194
Merkel cell tumors, 239 ff.
  enolase and, neuron-specific, 241
  study with case review, 242
  ultrastructure and immunocytochemistry, 239
Metastases
  lung, solitary, in high-risk melanoma patients, 215
  after melanoma excision, 208
  of melanoma, malignant, with unknown primary, 210

of melanoma, thin, 201 ff.
with death, 202
of skin carcinoma, basal cell, 224
Methotrexate
in psoriasis, severe, 310
8-Methoxypsoralen
photochemotherapy of psoriasis, 302
Methylprednisolone
pulse therapy in dermatomyositis, 88
Metronidazole
in rosacea, 37
Mibelli porokeratosis
5-fluorouracil in, 396
Miconazole
nitrate, for dandruff, 125
Microscopy
electron (*see* Electron microscopy)
light, in Gibert's pityriasis rosea, 373
Midfacial
epithelioma, curettage and electrodesiccation of, 222
Minoxidil
in alopecia areata, 171
Mitsuda-negative contacts
leprosy and, 178
Moist wound healing
under vapor permeable membrane, 335
Mole (*see* Melanoma, familial atypical multiple mole-melanoma syndrome)
Monoclonal antibodies
in atopic dermatitis, 104
fluorescent, in lymphogranuloma venereum, 49
^{131}I-, for melanoma imaging, 211
in study of polymorphic light eruption, 255
Monoclonal gammopathy
pyoderma gangrenosum and, 338
Monocyte
after colchicine, 313
Mononuclear
cells
in atopic dermatitis, 104
IgE production by, 106
inflammatory infiltrate in nevomelanocytes and malignant melanoma, 205
Mononucleosis
infectious, and cold urticaria, 328
Mouth (*see* Oral)
Mucocutaneous
candidiasis, ketoconazole in, 154
Mycobacterium leprae
in immunotherapy of leprosy, 178
Mycosis
fungoides
(*See also* Lymphoma, T cell)
carmustine in, topical, 237
lung cytology in, 232
systemic, ketoconazole in, 153
Myeloproliferative disorders
Sweet's syndrome and, 385

N

Nailfold
abnormalities in rheumatic disease, in children, 90
Neck
melanoma, incidence, 189
Necrosis, skin, 132 ff.
after coumadin, 132 ff.
heparin causing, 134
Necrotizing
granuloma, cutaneous extravascular, and systemic disease, 99
Neonatal (*see* Children, newborn)
Neoplasia (*see* Tumors)
Neuralgia
after herpes, pimozide in, 129
Neuroendocrine
carcinoma of skin (*see* Merkel cell tumors)
Neurofilaments
absence in pigmented nevi and malignant melanoma, 206
Neuroleptic
-induced parkinsonism, seborrheic dermatitis in, 142
Neuron
-specific enolase and Merkel cell tumors, 241
Neutrophil
chemotaxis in cystic acne, and isotretinoin, 23
after colchicine, 313
migration inhibition by etretinate, 298
Neutrophilic dermatosis
febrile (*see* Sweet's syndrome)
Nevi, 183 ff.
dysplastic, on scalp, of prepubertal children in melanoma-prone families, 184
of Jadassohn, verrucosebaceous, tumors of, 243
melanocytic
acquired, with malignant melanoma, favorable prognosis, 203
atypical, melanoma and, multiple, 183
dysplastic, with melanoma, 181
nevocellular, congenital, 185 ff.
patterns and histology, 186
treatment and case review, 185
pigmented, fibroblast-type intermediate filaments in, and neurofilaments absence in, 206
Nevocellular (*see* Nevi, nevocellular)

Nevomelanocytes
HLA and mononuclear inflammatory infiltrates in, 205
Newborn (*see* Children, newborn)
Newcastle disease virus oncolysate
melanoma and, stage II, 213
Nifedipine
in Raynaud's phenomenon, 95
Nitroglycerin
in Raynaud's phenomenon, 96
Nonrashes
as audible signs of cutaneous disease, 386
Nystatin
in diaper dermatitis, candidal, 156

O

Ocular disease
vitiligo and, 278
Oculocutaneous albinism
prenatal diagnosis, 286
Oncolysate
Newcastle disease virus, and stage II melanoma, 213
Ophthalmologic study
after PUVA, 303
Oral, 375 ff.
evening-primrose-seed oil in atopic eczema, 111
lichen planus, erosive, griseofulvin in, 377
manifestations of graft-vs.-host reaction, 375
mucosa in lichen planus, lymphocytotoxicity of, 375
pemphigus, features of, 55
Ovaries
polycystic ovary syndrome, hirsutism in, peripheral tissue events, 165
Oxytetracycline
in rosacea, 37

P

Palmoplantar pustulosis
etretinate in, 318 ff.
Palms
dermatitis, hyperkeratotic, PUVA in, 317
Papillomavirus, 345 ff.
frequency and distribution in warts, 345
type 1, immunity to, 346
type 5, DNA in skin cancer after immunosuppression, 217
Papulosis
lymphomatoid
clinicopathology, 390
PUVA in, 128
Para-aminobenzoic acid
sensitization of near-ultraviolet killing of mammalian cells by, 250
Parkinsonism
neuroleptic-induced, seborrheic dermatitis in, 142
Pemphigoid, 57, 61 ff.
antigens, heterogeneity of, 57
bullous
collagenase and elastase in blister fluid in, 61
lymphocytes in blister fluid in, 57
plasma exchanges in, 58
gliadin antibodies in, 62
Pemphigus, 53 ff.
epidemiologic study, 53
familial benign, etretinate in, 59
juvenile, 54
-like antigens in urine, 56
oral, features of, 55
transplacental transmission of, 53
D-Penicillamine
in rheumatoid arthritis, fatal myositis after, 140
Peritoneal dialysis
in psoriasis, 314
Peutz-Jeghers syndrome
in children, 273
Phlebotomy
in porphyria cutanea tarda, 259 ff.
Photochemotherapy
in alopecia areata, 168
in carcinoma of skin, 305
in dermatitis of palms, hyperkeratotic, 317
lentiginous eruption after, 270
long-term, in psoriasis, 307
8-methoxypsoralen, in psoriasis, 302
Photocopy paper
heat-activated, fumes causing hypersensitivity angiitis, 119
Phototherapy
coal tar, in psoriasis, 301
of pityriasis lichenoides, 263
Pigmentary incontinence
in fixed drug eruptions, 276
Pigmentation
in Addison's disease, 267
of comedones, open, ultrastructure, 35
Pigmented
actinic keratosis, spreading, 272
lesions, and photochemotherapy in psoriasis, 307
macule due to PUVA, 268
nevi, fibroblast-type intermediate filaments in, and neurofilaments absence in, 206
Pimozide
in postherpetic neuralgia, 129

Pityriasis, 263 ff.
  alba, study of, 114
  lichenoides, phototherapy of, 263
Pityriasis rosea, 371 ff.
  Gibert's
    histopathology, 371, 373
    light microscopy in, 373
    study of, 371
  respiratory tract infection and, upper, 372
  ultraviolet therapy of, 263
Placenta
  transplacental transmission of pemphigus, 53
Plaque
  dermatitis-like, in lentigo maligna melanoma, 197
  of pregnancy and pruritic urticarial papules, 388
Plasmapheresis
  in psoriasis, 315
Plasminogen activator
  epidermal, and psoriasis, 289
Podophyllin
  in anogenital warts, 352
Polyamines
  after etretinate in psoriasis, 289, 296
Polycystic ovary syndrome
  hirsutism in, peripheral tissue events in, 165
Polymorphic (*see* Light, eruption, polymorphic)
Polymyositis
  fatal, after D-penicillamine in rheumatoid arthritis, 140
  toxoplasmosis in, 89
Polyps
  colonic, skin tags for, 384
Porokeratosis of Mibelli
  5-fluorouracil in, 396
Poroma
  eccrine malignant, case review, 344
Porphyria, 258 ff.
  cutanea tarda, 259 ff.
    hydroxychloroquine in, 259
    phlebotomy in, 259 ff.
    uroporphyrinogen decarboxylase in, 260
  Günther's congenital erythropoietic, and carotenoids, 258
Porphyrin
  pattern after phlebotomy, 259
  -related disorder, bronze baby syndrome as, 262
Portal hypertension
  after vitamin A intoxication, 132
Prednisolone
  for acne vulgaris in women, 29
  in connective tissue disease, 87
Pregnancy
  Ehlers-Danlos syndrome type IV complicating, 157
  plaques of, and pruritic urticarial papules, 388
  with SLE, 76
  successive pregnancies, neonatal lupus in, 77
Prenatal
  diagnosis of oculocutaneous albinism, 286
  exclusion of Herlitz syndrome, 72
Proctitis
  hemorrhagic, due to lymphogranuloma venereum, 49
Propionibacteria
  in acne vulgaris, 31
Propionibacterium acnes
  resistance to antibiotics in acne, 30
Protein
  leakage after PUVA, 308
Pruritic urticarial papules
  plaques of pregnancy and, 388
Pruritus
  generalized, and systemic disease, 382
  in Hodgkin's disease, 234
Pseudomonas aeruginosa
  antifungal activity of, in gram-negative athlete's foot, 148
  serotype 0:9, in whirlpool-associated dermatitis, 43
Psoralen
  -containing sunscreen as tumorigenic (in mice), 253
  in dermatitis of palms, hyperkeratotic, 317
  genetic toxicity of, 264
  PUVA (*see* PUVA)
Psoriasis, 289 ff.
  cAMP in, 291
  anthralin in, 300
  arotinoid Ro 13-6298 in, 295 ff.
  benoxaprofen in, 312 ff.
  calmodulin elevation in, 290
  coal tar phototherapy in, 301
  colchicine in, 313
  dermatan sulfate and, 291
  dialysis in, peritoneal, 314
  dithranol in, irritant reactions to, 301
  epidermal plasminogen activator and, 289
  etretinate in, 296 ff.
    keratin polypeptide profile after, 297
    polyamine decrease after, 289
    study, 296
  glycosaminoglycans in irritant dermatitis of, 123
  cGMP in, 291
  Goeckerman regimen in, 299

growth hormone in, 316
HLA-DR antigen in, 293
khellin in, 311
Langerhans cells in, 293
8-methoxypsoralen photochemotherapy in, 302
photochemotherapy in, long-term, 307
plasmapheresis in, 315
PUVA in
arsenic carcinogenesis and, 306
with isotretinoin, 294
observations on, 309
retinoid in, aromatic, 293
severe, RePUVA, Ro 10–9359 and methotrexate in, 310
somatostatin in, 316
UVB in, 309
safety of, 305
virus-like particle associated with, 292
Psychiatric symptoms
in dermatology patients, 399
Psychoanalyist
-dermatologist's viewpoint, 397
Psychosomatic concepts
in dermatology, 397
Pustulosis
palmoplantar, etretinate in, 318 ff.
PUVA, 303 ff.
arsenic carinogenesis and, 306
in carcinoma of skin, 305
in dermatitis of palms, hyperkeratotic, 317
freckles after, 274
gray maculae after, ashen, 274
in light reaction, persistent, 256
long-term, ophthalmologic study in, 303
in papulosis, lymphomatoid, 128
pigmented macule due to, 268
protein leakage after, 308
in psoriasis (*see* Psoriasis, PUVA in)
RePUVA in severe psoriasis, 310
Pyoderma gangrenosum, 337 ff.
Crohn's disease and, 338
immunofluorescence in, direct, 337
monoclonal gammopathy and, 338
Pyogenic granuloma
-like acne during isotretinoin, 24

R

Radiation
(*See also* Radiotherapy)
dermatitis from radioactive gold jewelry, 380
ultraviolet (*see* Ultraviolet)
Radiotherapy
Favre-Racouchot syndrome and, 35
of keloids after excision, 380
in melanoma, nodular, 0–7–21, 216
Raynaud's phenomenon, 95 ff.
nifedipine in, 95
nitroglycerin, swinging arm maneuver and biofeedback training in, 96
Renal (*see* Kidney)
RePUVA
in psoriasis, severe, 310
Respiratory
tract infection, upper, and pityriasis rosea, 372
Reticulin
antibodies against, in dermatitis herpetiformis, 65
Reticuloid
actinic, etiology of, 254
Retinoic acid (*see cis*-retinoic acid)
Retinoid
aromatic
in psoriasis, 293
Ro 10–9359 (*see* Ro 10–9359)
aroretinoid Ro 13–6298 in psoriasis, 295 ff.
hyperostosis, 131
oral synthetic, anti-inflammatory activities of, 125
Retrovirus
-associated T cell lymphoma, 230
Rheumatic disease
nailfold abnormalities in, in children, 90
Rheumatoid arthritis
D-penicillamine in, fatal polymyositis after, 140
Ro 10–9359
cell-mediated immunity and, 298
in pemphigus, benign familial, 59
in psoriasis
keratin polypeptide profile after, 297
severe, 310
Ro 13–6298
in psoriasis, 295 ff.
Rosacea
metronidazole and oxytetracycline in, 37

S

Sarcoidosis
etretinate in viral warts and, 348
Sarcoma (*see* Kaposi's sarcoma)
Scabies, 368 ff.
eradication with single treatment schedule, 368
experimental canine, in humans, 369
Scalp
nevi, dysplastic, of prepubertal children from melanoma-prone families, 184

Scanning
of melanoma with ^{131}I-monoclonal antibodies, 211
Scissor excision
of anogenital warts, 352
Scleredema
adultorum, and diabetes, 101
Scleroderma, 91 ff.
with atrophy of left side of body and right side of face, 94
systemic, 91 ff.
in children, 91
fibroblasts synthesizing glycosaminoglycan in, 92
variants, and anticentromere antibody, 93
Sclerosis
progressive systemic (*see* Scleroderma, systemic)
tuberous, family studies in, 157
5-S-cysteinyldopa
after ultraviolet, 309
Seborrhea
contrasted with seborrheic dermatitis, 395
Seborrheic (*see* Dermatitis, seborrheic)
Sebum secretion
after 13-*cis*-retinoic acid, 22
sustainable rates in acne, 26
Selenium disulfide
for dandruff, 125
Sensitization
autoerythrocyte, 400
of near-ultraviolet killing of mammalian cells by para-aminobenzoic acid, 250
Serum sickness
zomepirac causing, 141
Sézary syndrome
cyclosporine in T cell lymphoma and, 235
Shock (*see* Toxic shock syndrome)
Sjögren-Larsson syndrome
ichthyosis of, etretinate for, 162
Skin
action of cyproterone acetate on, due to metabolite, 34
amebiasis, 51
amyloidosis, immunofluorescence and histochemistry of, 393
barrier properties, in newborn, 365
biopsy (*see* Biopsy, skin)
blastomycosis, 152
cancer, papillomavirus type 5 DNA in, after immunosuppression, 217
carcinoma (*see* Carcinoma, skin)
conditions after lithium, 139
disease
bullous, collagenase and elastase in blister fluid from, 61
gingivitis in, desquamative, 374
nonrashes as audible signs of, 386
work-related, epidemiology, 117
factors in malignant melanoma risk, 188
in hyperkeratosis, epidermolytic, 163
IgA deposits in, in alcoholic liver disease, 389
infiltrates of leprosy, 177
involvement in familial sea-blue histiocytosis, 160
lymphoma (*see* Lymphoma, skin)
manifestations of histiocytosis, malignant, 243
markings in malignant melanoma, 198
melanoma (*see* Melanoma, skin)
necrosis (*see* Necrosis, skin)
in necrotizing granuloma and systemic disease, 99
oculocutaneous albinism, prenatal diagnosis, 286
response to ultraviolet, 251
tags for colonic polyps, 384
tests, repeated delayed hypersensitivity, 121
thickness in acromegaly and Cushing's syndrome, 401
vasculitis, lymphomatous, and leukemia virus, 232
vessel leakage of proteins after PUVA, 308
xanthomatous eruption, in myelomonocytic leukemia, 384
Solar
keratosis, lichenoid, prevalence and immunology, 218
Solarium exposure
immunologic effects of, 248
Somatostatin
in psoriasis, 316
Spider bite
brown recluse, dapsone in, 128
Spirochetal etiology
of Lyme disease, 44
Sporotrichosis, 149 ff.
from a cat, 151
extracutaneous, 149
Staphylococcus aureus, 41 ff.
infection office treatment, in children, 42
toxic shock syndrome and lysogeny in, 41
Sulfametrole
in chancroid, 48

Sunburn
sensitivity, individual variations in, 249
Sunlight
exposure, T cell subset alterations after, 247
Sunscreen, 250 ff.
agent, para-aminobenzoic acid, 250
protection and erythema, 251
psoralen-containing, as tumorigenic (in mice), 253
Sweating
efficiency during exercise, 370
Sweet's syndrome
colchicine in, 378
elastase-like enzyme in, 389
myeloproliferative disorders and, 385
Swimming pools
brominated, and dermatosis, 122
Swinging arm maneuver
in Raynaud's phenomenon, 96
Sympathectomy
in leg ulcer, venous, 335
Syphilis
infectiousness of, study of, 44

T

Tags
skin, for colonic polyps, 384
T-cell, 12-3 ff., 230
leukemia virus, identification in patient, 232
lymphoma (*see* Lymphoma, T cell)
phenotypes in leprosy, 177
subsets, alteration after sunlight exposure, 247
unresponsiveness reversal in lepromatous leprosy, 176
Telangiectasia
unilateral dermatomal superficial, 341
Testes
Trichophyton dissemination to, 145
Testosterone
levels in acne in women, 27
Thymopoietin pentapeptide
in atopic dermatitis, 114
Thyroid autoimmunity
in urticaria and angioedema, 329
Tigason (*see* Etretinate)
Tinea
capitis, study of, 147
Tomography, computed
of lung metastases in high-risk melanoma patients, 215
Toxic shock syndrome, 41 ff.
dermatologic signs in, 41
Staphylococcus aureus in, 41
Toxicity
of 13-*cis*-retinoic acid in ichthyosis, 131
cytotoxicity, antibody-dependent, and colchicine, 313
genetic, of psoralen and ultraviolet radiation, 264
lymphotoxicity of oral mucosa in lichen planus, 375
Toxoplasmosis
in polymyositis-dermatomyositis, 89
TP–5
in atopic dermatitis, 114
Transplantation
kidney, immunosuppression for, papillomavirus type 5 DNA in skin cancer after, 217
Trauma
wheals in angioedema and, 323
Trichloroacetic acid
in anogenital warts, 352
Trichophyton
mentagrophytes granuloma, 145
tonsurans epidemic, 146
Trimethoprim
in chancroid, 48
Tuberous sclerosis
family studies in, 157
Tumorigenic
psoralen-containing sunscreen as (in mice), 253
Tumors
from endothelial cells, *Ulex europaeus* I lectin marking, 342
intraepidermal, laser in, 349
Merkel cell (*see* Merkel cell tumors)
on nevi of Jadassohn, verrucosebaceous, 243

U

Ulcer, 378 ff.
decubitus, and bacteremia, 379
leg, venous, sympathectomy in, 335
Marjolin's, experience with, 378
Ulex europaeus I lectin
marking tumors from endothelial cells, 342
Ultrastructure
in Gibert's pityriasis rosea, 371
in histiocytosis, familial sea-blue, 160
in hyperkeratosis, epidermolytic, 163
in Kaposi's sarcoma in homosexual men, 226
in lupus erythematosus, verrucous, 83
of Merkel cell tumors, 239, 242
of pigmentation of open comedones, 35
of pityriasis alba, 114

Ultraviolet, 250, 263
A
cellular hypersensitivity to, 254
hydroa vacciniforme and, 257
long-wave, topical protection against, 252
PUVA (*see* PUVA)
B
natural radiation from, 309
in psoriasis, 309
in psoriasis, safety of, 305
doses to produce erythemal response in normal skin, 249
erythemogenic, and coal tar, 301
genetic toxicity of, 264
in pityriasis rosea treatment, 263
5-S-cysteinyldopa after, 309
sensitization of near-ultraviolet killing of mammalian cells by para-aminobenzoic acid, 250
skin response to, 251
Uroporphyrinogen decarboxylase
in porphyria cutanea tarda, 260
Urticaria, 327 ff.
cold, and infectious mononucleosis, 328
hepatitis B virus in, 327
idiopathic
cimetidine in, 324
histologic studies, 331
natural course and etiology, in children, 330
pruritic papules, and plaques of pregnancy, 388
thyroid autoimmunity and, 329
UV (*see* Ultraviolet)
UVA (*see* Ultraviolet, A)
UVB (*see* Ultraviolet, B)
Uvea
in skin melanoma, 195

V

Vagina
candidiasis, clotrimazole and econazole in, 155
Vapor permeable membrane
moist wound healing under, 335
Vasculitis
skin lymphomatous, and leukemia virus, 232
Vein
leg ulcers, sympathectomy in, 335
Verrucosebaceous nevi of Jadassohn
tumors on, 243
Vertebra
Trichophyton dissemination to, 145
Vessels
skin, leakage of proteins after PUVA, 308
Vibration
-induced angioedema, 326
Vimentin
-type filaments in pigmented nevi and malignant melanoma, 206
Virology
of Gibert's pityriasis rosea, 371
Virus(es)
hepatitis B, in urticaria and angioedema, 327
herpes (*see* Herpes)
leukemia, T cell, identification in patient, 232
-like particle associated with psoriasis, 292
Newcastle disease virus oncolysate, and melanoma, stage II, 213
papillomavirus (*see* Papillomavirus)
retrovirus-associated T cell lymphoma, 230
warts due to, etretinate in, 348
Vitamin
A intoxication, portal hypertension and cirrhosis after, 132
K-dependent coagulation factors, and cholestasis, 133
Vitiligo, 276 ff.
cyclophosphamide in, 268
5-fluorouracil in, 281
generalized, after erythroderma, 282
HLA-DR4 and, 280
keratinocyte damage in, 279
-like leukoderma, electron microscopy of, 276
ocular disease and, 278
Vulva
condylomata acuminata, laser in, 349
warts, and cervical abnormalities, 347

W

Warts, 345, 351
anogenital, 352 ff.
scissor excision in, 352
trichloroacetic acid and podophyllin in, 352
bleomycin in, 353 ff.
locally injected, 354
recalcitrant warts, 353
interferon in, fibroblast, 351
papillomavirus frequency and distribution in, 345
papillomavirus type 1 in, immunity to, 346
virus, etretinate in, 348
vulva, and cervical abnormalities, 347
Wheals
in angioedema, and trauma, 323

Whirlpool-associated dermatitis
  Pseudomonas aeruginosa in, 43
Work-related skin disease
  epidemiology of, 117
Wound healing
  moist, under vapor permeable
    membrane, 355

X

Xanthomatous skin eruption
  in leukemia, myelomonocytic, 384
X-linked ichthyosis vulgaris, 161
X-ray (*see* Radiation)

Z

Zomepirac
  serum sickness due to, 141
Zoster
  acyclovir in, 355

Index to Authors

A

Abdel-Fattah, A., 311
Abemayor, E., 227
Abo-Darub, J. M., 217
Aboul-Enein, M. N., 311
Abramsohn, R., 371
Abramson, C., 148
Acheson, E. D., 97
Acuna, G., 356
Addis, B. J., 235
Aeppli, D., 355
Aftimos, B. G., 114
Agache, P., 346
Ahmed, A. R., 54, 56, 61, 81
Akimoto, T., 88
Albano, W. A., 182
Alber, R. L., 152
Albert, A., 273
Albert, D. M., 195, 276, 278
Allen, B. R., 313
Allen, R., 324
Alper, J. C., 332, 335
Altomare, G. F., 23
Alvarado, J., 178
Ambinder, R. F., 355
Amblard, P., 249
Ambrus, J. L., 209
Amer, M. A., 168
Andersen, E., 315
Anderson, P. C., 314
Anderson, T. F., 289
Andresen, R., 315
Angele, R., 306
Ansell, B. M., 87
Anton-Lamprecht, I., 72
Apfelberg, D. B., 394
Apisarnthanarax, P., 98, 272
Aranzazu, N., 178
Arlian, L., 369
Armstrong, B. K., 187
Arndt, K. A., 263
Arnett, F., 80
Arons, M., 186
Arons, M. S., 185
Arrick, B. A., 177
Arrue, C., 368
Åsbrink, E., 112
Ascari, E., 234
Aso, M., 127
Astarita, R. W., 222
Attardo-Parrinello, G., 234
Aufdemorte, T. B., 377
Austen, K. F., 57
Azzopardi, J. G., 241

B

Baadsgaard, O., 132
Babin, J. P., 258
Bacalu, L., 371
Bach, M. C., 41
Bahuth, N., 114
Balachandran, I., 232
Balch, C. M., 194
Balfour, H. H., Jr., 355
Balow, J. E., 85
Band, J. D., 43
Bangert, J. L., 60
Banks, P. M., 390
Barada, F. A., Jr., 93
Barber, K. A., 78
Barbet, M., 136
Barbour, A. G., 44, 46
Barneon, G., 316
Barnetson, R. St. C., 62, 175
Barnett, A. H., 267
Barr, L. H., 378
Barraclough, B. M., 399
Barrandon, Y., 243
Barsky, S., 146
Bart, R. S., 200, 201, 203
Bartlow, G. A., 222
Bauer, R., 125
Baviera, A., 136
Bazex, J., 91
Bean, B., 355
Beani, J., 249
Beastall, G. M., 316
Beattie, C. W., 207
Beaufils, M., 83
Becker, T., 47
Bégány, A., 255
Belehu, A., 176
Bell, D. M., 363
Bembe, M. L., 93
Benach, J. L., 46
Benezra, C., 120
Benoit, A. M., 22
Beral, V., 188
Berg, R. A., 51
Berger, H., 198
Bergfeld, W. F., 84
Berman, H., 380
Bernhard, J. D., 255, 386
Bernstein, J. E., 73, 134
Besser, G. M., 29
Bessone, E., 259
Bhan, A. K., 104, 205, 255
Bhawan, J., 279
Bhogal, B., 60
Bhutani, L. K., 279

Bias, W. B., 80
Billingham, R. P., 350
Binder, R. L., 142
Binkley, W., 84
Bisaccia, E., 236
Black, M. M., 60, 344
Blanc, D., 346
Blattner, W., 230
Blayney, D., 230
Bloch, K. J., 327
Bloch, P. H., 373
Blomberg, F., 106
Blumhagen, J. D., 157
Bodolay, E., 255
Bogaars, H., 332, 335
Bogokowsky, H., 371
Bolles, C., 239
Bolognesi, D. P., 232
Bonafé, J. L., 59, 371
Bondi, E. E., 198
Bonvalet, D., 243
Bordwell, B., 75
Borkovic, S. P., 197
Bosler, E. M., 46
Botcherby, P. K., 254
Boucheron, S., 238
Boulanger, A., 316
Bove, K. E., 90
Bowles, C., 153
Boyle, J., 348
Boylston, A. W., 71
Bradley, M., 248
Braun-Falco, O., 256
Breathnach, A., 33
Breathnach, S. M., 324
Bredberg, A., 264
Breeding, J., 301
Bressieux, J. M., 91
Briele, H. A., 207
Broadwater, J. R., 38
Broder, S., 230
Bronson, D. M., 146
Brown, J. P., 211
Brugo, M. A., 23
Bryan, C. S., 379
Bryant, R. L., 38
Bryson, Y. J., 356
Buckingham, R. B., 92
Buckley, D. B., 70
Bundino, S., 160
Bunn, P. A., Jr., 230
Burg, G., 120
Burgdorf, W. H. C., 171
Burgdorfer, W., 44, 46
Burgess, J., 239
Burke, B., 32

Burnett, A. K., 384
Burr, M. L., 110
Burton, J. L., 111, 395
Busse, W. W., 326
Byers, P. H., 157
Bystryn, J.-C., 57

C

Cainelli, T., 259, 259
Calcaterra, T. C., 227
Caldwell, E. H., 132
Campbell, A. N., 400
Camus, J.-P., 83
Cantoni, L., 259, 259
Canuel, C., 91
Caro, W. A., 243
Carrasquillo, J. A., 211
Carrey, Z., 208
Cartwright, L. E., 253
Casali, R. E., 38
Cassel, W. A., 213
Cassidy, S. B., 157
Catterall, M. D., 235
Cavalieri, S., 30
Center, D. M., 57
Chaintreul, J., 291
Chakmakjian, Z. H., 26
Chapman, M. D., 107
Chaudhuri, P. K., 207
Chen, J. T. T., 215
Cherry, J. D., 356
Chiorazzi, N., 79
Chowdhury, K. N., 389
Christ, M., 220
Christophers, E., 270
Christou, N. V., 121
Chuang, T.-Y., 372
Chung, P., 384
Ciftan, E., 391
Civatte, J., 243
Clark, W. H., Jr., 184, 198, 212
Claudy, A. L., 238
Clayton, R., 33
Clemmensen, O. J., 315
Clot, J., 316
Cloud, G., 153
Cobb, S. J., 108
Coburn, P. R., 300
Coggon, D., 97
Cohen, A. S., 75
Cohn, Z. A., 177
Coker, D. D., 224
Coleman, J. L., 46
Coller, J. A., 338
Colley, N. V., 347
Collins-Lech, C., 147
Colomb, D., 283
Conant, M. A., 226
Convit, J., 178
Coode, P. E., 235
Cook, L. J., 324
Cooper, P. H., 385
Copper, K. D., 114
Corbet, J.-P., 120
Cornwell, G. G., III, 393
Cosimi, A. B., 206
Coskey, R. J., 118
Coulter, C. A. E., 71
Courren, C., 58
Cox, E., 210
Craft, J. E., 44, 45
Crain, W. R., 237
Cram, D. L., 299
Cramers, M. K., 123, 291
Craven, P. C., 153
Creagan, E. T., 202
Creagh-Kirk, T., 356
Crosnier, J., 217
Crowe, W. E., 90
Cullison, D. A., 341
Culliton, M., 166
Cummings, B. J., 216
Cunliffe, W. J., 32
Cunningham, S., 166
Cunningham-Rundles, S., 228

D

Dahod, S., 24
Dale, B. A., 163
Dalen, A. B., 292
Dandona, P., 136
Danes, B. S., 182
Daniel, F., 136
Dann, J., 60
Danno, K., 302
Darley, C. R., 29
Das Gupta, T. K., 207
Davidson, T. M., 222
Davies, D. J. G., 250
Dawson, D. V., 391
Day, C. L., 181
Day, C. L., Jr., 206
D'Costa, L. J., 48
Dean, D., 357
Debreczeni, M., 255
Decker, J. L., 85
Denburg, J., 329
Deneau, D., 394
Denman, A. M., 87
de Paulet, A. C., 291
Desai, D. R., 146
DeSanna, E. T., 45
Desi, M., 94
De Villez, R. L., 377
Dew, C. E., 379
Dick, D. C., 348
Diffey, B. L., 309
Dillon, M., 356
Dinehart, S. M., 98
Di Padova, C., 259, 259
Di Prisco de Fuenmajor, M. C., 107
Dismukes, W. E., 153
Disney, F. A., 42
Divoux, D., 59
Dolovich, J., 104, 329
Donadio, D., 58
Donald, R. A., 267, 401
Dorsch, C. A., 80
Downing, D. T., 22, 26
Doyle, C. T., 70
Doyle, D. R., 140
Doyle, J. A., 149
Doyon, B., 249
Druker, D., 394
Drutz, D. J., 49
Dubertret, L., 298
Dubey, D., 103
Dubin, N., 221
Ducasse, M.-F., 217
Duell, E. A., 289
Duke, E. E., 129
Duncan, M. E., 175
Dunn, P. H., 232
Dupont, B., 230
Dutronquay, V., 217
Duvic, M., 391

E

Eady, E. A., 32
Eady, R. A. J., 286
Eckman, M. R., 152
Edens, B. L., 222
Edwards, A., 247, 248
Eisen, A. Z., 83
Eizaguirre, I., 273
Elder, D. E., 184, 198, 212
Elder, G. H., 260
El Garf, A., 168
Elias, J. M., 331
Ellis, C. N., 289
Ellison, R. H., 48
El-Menshawi, B., 311
Emeson, E. E., 363
English, J., 70
Enhamre, A., 380
Epstein, E. H., Jr., 237
Espiner, E. A., 267, 401
Esterly, N. B., 339
Estes, S. A., 369
Evans, D. H., 314
Evans, S., 104, 188
Exner, J. H., 24

F

Farrell, D. S., 332
Faure, M., 293
Faure, M. R., 297
Feder, H. M., Jr., 359
Fein, S., 228
Fekete, E., 176
Feldmann, U., 158
Felton, W. F., 44
Fenton, D. A., 171
Ferenczy, A., 349
Ferguson, J. K., 401
Ferguson, S. D., 366
Feucht, C. L., 341
Fiddian, A. P., 357, 358
Fields, B. T., Jr., 153
Finan, M. C., 99
Findlay, R. F., 364
Finlay, A. Y., 366
Finzi, A. F., 23

Fioroni, A., 23
Fischetti, V. A., 41
Fitzpatrick, T. B., 181, 206, 276
Flemetakis, A., 149
Fletcher, V., 226
Foged, E., 318
Foix, C., 136, 243
Foley, L. M., 280
Foley, S. M., 146
Fontan, B., 59
Forget, B., 195
Forget, B. M., 278
Forsbeck, M., 112
Forsum, U., 65
Fraki, J. E., 289
Fraser, M. C., 184
Freedman, M. H., 400
Freeman, R. G., 60
Fretzin, D., 243
Frick, P. G., 133
Friedland, G. H., 363
Friedman, R., 208
Friedman, R. J., 200, 201, 203, 206
Friedman, S. 35, 149
Frier, K., 108
Fries, J. F., 75
Fritz, K. A., 77
Fry, J. S., 71
Fry, L., 65, 66, 70, 71
Frye, A. J., 370
Fulton, R. A., 298
Fusaro, R. M., 181, 182

G

Gabriel, G., 44, 155, 352
Gallis, H. A., 153
Gallo, R. C., 230
Galosi, A., 256
Gantz, N. M., 50
Garner, A., 286
Gattass, C. R., 177
Gautron, R., 249
Gavaler, J., 384
Gaylarde, P. M., 126
Geha, R. S., 103, 330
Gehse, M., 31
Gellis, S., 106
Genner, J., 354
Ghorpade, A., 36
Giannelli, F., 254
Gibofsky, A., 79
Gieger, J. M., 295
Gieseker, D. R., 377
Gilgor, R. S., 289
Gilliam, J. N., 60
Ginsberg, M., 335
Gloor, M., 31
Gobbi, P. G., 234
Gockerman, J. P., 375
Godal, T., 176
Godfrey, H. P., 331
Goebelsmann, U., 165
Goellner, J. R., 242
Goerttler, K., 219
Gokhale, B. B., 280
Gold, J. W. M., 230
Goldman, L. I., 212
Goldman, M. A., 327
Goldschmidt, V. G., 152
Goldstein, N. G., 289
Gollack, J. M., 352
Gollnick, H., 21
Golomb, F. M., 206
Goodman, R. A., 43
Goos, M., 270
Goplerud, C. P., 76
Gori, G., 259, 259
Gorstein, F., 206
Graybill, J. R., 153
Greaves, M. W., 324
Green, A., 188, 190
Greene, M. H., 184
Greer, K. E., 385
Gregg, C. R., 153
Grekin, D. A., 237
Grekin, R. C., 289
Grever, M. R., 236
Grier, W. R. N., 201
Grimelius, L., 65
Grimwood, R., 360
Grodzicki, R. L., 44
Growdon, W., 356
Grubb, C., 347
Gu, J., 241
Guerry, D., IV, 198, 212
Guilhou, J. J., 58, 291, 316
Guillet, G., 258
Guillot, B., 58
Gulbas, N., 151
Gumpel, J. M., 87
Gumport, S. L., 201, 203, 206
Gunner, D. B., 286
Gustavii, B., 72

H

Hafez, G. R., 239
Haffenden, G., 65, 66
Haffenden, G. P., 70, 71
Hafiz, M. A., 224
Haftek, M., 293
Haghighi, P., 222
Hair, L. S., 177
Halasz, A. C. L. G., 257
Hall, R. P., 85
Hamada, T., 281
Hamanaka, K., 389
Hamblin, L. G., 399
Hammar, H., 380
Hanifin, J. M., 114
Hanke, C. W., 142
Hanrahan, J. P., 46
Hanson, V., 90
Happle, R., 169
Haran, G., 247, 248
Haregewoin, A., 176
Harpin, V. A., 365
Harris, A., 330
Harris, C., 363
Harris, H. H., 26
Harris, M. N., 201, 203, 206, 208
Harris, R., 27
Harris, T. J., 189
Harrist, T. J., 181, 205, 206, 255, 268, 361
Harwood, A. R., 216
Hasan, T., 320
Hasic, E., 247, 248
Hausen, B. M., 169
Haynes, B. F., 232
Head, E. S., 273
Heaston, D. K., 215
Hebert, A. A., 98
Heenan, P. J., 187
Heggers, J. P., 336
Heiberger, R. M., 212
Helin, H., 63
Hellgren, L., 292
Hellström, I., 211
Hellström, K. E., 211
Hemady, Z., 106
Hennessey, P., 206
Henry, J. C., 98
Herlin, T., 312, 313
Herndon, J. H., Jr., 26
Hersey, P., 247–248
Hietanen, J., 53, 55
Highsmith, A. K., 43
Hightower, A. W., 43
Hill, M., 252
Hinckley, D. M., 189
Hinds, M. W., 191
Hing, D. N., 336
Hironaga, M., 145
Höffler, U., 31
Hofmann, V., 133
Holborow, J., 65
Holbrook, K. A., 157, 163
Hollingworth, P., 87
Holm, P., 318
Holman, C. D. J., 187
Holman, R. C., 363
Holmes, R. C., 60
Holt, P. J. A., 366
Holthofer, H., 342
Hölzle, E., 256
Hönigsmann, H., 294
Horio, T., 302
Horkay, I., 255
Hornstein, O. P., 375
Horsburgh, C. R., Jr., 154
Horton, R., 165
Horwitz, M. A., 177
Horwitz, S. N., 151
Hoyer, H., 381
Huff, J. C., 77, 360
Hughes, J. E., 399
Huhta, K. E., 147
Humphrey, G. B., 171
Hunter, J. M., 352
Hunter, M. K., 363
Hurwitz, E. S., 363
Hurwitz, S., 185, 186
Huston, D. P., 85
Hutchinson, G. J., 45
Hutchinson, T. H., 361

I

Icart, J., 371
Igarashi, M., 284
Ihme, A., 158
Ilstrup, D. M., 372
Imanura, S., 302
Immerman, S. C., 220
Innes, D. J., Jr., 385
Inoue, F., 378
Ishizu, K., 389
Iversen, O.-J., 292

J

Jackson, R., 78
Jaffe, E., 230
Jagell, S., 162
Jahnberg, P., 303
James, D. C. O., 60
Jansén, C. T., 320
Janssen, P. A. J., 138
Jarratt, A. M., 252
Jenson, A. B., 345
Jibard, N., 346
Jimenez, J., 273
Johanson, C. R., 216
Johnson, B. L., 356
Johnson, E., 44
Jonelis, F. J., 142
Jones, D. P. H., 397
Jones, S. E., 239
Jonsson, J., 65
Jori, G., 262
Jorizzo, J. L., 98, 272
Josse, R. G., 329
Jung, E. G., 306
Jung, H.-D., 193
Jurecka, W., 60
Juvakoski, T., 274, 319

K

Kagen, L. J., 89
Kalimo, K., 63, 64
Kamon, E., 370
Kanerva, L., 274, 319
Kang, K., 114
Kantor, G. R., 382
Kaplan, A. P., 331
Kaplan, G., 177
Kaplan, R. P., 296
Kaplowitz, L. G., 153
Karakousis, C. P., 209
Karasira, P., 48
Kastrup, W., 85
Katsambas, A., 149
Kavin, H., 389
Keczkes, K., 101
Keeney, R., 356
Keeney, R. E., 355
Keil, J. E., 117
Kempson, G. E., 97
Kendricks, F., 384
Kerkering, T. A., 153
Kerr, R. E. I., 108, 109
Kessler, J. F., 239
Khabbaz, R. F., 43
Kiani, R., 141
Kieffer, M., 62
Kienzler, J. L., 346
Kietzmann, H., 270
Kiistala, U., 61
Kimberling, W. J., 181, 182
King, L. E., Jr., 128
Kingston, T., 301
Kirby, J. D., 29
Kirk, L. E., 355
Kirkpatrick, C. H., 154
Kirkwood, J., 195, 278
Klein, I., 389
Klein, R. S., 363
Kligman, A. M., 30
Klippel, J. H., 85
Klotz, S. A., 49
Klövekorn, G., 393
Klövekorn, W., 393
Knox, K. L., 220
Knudsen, L., 113
Koblenzer, C. S., 397
Koenig, R., 203
Koh, H. K., 276
Koike, T., 88
Kolonel, L. N., 191
Kongsholm, H., 354
Kopf, A. W., 200, 201, 203, 206, 208, 221
Kornblatt, A. N., 44
Korobkin, M., 215
Koudsi, H., 301
Kouki, F., 83
Koumentaki, E., 149
Kövary, P. M., 161
Koziner, B., 228
Kraemer, K. H., 184
Kragballe, K., 312, 313
Krajczár, J., 247
Kreis, H., 217
Krieg, T., 158
Krigel, R. L., 229
Krishman, J., 234
Kromann, N., 381
Krown, S. E., 228
Kruse, K., 158
Kuehln-Petzold, C., 198
Kumagai, A., 88
Kummel, B., 369
Kunkel, H. G., 79
Kurban, A. K., 114
Kurland, L. T., 372
Kushner, M., 141

L

Lagerholm, B., 307
Lahita, R. G., 79
Laidet, B., 91
Lancaster, W. D., 345
Larkö, O., 305, 309
Laros, R. K., Jr., 53
LaRossa, D., 212
Larrègue, M., 91
Larsen, P. Ø., 318
Larson, D. M., 152
Larson, S. M., 211
Lash, H., 394
Laskaris, G., 374
Laskin, O. L., 355
Lassus, A., 274, 319
Lattanzio, G., 234
Laubenstein, L. J., 229
Laude, T. A., 147
Lauharanta, J., 274, 319
Laurberg, G., 318
Laurent, R., 346
Lavin, P. T., 195
Lawley, T. J., 85
Lazarus, G. S., 289
Leach, E. E., 257
Leavitt, J., 384
Lebreton, C., 298
Lee, L. A., 77
Lehto, V.-P., 206, 342
Lemish, W. M., 187
Lemoine, M. T., 346
Leonard, J., 65
Leonard, J. N., 66, 70, 71
Le Petit, J. C., 238
Lepresle, J., 94
Lerner, A. B., 278
Leung, D. Y. M., 103, 104
Levenstein, M., 200, 203
Levine, J., 203
Levine, J. L., 200
Levine, L. E., 73, 134
LeVine, M. J., 263
Levine, N., 239
Levinson, J. E., 90
Levis, W. R., 177
Lew, R., 203
Lew, R. A., 206
Lewis, F. G., 350
Leyden, J. J., 30
Leznoff, A., 329
Li, C.-Y., 234
Lidén, S., 162
Lieblich, L., 203
Lillis, P. J., 77
Linder, E., 63
Lindskov, R., 113, 305
Link, C. C., Jr., 345
Littlewood, S. M., 313
Ljunghall, K., 65, 67, 85
Lloyd, R. V., 239
Lobo, R. A., 165
Löfberg, H., 85
Löfberg, L., 72
Long, S. S., 359
Lööf, L., 65
Lookingbill, D. P., 382
Lovett, M., 356
Lowe, D., 344
Lowe, N. J., 280, 296, 301
Lucky, A. W., 28
Lucky, P. A., 28
Ludwig, R. A., 232
Luria, L. W., 380
Lutzner, M. A., 217
Lydahl, E., 303

Lynch, H. T., 181, 182
Lynch, J. F., 181, 182
Lynch, P. J., 239
Lynd, J., 361
Lynfield, Y., 147
Lyons, F., 34

M

Mabry, C. D., 38
McCaffree, D. L., 26
McCarthy, W. H., 194, 248
McCarty, G. A., 93
McCarty, K. S., 210
McCauley, R. L., 336
McClure, P. D., 400
McCrea, E. S., 224
McCurley, T. L., 140
McDaniel, W. E., 224
McDonald, G. A., 384
McDonald, S. G., 396
McGinley, K. J., 30
McGovern, V. J., 194
McGuide, J., 28
McKee, P. H., 344
McKenna, T. J., 166
MacKenzie, L. A., 249
MacKie, R. M., 108, 109, 183, 217, 316, 348
McKinley, T. W., 43
Maclean, I. W., 48
McMinn, R., 65
McMinn, R. M. H., 66, 71
McNaughton, F., 101
McNutt, N. S., 226, 237
McShane, D. J., 75
Maddox, W. A., 194
Magee, F., 166
Magid, S. K., 89
Magnus, I. A., 254
Maguire, J. H., 50
Maguire, P., 335
Mahood, J. M., 392
Malawista, S. E., 44, 45
Maleville, J., 258
Malt, R. A., 206
Mansfield, L. E., 325, 326
Marangos, P. J., 241
Marchase, P., 289
Marchesi, L., 259, 259
Marier, R. L., 153
Marimo, B., 254
Marino, C., 81
Marks, J., 300
Marks, R., 218, 251, 301
Marsden, J. R., 300
Martin, C., 258
Marynick, S. P., 26
Maser, M. R., 394
Mashkilleysson, A. L., 310
Mashkilleysson, N. A., 310
Masi, A. T., 75
Massey, D. A., 46
Masu, S., 276
Matozzo, I., 212
Matsumoto, K., 378
Matthews, M. J., 230
Meakins, J. L., 121
Medenica, M. M., 73, 134
Medoff, G., 153
Medsger, T. A., Jr., 94
Meehan, R. T., 76
Meigel, W., 21
Melsom, R., 175
Ménard, J., 136
Menard, J. W., 378
Menezas-Brandao, F., 120
Menter, A., 299
Menzel, S., 175
Mertin, J., 87
Mesko, W., 328
Metz, E. N., 236
Metzgar, R. S., 232
Meyers, J. D., 355
Meynadier, J., 58, 291, 316
Meyskens, F. L., Jr., 239
Michaëlsson, G., 72
Michalopoulos, M., 149
Michel, B., 291
Middleton, D., 361
Mier, A., 136
Miettinen, A., 342
Miettinen, M., 206, 342
Mignon, F., 83
Mihm, M. C., 276
Mihm, M. C., Jr., 181, 205, 206, 255, 361
Miller, S. E., 232
Mills, O. H., 30
Milner, R., 104
Milton, G., 188
Milton, G. W., 194
Mintzis, M. M., 200, 206
Misheloff, E., 280
Mishra, V., 389
Mitchell, E. B., 107
Mittelman, A., 228
Mobacken, H., 85, 317
Moll, B., 363
Mollard, S., 258
Molloy, W., 70
Momtaz-T, K., 268
Moore, A., 166
Moore, J. O., 232
Moore, J. W., 29
Moore, R., 209
Moragas, J. M., 388
Morandotti, A., 23
Morel-Maroger, L., 83
Moreno, A., 388
Morens, D. M., 363
Morgan, N. E., 243
Moschella, S., 50
Moss, S. H., 250
Mottaz, J. H., 35
Muggia, F. M., 229
Muhlbauer, J. E., 255
Müller, P. K., 158
Muller, S. A., 390
Munkvad, M., 372
Munro, D. D., 29
Munz, D., 156
Murad, T. M., 194
Murahata, R. I., 56
Murdoch, W., 393
Murray, D. R., 213
Mustafa, A. S., 176
Myskowski, P. L., 228, 230

N

Nabarro, J. M., 358
Nakagawa, H., 276
Natbony, S. F., 331
Nawata, Y., 88
Nazzaro-Porro, M., 33
Negri, M., 371
Neidhart, J. A., 236
Nelson, H. S., 325
Newton, K. A., 214
Nicholson, E., 215
Nielsen, P. G., 37
Niemi, K.-M., 274
Niimura, M., 351
Nilsson, L.-Å., 85
Nimrod, C., 157
Nogueira, N., 177
Noguera, J., 388
Nolph, K. D., 314
Nordlund, J. J., 195, 278
Nordmann, Y., 258
Norén, P., 393
Norris, D. A., 77
Novey, H. S., 119
Nozaki, T., 88
Nsanze, H., 48
Nusbaum, B. P., 151

O

Odom, R. B., 364
O'Donnell, J. R., 384
Oettgen, H. F., 228
Oikarinen, A. I., 61
Oka, M., 239
Okazaki, N., 145
O'Keefe, E. J., 353
Oksman, F., 371
Orfanos, C. E., 125, 295
Oriel, J. D., 347
Orth, G., 217, 346
Osgood, P. J., 250
Ott, F., 295
Ozaki, M., 302

P

Pagon, R. A., 157
Pai, C. H., 156
Paladugu, R. R., 196, 202
Palker, T. J., 232
Palosuo, T., 64
Pan, S. C., 50
Pandey, J., 230
Panizzon, R., 373
Papageorgiou, C., 120
Parakh, A. P., 280
Parker, J. D., 358
Parrish, J. A., 263

Pass, F., 345
Passi, S., 33
Pasternack, A., 63
Patman, R. D., 335
Paul, B. S., 263
Payling-Wright, C., 345
Payne, J. P., 126
Pearse, A. D., 251
Pearse, A. G. E., 241
Pearson, J. M. H., 175
Pecegueiro, M., 120
Penny, P. T., 122
Pepin, M., 157
Perpère, M., 371
Perry, H. O., 337, 338, 372
Pester, J., 182
Peterka, E. S., 396
Peters, G. E., 341
Peterson, B. H., 328
Peterson, L. L., 96
Petrino, R. A., 38
Phillips, H. S., 213
Phillips, M. E., 331
Picardo, M., 33
Pichichero, M. E., 42
Pieraggi, M. T., 59
Pietsch, J. B., 121
Pigatto, P. D., 23
Pinardi, M. E., 178
Pinkus, H., 393
Pittelkow, M. R., 390
Pitts, J. D., 217
Pittsley, R. A., 131
Platts-Mills, T., 87
Platts-Mills, T. A. E., 107
Plewig, G., 21, 256, 393
Plouin, F., 136
Plummer, F. A., 48
Pochi, P. E., 24
Podenzani, S. A., 259, 259
Poh-Fitzpatrick, M. B., 257
Polak, J. M., 241
Pollack, M. S., 230
Postel, A., 206
Poulsen, J. H., 123, 291
Powell, F. C., 337, 338
Powell, K. R., 156
Priestman, T. J., 214
Prince, R. K., 92
Prioleau, P. G., 83
Provost, T. T., 80
Przybilla, B., 120
Pulverer, G., 31
Putman, C. E., 215
Puzik, A., 47
Pye, R. J., 395

Q

Quirt, I., 216

R

Ragaz, A., 203
Rahn, D. W., 45
Raimer, S. S., 98
Raker, J. W., 206
Ramdené, P., 91
Rand, C., 104
Rapini, R. P., 22
Rauls, D. O., 326
Ravin, C. E., 215
Real, F. X., 228
Reano, A., 297
Reddi, E., 262
Reed, K. H., 49
Rees, R. S., 128
Reimann, B. E. F., 326
Reimer, G., 375
Reinarz, J. A., 98
Reintgen, D. S., 210
Reisner, E. G., 391
Retsas, S., 214
Reunala, T., 63, 64
Reveille, J. D., 80
Reyes, O., 178
Reymann, F., 318, 381
Reymond, J., 249
Reynolds, K. L., 379
Rhodes, A. R., 103, 181, 268
Rice, J. R., 93
Rich, B. H., 28
Richet, G., 83
Ridley, D. S., 179
Ridley, M. J., 179
Rietschel, R. L., 27
Rigel, D., 206, 208
Rigel, D. S., 200, 201, 203
Rimsza, M. E., 51
Ring, N., 66
Risteli, J., 158
Risteli, L., 158
Riva, F., 23
Rivera, A., 368
Rizzardini, M., 259
Rizzo, S. C., 234
Robert-Guroff, M., 230
Robinson, J. K., 142
Robson, M. C., 336
Rocklin, R. E., 106
Rodan, B. A., 215
Rodeck, C. H., 286
Rodeheffer, R. J., 95
Rodnan, G. P., 92, 94
Rodriquez-Rigau, L. J., 341
Rodu, B., 375
Roesdahle, K., 318
Rogers, G. S., 200
Rommer, J. A., 95
Ronald, A. R., 48
Ronan, S. G., 207
Rönnerfält, L., 303
Rorsman, H., 267
Ros, A.-M., 307
Rosdahl, I., 267
Rosén, K., 319
Rosenfield, R. L., 28
Roses, D. F., 203, 206, 208
Roth, W. I., 368
Rothfield, N., 81
Rothfield, N. F., 75, 75
Rouchouse, B., 238
Rovagnati, P., 259, 259
Rowntree, S., 107
Royer, E., 291
Rubaltelli, F. F., 262
Rudd, N. L., 157
Ruiter, D. J., 205
Russell, D. H., 296
Rutter, N., 365
Rycroft, R. J. G., 122

S

Safai, B., 228, 230
Sagebiel, R. W., 163
Saito, K., 145
Salasche, S. J., 222
Salm, M., 54
Salo, O. P., 53
Sampson, H. A., 110
Sanchez, N. P., 242, 390
Santa Cruz, D. J., 83
Sarantidis, D., 139
Sarkany, I., 126
Sarno, E. N., 177
Sarosi, G. A., 153
Satchidanand, S., 380
Sato, S., 284
Scanlon, E. F., 220
Scarborough, D. A., 236
Schaller, J. G., 75, 90
Schardt, M., 375
Schechter, G. P., 230
Scheithauer, B. W., 242
Scheynius, A., 65
Schiavone, F. E., 27
Schilling, W., 65
Schlesinger, M., 90
Schmid, G. P., 44
Schmitt, D., 293
Schneeberger, E. E., 104
Schneider, B., 306
Schober, P. C., 44
Schoetz, D. J., Jr., 338
Schriewer, H., 161
Schroeter, A. L., 242, 337, 338
Schutzer, S. E., 41
Schwartz, R. A., 197, 282
Schwebig, A., 136
Schweizer, J., 219
Searl, S. S., 195
Segreti, A. C., 355
Sehgal, V. N., 36
Seibold, J. R., 94
Seigler, H. F., 210, 215
Seiji, M., 276, 284
Sergent, J. S., 140
Sgoutas, D., 27
Shadomy, S., 153
Shah, B. R., 147
Shaw, H., 188
Shaw, H. M., 194
Shaw, M., 344
Sheppard, D. M., 260
Sheth, R. A., 125
Shmunes, E., 117
Shornick, J. K., 60

Shumer, S. M., 353
Shuster, S., 34, 300, 324
Sidgwick, A., 70
Sigal, L. H., 45
Simon, M., Jr., 375
Sindhuphak, W., 167
Singer, K. H., 289
Siskind, V., 190
Sklavounou, A., 374
Skog, E., 112
Slatford, K., 352
Slutzki, S., 371
Small, C. C. B., 363
Smiles, K., 252
Smith, C. R., 95
Smith, D. S., 87
Smith, E. B., 272
Smith, J. A., 325
Smith, J. G., Jr., 341
Smith, J. L., 235
Sober, A. J., 181, 205, 206, 276
Sohnle, P. G., 147
Soltani, K., 73, 134
Sommer, S., 345
Songsiridej, V., 326
Soong, S.-J., 194
Soter, N. A., 361
Soule, E. H., 202
Souteyrand, P., 298
Spence, B., Jr., 394
Spencer-Green, G., 90
Spigland, I., 345
Staberg, B., 308, 354
Stafford, T. J., 126
Stamm, A. M., 153
Staquet, M. J., 297
Starsnic, J., 84
Steere, A. C., 44, 45
Steigbigel, N. H., 363
Stein, R., 104
Steinberg, A. D., 85
Steinman, R. M., 177
Steinmetz, R., 148
Stenn, K. S., 186
Stern, R. S., 263
Stevens, D. A., 153
Steward, M. E., 26
Stewart, M. E., 22
Stewart, S., 132
Stiller, R. L., 153
Stone, B., 75
Stranieri, A. M., 22
Stratigos, I., 149
Strauss, J. S., 22, 26
Strottmann, M. P., 76
Stubbings, R., 357
Su, W. P. D., 35, 68, 234, 337, 338
Subrt, P., 98, 272
Suehisa, S., 378
Sueishi, M., 88
Svensson, A., 85
Swain, A. F., 70, 71
Swain, F., 65, 66
Swanbeck, G., 305, 317
Swanson, N. A., 289
Swerdlow, M. A., 389
Sybert, V. P., 163
Symoens, J. E., 138
Syrop, C. H., 76

T

Tagami, H., 378
Tait, K. A., 43
Takasugi, S., 389
Takematsu, H., 284
Talal, N., 75
Tam, M. R., 49
Tan, C. Y., 218
Tan, E. M., 75
Tan, O. T., 126
Tansey, P., 384
Taplin, D., 368
Tardieu, J. C., 316
Taylor, L., 301
Taylor, S., 356
Tedla, T., 176
Tegner, E., 309
Tejerina, A., 347
Temple, D. F., 209
Tencati, J. R., 119
Tenekjian, K. K., 114
Thieme, C., 120
Thin, R. N., 44, 358
Thin, R. N. T., 155, 352
Thivolet, J., 293, 297, 298
Thomas, J. R., III, 68, 242
Thompson, C. J., 212
Thomsen, K., 128
Thomsen, N. H., 132
Thomson, J., 384
Thomson, J. A., 316
Thyresson-Hök, M., 303
Tibbetts, C., 75
Tilsey, C., 126
Timlin, D., 60
Ting, S., 326
Tiwari, J. L., 280
Tjernlund, U., 67, 85
Toki, N., 389
Tomioka, H., 88
Tonnesen, M. G., 361
Touraine, R., 298
Tovar, J. A., 273
Tovey, J. A., 260
Trau, H., 201, 203
Traupe, H., 161
Trotter, M. G., 282
Tsambaos, D., 295
Tsuji, T., 281
Tucker, M. A., 184
Tucker, W., 65
Tucker, W. F. G., 66, 70, 71
Twarog, F. J., 330
Tyndall, A. D., 87

U

Uitto, J., 61, 83
Ullman, S., 318
Ulrich, M., 178
Uno, H., 239
Unsworth, D. J., 70
Unsworth, J., 65
Urguhart, A. J., 260

V

Vaida, G. A., 327
Vainio, E., 64
Valenzuela, R., 84
van de Kerkhof, P. C. M., 290
van Erp, P. E. J., 290
Van Horn, M., 212
Van Noorden, S., 241
VanThiel, D. H., 384
Van Voorhis, W. C., 177
Variakojis, D., 243
Varner, M. W., 76
Veidenheimer, M. C., 338
Viac, J., 297
Viander, M., 64
Vibhagool, A., 167
Vic, P., 316
Vincent, J., 292
Virtanen, I., 206, 342
Vivoux, D., 371
Voorhees, J. J., 289
Vorhies, C., 96

W

Wade, J. C., 355
Wagner, G., 198
Wagoner, M. D., 278
Waldo, E., 203
Walker, J. G., 368
Walker, P. G., 347
Walter, J. F., 253
Walther, R. R., 257
Wantzin, G. L., 128
Ward, A. M., 324
Warin, R. P., 323
Warner, T. F. C. S., 239
Wassel, G., 311
Wasserman, S. I., 94
Wasserstrum, N., 53
Watanabe, S., 145
Waters, B., 139
Weber, K., 47
Webster, G. F., 30
Weerakoon, J., 136
Wei, N., 85
Weinstein, A., 75
Welch, E. A., 332, 335
Wennersten, G., 303, 307
Westbrook, K. C., 38
Westbury, G., 214
Westermark, P., 393
Weston, T. S., 401
Weston, W. L., 77, 360
Wheeland, R. G., 171
Whelton, M. J., 70
White, J. E., 399
White, P., 44
Whittier, F. C., 314

Wick, M. R., 242
Wiebelt, H., 198
Wiesmeier, E., 356
Wiesner-Menzel, L., 169
Wigley, F., 95
Wilkin, J. K., 341
Wilkinson, J. D., 171
Winberg, C. D., 196
Winchester, R. J., 75, 79
Winkelmann, R. K., 99, 390
Winkelstein, J. A., 80
Winter, H., 219
Wintroub, B. U., 51, 361
Wokalek, H., 21
Wolff, K., 294
Wood, N., 103
Wood, W. C., 206
Woodard, B., 210
Woods, J. E., 202
Workman, S., 81
Wortzman, M. S., 301
Wright, P. W., 211
Wright, S., 111
Wu, L. Y. F., 328

Y

Yanagisawa, T., 88
Yates, V. M., 108, 109
Yemaneberhan, T., 176
Yeo, J. M., 357
Yoder, F. W., 131
Yonemoto, R. H., 196, 202
Yoshikuni, K., 378
Young, R. C., 230
Yung, C. W., 73, 134

Z

Zabriskie, J. B., 41
Zachariae, H., 313
Zackheim, H. S., 237
Zaia, J. A., 355
Zaynoun, S. T., 114
Zelickson, A. S., 35
Zhu, X.-J., 57
Zina, A. M., 160
Zina, G., 33
Zissis, N. P., 149
Zone, J. J., 61